Legal Aspects of Health Care Administration

Tenth Edition

George D. Pozgar, MBA, CHE
Consultant and Hospital Surveyor
Gp Health Care Consulting, International
Annapolis, Maryland
Surveyor
The Joint Commission
Oakbrook Terrace, Illinois

Legal Review

Nina M. Santucci
General Counsel
Essex Corporation
Columbia, Maryland

JONES AND BARTLETT PUBLISHERS
Sudbury, Massachusetts
BOSTON   TORONTO   LONDON   SINGAPORE

World Headquarters

Jones and Bartlett Publishers
40 Tall Pine Drive
Sudbury, MA 01776
978-443-5000
info@jbpub.com
www.jbpub.com

Jones and Bartlett Publishers
Canada
6339 Ormindale Way
Mississauga, Ontario
L5V 1J2
CANADA

Jones and Bartlett Publishers
International
Barb House, Barb Mews
London W6 7PA
UK

Jones and Bartlett's books and products are available through most bookstores and online booksellers. To contact Jones and Bartlett Publishers directly, call 800-832-0034, fax 978-443-8000, or visit our website at www.jbpub.com.

Substantial discounts on bulk quantities of Jones and Bartlett's publications are available to corporations, professional associations, and other qualified organizations. For details and specific discount information, contact the special sales department at Jones and Bartlett via the above contact information or send an email to specialsales@jbpub.com.

This publication is designed to provide accurate and authoritative information in regard to the subject matter covered. It is sold with the understanding that the publisher is not engaged in rendering legal, accounting, or other professional service. If legal advice or other expert assistance is required, the service of a competent professional person should be sought.

Library of Congress Cataloging-in-Publication Data

Pozgar, George D.
    Legal aspects of health care administration / George D. Pozgar.—10th ed.
        p. cm.
    Includes bibliographical references and index.
    ISBN-13: 978-0-7637-3927-0
    ISBN-10: 0-7637-3927-8
    1. Medical laws and legislation—United States.   2. Medical personnel—Malpractice—United States.   I. Title.
    KF3821.P69 2007
    344.7304'1—dc22
                                                                2006021306

6048

Production Credits
Publisher: Michael Brown
Production Director: Amy Rose
Associate Production Editor: Rachel Rossi
Marketing Manager: Sophie Fleck
Manufacturing Buyer: Therese Connell
Composition: Circle Graphics
Cover Design: Timothy Dziewit
Printing and Binding: Transcontinental Gagne
Cover printing: Transcontinental Gagne

Printed in Canada
11 10 09 08 07   10 9 8 7 6 5 4 3 2

Contents

Preface

Welcome to the tenth edition of *Legal Aspects of Health Care Administration*. Whether the reader is a student or a seasoned professional, the topics presented in the following chapters, as with previous editions, lay a strong foundation in health law. The tenth edition presents a wide range of health law topics in an interesting and understandable format, leading the reader through the complicated maze of the legal system. This book describes how common medical errors which have consistently been repeated over time continue to have a negative impact on the reputations and financial well-being of health care professionals, their employers, and more importantly, the health and lives of their patients.

The news media continues to paint a grim picture of the health care industry by featuring distressing headlines that sensationalize medical errors. The following are some of the more recent examples of headlines in the media:

- Third Baby Dies after Error at Indiana Hospital

    ". . . infant was one of six premature babies who received adult doses of the anti-clotting drug heparin. . . ."

    —*USA Today*, September 1, 2006

- ERs Swamped Despite New Beds and Strategies

    "The demands on emergency medicine that last week brought warnings of a national system in crisis are as intense locally as almost anywhere in the country."

    —*The Washington Post*, June 18, 2006

- When Doctors Make Mistakes

    "I wouldn't have sued if I'd been shown the smallest bit of human compassion. . . ."

    —*SELF,* May 2006

- "They're Here"

    "Previously, hospitals were told well in advance of when the JCAHO surveyors were scheduled to arrive for on-site inspections, and facilities spent months preparing for the visit. Prompted by criticism that the visits were being stage-managed, the JCAHO switched to unannounced inspections. . . . Now, hospitals only know that surveyors will show up. . . ."

    —*Modern Hospital*, April 24, 2006

- What Doctors Hate About Hospitals

    "It requires almost a stroke of luck to enter a U.S. hospital and receive precisely the right treatment—no more and no less."

    —*TIME*, May 1, 2006

- Illegal Trade in Bodies Horrifies Loved Ones

    "Over the past 19 years, more than 16,800 families have been represented in lawsuits claiming loved ones' body parts were stolen for profit."

    —*USA TODAY,* April 27, 2006

- Hospitals Save Money but Safety is Questioned

    "A growing number of hospitals . . . are saving money by reusing medical devices designated for one time use, ignoring the warnings of manufacturers, which will not vouch for the safety of their reconditioned products. . . ."

    —*The Washington Post*, December 11, 2005

- 11,600 Patients Got Infections in PA Hospitals

  "Pennsylvania . . . the first state to publicly report the toll hospital infections take, saying that more than 11,600 patients got infections last year."

  —*USA TODAY,* July 13, 2005

- Life and Death Politics

  "The Schiavo case is just the latest front in a much nastier war. It is an American tragedy for the modern media age–litigious, polarizing, personal, political, and televised round the clock. . . ."

  —*U.S. News and World Report,* April 4, 2005

- When a Heart Attack Goes Undiagnosed

  ". . . one in 50 heart attack victims are mistakenly sent home by emergency room doctors . . . Connie Gustafson, who won her own battle with breast cancer, says her husband's fight to survive reminded her 'how vigilant you have to be in taking care of yourself in hospitals. The system is very precarious, and it is easy for mistakes to be made.'"

  —*USA TODAY,* October 25, 2006

- Top 100 Verdicts of 2004

  "Resident left unattended drowned in bathtub . . . Brain damage blamed on delayed response to early labor emergency situation . . . Nurse failed to inform physician of irregular heart rate . . . Doctor cut one duct too many during gallbladder removal. . . ."

  —*National Law Journal,* February 21, 2005

- Fatal Medical Errors Said to be More Widespread

  ". . . the number of patients who died from medical errors is more than double the findings in a 1999 report that sparked widespread concern."

  —*The Wall Street Journal,* July 27, 2004

- Public Opinion on Medical Care

  "Nearly half the public say they are very concerned about an error resulting in injury happening to themselves or their family when they receive health care in general. . . ."

  —*Kaiser Family Foundation,* July/August 2003.

Because the law is continually evolving, it is important that the reader possess a basic understanding of how and when the law relates to the heath care field in general, and the reader's specific area of responsibility in particular. This book answers that need by serving as both a text in the classroom and as a reference for the practitioner. To assist the reader in applying the substantive material in this book, actual court cases are presented. The decisions in cases discussed are generally governed both by applicable state and federal statutes and common-law principles. When reviewing a case, the reader must keep in mind that the case law and statutes of one state are not binding in another state.

This edition begins with a chapter that provides some historical perspective on the development of hospitals, illustrating both their progress and failures through the centuries. There is broad discussion of the legal system, including the sources of law. The text continues with a basic review of tort law, criminal issues, contracts, anti-trust, civil procedure, and a wide range of real life legal and ethical dilemmas that caregivers have faced as they wound their way through the courts. The final chapters provide an overview of various ways to improve the quality and delivery of health care.

Although the court cases relating examples of malpractice are often mirror images of the failures of medicine, this tenth edition presents a book of lessons from which the reader can understand where the medical and legal worlds collide. Taken as a whole, the content of this book serves as a reminder to its readers that they must learn from the mistakes and tragedies experienced by others to avoid repeating them. The legal cases and resulting headlines should be a reminder as to the responsibility the caregiver has to the profession he or she has chosen, and to use the knowledge gained from studying this book to help prevent himself or herself from becoming the next headline.

IT'S YOUR GAVEL

"It's Your Gavel" boxes provide the reader an opportunity to make decisions about actual court cases. Most chapters begin with a case that has been reviewed by the courts in state or federal jurisdictions. After reviewing each case and subsequent relevant material, readers can take on the role of the fact finder and render a decision. Then, at the end of the respective chapters, the actual court findings and reasoning for each case are given in "The Court's Decision" box.

CASE PRESENTATION FORMAT

When reviewing the various cases in this book, the reader should consider what happened, why things went wrong, what the relevant legal issues are, and how the event could have been prevented. The reader should also consider if one fact in a particular case changed, how the outcome might have been different. What would the fact be? The cases presented in the text have been chosen because of their frequency of occurrence.

The general format for each boxed case review is as follows:

Title: Each case has a title that signals the type of case to be reviewed.

Case Citation: describes where a court's opinion in a particular case can be located. It identifies the parties in the case, the text in which the case can be found, the court writing the opinion, and the year in which the case was decided. For example, the case citation "Bouvia v. Superior Court (Glenchur), 225 Cal. Rptr. 297 (Ct. App. 1986)" is described as follows:

* Bouvia v. Superior Court (Glenchur): identifies the basic parties involved in the lawsuit.

* 225 Cal. Rptr. 297: identifies the case as being reported in volume 225 of the California Reporter on page 297.

* Cal. Ct. App. 1986: identifies the case as being decided in the California Court of Appeals in 1986.

Students who wish to research a specific case should visit a law school library, which will contain various state and regional reporters.

Facts: A review of the material facts of the case is presented.

Issues: This is the disputed point or question the judge or jury must decide. The issues discussed in any given case are selected for review on the basis of medical and legal pertinence to the health care professional. Although any one case in this text may have multiple issues, emphasis is placed on those issues considered to be more relevant for the reader in the context of the topic being discussed.

Holding: The court's ruling based on the facts, issues, and applicable laws pertaining to a case is summarized.

Reason: The rationale for the court's decision based on the facts, issues, and relevant laws surrounding a case is presented.

Discussion: Discussion questions, although prompted by a particular case, may not necessarily be germane to the facts of the case. The questions are merely presented as opportunities for discussion and in no way add to the facts of a specific case decision.

Author's Note: This text is educational in nature and should not be considered a substitute for legal advice on any particular issue. Moreover, each chapter presents an overview, rather than an exhaustive treatment, of the various topics.

The author, legal reviewers, and/or publisher cannot be responsible for any errors or omissions, including: additions to, interpretations of, and/or changes in the regulations presented in this book.

Acknowledgments

I am grateful to the very special people in the more than 600 hospitals in forty states with whom I have consulted, surveyed, and provided education over the past 15 years. Their shared experiences have served to remind me of the importance to make this book more valuable in the classroom and as a reference for practicing health care professionals.

To my students in health care law classes at the New School for Social Research, Molloy College, Long Island University-C.W. Post College, Saint Francis College, Saint Joseph's College, my intern from Brown University, and my resident in hospital administration, while I was an on-site faculty member of the George Washington University in Washington, D.C., as well as those I have instructed through the years at various seminars, I will always be indebted for your inspiration.

Special thanks to the Physicians' Record Company for granting permission to use the chapter "Historical Perspective," as adapted from the book Hospital Organization and Management by Malcolm T. MacEachern, M.D., C.M., D.Sc. (Hon.), LL.D. (Hon.), F.A.C.S., F.A.C.P., F.A.C.H.A., F.A.I.H.A. (Australia).

Many thanks are also extended to all those special people at the National Library of Medicine and the Library of Congress for their guidance over the years in locating research materials.

The author especially acknowledges the staff at Jones and Bartlett Publishers, Inc., whose guidance and assistance was so important in making this Tenth Edition a reality. Special thanks to Mike Brown, and Rachel Rossi.

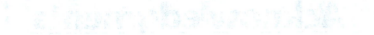

CHAPTER 1

Historical Perspective

History is relevant to understanding the past, defining the present, and influencing the future.

Author Unknown

This chapter provides the reader with a brief overview of the advance of civilization as disclosed in the history of hospitals. A study of the past often reveals errors that then can be avoided, customs that persist only because of tradition and practices that have been superseded by others more effectual. The past may also bring to light some long-abandoned procedures, which may be revived to some advantage. The story of the birth and evolution of the hospital portrays the triumph of civilization over barbarism, and the progress of civilization toward an ideal characterized by an interest in the welfare of the community.

EARLY HINDU AND EGYPTIAN HOSPITALS

Two ancient civilizations, India and Egypt, had crude hospitals. Hindu literature reveals that in the 6th century B.C., Buddha appointed a physician for every 10 villages and built hospitals for the crippled and the poor. His son, Upatiso, built shelters for the diseased and for pregnant women. These examples probably moved Buddha's devotees to erect similar hospitals. Despite a lack of records historians agree that hospitals existed in Ceylon as early as 437 B.C.

During his reign from 273 to 232 B.C., King Asoka built 18 hospitals that hold historical significance because of their similarities to the modern hospital. Attendants gave gentle care to the sick, provided patients with fresh fruits and vegetables, prepared their medicines, gave massages, and maintained their personal cleanliness. Hindu physicians, adept at

surgery, were required to take daily baths, keep their hair and nails short, wear white clothes, and promise that they would respect the confidence of their patients. Although bedside care was outstanding for those times, medicine was only beginning to find its way.

Egyptian physicians were probably the first to use drugs such as alum, peppermint, castor oil, and opium. In surgery, anesthesia consisted of hitting the patient on the head with a wooden mallet to render the patient unconscious. Surgery was largely limited to fractures, and medical treatment was usually given in the home. Therapy away from home was often available in temples, which functioned as hospitals.

GREEK AND ROMAN HOSPITALS

The term *hospital* derives from the Latin word *hospitalis,* which relates to guests and their treatment. The word reflects the early use of these institutions not merely as places of healing but as havens for the poor and weary travelers. Hospitals first appeared in Greece as *aesculapia,* named after the Greek god of medicine, Aesculapius. For many centuries, hospitals developed in association with religious institutions, such as the Hindu hospitals opened in Sri Lanka in the 5th century B.C. and the monastery-based European hospitals of the Middle Ages (5th century to 15th century). The Hotel-Dieu in Paris, a monastic hospital founded in 660, is still in operation today.

In early Greek and Roman civilization, when medical practices were rife with mysticism and superstitions, temples

Note: This chapter, "Historical Perspective," is adapted from the book *Hospital Organization and Management* by Malcolm T. MacEachern, M.D., C.M., D.Sc. (Hon.), LL.D. (Hon.), F.A.C.S., F.A.C.P., F.A.C.H.A., F.A.I.H.A. (Australia), with permission from the Physician's Record Company.

were also used as hospitals. Every sanctuary had a sacred altar before which the patient, dressed in white, was required to present gifts and offer prayers. If a patient was healed, the cure was credited to miracles and divine visitations. If the patient remained ill or died, he or she was considered to be lacking in purity and unworthy to live.

Greek temples provided refuge for the sick. One of these sanctuaries, dedicated to Aesculapius, is said to have existed as early as 1134 B.C. at Titanus. Ruins attest to the existence of another, more famous Greek temple built several centuries later in the Hieron, or sacred grove, at Epidaurius. Here physicians ministered to the sick holistically in body and soul. They prescribed medications such as salt, honey, and water from a sacred spring. They gave patients hot and cold baths to promote speedy cures and encouraged long hours of sunshine and sea air, combined with pleasant vistas, as an important part of treatment. The temple hospitals housed libraries and rooms for visitors, attendants, priests, and physicians. The temple at Epidaurius even boasted what might be described as the site of the first clinical records. The columns of the temple were inscribed with the names of patients, brief histories of their cases, and comments as to whether or not they were cured.

The Aesculapia spread rapidly throughout the Roman Empire as well as through the Greek world. Although some hospitals were simply spas, others followed the therapy outlined by the leading physicians of the day. Hippocrates, for example, a physician born about 460 B.C., advocated medical theories, which have startling similarity to those of the present day. He employed the principles of percussion and auscultation, wrote intelligently on fractures, performed numerous surgical operations, and described such conditions as epilepsy, tuberculosis, malaria, and ulcers. He also kept detailed clinical records of many of his patients. Physicians like Hippocrates not only cared for patients in the temples, but also gave instruction to young medical students.

HOSPITALS OF THE EARLY CHRISTIAN ERA

Christianity and the doctrines preached by Jesus stressing the emotions of love and pity gave impetus to the establishment of hospitals, which, with the advance of Christianity, became integral parts of the church institution. These Christian hospitals replaced those of Greece and Rome and were devoted entirely to care of the sick, and they accommodated patients in buildings outside the church proper.

The decree of Constantine in 335 closed the Aesculapia and stimulated the building of Christian hospitals, which, during the 4th and 5th centuries, reached the peak of their development. Many were erected by the rulers of the period or by wealthy Romans who had converted to Christianity. By the year 500, most large towns in the Roman empire had

erected hospitals. Nursing, inspired by religion, was gentle and considerate, but soon began to discard the medical precepts of Hippocrates, Antyllus, and other early Greek physicians because of their pagan origins. Instead, health care turned toward mysticism and theurgy (the working of a divine agency in human affairs) as sources of healing.

Hospitals rarely succeeded during the centuries leading to the Middle Ages; only a few existed outside Italian cities. Occasional almshouses in Europe sheltered some of the sick, while inns along the Roman roads housed others. No provision appears to have been made for care of the thousands of helpless paupers who had been slaves and were later set free when Christianity was introduced into the Roman Empire.

MOHAMMEDAN HOSPITALS

The followers of Mohammed were almost as zealous as the Christians in caring for the sick. In Baghdad, Cairo, Damascus, Cordova, and many other cities under their control, luxurious hospital accommodations were frequently provided. Harun al-Rashid, the glamorous *caliph* (a title for a religious or civil ruler claiming succession from Muhammad) of Baghdad (786–809), built a system of hospitals, paying the physicians himself. Medical care in these hospitals was free. About four centuries later, in 1160, a Jewish traveler reported that he had found as many as 60 dispensaries and infirmaries in Baghdad alone. The Persian physician Rhazes, who lived from about 850 to 923, was skilled in surgery. He was probably the first to use the intestines of sheep for suturing and cleansed patient wounds with alcohol. He also gave the first rational accounts of smallpox and measles.

Mohammedan physicians like Rhazes received much of their medical knowledge from the persecuted Christian sect known as the Nestorians. Nestorius, driven into the desert with his followers after having been appointed patriarch of Constantinople, took up the study of medicine. The school at Edessa in Mesopotamia, with its two large hospitals, eventually came under the control of the Nestorians in which they established a remarkable teaching institution. Eventually driven out of Mesopotamia by the orthodox bishop Cyrus, they fled to Persia, establishing the famous school at Gundishapur, which is conceded to be the true starting point of Mohammedan medicine. Gundishapur was home to the world's oldest known teaching hospital and also comprised a library and a university. It was located in the present-day province of Khuzestan, in the southwest of Iran, not far from the Karun river.

Mohammedan medicine flourished up to about the 15th century. Mohammedan physicians were acquainted with the possibilities of inhalation anesthesia. They instituted precautions against adulteration of drugs and developed a vast number of new drugs. Mohammedan countries also built asylums for the mentally ill a thousand years before such institutions appeared in Europe. The people of Islam made a brilliant start in medicine, but never fulfilled the great promise that glowed in their early work in medical arts, and hospitalization was never fulfilled. Wars, politics, superstitions, and a non-progressive philosophy stunted the growth of a system that had influenced the development of hospitals.

EARLY MILITARY HOSPITALS

Engraved on a limestone pillar dating back to the Sumerians (2920 B.C.) are pictures, which, among other military procedures, show the assemblage of the wounded. The book of Deuteronomy in the Bible records that Moses laid down outstanding rules of military hygiene. Out of the urgency of care for the wounded in battle came much of the impetus for medical progress. Hippocrates is quoted as saying that war is the only proper school for a surgeon. Under the Romans, surgery advanced largely because of experience gained through gladiatorial and military surgery.

MEDIEVAL HOSPITALS—THE DARK AGES

Religion continued to dominate the establishment of hospitals during the Middle Ages. Although physicians cared for physical ailments to afford relief, they rarely attempted to cure the sick. Dissection of a human body would have been sacrilege, because the body was created in the image of God.

Notwithstanding concern for the soul and a disregard of the body, religion continued to be the most important factor in the establishment of hospitals during the Middle Ages. A number of religious orders created *hospitia,* or travelers' rests and infirmaries adjacent to monasteries that provided food and temporary shelter for weary travelers and pilgrims. One of these, the famous Alpine hospice of St. Bernard, founded in 962, gave comfort to the weary and sent its renowned dogs to the rescue of lost mountain climbers.

The hospital movement grew rapidly during the Crusades, which began in 1096. Military hospital orders sprang up, and accommodations for sick and exhausted crusaders were provided along all traveled roads. One body of crusaders organized the Hospitalers of the Order of St. John, which in 1099 established in the Holy Land a hospital capable of caring for 2000 patients. Knights of this order took personal charge of service to patients and often denied themselves so that the sick might have food and medical care. For years these institutions were the best examples of hospitals of that period.

Finally, an active period of hospital growth came during the late 12th and early 13th centuries. In 1198, Pope Innocent III urged that hospitals of the Holy Spirit be subscribed for by the citizenry of many towns. He set an example by founding a model hospital in Rome, known as Santo Spirito in Sassia. Built in 1204, it survived until 1922, when it was destroyed by fire. In Rome, nine other hospitals were founded shortly after completion of the one in Sassia; it is estimated that in Germany alone 155 towns had hospitals of the Holy Spirit during early medieval times.

Although most hospitals erected during the Middle Ages were associated with monasteries or founded by religious groups, a few cities, particularly in England, built municipal institutions. Like all hospitals of the period, the buildings were costly, often decorated with colorful tapestries and stained glass windows, but the interiors often consisted of large, drafty halls with beds lining each side. A few of the better institutions were arranged on the ward plan, usually built in the shape of a cross. Floors were made of red brick or stone and the only ventilation came from the cupola in the ceiling.

With the spread of leprosy during the 12th and 13th centuries, lazar houses sprang up, supplying additional hospital facilities. Crude structures, lazar houses were usually built on the outskirts of towns and maintained for the segregation of lepers rather than for their treatment. Special groups of attendants including members of the Order of St. Lazar nursed the patients. The group represented an important social and hygienic movement, because their actions served to check the spread of epidemics through isolation. The group is credited for virtually stamping out leprosy.

During the same period of hospital growth, three famous London institutions were established: St. Bartholomew's in 1137; St. Thomas's before 1207, and St. Mary of Bethlehem in 1247. St. Bartholomew's, founded by Rahere (the reported court jester of Henry I), cared for the sick poor, but unlike like many hospitals of that day, was well organized. St. Thomas's Hospital was founded by a woman, later canonized as St. Mary Overie. It burned in 1207, was rebuilt six years later, and constructed again on a new site in 1228. St. Mary of Bethlehem was the first English hospital to be used exclusively for the mentally ill.

The Hotel-Dieu of Paris was probably typical of the better hospitals of the Middle Ages. Built at the beginning of the 13th century, the hospital provided four principal rooms for patients in various stages of disease, as well as a room for convalescents and another for maternity patients. Illustrations by artists of the time show that two persons generally shared one bed. Heavy curtains sometimes hung from canopies over the bed to afford privacy, but this advantage was more than offset by the fact that the draperies, never washed, spread infection and prevented free ventilation. The institution was self-contained, maintaining a bakery, herb garden, and farm. Often, patients who had fully recovered remained at the hospital to work on the farm or in the garden for several days in appreciation for the care they had received.

The "Dark Age" of Hospitals

Most hospitals during the Middle Ages, however, were not all as efficiently managed as the Hotel-Dieu of Paris. Pictures and records prove that many hospitals commonly crowded several patients into one bed regardless of the type or seriousness of illness. A mildly ill patient might be placed in the same bed as an occupant suffering from a contagious disease.

Medical care was deplorable during this dark age of hospitals. A notable exception to the general deterioration in medicine during this era was the conscientious effort of those monks who copied by hand and preserved the writings of Hippocrates and other ancient physicians.

The great Al-Mansur Hospital, built in Cairo in 1276, struck a contrast to the European institutions of the Middle Ages. It was equipped with separate wards for the more serious diseases and outpatient clinics. The handful of hospitals like Al-Mansur would lay the groundwork for hospital progress to come in later centuries.

HOSPITALS OF THE RENAISSANCE

During the revival of learning around the close of the 14th century, hundreds of medical hospitals in Western Europe received the new, more inquiring surgeons that the Renaissance produced. New drugs were developed, and anatomy became a recognized study. Ancient Greek writings were printed, and dissection was performed by such masters as Leonardo da Vinci, known as the originator of cross-sectional anatomy, and Vesalius. Hospitals also became more organized. Memoranda from 1569 describe the duties of the medical staff in the civil hospital of Padua, a city that was home to the most famous medical school during the 16th century. These read:

> There shall be a doctor of physic upon whom rests the duty of visiting all the poor patients in the building, females as well as males; a doctor of surgery whose duty it is to apply ointments to all the poor people in the hospital who have wounds of any kind; and a barber who is competent to do, for the women as well as the men, all the other things that a good surgeon usually does.

The practice of surgery during the Renaissance became more scientific and progressive. Operations for lithotomy and hernioplasty were undertaken without the use of anesthetics. Surgery was practiced by the *long-robe surgeons,* a small group who were educated in the universities and permitted to perform all types of operations, and by the *short-robe surgeons,* the barbers who in most communities were

allowed only to leech and shave the patient, unless permission was granted to extend the scope of treatment. Both groups were regarded as inferior to physicians.

In 1506, a band of long-robe surgeons organized the Royal College of Surgeons of Edinburgh. By 1540, both the long- and the short-robe surgeons in England joined to form the Company of Barber-Surgeons of London. In 1528, English physicians were organized by Thomas Linacre, physician to Henry VIII, as the Royal College of Physicians of England.

During the 16th century, Henry VIII of England ordered that hospitals associated with the Catholic church be given over to secular uses or destroyed. The sick were turned into the streets. Conditions in hospitals became so intolerable that the king was petitioned to return one or two buildings for the care of patients. Henry consented and restored St. Bartholomew's in 1544. Practically the only hope for the sick poor among outlying towns was to journey many miles to London.

The dearth of hospitals in England continued throughout the 17th century, when the medical school was developed. The French and the English quickly accepted what had originated in Italy; the first attempt to make medical instruction practical. St. Bartholomew's took the lead in education by establishing a medical library in 1667 and permitted apprentices to walk the wards for clinical teaching under experienced surgeons.

In 1634, an outstanding contribution was made to nursing by the founding of the order of the Daughters of Charity of St. Vincent de Paul. Originating at the Hotel-Dieu of Paris as a small group of village girls who were taught nursing by the nuns, the order grew rapidly and was transplanted to the United States by Mother Seton in 1809.

HOSPITALS OF THE 18TH CENTURY

During the 18th century, the building of hospitals revived partially. Because of poverty, at first the movement made slow progress in England, but a few hospitals were built and supported jointly by parishes. By 1732, there were 115 such institutions in England, some of them a combination of almshouse and hospital. As hospitals grew in number, new advances in health care began.

The Royal College of Physicians established a dispensary where medical advice was given free and medicines were sold to the needy at cost. Controversies and lawsuits, however, brought an untimely end to this early clinic. Not discouraged by this experience, the Westminster Charitable Society created a similar dispensary in 1715. The same organization in 1719 founded Westminster Hospital, an infirmary built by voluntary subscription, in which the staff gave its services gratuitously. Ten years later, the Royal College of Physicians in Edinburgh opened the Royal Infirmary. London Hospital, another notable, had its origin in 1740. Admission of charity patients to the London Hospital was apparently by ticket, because among its historical relics is an admission card. On the back of that card is a representation of a Biblical scene drawn by the artist Hogarth.

As hospitals worked to provide services to more people, scientists worked to provide better services. Filling a need in hospitals at the time was Desaguliers's invention in 1727 of a machine for pumping fresh air into and foul air out of rooms. Used at first for prisons and public buildings, it later was installed in hospitals.

In the Elizabethan period, however, the deterioration of hospital service that had set in under Henry VIII continued. Despite advances made during the 18th century and the steady growth in population and wealth, hospital progress was uneventful.

Antony van Leeuwenhoek (1632–1723) succeeded in making some of the most important discoveries in the history of biology. Although Leeuwenhoek did not invent the first microscope, he was able to perfect it. Many of his discoveries included bacteria, free-living and parasitic microscopic protists, sperm cells, blood cells, and microscopic nematodes. His research opened up an entire world of microscopic life. Leeuwenhoek had a pronounced influence on the creation of the sciences of cytology, bacteriology, and pathology. His discoveries have forever affected the delivery of health care not only in hospitals but in the way health care is delivered in all settings.

EARLY HOSPITALS IN THE UNITED STATES

Manhattan Island claims the first account of a hospital in the New World; a hospital that was used in 1663 for sick soldiers. Fifty years later, in Philadelphia, William Penn founded the first almshouse established in the American colonies. The Quakers supported the almshouse, which was open only to members of that faith. However, Philadelphia was rapidly growing and also in need of a public almshouse. Such an institution for the aged, the infirm, and the mentally ill was established in 1732. The institution later became the historic Old Blockley, which in turn evolved into the Philadelphia General Hospital.

Philadelphia was the site of the first incorporated hospital in America, the Pennsylvania Hospital. Dr. Thomas Bond wished to provide a place where Philadelphia physicians might treat their private patients. With the aid of Benjamin Franklin, Bond sought a charter for the Pennsylvania Hospital, which was granted by the crown in 1751. Franklin helped design the structure, and in 1755, the hospital, quite modern in plan with a central administration unit and two wings, was opened to the public. The first staff consisted of Dr. Phineas Bond, Dr. Lloyd Zachary, and the founder, Dr. Thomas Bond, all of whom gave their services without remuneration for three years.

Rich in the history of hospitals, Philadelphia must also be credited with the first quarantine station for immigrants (created in 1743) and the first lying-in hospital (established in 1762), a private institution owned by the noted obstetrician William Shippen. Quality in American health care seemed to be improving.

Dr. John Jones, an American, published a book in 1775 calling attention to frightful conditions existing in hospitals. He charged that hospitals abroad were crowded far beyond capacity, that Hotel-Dieu of Paris frequently placed three to five patients in one bed—the convalescent with the dying and fracture cases with infectious cases. He estimated that one fifth of the 22,000 patients cared for at Hotel-Dieu died each year. Wounds were washed daily with a sponge that was carried from patient to patient. The infection rate was said to be 100 percent. Mortality after amputation was as high as 60 percent. Jones's call to action had a positive effect on American health care.

As late as 1769, New York City, with nearly 300,000 inhabitants, was without hospitals. In 1771, a small group of citizens, Dr. Jones among them, formed the Society of the New York Hospital and obtained a grant to build. The society purchased a five acre site and made plans for a model structure that would allow a maximum of eight beds per ward and provide good ventilation. The hospital fell into the hands of the British troops during the Revolution and was used as a barracks and military hospital.

During postwar reconstruction, the New York Hospital broadened its services. Under the supervision of Dr. Valentine Seaman, the hospital began providing instruction in nursing, and in 1779, it introduced vaccination in the United States and established an ambulance service.

Other early American hospitals of historic interest include the first psychiatric hospital in the New World, founded at Williamsburg, Virginia, in 1773 and a branch of federal hospitals created by passage of the U.S. Marine Hospital Service Act in 1798. Under this act, two marine hospitals were established in 1802; one in Boston and another in Norfolk, Virginia.

The Massachusetts General Hospital, which pioneered many improvements in medicine, originated in Boston. Its first patient, admitted in 1821, was a 30-year-old sailor.

More than a decade earlier, two Boston doctors had appealed to the city's "wealthiest and most influential citizens" to establish a general hospital. The War of 1812 delayed the dream, but on July 4, 1818, the cornerstone was finally laid. The original building, designed by Boston's leading architect Charles Bulfinch, is still in use. One of the world's leading centers of medical research and treatment has grown up around it. The original domed operating amphitheater, where anesthesia was first publicly demonstrated in 1846, is now a Registered National Historic Landmark.

MGH has achieved countless medical milestones, including the first successful reattachment of a human limb.[1]

In 1832, the Boston Lying-In Hospital opened its doors to women unable to afford in-home medical care. It was one of the nation's first maternity hospitals, made possible because of fundraising appeals to individuals and charitable organizations.

Despite the increased volume of institutions for care of the sick, the first half of the 19th century stands as a dark period in hospital history. Surgeons of the day had sufficient knowledge of anatomy to lead them to perform many ordinary operations, and as a result more surgery was probably undertaken than during any previous era. However, there was one important aspect: while the medieval and ancient surgeons had sought to keep wounds clean, even using wine in an attempt to accomplish this purpose, 19th-century surgeons believed *suppuration* (the production and discharge of pus) to be desirable and encouraged it. Hospital wards were filled with discharging wounds, which made the atmosphere offensive enough to warrant the use of perfume. Nurses of that period are said to have used snuff to make conditions tolerable. Surgeons wore their operating coats for months without washing. The same bed linens served several patients. Pain, hemorrhage, infection, and gangrene infested the wards. Mortality from surgical operations rated as high as 90 to 100 percent. Nathan Smith, in the second decade of that century, advocated a bichloride of mercury solution for reducing infection, but his ideas were ignored.

LATE 19TH-CENTURY RENAISSANCE

To the modern health care worker who takes for granted hospital cleanliness and the kindly treatment of the sick, the magnitude of Florence Nightingale's service may be incomprehensible. The famous English nurse began her career by training at Kaiserswerth on the Rhine in a hospital and deaconess home established in 1836 by Theodor Fliedner and his wife. Florence Nightingale wrote disparagingly of her training there, particularly of the hygiene practiced. Returning to England, she put her own ideas of nursing into effect and rapidly acquired a reputation for efficient work.

By 1854, during the Crimean War, the English government, disturbed by reports of conditions among the sick and wounded soldiers, selected Florence Nightingale as the one person capable of improving patient care. Upon her arrival at the military hospital in Crimea with a small band of nurses whom she had assembled, she found that the sick were lying on canvas sheets in the midst of dirt and vermin. There was neither laundry nor hospital clothing and beds were made of straw. She proceeded to establish order and cleanliness. She organized diet kitchens, a laundry service, and departments of supplies, often using her own funds to finance her projects. Ten days after her arrival, the newly established kitchens were feeding 1000 soldiers. Within three months, 10,000 soldiers were receiving clothing, food, and medicine. As a result of her work, the death rate substantially declined. She has been credited with observing:

> A good nursing staff will perform their duties more or less satisfactorily under every disadvantage. But while doing so, their head will always try to improve their surroundings, in such a way as to liberate them from subsidiary work, and enable them to devote their time more exclusively to the care of the sick.[2]

Because of her organizational skills, many consider Florence Nightingale to be the first true health care administrator. Later she extended her administrative duties to include planning the details of sanitary engineering in a new military hospital.

As the field of nursing continued to progress, so did medicine. Crawford Long, for example, first used ether as an anesthetic in 1842 to remove a small tumor from the neck of a patient. He did not publish any accounts of his work until later, however, so the discovery is often attributed to W. T. G. Morgan, a dentist who developed sulfuric ether and arranged for the first hospital operation under anesthesia at Massachusetts General Hospital in 1846. Although not put to practical use immediately, ether soon took away some of the horror that hospitals had engendered in the public mind. Chloroform was first used as an anesthetic in 1847 for an obstetrical case in England by Sir James Simpson.

The year 1847 also brought about the founding of the American Medical Association (AMA) under the leadership of Dr. Nathan Smith Davis. The association, among its main objectives, strived to improve medical education, but most of the organization's tangible efforts in education began at the close of the century. The AMA was a strong advocate for establishing a code of ethics, promoting public health measures, and improving the status of medicine.

The culmination of Florence Nightingale's work came in 1860, after her return to England. There she founded the Nightingale School of Nursing at the St. Thomas Hospital. From this school, a group of 15 nurses graduated in 1863. They later became the pioneer heads of training schools throughout the world.

In 1886, the Royal British Nurses' Association (RBNA) was formed. The RBNA worked toward establishing a standard of technical excellence in nursing. A charter granted to the RBNA in 1893 denied nurses a register, although it did agree to maintain a list of persons who could apply to have their name entered thereon as nurses.[3]

The first formally organized American nursing schools were established in 1872 at the New England Hospital for Women and Children in Boston (Brigham and Women's

Hospital), and then in 1873 at Bellevue, New Haven, and Massachusetts General Hospital. In 1884, Alice Fisher was appointed as the first head of the nurse training at Philadelphia Hospital's (renamed as the Philadelphia General Hospital in 1902) nurses training school. She had the distinction of being the first Nightingale-trained nurse recruited to Philadelphia upon recommendation by Florence Nightingale.

Mrs. Bedford Fenwick, a nurse leader in the English nurse registration movement, traveled to Chicago in 1893 to arrange the English nursing exhibit to be displayed in the women's building at the World's Fair. As part of the Congress on Hospitals and Dispensaries, a nursing section included papers on establishing standards in hospital training schools, the establishment of a nurses association, and nurse registration. The group formulated plans to improve nursing curriculum and hospital administration in the first concerted attempt to improve hospitals through a national organization.

Progress in Infection Control

Ignatz Philipp Semmelweiss of Vienna, Austria, unknowingly laid the foundation for Pasteur's later work. In 1847, at the Vienna Lying-in Hospital, Europe's largest teaching obstetrical department, he boldly declared that the alarming number of deaths from puerperal fever was due to infection transmitted by students who came directly from the dissecting room to take care of maternity patients. Semmelweiss noted that Division 1 of the hospital was a medical student teaching service; Division 2 was utilized for midwife trainees. Maternal deaths for Division 1 averaged 10 percent; Division 2 averaged 3 percent. Medical students performed autopsies; midwives did not. As a result of these findings, an order was posted on May 15, 1847, requiring all students to scrub their hands in chlorinated lime until the cadaver smell was gone. The order was later revised to include hand washing between patients.

Despite having made bitter enemies, Semmelweis had the satisfaction of seeing the mortality rate in his obstetrical cases drop from 9.92 percent to 1.27 percent in little more than a year as a result of an aseptic technique that he devised. A few years later, Louis Pasteur demonstrated the scientific reason for Semmelweis' success when he proved that bacteria were produced by reproduction and not by spontaneous generation, as was then generally believed. From his work came the origin of modern bacteriology and clinical laboratories.

Also of great importance to hospitals and infection control was Bergmann's introduction of steam sterilization in 1886 and William Stewart Halstead's introduction of rubber gloves in 1890.

By the end of the century, Lister carried Pasteur's work a step further and showed that wound healing could be has-

tened by using antiseptics to destroy disease-bearing organisms and by preventing contaminated air from coming into contact with these wounds. Lister was not content with obtaining better results in his own surgical cases; he devoted his life to proving that suppuration is dangerous and that it should be prevented or reduced by use of antiseptics. Despite his successful work and eloquent pleas, his colleagues persisted in following their old methods. Years after his discovery, they continued to deride him and his technique, which consisted of spraying carbolic solution so profusely about the operating room that both surgeons and patients were drenched. As time went on and antiseptics and the techniques of using them were improved, even the skeptical were impressed by the clinical results. Surgeons, at last, realized that they could undertake major operations without the fear of morbidity and mortality.

Discovery of Anesthesia

As the 19th century neared its close, surgery was becoming more frequent. The discovery of anesthesia and the principle of antiseptics are to be regarded as two of the most significant influences in the development of surgical procedures and the modern hospital. Anesthesia improved pain control and improved hygiene practices helped reduce the incidence of surgical site infections.

Modern Hospital Laboratory

The study of cytology originated about the middle of the 19th century and influenced the development of the modern hospital clinical laboratory. The cell theory was first advanced in 1839 by the German anatomist Theodor Schwann and was further developed by Jacob Henle, whose writings on microscopic anatomy appeared about 1850. Rudolph Virchow was the most eminent proponent of the cell theory. His studies in cellular pathology speeded research in the etiology of disease.

Changing Hospital Structure

With nursing, anesthesia, infection control, and cytology under way, a change in hospital structure began in the last quarter of the 19th century. Buildings of the Civil War days continued with as many as 25 to 50 beds in a ward, with little provision for segregation of patients. In New York City in 1871, construction of Roosevelt Hospital, built on the lines of a one-story pavilion with small wards, set the style for a new type of architecture that came to be known as the American plan. A noteworthy feature was ventilation by means of openings in the roof, a definite improvement upon earlier hospitals that were characterized by a lack of provision for ventilation. Dr. W. G. Wylie, writing in 1877, said he favored this type of building, but he advocated that it be a temporary structure only, to be destroyed when it became infected.

Changing Hospital Function

Promoted by the wealth of bacteriological discoveries, hospitals began to care for patients with communicable diseases. During the decade 1880 to 1890, the tubercle bacillus was discovered; Pasteur vaccinated against anthrax; Koch isolated the cholera bacillus; diphtheria was first treated with antitoxin; the tetanus bacillus and the parasite of malarial fever were isolated; and inoculation for rabies was successful. Treatment of patients with some of the infections necessitated isolation, and hospitals were the logical place for observation of communicable diseases. Consequently, at the end of the century, in addition to their many surgical cases, hospitals were crowded with large numbers of patients suffering from scarlet fever, diphtheria, typhoid, and smallpox.

Discovery of the X-Ray

Wilhelm Konrad Roentgen's discovery of the X-ray in 1895 was a major scientific achievement. The first use of the X-ray symbolizes the beginning of the period that necessitated equipment so costly that the average practitioner could not afford to install it. The natural result was the founding of community hospitals in which physicians could jointly use such equipment. Nineteenth-century inventions also included the clinical thermometer, the laryngoscope, the Hermann Helmholtz ophthalmoscope, and innumerable other aids to accurate diagnosis.

Although the medical and nursing professions of the later half of the 19th century did not reap the full reward of their discoveries, they provided the 20th century with a firm foundation upon which to build.

20TH-CENTURY PROGRESS

The treatment of metabolic diseases, nutritional deficiencies, the importance of vitamins, and the therapy of glandular extracts played an important role in the advancement of medicine in the 20th century. As early as 1906, Gowland Hopkins began investigations of vitamins. Two years later, Carlos Finlay produced experimental rickets by means of a vitamin-deficient diet. This, in turn, was followed by Kurt Huldschinsky's discovery that rickets could be treated successfully with ultraviolet light. In quick succession came Casimir Funk's work with vitamins, Elmer McCollum's discovery of vitamins A and B, Joseph Goldberger's work in the prevention of pellagra, and Harry Steenbock's irradiation of foods and oils. Other outstanding contributions to the science of nutrition include Frederick Banting's introduction of insulin in 1922, the studies in anemia carried out by George Hoyt Whipple and Frieda Robscheit-Robbins, and the Minot and Murphy liver extract.

Einthoven's invention of the electrocardiograph in 1903 marked the beginning of an era of diagnostic and therapeutic aids. Shortly after that invention came the first basal metabolism apparatus, then the Wassermann (August Von) test in 1906, and tests for pancreatic function. Invention of the fluoroscopic screen followed in 1908. Subsequently, the introduction of blood tests and examinations of numerous body secretions required well-equipped and varied laboratories. Concurrent with this progress in the field of internal medicine was the introduction of radium for the treatment of malignant growths, increasing the use of the clinical laboratory for microscopic examination of pathological tissue and developments in antibiotics. The result of these many new aids was the conquest of diseases formerly regarded as incurable, which in turn resulted in improved public confidence in hospitals.

The 20th century is also characterized by rapid growth in nursing education. The earlier schools were maintained almost entirely for the purpose of securing nursing service at a low cost. The nurse's duties were often menial, the hours long, and classroom and laboratory study almost entirely lacking. Nurses themselves had begun to organize for educational reforms. By 1910, training increasingly emphasized theoretical studies. This movement was largely due to the work of organizations such as the American Nurses Association and the National League for Nursing, along with the organization of the Committee on the Grading of Nursing Schools. In 1943, the U.S. Cadet Nurse Corps was organized to spur enrollment of student nurses in nursing schools to help meet the shortages due to enlistment of graduate nurses for military service. As a result, efforts increased to train practical nurses and nurses' aides in order to relieve the shortage of graduate nurses.

Reform in medical education began early in the century and was due almost wholly to the efforts of the Council on Medical Education and Hospitals, which was established in 1905 by the American Medical Association. Immediately after its organization, this council began inspection of medical schools. The council, by establishing standards and by grading the schools, brought about gradual elimination of most of the unethical, commercial, and unqualified institutions.

A great stimulus to the profession of hospital administration has been the work of the American Hospital Association. Organized in 1899 as the Association of Hospital Superintendents, it took its present name in 1907. Since its inception, the organization has concerned itself particularly with the problems of hospital management. As early as 1910, the association held educational programs for hospital chief executive officers and trustees.

The American College of Surgeons was founded in 1913 under the leadership of Dr. Franklin H. Martin, the first director general of the organization. One of the most dramatic of the achievements of the American College of Surgeons was the hospital standardization movement begun in 1918. The founders drew up what was known as the "minimum standard," a veritable constitution for hospitals, setting forth requirements for the proper care of the sick. An annual survey of all hospitals having 25 or more beds made the standard effective. In 1918, when the first survey was conducted, only 89 hospitals in the United States and Canada could meet the requirements.

The hospital standardization movement focused all efforts on the patient, with the goal of providing the patient with the best professional, scientific, and humanitarian care possible. The growth of this movement is remarkable, especially given that participation in the hospital standardization (now referred to as The Joint Commission) program is voluntary.

The years following 1929 will long be remembered as one of the most trying periods in the history of hospitals. Due to critical economic conditions, many institutions found it difficult to keep their doors open. Lowered bed occupancy and increased charity load, coupled with steadily decreasing revenues from endowments and other sources of income, worked hardships on private institutions. Fortunately, however, every economic crisis brings forth new ideas and means and methods of organization to benefit mankind.

In the later half of the 20th century, competition among hospitals began to grow as for-profit hospital chains began to spring up and compete with nonprofit organizations. Advances in medical technology, such as CT, MRI, and PET scanners and robotic surgery, as well as an ever-growing list of new medications, have revolutionized the practice of medicine. Less-invasive surgical procedures and a trend toward care in outpatient settings have reduced the need for lengthy in-hospital stays.

HEALTH CARE AND HOSPITALS IN THE 21ST CENTURY

The modern hospital is a complex health care organization, which continues to be the revolutionary product of a long and arduous struggle. The challenges of health care are enormous and continue to test health care organizations. Some of today's health care challenges include exorbitant malpractice awards; skyrocketing insurance premiums; high expectations of society for miracle drugs and miracle cures; balancing fairly the mistakes of caregivers with the hundreds of thousands of successful events that occur each year

across the nation; negative press that increases public fear; the ethical dilemmas of abortion and human cloning; the exponential growth of information and medical technology; and the ever-increasing shortage of nurses, physicians, pharmacists, physical therapists, and the like. In addition, the ability to provide affordable access to health care services to even the insured is an ongoing challenge. The ever-increasing number of uninsured (those who have no health insurance) and underinsured (those with inadequate health insurance and often unable to pay for catastrophic illness) continue to be a national issue of grave concern. In addition, with employer-based coverage declining, many working families are left with decreasing health benefits. Unfortunately, there is little evidence that the U.S. Congress is able to reach any consensus for effectively addressing the issue. The greatest challenge of the 21st century requires that each member of society assume a more proactive role in his or her health care.

JUST A BEGINNING

Because history often repeats itself, society must learn from its many lessons; otherwise, it will be doomed for a return to the dark ages of medicine. Early discoveries should not be forgotten or taken for granted. To this day, for example, clean hands and the use of surgical gloves are two of the most effective infection-control practices. Caregivers all too often jeopardize patient safety by failing to observe appropriate hand hygiene, representing a failure to learn from past mistakes. As a result, accreditation agencies, such as The Joint Commission, have found it necessary to make good hand hygiene a national patient safety goal. Let us not forget how to practice safe medicine:

> *Where we were,*
> *What we have come to expect, and*
> *Our future directions,*
> *Have been influenced by what has preceded us.*

Author Unknown

The pinnacle of hospital evolution has not been reached nor has the final page of its colorful history been written. As long as there remains a humanitarian impulse, as long as a society feels compassion, love, and sympathy for its neighbors, there will be hospitals. In the past, hospitals changed as conditions changed. In the future, they will continue to change to meet the needs of their communities. Leaders of the 21st century understand the historical value of knowing the past, have the vision to preserve the good, and have the passion to create an even better health care system.

CHAPTER REVIEW

1. In its evolution, the hospital climbed a long, tortuous road and struggled along a hazardous path from India and Egypt to Greece and Rome, to the Islamic countries, to England, France, Germany, Spain, Italy, and on to America. The existence of hospitals is evidence of a high degree of civilization in which people are interested not only in the well-being of themselves and their families, but also in the community.

2. Religion played an important role in the development of hospitals. Faith healing was practiced in India and Egypt many centuries before Christ. *Aesculapia* (hospital temples) were numerous in ancient Greece and Rome and were dedicated to the god of medicine. Hospitals in the early Christian era and in the Middle Ages were an integral part of the church. Not until abuses crept into their administration under ecclesiastical authority in the 15th and 16th centuries were some of them taken over and managed by civil bodies.

3. The development of the hospital has not been a smooth and easy advance. Centuries of experiments, scientific discoveries, and public enlightenment were necessary to break down the barriers of ignorance and prejudice. The evolution was accomplished in cycles, with alternating dark and golden ages. However, never has the hospital possessed the quality and quantity of scientific care for the sick that it has today; never before has its influence been so extensive and so widespread; never before has it played such an important role in the life of the community. In all of this growth and development, hospitals benefited by the technical as well as scientific developments that occurred during the various periods.

4. Although patients often approach the hospital with some reluctance, apprehension, and fear of death, there continues to be confidence and hope of improved health with a longer, healthier, happier, and productive life.

5. The primary function of the hospital—the one that has been constant throughout its evolution—is to care for the sick and injured. The scope of services offered by hospitals continues to change as they take on the role of not only treating the sick and injured, but also preventing illness and prolonging purposeful, productive lives.

6. Although this chapter is but a short synopsis of the history of hospitals, students wishing to expand their knowledge in this area should access the National Library of Medicine's Web site at www.nlm.nih.gov. The NLM has the world's largest medical library. The library's collections contain more than 6 million items, including books, journals, photographs, and images. Housed within the library is one of the world's finest medical history collections of old and rare medical books.

REVIEW QUESTIONS

1. Who is often recognized as being the first hospital administrator?
2. Which invention attributed to Van Leeuwenhoek had a pronounced influence on the creation of the sciences of cytology, bacteriology, and pathology?
3. What issue did Florence Nightingale identify in the 1800s as being a major source/vehicle for the spread of infection and continues to be so today?
4. What data did Semmelweis collect? What was the significance of that data as related to performance improvement in the present-day hospital?
5. What were two of the greatest influences in the development of present-day hospitals?
6. Describe how you think history is repeating itself in today's health care system.

WEB SITE RESOURCES

American Hospital Association   www.hospitalconnect.com/

Centers for Medicare and Medicaid Services   www.hcfa.gov/stats/nhe-oact

Helen Hayes Hospital	www.helenhayeshospital.org/hist.htm
History of Pennsylvania Hospital	www.uphs.upenn.edu/paharc/tour/tour2.html
HospitalLink.com [over 6,000 hospitals]	www.hospitallink.com
Internet Resources	www.people.fas.harvard.edu/~burchst/HSbibMed.html#Internet
Johns Hopkins Medicine	www.johnshopkinsmedicine.org
Massachusetts General Hospital	www.mgh.harvard.edu
Museum of Medical Research	http://history.nih.gov
Mombasa Hospital	www.mombasahospital.com/history.html
National Library of Medicine	www.nlm.nih.gov
National Health Museum	www.accessexcellence.com
Sinai-Grace Hospital	www.sinaigrace.org
Widener University School of Law Library	www.law.widener.edu/Law-Library
Wills Eye Hospital Society	www.wehsociety.org/history.html

NOTES

1. Mass Moments, *Massachusetts General Hospital Admits First Patient, September 3, 1821,* June 21, 2006 [www.massmoments.org/moment.cfm?mid=256].

2. Byrnes, *Non-Nursing Functions: The Nurses State Their Case,* 82 AM. J. NURSING 1089 (1982).

3. C. Howse, 85 (49) NURSING TIMES, Dec. 6, 1989, at 32.

Introduction to Law

Laws are the very bulwarks of liberty; they define every man's rights, and defend the individual liberties of all men.

J. G. Holland

This chapter introduces the health care professional to the development of U.S. law, the functioning of the legal system, and the roles of the different branches of government in creating, administering, and enforcing the law. It is important to understand the foundation of the U.S. legal system before one can appreciate or comprehend the specific laws and principles relating to health care.

U.S. Supreme Court Justice Oliver Wendell Holmes said that the law "is a magic mirror, wherein we see reflected not only our own lives but also the lives of those who went before us."[1] Chief Justice Marshall in delivering his opinion to the Court in *Marbury v. Madison* said "The very essence of civil liberty certainly consists in the right of every individual to claim the protection of the laws, whenever he receives an injury. One of the first duties of government is to afford that protection. [The] government of the United States has been emphatically termed a government of laws, and not of men. It will certainly cease to deserve this high appellation, if the laws furnish no remedy for the violation of a vested right."[2]

Most define the law as a system of principles and processes by which people in a society deal with disputes and problems, seeking to solve or settle them without resorting to force. Simply stated, laws are rules of conduct enforced by government, which imposes penalties when prescribed laws are violated.

Laws govern the relationships between private individuals and organizations and between both of these parties and government. *Public law* deals with relationships between individuals and government; *private law* deals with relationships among individuals.

The thrust of most public law is to attain what society deems to be valid public goals. One important segment of public law, for example, is criminal law, which prohibits conduct deemed injurious to public order and provides for punishment of those proven to have engaged in such conduct.

In contrast, private law is concerned with the recognition and enforcement of the rights and duties of private individuals. Tort and contract actions are two basic types of private law. In a *tort action,* one party asserts that the wrongful conduct of another has caused harm, and the injured party seeks compensation for the harm suffered. A *contract action* usually involves a claim by one party that another party has breached an agreement by failing to fulfill an obligation. Either remuneration or specific performance of the obligation may be sought as a remedy. Without an organized, clear system of laws that regulate society, anarchy would clearly arise.

SOURCES OF LAW

The sources of law are:

1. *common law,* which is derived from judicial decisions

2. *statutory law,* which emanates from federal and state legislatures

3. *administrative law,* prescribed by administrative agencies

In those instances in which written laws are silent, vague, or contradictory to other laws, the judicial system is called on to resolve those disputes. The following sections discuss the sources of law that formed the foundation of the U.S. legal system.

Common Law

Common law refers to the body of principles that evolved and expanded from judicial decisions that arise during the trial of court cases. Many of the legal principles and rules applied today by courts in the United States have their origins in English common law.

Because a law could never cover every potential human event that might occur in society, the judicial system is doubly necessary. It not only serves as a mechanism for reviewing legal disputes that arise in the written law, but it is also an effective review mechanism for those issues on which the written law is silent or in instances of a mixture of issues involving both written law and common-law decisions. For example, in the *Cruzan* case, discussed in Chapter 17, the U.S. Supreme Court based its decision on the consideration of existing statutory law and prior judicial decisions.[3]

Common Law in England

> Law reflects to a large degree the civilization of those that live under it. Its progress and development are mirrors not merely of material prosperity but of the method of thought and of the outlook of the age.[4]

The common law of England is much like its language. It is as varied as the nations that peopled its land in different locations and different periods. Some common law is derived from the Britons, the Romans, the Saxons, the Danes, and the Normans.

> To recount what innovations were made by the succession of these different nations, or estimate what proportion of the customs of each go to the composing of our body of common law, would be impossible at this distance of time. As to a great part of this period, we have no monuments of antiquity to guide us in our inquiry; and the lights which gleam upon the other part afford but dim prospect. Our conjectures can only be assisted by the history of the revolutions effected by these several nations.[5]

The Romans governed the island as a province from the time of Claudius (A.D. 43) until A.D. 448. It was a time of peace and cultivation of the arts. Roman laws were administered as laws of the country. When the Romans left Britain to attend to their own domestic safety, the Picts and the Scots clashed with inhabitants of southern England. Unable to oppose the attack, these southern inhabitants appealed to the Saxons for assistance. The Saxons, who came from German lands, drove the northern invaders back inside their own borders.[6] The Saxons contended with Danish raiders from the 8th to the 11th centuries.

The law in England before the Norman Conquest in 1066 was dispensed primarily by tradition and local customs and mostly dealt with violent crimes. The kings during this period were concerned more with enforcing customary law than with amending it. The courts mainly consisted of open-air meetings where no records were maintained. "For the Anglo-Saxons justice was a local matter, administered chiefly in the shire courts, and was largely dependent upon local customs, preserved in the memory of those persons who declared the law in the court."[7] The Saxons operated with the goal of exterminating the Britons and destroying all their monuments and establishments. Subsequently, the native Briton customs and laws fell out of favor. The Britons were forced into the mountains of Wales, dividing the remainder of the dominion into seven independent kingdoms.[8]

These kingdoms were, for a time, independent of one another. A variety of laws grew among the Saxons themselves, as well as among the Danes, who following a treaty in Northumberland, were considered in some measure to be part of the nation. Toward the later part of Saxon times, the kingdom was governed by a variety of laws (Mercian Law, West-Saxon Law, and Danish Law) and local customs. All British and Roman customs that survived the times were buried within one of the three laws, which governed all of England.[9]

Following their conquest in 1066, the Normans had little regard for Anglo-Saxon laws. They considered themselves apart from such laws.

> It is obviously impossible to attempt an adequate picture of Anglo-Saxon life. It was a wild time. Men lived in terror of the vast forests, where it was easy to be lost and succumb to starvation, of their fellow man who would plunder and slay, and above all of the Unknown, whose inscrutable ways seemed constantly to be bringing famine and disaster. The uncertainties of modern life pale into insignificance when regarded from the standpoint of these men. It is natural, therefore, that their law should reflect their reaction against the environment. It was conservative and harsh. Violence, robbery and death formed its background.[10]

The principal change introduced by the Norman Conquest was that the king's court opened for disputes about land-tenure. Land disputes involved the Saxons who held the land before the conquest and the Normans who dispossessed them. Evidence in such disputes was often the result of oral testimony from neighboring landowners. Although no professional judiciary yet existed, trials were held before the county courts by the king's representatives and a cleric often presided.

Soon, a system of national law began to develop based on custom, foreign literature, and the rule of strong kings. The first royal court was established in 1178. This court, enlisting the aid of a jury, heard the complaints of the kingdom's subjects. Because there were few written laws, a body of principles evolved from these court decisions, which became known as common law. Judges used these court decisions to decide subsequent cases. As Parliament's power to legislate grew, the initiative for developing new laws passed from the king to Parliament.

Common Law in the United States

During the colonial period, English common law began to be applied in the colonies. In the vast new country with its abundance of natural resources, English common law could not be adopted exactly; the law was thus adapted to meet the needs of the new land. Compared to England, the New World glistened with land, timber, and minerals, so the law would have to aid the new society in mastering the land.

In an 1829 U.S. Supreme Court decision, Joseph Story wrote, "The common law of England is not to be taken in all respects to be that of America. Our ancestors brought with them its general principles, and claimed it as their birthright but they brought with them and adopted only that portion which was applicable to their situation."[11]

After the Revolution, each state, with the exception of Louisiana, adopted all or part of the existing English common law and added to it as needed. Louisiana civil law is based to a great extent on the French and Spanish laws and, especially, on the Code of Napoleon. As a result there is no national system of common law in the United States and common law on specific subjects may differ from state to state.

> Case law court decisions did not easily pass from colony to colony. There were no printed reports to make transfer easy, though in the 18th century some manuscript materials did circulate among lawyers. These could hardly have been very influential. No doubt custom and case law slowly seeped from colony to colony. Travelers and word of mouth spread knowledge of living law. It is hard to say how much; thus it is hard to tell to what degree there was a common legal structure.[12]

Judicial review became part of the law in the decade before the federal Constitution was adopted. Courts began to assert their power to rule on the constitutionality of legislative acts and to void unconstitutional statutes.

Today, cases are tried applying common-law principles unless a statute governs. Even though statutory law has affirmed many of the legal rules and principles initially established by the courts, new issues continue to arise, especially in private-law disputes, which require decision making according to common-law principles. Common-law actions are initiated mainly to recover money damages or possession of real or personal property.

When a higher state court has enunciated a common-law principle, the lower courts within the state where the decision was rendered must follow that principle. A decision in a case that sets forth a new legal principle establishes a precedent. Trial courts or those on equal footing are not bound by the decisions of other trial courts. Also, a principle established in one state does not set precedent for another state. Rather, the rulings in one jurisdiction may be used by the courts of other jurisdictions as guides to the legal analysis of a particular legal problem. Decisions found to be reasonable will be followed.

The position of a court or agency, relative to other courts and agencies, determines the place assigned to its decision in the hierarchy of decisional law. The decisions of the U.S. Supreme Court are highest in the hierarchy of decisional law with respect to federal legal questions. Because of the parties or the legal question involved, most legal controversies do not fall within the scope of the Supreme Court's decision-making responsibilities. On questions of purely state concern—such as the interpretation of a state statute that raises no issues under the U.S. Constitution or federal law—the highest court in the state has the final word on proper interpretation. The following are explanations of some of the more important common-law principles:

- *Precedent.* A *precedent* is a judicial decision that may be used as a standard in subsequent similar cases. A precedent is set when a court decision is rendered that serves as a rule for future guidance when deciding similar cases.

- *Res Judicata.* In common law, the term *res judicata*— which means the thing is decided—refers to that which has been previously acted on or decided by the courts. According to *Black's Law Dictionary,* it is a rule where "a final judgment rendered by a court of competent jurisdiction on the merits is conclusive as to the rights of the parties and their privies, and, as to them, constitutes an absolute bar to subsequent action involving the same claim, demand, or cause of action."[13]

- *Stare Decisis.* The common-law principle *stare decisis* (let the decision stand) provides that when a decision is rendered in a lawsuit involving a particular set of facts, another lawsuit involving an identical or substantially similar situation is to be resolved in the same manner as the first lawsuit. The resolution of future lawsuits is arrived at by applying rules and principles of preceding cases. In this manner, courts arrive at comparable rulings. Sometimes slight factual differences may provide a basis for recognizing distinctions between the precedent and the current case. In some cases, even when such differences are absent, a court may conclude that a particular common-law rule is no longer in accord with the needs of society and may depart from precedent. Principles of law are subject to change, whether they originate in statutory or in common law. Common-law principles may be modified, overturned, abrogated, or created by new court decisions in a continuing process of growth and development to reflect changes in social attitudes, public needs, judicial prejudices, or contemporary political thinking.

Medical Malpractice

The first common-law case in the United States in which a physician was held legally responsible for a negligence-related action occurred as early as 1794. In *Cross v. Guthery,* 2 Root 90, 92 (Conn. 1794), the court heard that when Mrs. Cross complained that there was something wrong with her breast, her husband sent for Dr. Guthery. The doctor examined Mrs. Cross, diagnosed her ailment, and amputated her breast. Shortly after the surgery, she bled to death. Guthery expressed his regrets to her husband and then sent him a bill for 15 pounds. Cross hired a lawyer, who persuaded a jury to dismiss Guthery's bill and awarded Cross 40 pounds as compensation for the loss of his wife's companionship. Since that time, physicians have experienced recurring periods of substantial increases in the number of malpractice cases. The first such increase occurred in the 15 years prior to the Civil War.[14] Increases in malpractice cases and concern about them occurred at the beginning of this century and also in the years before World War II.

By 1941, *The Journal of the American Medical Association* published studies showing that 1,296 malpractices had occurred between 1900 and 1940, with more than 500 between 1930 and 1940. The increases in malpractice cases were attributed to opinions expressed about the current malpractice situation involving high patient expectations, new diagnostic procedures, and erosion of the physician-patient relationship.[15]

The Harvard Medical Malpractice Study, commissioned by the state of New York to determine the rate of medical injury in New York hospitals, revealed that 3.7 percent of patients entering New York hospitals in 1984 were injured by the care provided. A tenth of those who were treated negligently filed malpractice suits.[16] The research group conducting the study suggested that "only one claim makes its way into the tort system for every eight cases of injury caused by medical negligence."[17] The study, which cost $3.1 million and ran 1,200 pages, was funded by the state and a grant from the Robert Wood Johnson Foundation. It involved four years of research and included the review of more than 30,000 medical records.[18]

The number of malpractice suits is staggering. Critics say that the system fails by making too little information known.[19]

A report by the Physicians Insurers of America, which represents 50 malpractice insurance companies covering 50 percent of private physicians in the United States, claims that breast cancer accounts for more medical malpractice claims than any other medical condition. Delayed diagnosis is common among both younger and older women. The report focuses on 487 lawsuits in which damages were awarded for delayed diagnosis. The most common reasons for delay were misdiagnosis, failure to follow up, and false negative mammograms. The next most common medical diagnoses involving malpractice suits were infant brain damage, pregnancy, and heart attacks.[20] Nothing much has changed since this study was conducted. Misdiagnosis and failure to follow up remain high on the list of common malpractice claims.

Statutory Law

Statutory law is written law emanating from a legislative body. Although a statute can abolish any rule of common law, it can do so only by express words. The principles and rules of statutory law are set in hierarchical order. The Constitution of the United States adopted at the Constitutional Convention in Philadelphia in 1787 is highest in the hierarchy of enacted law. Article VI of the Constitution declares:

> This Constitution, and the Laws of the United States which shall be made in Pursuance thereof; and all Treaties made, or which shall be made, under the Authority of the United States, shall be the supreme Law of the Land; and the Judges in every State shall be bound thereby, any Thing in the Constitution or Laws of any State to the Contrary notwithstanding.[21]

The clear import of these words is that the U.S. Constitution, federal law, and federal treaties take precedence over the constitutions and laws of specific states and local jurisdictions.

Statutory law may be amended, repealed, or expanded by action of the legislature. States and local jurisdictions can only enact and enforce laws that do not conflict with federal law. Statutory laws may be declared void by a court; for example, a statute may be found unconstitutional because it does not comply with a state or federal constitution, because it is vague or ambiguous, or, in the case of a state law, because it is in conflict with a federal law.

In many cases involving statutory law, the court is called on to interpret how a statute applies to a given set of facts. For example, a statute may state merely that no person may discriminate against another person because of race, creed, color, or sex. A court may then be called on to decide whether certain actions by a person are discriminatory and therefore violate the law.

Administrative Law

Administrative law is the extensive body of public law issued by either state or federal agencies to direct the enacted laws of the federal and state governments. It is the branch of law that controls the administrative operations of government. Congress and state legislative bodies realistically cannot oversee their many laws; therefore, they delegate implementation and administration of the law to an appropriate administrative agency. Health care organizations in particular are inundated with a proliferation of administrative rules and regulations affecting every aspect of their operations.

The *Administrative Procedures Act*[22] describes the different procedures under which federal administrative agencies must operate.[23] The act prescribes the procedural responsibilities and authority of administrative agencies and provides for legal remedies for those wronged by agency actions. The regulatory power exercised by administrative agencies includes power to license, power of rate setting (e.g., Centers for Medicare and Medicaid Services [CMS]), and power over business practices (e.g., National Labor Relations Board [NLRB]).

Rules and Regulations

Administrative agencies have legislative, judicial, and executive functions. They have the authority to formulate rules and regulations considered necessary to carry out the intent of legislative enactments. Regulatory agencies have the ability to legislate, adjudicate, and enforce their own regulations in many cases.

Rules and regulations established by an administrative agency must be administered within the scope of authority delegated to it by Congress. Although an agency must comply with its own regulations, agency regulations must be consistent with the statute under which they are promulgated. An agency's interpretation of a statute cannot supersede the language chosen by Congress. An executive regulation that defines some general statutory term in a too-restrictive or unrealistic manner is invalid. Agency regulations and administrative decisions are subject to judicial review when questions arise as to whether an agency has overstepped its bounds in its interpretation of the law.

§702: Right to Review

A person suffering legal wrong because of agency action, or adversely affected or aggrieved by agency action within the meaning of a relevant statute, is entitled to judicial review thereof. . . .[24]

§706: Scope of Review

To the extent necessary . . . the reviewing court shall decide all relevant questions of law, interpret constitutional and statutory provisions, and deter-

mine the meaning or applicability of the terms of an agency action. The reviewing court shall

(1) compel agency action unlawfully withheld or unreasonably delayed; and

(2) hold unlawful and set aside agency action, findings, and conclusions found to be

    (A) arbitrary, capricious, an abuse of discretion, or otherwise not in accordance with law;

    (B) contrary to constitutional right, power, privilege, or immunity;

    (C) in excess of statutory jurisdiction, authority, or limitations, or short of statutory right;

    (D) without observance of procedure required by law;

    (E) unsupported by substantial evidence in a case subject to sections 556 and 557 of this title or otherwise reviewed on the record of an agency hearing provided by statute; or

    (F) unwarranted by the facts to the extent that the facts are subject to trial de novo by the reviewing court.

In making the foregoing determinations, the court shall review the whole record or those parts of it cited by a party, and due account shall be taken of the rule of prejudicial error.[25]

Recourse to an administrative agency for resolution of a dispute is generally required prior to seeking judicial review. The Pennsylvania Commonwealth Court held in *Fair Rest Home v. Commonwealth, Department of Health*[26] that the department of health was required to hold a hearing before it ordered revocation of a nursing home's operating license. The department of health failed in its responsibility when "in a revocation proceeding it [did] not give careful consideration to its statutorily mandated responsibility to hear testimony."[27]

Regulations and decisions of administrative agencies reviewed by the courts may be upheld, modified, overturned, or reversed and remanded for further proceedings. For example, the owner and operator of a licensed residential care facility brought an action challenging regulations governing administration of medicines in residential care facilities, promulgated by the U.S. Department of Health and Human Services (DHHS) through its Office of Long-Term Care (OLTC).[28] The owner challenged two OLTC regulations that required:

3. Under no circumstances shall an operator or employee or anyone solicited by an operator or employee be permitted to administer any oral medications, injectable medications, eye drops,

ear drops, or topical ointments (both prescription and nonprescription drugs).

4. In addition, any owner and/or operator of a Residential Care Facility who is a licensed nurse who administers any medication to a resident will be in violation of operating an unlicensed nursing home.[29]

The circuit court in this case held that the regulations were invalid and DHHS appealed. The Supreme Court, reversing the circuit court's decision, held that the regulations were reasonable in light of the distinctions between residential care facilities and nursing homes.

Conflict of Laws

The following case illustrates how federal and state laws may be in conflict. The plaintiff in *Dorsten v. Lapeer County General Hospital*[30] brought an action against a hospital and certain physicians on the medical board alleging wrongful denial of her application for medical staff privileges. The plaintiff asserted claims under the U.S. Code for sex discrimination, violations of the Sherman Antitrust Act, and the like. The plaintiff filed a motion to compel discovery of peer-review reports to support her case. The U.S. District Court held that the plaintiff was entitled to discovery of peer-review reports despite a Michigan state law purporting to establish an absolute privilege for peer-review reports conducted by hospital review boards.

GOVERNMENT ORGANIZATION

The three branches of the federal government are the legislative, executive, and judicial branches (Figure 2–1). Figure 2–2 illustrates a typical example of a state government organization. A vital concept in the constitutional framework of government on both federal and state levels is the separation of powers. Essentially, this principle provides that no one branch of government is clearly dominant over the other two; however, in the exercise of its functions, each may affect and limit the activities, functions, and powers of the others.

Legislative Branch

On the federal level, legislative powers are vested in the Congress of the United States, which consists of the Senate and the House of Representatives. The function of the legislative branch is to enact laws that may amend or repeal existing legislation and to create new legislation. The legislature determines the nature and extent of the need for new laws and for changes in existing laws. Committees of both houses of Congress are responsible for preparing federal legislation. There are 16 standing committees in the Senate and 19 in the House of Representatives, all of whose membership are appointed by a vote of the entire body.

Legislative proposals are assigned or referred to an appropriate committee for study. The committees conduct investigations and hold hearings where interested persons may present their views regarding proposed legislation. These proceedings provide additional information to assist committee members in their consideration of proposed bills. A bill may be reported out of a committee in its original form, favorably or unfavorably; it may be reported out with recommended amendments; or the bill might be allowed to lie in the committee without action. Some bills eventually reach the full legislative body, where, after consideration and debate, they may be approved or rejected.

The U.S. Congress and all state legislatures are *bicameral* (consisting of two houses), except for the Nebraska legislature, which is unicameral. Both houses in a bicameral legislature must pass identical versions of a legislative proposal before the legislation can be brought to the chief executive.

Executive Branch

The primary function of the executive branch of government on the federal and state level is to administer and enforce the law. The chief executive, either the President of the United States or the governor of a state, also has a role in the creation of law through the power to approve or veto legislative proposals.

The U.S. Constitution provides that the President of the United States of America holds the executive power. The president serves as the administrative head of the executive branch of the federal government. The executive branch includes 15 executive departments (see Figure 2–1), as well as a variety of agencies, both temporary and permanent.

The cabinet is composed of the 15 executive department heads.[31] Each department is responsible for a different area of public affairs, and each enforces the law within its area of responsibility. For example, the DHHS administers much of the federal health law enacted by Congress. Most state executive branches are also organized on a departmental basis. These departments administer and enforce state law concerning public affairs.

On a state level, the governor serves as the chief executive officer. The responsibilities of a state governor are provided for in the state's constitution. The Massachusetts State Constitution, for example, describes the responsibilities of the governor as:[32]

- presenting an annual budget to the state legislature

- recommending new legislation

- vetoing legislation

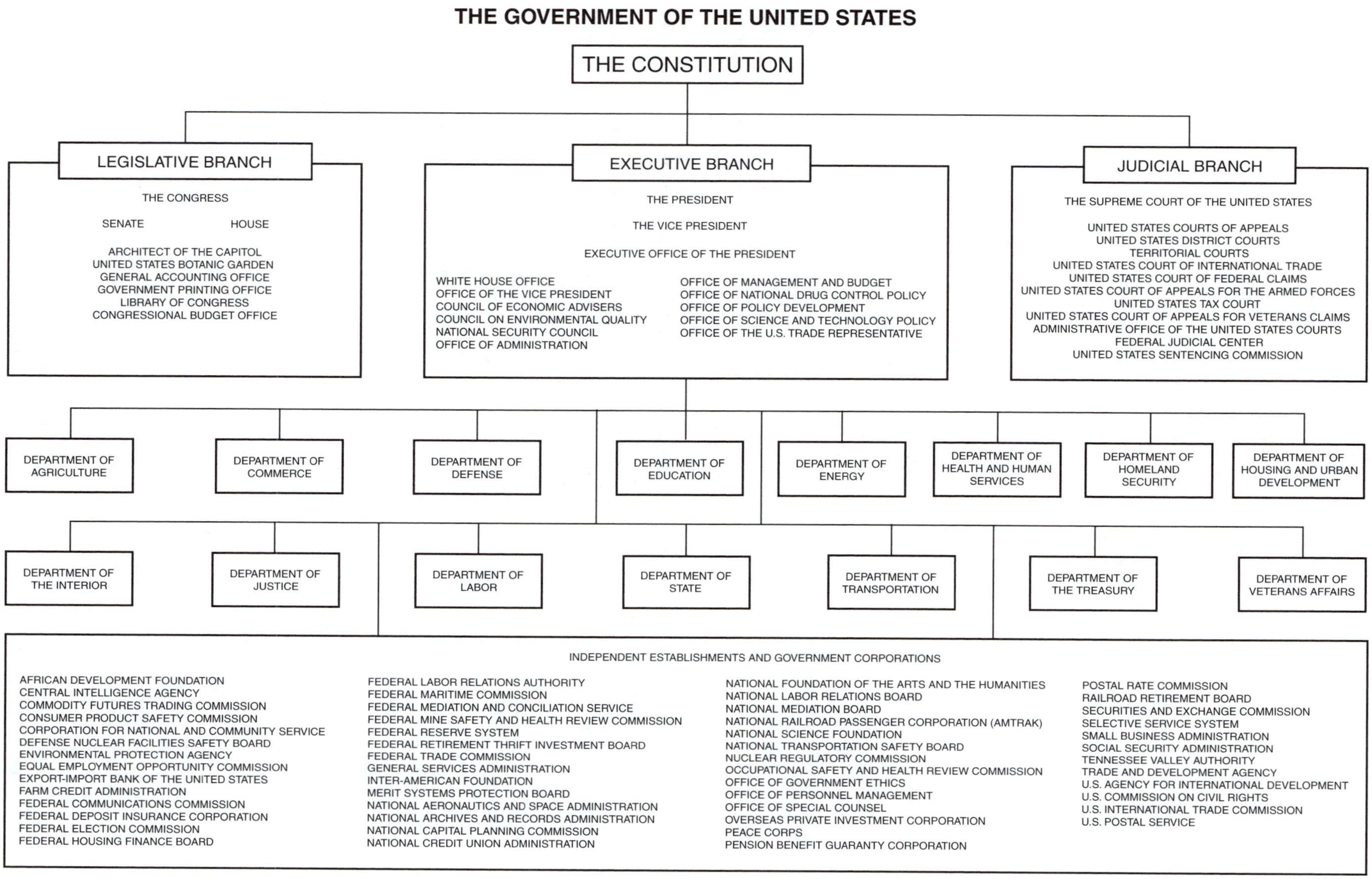

THE GOVERNMENT OF THE UNITED STATES

THE CONSTITUTION

LEGISLATIVE BRANCH

THE CONGRESS

SENATE   HOUSE

ARCHITECT OF THE CAPITOL
UNITED STATES BOTANIC GARDEN
GENERAL ACCOUNTING OFFICE
GOVERNMENT PRINTING OFFICE
LIBRARY OF CONGRESS
CONGRESSIONAL BUDGET OFFICE

EXECUTIVE BRANCH

THE PRESIDENT

THE VICE PRESIDENT

EXECUTIVE OFFICE OF THE PRESIDENT

WHITE HOUSE OFFICE
OFFICE OF THE VICE PRESIDENT
COUNCIL OF ECONOMIC ADVISERS
COUNCIL ON ENVIRONMENTAL QUALITY
NATIONAL SECURITY COUNCIL
OFFICE OF ADMINISTRATION

OFFICE OF MANAGEMENT AND BUDGET
OFFICE OF NATIONAL DRUG CONTROL POLICY
OFFICE OF POLICY DEVELOPMENT
OFFICE OF SCIENCE AND TECHNOLOGY POLICY
OFFICE OF THE U.S. TRADE REPRESENTATIVE

JUDICIAL BRANCH

THE SUPREME COURT OF THE UNITED STATES

UNITED STATES COURTS OF APPEALS
UNITED STATES DISTRICT COURTS
TERRITORIAL COURTS
UNITED STATES COURT OF INTERNATIONAL TRADE
UNITED STATES COURT OF FEDERAL CLAIMS
UNITED STATES COURT OF APPEALS FOR THE ARMED FORCES
UNITED STATES TAX COURT
UNITED STATES COURT OF APPEALS FOR VETERANS CLAIMS
ADMINISTRATIVE OFFICE OF THE UNITED STATES COURTS
FEDERAL JUDICIAL CENTER
UNITED STATES SENTENCING COMMISSION

DEPARTMENT OF AGRICULTURE

DEPARTMENT OF COMMERCE

DEPARTMENT OF DEFENSE

DEPARTMENT OF EDUCATION

DEPARTMENT OF ENERGY

DEPARTMENT OF HEALTH AND HUMAN SERVICES

DEPARTMENT OF HOUSING AND URBAN DEVELOPMENT

DEPARTMENT OF THE INTERIOR

DEPARTMENT OF JUSTICE

DEPARTMENT OF LABOR

DEPARTMENT OF STATE

DEPARTMENT OF TRANSPORTATION

DEPARTMENT OF HOMELAND SECURITY

DEPARTMENT OF THE TREASURY

DEPARTMENT OF VETERANS AFFAIRS

INDEPENDENT ESTABLISHMENTS AND GOVERNMENT CORPORATIONS

AFRICAN DEVELOPMENT FOUNDATION
CENTRAL INTELLIGENCE AGENCY
COMMODITY FUTURES TRADING COMMISSION
CONSUMER PRODUCT SAFETY COMMISSION
CORPORATION FOR NATIONAL AND COMMUNITY SERVICE
DEFENSE NUCLEAR FACILITIES SAFETY BOARD
ENVIRONMENTAL PROTECTION AGENCY
EQUAL EMPLOYMENT OPPORTUNITY COMMISSION
EXPORT-IMPORT BANK OF THE UNITED STATES
FARM CREDIT ADMINISTRATION
FEDERAL COMMUNICATIONS COMMISSION
FEDERAL DEPOSIT INSURANCE CORPORATION
FEDERAL ELECTION COMMISSION
FEDERAL HOUSING FINANCE BOARD

FEDERAL LABOR RELATIONS AUTHORITY
FEDERAL MARITIME COMMISSION
FEDERAL MEDIATION AND CONCILIATION SERVICE
FEDERAL MINE SAFETY AND HEALTH REVIEW COMMISSION
FEDERAL RESERVE SYSTEM
FEDERAL RETIREMENT THRIFT INVESTMENT BOARD
FEDERAL TRADE COMMISSION
GENERAL SERVICES ADMINISTRATION
INTER-AMERICAN FOUNDATION
MERIT SYSTEMS PROTECTION BOARD
NATIONAL AERONAUTICS AND SPACE ADMINISTRATION
NATIONAL ARCHIVES AND RECORDS ADMINISTRATION
NATIONAL CAPITAL PLANNING COMMISSION
NATIONAL CREDIT UNION ADMINISTRATION

NATIONAL FOUNDATION OF THE ARTS AND THE HUMANITIES
NATIONAL LABOR RELATIONS BOARD
NATIONAL MEDIATION BOARD
NATIONAL RAILROAD PASSENGER CORPORATION (AMTRAK)
NATIONAL SCIENCE FOUNDATION
NATIONAL TRANSPORTATION SAFETY BOARD
NUCLEAR REGULATORY COMMISSION
OCCUPATIONAL SAFETY AND HEALTH REVIEW COMMISSION
OFFICE OF GOVERNMENT ETHICS
OFFICE OF PERSONNEL MANAGEMENT
OFFICE OF SPECIAL COUNSEL
OVERSEAS PRIVATE INVESTMENT CORPORATION
PEACE CORPS
PENSION BENEFIT GUARANTY CORPORATION

POSTAL RATE COMMISSION
RAILROAD RETIREMENT BOARD
SECURITIES AND EXCHANGE COMMISSION
SELECTIVE SERVICE SYSTEM
SMALL BUSINESS ADMINISTRATION
SOCIAL SECURITY ADMINISTRATION
TENNESSEE VALLEY AUTHORITY
TRADE AND DEVELOPMENT AGENCY
U.S. AGENCY FOR INTERNATIONAL DEVELOPMENT
U.S. COMMISSION ON CIVIL RIGHTS
U.S. INTERNATIONAL TRADE COMMISSION
U.S. POSTAL SERVICE

Figure 2–1 The Government of the United States

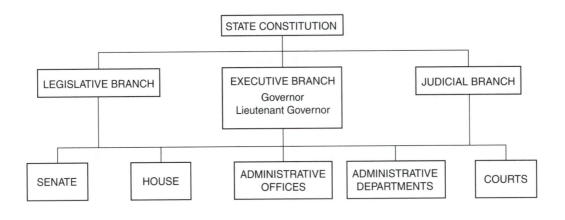

Figure 2–2 State Government Organizations

- appointing and removing department heads
- appointing judicial officers
- acting as Commander-in-Chief of the state's military forces (the Massachusetts National Guard)

Judicial Branch

As I have said in the past, when government bureaus and agencies go awry, which are adjuncts of the legislative or executive branches, the people flee to the third branch, their courts, for solace and justice.[33]

Justice J. Henderson,
Supreme Court of South Dakota

The function of the judicial branch of government is *adjudication*—resolving disputes in accordance with law. As a practical matter, most disputes or controversies that are covered by legal principles or rules are resolved without resort to the courts.

Alexis de Tocqueville (1805–1859), a foreign observer commenting on the primordial place of the law and the legal profession, stated, "Scarcely any political question arises in the United States that is not resolved, sooner or later, into a judicial question."[34]

The decision as to which court has *jurisdiction*—the legal right to hear and rule on a particular case—is determined by such matters as the locality in which each party to a lawsuit resides and the issues of a lawsuit. Each state in the United States provides its own court system, which is created by the state's constitution and statutes. Most of the nation's judicial business is reviewed and acted on in state courts. Each state maintains a level of trial courts that have

original jurisdiction, meaning the authority of a court to first conduct a trial on a specific case as distinguished from a court with *appellate jurisdiction,* where appeals from trial judgments are held. This jurisdiction may exclude cases involving claims with damages less than a specified minimum, probate matters (i.e., wills and estates), and workers' compensation. Different states have designated different names for trial courts (e.g., superior, district, circuit, or supreme courts). Also on the trial court level are minor courts such as city, small claims, and justice of the peace courts. States such as Massachusetts have consolidated their minor courts into a statewide court system.

Each state has at least one appellate court. Many states have an intermediate appellate court between the trial courts and the court of last resort. Where this intermediate court is present, there is a provision for appeal to it, with further review in all but select cases. Because of this format, the highest appellate tribunal is seen as the final arbiter in cases that possess importance in themselves or for the particular state's system of jurisprudence. Figure 2–3 depicts a typical state court system.

The trial court of the federal system is the U.S. District Court. There are 89 district courts in the 50 states (the larger states having more than one district court) and one in the District of Columbia. The Commonwealth of Puerto Rico also has a district court with jurisdiction corresponding to that of district courts in the different states. Generally, only one judge is required to sit and decide a case, although certain cases require up to three judges. The federal district courts hear civil, criminal, admiralty, and bankruptcy cases.

The U.S. Courts of Appeals are appellate courts for the 11 judicial circuits. Their main purpose is to review cases tried in federal district courts within their respective circuits, but they also possess jurisdiction to review orders of designated administrative agencies and to issue original writs in appropriate cases. These intermediate appellate courts were created to relieve the U.S. Supreme Court of deciding all cases appealed from the federal trial courts.

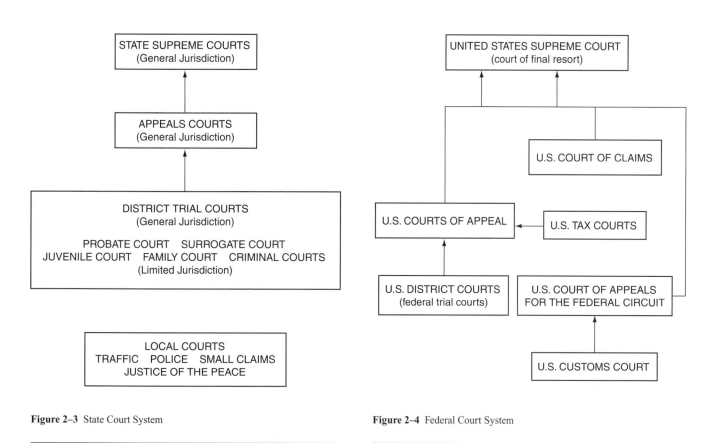

Figure 2–3 State Court System

Figure 2–4 Federal Court System

The Supreme Court, the nation's highest court, is the only federal court created directly by the Constitution. Eight associate justices and one chief justice sit on the Supreme Court. The court has limited original jurisdiction over the lower federal courts and the highest state courts. In a few situations, an appeal will go directly from a federal or state court to the Supreme Court, but in most cases, review must be sought through the discretionary writ of certiorari, an appeal petition. In addition to the aforementioned courts, special federal courts have jurisdiction over particular subject matters. The U.S. Court of Claims, for example, has jurisdiction over certain claims against the government. The U.S. Court of Appeals for the Federal Circuit has appellate jurisdiction over certain customs and patent matters. The U.S. Customs Court reviews certain administrative decisions by customs officials. Also, there is a U.S. Tax Court and a U.S. Court of Military Appeals. The federal court system is illustrated in Figure 2–4.

Separation of Powers

The concept of separation of powers, a system of checks and balances, is illustrated in the relationships among the branches of government with regard to legislation. On the federal level, when a bill creating a statute is enacted by Congress and signed by the president, it becomes law. If the president vetoes a bill, it takes a two thirds vote of each house of Congress to override the veto. The president also

can prevent a bill from becoming law by avoiding any action while Congress is in session. This procedure, known as a *pocket veto,* can temporarily stop a bill from becoming law and may permanently prevent it from becoming law if later sessions of Congress do not act on it favorably.

A bill that has become law may be declared invalid by the Supreme Court if the law violates the Constitution. "It is not entirely unworthy of observation, that in declaring what shall be the Supreme law of the land, the Constitution itself is first mentioned; and not the laws of the United States generally, but those only made in pursuance to the Constitution, have that rank."[35]

Even though a Supreme Court decision is final regarding a specific controversy, Congress and the president may generate new, constitutionally sound legislation to replace a law that has been declared unconstitutional. The procedures for amending the Constitution are complex and often time consuming, but they can serve as a way to offset or override a Supreme Court decision.

DEPARTMENT OF HEALTH AND HUMAN SERVICES

The DHHS (Figure 2–5), a cabinet-level department of the executive branch of the federal government, is concerned with people and is most involved with the nation's human concerns. The DHHS is responsible for developing and implementing

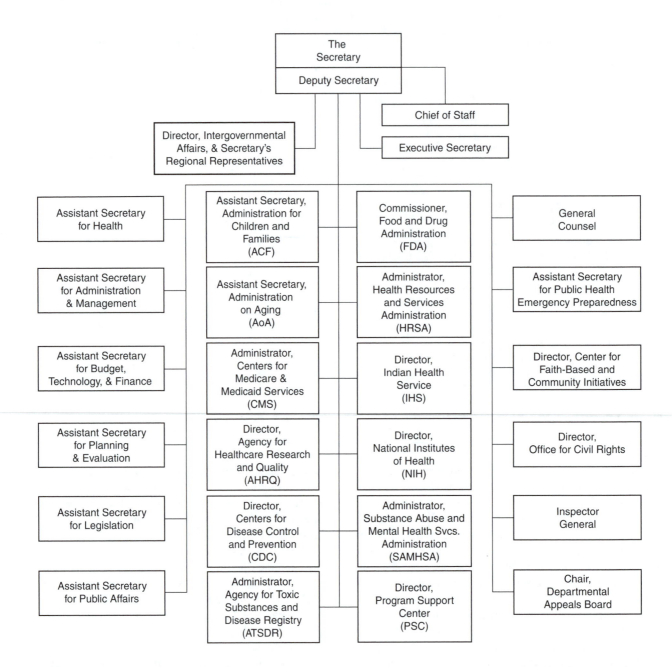

Figure 2–5 Department of Health and Human Services. *Source:* Reprinted from *U.S. Government Manual*, Department of Health and Human Services.

appropriate administrative regulations for carrying out national health and human services policy objectives. It is also the main source of regulations affecting the health care industry. The secretary of the DHHS, serving as the department's administrative head, advises the president with regard to health, welfare, and income security plans, policies, and programs.

The DHHS also is responsible for many of the programs designed to meet the needs of senior citizens, including Social Security benefits (e.g., retirement, survivors, and disability), Supplemental Security Income (which ensures a minimum monthly income to needy persons and is adminis-

tered by local Social Security offices), Medicare, Medicaid, and programs under the Older Americans Act (e.g., in-home services, such as home health and home-delivered meals, and community services such as adult day care, transportation, and ombudsman services in long-term care facilities).

Administration on Aging

The Administration on Aging (AOA) is the principal agency designated to carry out the provisions of the Older Americans Act of 1965, which as amended focuses on improving the lives of senior citizens in areas of income, housing, health, employment, retirement, and community services. The AOA develops policies, plans, and programs designed to promote the welfare of the elderly. It promotes their needs by planning programs and developing policy, procedural direction, and technical assistance to states and Native American tribal governments.

The Centers for Disease Control and Prevention

The Centers for Disease Control and Prevention (CDC) is recognized as the lead federal agency for protecting the health and safety of people at home and abroad, providing credible information to enhance health decisions and promoting health. The CDC serves as the national focus for developing and applying disease prevention and control, environmental health, and health promotion and education activities designed to improve the health of the people of the United States.

The Centers for Medicare and Medicaid Services

The Centers for Medicare and Medicaid Services (CMS), formerly the Health Care Financing Administration, was created to combine under one administration the oversight of the Medicare program, the federal portion of the Medicaid program, the State Children's Health Insurance Program, and related quality-assurance activities.

Medicare

Medicare is a federally sponsored health insurance program for persons older than 65 years of age and certain disabled persons. It has two complementary parts: Medicare Part A helps cover the costs of inpatient hospital care and, with qualifying preadmission criteria, skilled nursing facility care, home health care, and hospice care. Medicare Part B Medical Insurance helps pay for physicians' services, outpatient hospital services, and so forth.

Medicare is funded through Social Security contributions (Federal Insurance Contributions Act payroll taxes), premiums, and general revenue. The program is administered through private contractors, referred to as *intermediaries* under Part A and *carriers* under Part B. The financing of the Medicare program has received much attention by Congress because of its rapidly rising costs and drain on the nation's economy.

Medicaid

The Medicaid program, Title XIX of the Social Security Act Amendments of 1965, is a government program admin-istered by the states providing medical services (both institutional and outpatient) to the medically needy. Federal grants, in the form of matching funds, are issued to those states with qualifying Medicaid programs. In other words, Medicaid is jointly sponsored and financed by the federal government and several states. Medical care for needy persons of all ages is provided under the definition of need established by each state. Each state has set its own criteria for determining eligibility for services under its Medicaid program.

The Health Insurance Portability and Accountability Act of 1996

The CMS is responsible for implementing various provisions of the Health Insurance Portability and Accountability Act of 1996 (HIPAA). The administrative simplification provisions of HIPAA require that the DHHS establish national standards for electronic health care transactions and national identifiers for providers, health plans, and employers. It also addresses the privacy of health data.

Public Health Service

The mission of the Public Health Service (PHS) is to promote the protection of the nation's physical and mental health. The PHS accomplishes its mission by coordinating with the states in setting and implementing national health policy and pursuing effective intergovernmental relations; generating and upholding cooperative international health-related agreements, policies, and programs; conducting medical and biomedical research; sponsoring and administering programs for the development of health resources, the prevention and control of diseases, and alcohol and drug abuse; providing resources and expertise to the states and other public and private institutions in the planning, direction, and delivery of physical and mental health care services; and enforcing laws to ensure drug safety and protection from impure and unsafe foods, cosmetics, medical devices, and radiation-producing objects.

Within the PHS are smaller agencies responsible for carrying out the purpose of the division and DHHS, and include the following:

- *Agency for Healthcare Research and Quality*

  The Agency for Healthcare Research and Quality (AHRQ) research provides evidence-based information on health care outcomes, quality, cost, use, and access. Information from AHRQ's research helps people make more informed decisions and improve the quality of health care services.

• *Food and Drug Administration*

The Food and Drug Administration (FDA) supervises and controls the introduction of drugs, foods, cosmetics, and medical devices into the marketplace and protects society from impure and hazardous items. The FDA regulates nearly every consumer product.

• *National Institutes of Health*

The National Institutes of Health (NIH) is the principal federal biomedical research agency. It is responsible for conducting, supporting, and promoting biomedical research.

CHAPTER REVIEW

1. A *law* is a general rule of conduct that is enforced by the government. When a law is violated, the government imposes a penalty.

   • *Public laws* deal with the relationships between individuals and the government.

   • *Private laws* deal with relationships among individuals. Two types of private law are tort and contract actions. In a tort action, one person holds that wrongful conduct caused another person and the victim seeks compensation. Contract action deals with the accusation of a breach of agreement between two parties. Compensation can come in the form of remuneration or performance of the contracted obligation.

2. *Common law* is derived from judicial decisions. U.S. common law has as its roots the English common-law system. The first English royal court was established in 1178. There were few written laws at the time, and a collection of principles evolved from the decisions of the court. These principles, known as common law, were used to decide subsequent cases. During the colonial period, the United States based its law on English common law, but states had the authority to modify their legal systems. As a result, there is no uniform system of common law among the states.

3. A common-law principle established in a higher state court must be followed by the lower courts in that state. However, trial courts or those otherwise on equal footing are not bound by the decisions of other trial courts, and a principle established in one state does not set precedent within another state. Common-law principles can be modified, overturned, abrogated, or created by new court decisions. These changes help the law keep pace with changes in society.

4. *Statutory law* is written law that emanates from legislative bodies. Using express words, a statute can abolish any rule of common law. The Constitution is the highest level of enacted law; it takes precedence over the constitutions and laws of specific states and local jurisdictions.

5. Statutory law can be amended, repealed, or expanded by the legislature. States and local jurisdictions can enact and enforce only laws that do no conflict with federal laws.

6. *Administrative law* is public law issued by administrative agencies to administer the enacted laws of the federal and state governments. This branch of law controls the administrative operations of the government.

7. Administrative agencies implement and administer the administrative law. The rules and regulations established by an agency must be administered within the scope of the authority delegated to the agency by Congress. Agency regulations and decisions can be subject to judicial review.

8. Each state has its own system of administrative law.

9. The concept of *separation of powers* provides that no one branch of the government—legislative, executive, or judicial—will be clearly dominant over the other two. The *legislative branch* enacts, amends, and/or repeals existing laws. The *executive branch* administers and enforces the law. The *judicial branch* resolves disputes in accordance with the law.

10. The Department of Health and Human Services develops and implements administrative regulations for carrying out national health and human services policy objectives.

REVIEW QUESTIONS

1. Define the term *law* and describe the sources from which law is derived.
2. Define the legal terms *precedent, res judicata, stare decisis, original jurisdiction,* and *appellate jurisdiction.*

3. Describe the function of each branch of government.
4. What is the meaning of separation of powers?
5. What is the function of an administrative agency?
6. Describe the responsibilities of the DHHS.

NOTES

1. B. Schwartz, The Law in America 1 (1974).

2. 5 U.S. (Cranch) 137, 163 (1803).

3. *Cruzan v. Director of the Mo. Dept. of Health,* 496 U.S. 261, 110 S.Ct. 2841 (1990).

4. A. K. R. Kiralfy, Potter's Historical Introduction to English Law 9 (1962).

5. J. Reeves, History of the English Law 2 (1814).

6. *Id.*

7. G. W. Keeton, English Law 70 (1974).

8. *Id.*

9. *Id.*

10. Kiralfy, *supra* note 4, at 9–10.

11. Schwartz, *supra* note 1, at 29.

12. L. Friedman, A History of American Law 92 (1985).

13. Black's Law Dictionary 1305 (6th ed. 1990).

14. U.S. Dept. of Health & Human Services, Task Force on Medical Liability and Malpractice 3 (1987).

15. *Id.*

16. Zinman, *Study Finds Hospitals "Harm" Some,* NEWSDAY, March 1, 1990, at 17.

17. The Robert Wood Johnson Foundation, *The Tort System for Medical Malpractice: How Well Does It Work, What Are the Alternatives?,* ABRIDGE, Spring 1991, at 2.

18. The Robert Wood Johnson Foundation, *Negligent Medical Care: What Is It, Where Is It, and How Widespread Is It?,* ABRIDGE, Spring 1991, at 6.

19. D. Sharp, *Errors Renew the Call for Doctor Review,* USA TODAY, March 27, 1995, at 2.

20. K. Painter, *Breast Cancer Top Cause of Malpractice Complaints,* USA TODAY, June 15, 1996, at 1.

21. U.S. CONST. art. VI, § 1, cl. 2.

22. 5 U.S.C.S. §§ 500–576 (Law. Co-op. 1989).

23. An "agency means each authority of the Government of the United States, . . . but does not include (A) the Congress; the Courts of the United States; . . ." 5 U.S.C.S. § 551(1) (Law. Co-op. 1989).

24. 5 U.S.C.S. § 702 (Law. Co-op. 1989).

25. 5 U.S.C.S. § 706 (Law. Co-op. 1989).

26. 401 A.2d 872 (Pa. Commw. Ct. 1979).

27. *Id.* at 873.

28. *Department of Human Serv. v. Berry,* 764 S.W.2d 437 (Ark.1989).

29. *Id.* at 439.

30. 88 F.R.D. 583 (E.D. Mich. 1980).

31. http://dir.yahoo.com/Government/U_S_Government/Executive_Branch/Departments_and_Agencies/.

32. D. Levitan, Your Massachusetts Government 14 (10th ed. 1984).

33. *Heritage of Yankton, Inc. v. South Dakota Dep't. of Health,* 432 N.W.2d 68, 77 (S.D. 1988).

34. Schwartz, *supra* note 1, at 15.

35. *Marbury v. Madison,* 5 U.S. (Cranch) 137, 180 (1803).

Tort Law

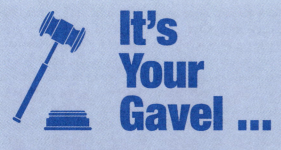

It's Your Gavel ...

THE COURT WAS APPALLED

The plaintiff, while in the custody of the defendant penal institution, alleged that because the defendant's employees failed to timely diagnose her breast cancer, her right breast had to be removed. The defendant contended that even if its employees were negligent, the plaintiff's cancer was so far developed when discovered that it would nevertheless have required removal of her breast.[1]

Pursuant to the defendant's policy of medically evaluating all new inmates, on May 26, 1989, Dr. Evans gave the plaintiff a medical examination. He testified that his physical evaluation included an examination of the plaintiff's breasts. However, he stated that his examination was very cursory.

The day following her examination, the plaintiff examined her own breasts. At that time she discovered a lump in her right breast, which she characterized as being about the size of a pea.

The plaintiff then sought an additional medical evaluation at the defendant's medical clinic. Testimony indicated that fewer than half of the inmates who sign the clinic list are actually seen by medical personnel the next day. Also, those not examined on the day for which the list is signed are given no preference in being examined on the following day. Their names are simply deleted from the daily list and their only recourse is to continually sign the list until they are examined. The evidence indicated that after May 27, the plaintiff constantly signed the clinic list and provided the reason she was requesting medical care.

A nurse finally examined the plaintiff on June 21. The nurse noted in her nursing notes that the plaintiff had a "moderate large mass in right breast." The nurse recognized that the proper procedure was to measure such a mass but she testified that this was impossible because no measuring device was available. The missing measuring device to which she alluded was a simple ruler. The nurse concluded that Evans should again examine the plaintiff.

On June 28, Evans again examined the plaintiff. He recorded in the progress notes that the plaintiff had "a mass on her right wrist. Will send her to hospital and give her Benadryl for allergy she has."[2] Evans meant to write "breast" not "wrist."

He again failed to measure the size of the mass on the plaintiff's breast.

The plaintiff was transferred to the Franklin County Prerelease Center (FCPR) on September 28. On September 30, a nurse at FCPR examined the plaintiff; the nurse recorded that the plaintiff had a "golf-ball"–sized lump in her right breast. The plaintiff was transported to the hospital on October 27, where Dr. Walker treated her. The plaintiff received a mammogram examination, which indicated that the tumor was probably malignant. This diagnosis was confirmed by a biopsy performed on November 9. The plaintiff was released from confinement on November 13.

On November 16, Dr. Lidsky, a surgeon, examined the plaintiff. Lidsky noted the existence of the lump in the plaintiff's breast and determined that the size of the mass was approximately 4 to 5 centimeters and somewhat fixed. He performed a modified radical mastectomy upon the plaintiff's right breast, by which nearly the plaintiff's entire right breast was removed.

WHAT IS YOUR VERDICT?

Every instance of a man's suffering the penalty of the law is an instance of the failure of that penalty in effecting its purpose, which is to deter from transgression.

Whately

This chapter introduces the reader to the study of tort law. A *tort* is a civil wrong, other than a breach of contract, committed against a person or property (real or personal) for which a court provides a remedy in the form of an action for damages. Tort actions touch an individual both on a personal and a professional level, which is why those involved in the health care field should be armed with the knowledge necessary to make them aware of their rights and responsibilities.

The basic objectives of tort law are preservation of peace between individuals by providing a substitute for retaliation; *culpability* (to find fault for wrongdoing); deterrence to discourage the wrongdoer (tort-feasor) from committing future torts; and compensation to indemnify the injured persons of wrongdoing.

Compensation for adverse medical outcomes typically takes the form of financial damages. When finding fault, the court must determine who should bear the cost of an unfavorable outcome—the patient-plaintiff or the provider-defendant. The plaintiff must prove negligence by the defendant. Conversely, the defendant argues a case to avoid fault determination. Underlying this adversarial proceeding is the assumption that when a defendant bears the cost of a negligent act, there will be a decline in similar acts. Although professional liability insurance helps to insulate a provider from financial loss, the fear is ever present that the monetary award may exceed coverage limits, thus resulting in out-of-pocket expenses for the provider.

Incidents that raise issues of liability fall under three basic categories of tort law. In the context of the first category, patient care, negligent torts occur most commonly. The next, intentional torts, includes assault, battery, false imprisonment, invasion of privacy, and infliction of mental distress. Finally, strict liability, irrespective of fault, may be imposed in certain situations in which the activity, regardless of intentions or negligence, is so dangerous to others that public policy demands absolute responsibility on the part of the tort-feasor.

NEGLIGENCE

Negligence is a tort; a civil or personal wrong. It is the unintentional commission or omission of an act that a reasonably prudent person would or would not do under the same or similar circumstances. It is the failure to use ordinary or reasonable care. Ordinary or reasonable care is that care which persons of ordinary prudence would use.

Commission of an act would include, for example:

- Administering the wrong medication
- Administering the wrong dosage of a medication
- Administering medication to the wrong patient
- Performing a surgical procedure without patient consent
- Performing a surgical procedure on the wrong patient
- Performing the wrong surgical procedure

Omission of an act would include, for example:

- Failing to conduct a thorough history and physical examination

- Failing to assess and reassess a patient's nutritional needs
- Failing to administer medications
- Failing to order diagnostic tests
- Failing to follow up on abnormal test results

Negligence is a form of conduct caused by heedlessness or carelessness that constitutes a departure from the standard of care generally imposed on reasonable members of society. It can occur when after considering the consequences of an act, a person does not exercise the best possible judgment; where one fails to guard against a risk that should be appreciated; or where one engages in behavior expected to involve unreasonable danger to others. Negligence or carelessness of a professional person is classified as *malpractice,* whereas *criminal negligence* is the reckless disregard for the safety of another (e.g., willful indifference to an injury that could follow an act).

Malpractice suits may allege various mistakes made by doctors or other medical professionals, including misdiagnosis, mistreatment, delayed diagnosis, failure to diagnose, surgical errors, medical errors, or various types of negligence. Not all errors in medical diagnosis and treatment are necessarily malpractice, because there are certain risks and margins for error that arise inherently in the practice of medicine.[3]

Forms of Negligence

The three basic forms of negligence are:

1. *Malfeasance:* performance of an unlawful or improper act (e.g., performing an abortion in the third trimester when such is prohibited by state law)
2. *Misfeasance:* improper performance of an act, resulting in injury to another (e.g., wrong-sided surgery)
3. *Nonfeasance:* failure to act, when there is a duty to act as a reasonably prudent person would in similar circumstances (e.g., failing to order diagnostic tests or prescribe medications that should have been ordered or prescribed under the circumstances)

Degrees of Negligence

There are two degrees of negligence:

1. *Ordinary negligence:* failure to do what a reasonably prudent person would or would not do, under the circumstances of the act or omission in question
2. *Gross negligence:* intentional or wanton omission of care that would be proper to provide or the doing of that which would be improper to do

Elements of Negligence

The elements that must be present in order for a plaintiff to recover damages caused by negligence are:

1. Duty to care
   - There must be an obligation to conform to a recognized standard of care.
2. Breach of duty
   - There must be a deviation from the recognized standard of care.
   - There must be a failure to adhere to an obligation.
3. Injury
   - Actual damages must be established.
   - If there are no injuries, no damages are due.
4. Causation
   - The departure from the standard of care must be the cause of the plaintiff's injury.
   - The injury must be foreseeable.

All four elements must be present in order for a plaintiff to recover damages suffered as a result of a negligent act. When the four elements of negligence have been proven, the plaintiff is said to have presented a *prima facie case of negligence,* which will enable the plaintiff to prevail in the lawsuit.

The *burden of proof* in a negligence case is not as great as the beyond-a-reasonable-doubt standard borne by a prosecutor in a criminal case. Therefore, if a plaintiff supports a negligence claim with evidence sufficient to outweigh the evidence presented by the defendant, the defendant will be found liable for the negligent act. The defendant then will be ordered by the court, in accordance with the verdict rendered by the jury or by the court itself, to compensate the plaintiff monetarily for the harm that the plaintiff suffered. *Compensatory damages* seek to restore the injured party's financial situation to match the party's financial state before suffering harm. *Punitive damages* can also be awarded to the plaintiff for pain and suffering caused by conduct that would be considered egregious.

Duty to Care

To establish negligence, the plaintiff must first prove the existence of a legal relationship between himself or herself and the defendant. *Duty* is defined as a legal obligation of care, performance, or observance imposed on one to safeguard the rights of others. Duty may arise from a special relationship such as that between a physician and a patient.

The existence of the relationship implies that a physician-patient relationship was in effect at the time an alleged injury occurred. The duty to care can arise from a simple telephone conversation or out of a physician's voluntary act of assuming the care of a patient. Duty also can be established by statute or contract between the plaintiff and the defendant. Where there is a contractual duty of care and an injury occurs, patients have a choice of theories to use to determine which type of lawsuit to pursue—breach of contract or tort. In some jurisdictions, the statute of limitations for breach of contract is longer than for negligence actions. In such cases, the existence of a contractual duty of care may extend the liability of a health care provider for several years.

In *O'Neill v. Montefiore Hospital*,[4] the duty owed to a patient was clear. The plaintiff sought recovery against the hospital for failure to render necessary emergency treatment and against a physician for his failure and refusal to treat her spouse. The deceased, Mr. O'Neill, while experiencing pains in his chest and arms, walked with his wife to the hospital at 5:00 A.M. He claimed that he was a member of the Hospital Insurance Plan (HIP). The emergency department nurse stated that the hospital had no connection with HIP and did not take HIP patients. The nurse indicated that she would try to get a HIP physician for O'Neill. The nurse called Dr. Graig, an HIP physician, and explained the patient's symptoms to the doctor. It was suggested by Graig that O'Neill see a HIP physician at 8:00 A.M. The nurse then handed the phone to O'Neill, who said, "Well, I could be dead by 8 o'clock." O'Neill concluded his phone conversation and spoke to the nurse, indicating that he had been told to go home and come back when HIP was open. Mrs. O'Neill asked that a physician see her husband. The nurse again requested that they return at 8:00. O'Neill again commented that he could be dead by 8:00. He then left with his wife to return home, pausing occasionally to catch his breath. Shortly after arriving at home, O'Neill suddenly fell to the floor and died. Graig claimed that he had offered to come to the emergency department, but that O'Neill had said that he would wait and see another HIP physician at 8:00 that morning.

The New York Supreme Court for Bronx County entered a judgment dismissing the complaint, and the plaintiff appealed. The New York Supreme Court, Appellate Division, reversed the lower court and held that a physician who abandons a patient after undertaking examination or treatment can be held liable for malpractice. The proof of the record in this case indicated that the physician undertook to diagnose the ailments of the deceased by telephone, thus establishing at least the first element of negligence—duty to use due care. The finding of the trial court was reversed, and a new trial was ordered.

In a similar case, the surviving parents in *Hastings v. Baton Rouge Hospital*[5] brought a medical malpractice action for the wrongful death of their 19-year-old son. The action was brought against the hospital; the emergency department physician, Dr. Gerdes; and the thoracic surgeon on call, Dr. McCool. The patient had been brought to the emergency department at 11:56 P.M. because of two stab wounds and weak vital signs. Gerdes decided that a thoracotomy had to be performed. He was not qualified to perform the surgery and called McCool, who was on call that evening for thoracic surgery. Gerdes described the patient's condition, indicating he had been stabbed in a major blood vessel. At trial, McCool claimed that he did not recall Gerdes saying that a major blood vessel could be involved. McCool asked Gerdes to transfer the patient to the Earl K. Long Hospital. Gerdes said, "I can't transfer this patient." McCool replied, "No. Transfer him." Kelly, an emergency department nurse on duty, was not comfortable with the decision to transfer the patient and offered to accompany him in the ambulance. Gerdes reexamined the patient, who exhibited marginal vital signs, was restless, and was draining blood from his chest. The ambulance service was called at 1:03 A.M., and by 1:30 A.M. the patient had been placed in the ambulance for transfer. The patient began to fight wildly, the chest tube came out, and the bleeding increased. An attempt to revive him from a cardiac arrest was futile, and the patient died after having been moved back to the emergency department. The patient virtually bled to death.

The duty to care in this case cannot be reasonably disputed. Louisiana, by statute, imposes a duty on hospitals licensed in Louisiana to make emergency services available to all persons residing in the state regardless of insurance coverage or economic status. The hospital's own bylaws provide that patient transfer should never occur without due consideration for the patient's condition. The 19th Judicial District Court directed a verdict for the defendants, and the plaintiffs appealed. The court of appeals affirmed the district court's decision. On further appeal, the Louisiana Supreme Court held that the evidence presented to the jury could indicate the defendants were negligent in their treatment of the victim. The findings of the lower courts were reversed, and the case was remanded for trial.

As in *Hastings v. Baton Rouge Hospital*, some duties are created by statute, which occurs when a statute specifies a particular standard that must be met. Many such standards are created by administrative agencies under the provisions of a statute. To establish liability based on a defendant's failure to follow the standard of care outlined by statute, the following elements must be present:

1. the defendant must have been within the specified class of persons outlined in the statute
2. the plaintiff must have been injured in a way that the statute was designed to prevent
3. the plaintiff must show that the injury would not have occurred if the statute had not been violated

Duties may also be created by an institution through its internal rules and regulations. The courts hold that such internal rules are indicative of the organization's knowledge of the proper procedure to follow and, hence, create a duty. Thus, if an employee fails to follow an operating rule of that organization and, as a result, a patient is injured, then the employee who violated the rule would be considered negligent.

Texas courts, for example, recognize that an employer has a duty to hire competent employees, especially if they are engaged in an occupation that could be hazardous to life and limb and requires skilled or experienced persons. For example, the appellant in *Deerings West Nursing Center v. Scott*[6] was found to have negligently hired an incompetent employee that it knew or should have known was incompetent, thereby causing unreasonable risk of harm to others. In this case, an 80-year-old visitor had gone to Deerings to visit her infirm older brother. During one visit, Nurse Hopper, a 6-foot-4-inch male employee of Deerings, confronted the visitor to prevent her from visiting. The visitor recalled that he was angry and just stared. She stated that upon his approach she had thrown up her hands to protect her face, but he hit her on the chin, slapped her down on the concrete floor, and got on top of her, pinning her to the floor.

Hopper testified that he was hired sight unseen over the telephone by Deerings' director of nursing. Even though the following day, Hopper completed an application at the nursing facility, he still maintained that he was hired over the phone. In his application, he falsely stated that he was a Texas licensed vocational nurse (LVN). Additionally, he claimed that he had never been convicted of a crime. In reality, he had been previously employed by a bar, was not a LVN, had committed more than 56 criminal offenses of theft, and was on probation at the time of his testimony.

The trial court awarded the plaintiff a judgment of $35,000 for actual damages and $200,000 in punitive damages. The court of appeals held that there was evidence supporting findings that the employee's failure to obtain a nursing license was the proximate cause of the visitor's damages and that the hiring was negligent, and also showed a heedless and reckless disregard of the rights of others.

> It is common knowledge that the bleakness and rigors of old age, drugs, and the diseases of senility can cause people to become confused . . . and cantankerous. It is predictable that elderly patients will be visited by elderly friends and family. It is reasonable to anticipate that a man of proven moral baseness would be more likely to commit a morally base act on an 80-year-old woman. Fifty-six convictions for theft is some evidence of mental aberration. Hopper was employed not only to administer medicine but also to contend with the sometimes erratic behavior of the decrepit. The investigative process necessary to the procurement of a Texas nursing license would have precluded the licensing of Hopper. In the hiring of an unlicensed and potentially mentally and morally unfit nurse, it is reasonable to anticipate that an injury would result

as a natural and probable consequence of that negligent hiring.[7]

Deerings West Nursing Center v. Scott showed a clear duty of care. The appellant violated the very purpose of Texas licensing statutes by failing to verify whether Hopper held a current LVN license. The appellant then placed him in a position of authority, allowed him to dispense drugs, and made him a shift supervisor. This negligence eventually resulted in the inexcusable assault on an elderly woman.

Standard of Care

A duty of care carries with it a corresponding responsibility not only to provide care, but also to provide it in an acceptable manner. The plaintiff must show that the defendant failed to meet the prevailing standard of care. The fact that an injury is suffered is not sufficient for imposing liability without proof that the defendant deviated from the standard practice of competent fellow professionals. A nurse, for example, who assumes the care of a patient has the duty to exercise that degree of skill, care, and knowledge ordinarily possessed and exercised by other nurses. The standard of care describes the conduct expected of an individual in a given situation. The general standard of care that must be followed is that which a "reasonably prudent person" would exercise acting under the same or similar circumstances. The reasonably prudent person represents the conduct of the average person in the community under the circumstances facing the defendant at the time of the alleged negligence. The reasonableness of conduct is judged in light of the circumstances apparent at the time of injury and by reference to different characteristics of the actor (e.g., age, sex, physical condition, education, knowledge, training, mental capacity). The actual performance of an individual in a given situation will be measured against what a reasonably prudent person would or would not have done. Deviation from the standard of care will constitute negligence if there are resulting damages.

> The standard of conduct of a reasonable person may be: (a) established by a legislative enactment or administrative regulation which so provides, (b) adopted by the court from a legislative enactment or an administrative regulation which does not so provide, or (c) established by judicial decision, or, (d) applied to the facts of the case by the trial judge or jury, if there is no such enactment, regulation or decision.[8]

Traditionally, in determining how a reasonably prudent person should perform in a given situation, the courts often rely on the testimony of an expert witness as to the standard of care required in the same or similar communities. The plaintiff's expert witness in *Stogsdill v. Manor Convalescent Home, Inc., and Hiatt, MD,*[9] who practiced about 12 miles from the convalescent home where the defendant physician treated the plaintiff, was found competent to testify. The defendant objected, stating the expert never practiced in the county where the malpractice occurred. The court overruled this objection on the grounds that locality cannot be construed so narrowly as to be determined by county lines.

Expert testimony like that in *Stogsdill v. Manor Convalescent Home, Inc., and Hiatt, MD* is necessary when the jury is not trained or qualified to determine what the reasonably prudent professional's standard of care would be under similar circumstances. Most states hold those with special skills (e.g., physicians, nurses, and dentists) to a standard of care that is reasonable in the light of their special abilities and knowledge. For example, the plaintiff, in *Kowal v. Deer Park Fire District*[10] submitted affidavits from two doctors who stated that, to a reasonable degree of medical certainty, the death of the plaintiff's decedent "was caused by severe and extensive cerebral anoxia caused by . . . incorrect intubation," that the incorrect intubation of the decedent constituted medical malpractice, and that the failure to recognize that she had been improperly intubated constituted a gross departure from good and accepted practice of what is "a common place medical technique. Assuming that the deposition testimony of the defendants established prima facie evidence that they were not grossly negligent, the sworn opinion of the plaintiff's experts established that there were issues of fact that precluded the granting of summary judgment.

The courts have been moving away from reliance on a community standard and have applied an industry or national standard. This trend has developed as a result of a more reasonable belief that the standard of care should not vary with the locale where an individual receives care. It would be unreasonable for any one health care facility and/or health care professional to set the standard simply because there is no local basis for comparison. Geographic proximity rules have increasingly given way to a national standard, with the standard in the professional's general locality becoming a factor in determining whether the professional has exercised that degree of care expected of the average practitioner in the class to which he or she belongs.

The ever-evolving advances in medicine and mass communications, the availability of medical specialists, the development of continuing education programs, and the broadening scope of government regulations continue to raise the standard of care required of health care professionals and organizations. Many courts have adopted the view that the practice of medicine should be national in scope. In *Dickinson v. Mailliard,* the court stated:

> Hospitals must now be licensed and accredited. They are subject to statutory regulation. In order to obtain approval they must meet certain standard requirements. . . . It is no longer justifi-

able, if indeed it ever was, to limit a hospital's liability to that degree of care which is customarily practiced in its own community. . . . [M]any communities have only one hospital. Adherence to such a rule, then, means the hospital whose conduct is assailed, is to be measured only by standards which it has set for itself.[11]

The Court of Appeals of Maryland, in *Shilkret v. Annapolis Emergency Hospital Association,* stated:

> [A] hospital is required to use that degree of care and skill which is expected of a reasonably competent hospital in the same or similar circumstances. As in cases brought against physicians, advances in the profession, availability of special facilities and specialists, together with all other relevant considerations, are to be taken into account.[12]

Evidence of the standard of care applicable to professional activities may be found in a variety of documents, such as regulations of government agencies (e.g., state licensure laws) and standards established by private organizations, such as The Joint Commission.

While the courts tend to prefer a broader standard of care, the community standard can be extremely important in any given situation.

> Assume for a moment that the question is whether a doctor in a remote area of Alaska has placed patients at an unnecessarily high risk by receiving telephone inquiries from nurses in Eskimo villages at even more remote areas and attempting to prescribe by phone. Clearly, such conduct would violate the standard of care in San Francisco and, in San Francisco, would place his patients in an "unnecessarily" high-risk situation. For the doctor in Alaska, on the other hand, this method of consultation may be the only possible one, and thus not at all unnecessary or a gross and flagrant violation.[13]

The parents in *Wickliffe v. Sunrise Hospital*[14] sued the hospital for the wrongful death of their teenage daughter who suffered respiratory arrest while recovering from surgery. The Nevada Supreme Court held that the level of care to which the hospital must conform is a nationwide standard. The hospital's level of care is no longer subject to narrow geographic limitations under the so-called locality rule; rather, the hospital must meet a nationwide standard.

Further, the Georgia Court of Appeals in *Hodges v. Effingham*[15] held that application of the locality rule was erroneous in an action against the hospital. The alleged failure of nurses to take an accurate medical history of the patient's serious condition and convey the information to the physician drew into question the professional judgment of the nurses. The jury should have been instructed as to the general standard of nursing required.

> There are no degrees of care in fixing responsibility for negligence, but the standard is always that care which a prudent person should use under like circumstances. The duty to exercise reasonable care is a standard designed to protect a society's members from unreasonable exposure to potentially injurious hazards; negligence is conduct that falls short of the reasonable care standard. Perfection of conduct is humanly impossible, however, and the law does not exact an unreasonable amount of care from anyone.[16]

Specialists

Specialists in particular are held to a higher standard of care than nonspecialists. Generally, the reliance of the public upon the skills of a specialist and the wealth and sources of his or her knowledge are not limited to the geographic area in which he or she practices. Rather, his or her knowledge is a specialty; a person specializes to keep abreast. Any other standard for a specialist would negate the fundamental expectations and purpose of a specialty.

Breach of Duty

Once a duty to care has been established, the plaintiff must demonstrate that the defendant breached that duty by failing to comply with the accepted standard of care. *Breach of duty* is the failure to conform to or the departure from a required duty of care owed to a person. The obligation to perform according to a standard of care may encompass either doing or refraining from doing a particular act.

The court in *Hastings v. Baton Rouge Hospital,*[17] discussed earlier, found a severe breach of duty when a patient did not receive adequate care. Hospital regulations provided that when a physician cannot be reached or refuses a call, the chief of service must be notified so that another physician can be obtained. This was not done. A plaintiff need not prove that a patient would have survived if proper treatment had been administered, but only that the patient would have had a chance of survival. As a result of Dr. Gerdes' failure to make arrangements for another physician and Dr. McCool's failure to perform the necessary surgery, the patient had no chance of survival. The duty to provide for appropriate care under the circumstances was breached.

In *Dunahoo v. Brooks,*[18] the nursing facility was found to have breached its duty when a patient tripped over an obvi-

ously ill-placed light cord. The court stated that because the defendant nursing facility operator had been aware of the 94-year-old plaintiff's infirmities and had agreed to provide her nursing care, the nursing facility assumed an obligation to exercise care commensurate with her physical condition. While the plaintiff was getting out of bed, she tripped and fell over a light cord that was loose on the floor in an area that the defendant knew the plaintiff frequently used. The cord was plugged into a socket on the floor 5 inches from the baseboard. The court was impressed with the ease with which the situation could have been corrected, noting that the cord could have been fastened down with a few nails and the outlet placed on the baseboard instead of nearly in the middle of the floor.

Another nursing facility was found negligent in *Booty v. Kentwood Manor Nursing Home, Inc.,*[19] when a 90-year-old resident wandered outside the facility, fell, and suffered a hip fracture. The resident's physical condition deteriorated and he eventually died. The staff were aware of the resident's confusion and tendency to stray. The court found that the facility was responsible for taking reasonable steps to prevent injury to a mentally confused and physically fragile resident. The facility's alarm system might have alerted the staff of unauthorized resident departures, but it had been deactivated, and the doors were propped open for the convenience of the staff. The record demonstrated that inadequate supervision of the resident had been the cause of his departure and that he probably would not have suffered injury but for the nursing facility's breach of duty owed to the resident.

Injury/Actual Damages

A defendant may be negligent and still not incur liability if no injury or actual damages result to the plaintiff. Without harm or injury, there is no liability. *Injury* includes physical harm, pain, suffering, and loss of income or reputation.

The mere occurrence of an injury "does not establish negligence for which the law imposes liability, since the injury may be the result of an unavoidable accident, or an act of God, or some cause so remote to the person sought to be held liable for negligence that he cannot be charged with responsibility for the injury."[20]

Injury was obvious in *Lucas v. HCMF Corp.,*[21] where the patient had been transferred to a nursing facility following hospitalization for several ailments, including early decubitus ulcers. The resident was returned to the hospital 24 days later. "At that time the ulcer on her hip had become three large ulcers that reached to the bone and tunneled through the skin to meet one another. The ulcer on her buttocks had grown from one inch in diameter to eight inches in diameter and extended to the bone. Additional ulcers had developed on each of her ribs, on her left arm and wrist, and on the left side of her face."[22] The standard of care required in preventing and treating decubitus ulcers required that the resident be mobilized and turned every two hours to prevent deterioration of tissue. The treatment records reflected that the resident was not turned at all from September 22 through October 1, nor was she turned on October 4, 7, or 12. Failure to periodically turn the resident and move her to a chair had caused the deterioration in her condition.

Causation

The fourth element necessary to establish negligence requires that there be a reasonable, close, and causal connection or relationship between the defendant's negligent conduct and the resulting damages suffered by the plaintiff. In other words, the defendant's negligence must be a substantial factor causing the injury. *Proximate cause* is a term referring to the relationship between a breached duty and the injury. The breach of duty must be the proximate cause of the resulting injury. The mere departure from a proper and recognized procedure is not sufficient to enable a patient to recover damages unless the plaintiff can show that the departure was unreasonable and the proximate cause of the patient's injuries. Causation in the *Hastings v. Baton Rouge Hospital*[23] case was well established. In the ordinary course of events, Hastings would not have bled to death in a hospital emergency department over a two-hour period without some surgical intervention to save his life.

Negligent Misreading of CT Scan

On November 2, 1995, the plaintiff was admitted into the Brooklyn Hospital Center complaining of a severe headache, an inability to open her eyes, and the absence of feeling in her legs. A CT scan was administered, which the defendant conceded was misread by its staff physician as normal. After discharging the plaintiff from its care, the defendant's radiologist reviewed the CT scan and concluded it was, in fact, not normal. The defendant did not contact the plaintiff to alert her to the revised finding. After the hospital conceded that its employee's initial misreading of the CT scan and its failure to alert the plaintiff to the misreading were departures from accepted medical practice, the jury properly found that those conceded departures were the proximate causes of the plaintiff's injury. The evidence adduced at trial was legally sufficient to support the jury's verdict on causation.[24]

Failure to Refer

In *Robinson v. Group Health Association, Inc.,*[25] the District of Columbia Court of Appeals held that there was a genuine issue of material fact as to whether the failure of a group health provider to treat a patient's diabetes aggressively resulted in the amputation of his leg below the knee. The testimony of the plaintiff's expert, as it related to the issue of proximate cause, was sufficient to allow the case to go to the jury. According to the expert witness, the failure of the provider to refer the patient for vascular evaluation resulted in his below-the-knee amputation. The expert testified to a reasonable degree of medical certainty, which he equated to a greater than 50 percent chance, that if there had been an early vascular consult, followed by an angioplasty and perhaps a partial foot amputation, a below-the-knee amputation could have been avoided. Although the provider presented contrary testimony, the plaintiff's expert testimony was found sufficient to permit a reasonable juror to find that there was a direct and substantial causal relationship between the provider's breach of the standard of care and the patient's injuries.

> The primary wrong upon which a cause of action for negligence is based consists in the breach of a duty on the part of one person to protect another against injury, the proximate result of which is an injury to the person to whom the duty is owed. These elements of duty, breach, and injury are essentials of actionable negligence, and in fact most judicial definitions of the term "negligence" or "actionable negligence" are couched in those terms. In the absence of any one of them, no cause of action for negligence will lie.[26]

Eliminating Causes

Another way to establish the causal relationship between the particular conduct of a defendant and a plaintiff's injury is through the process of eliminating causes other than the defendant's conduct. For example, in *Shegog v. Zabrecky,*[27] Mr. Pereyra sought treatment for back pain from Dr. Zabrecky, a chiropractor at the Life Extension Center, in January 1987. Zabrecky ordered X-rays. The X-rays revealed that Pereyra was suffering from a fractured vertebra caused by a malignant tumor. Pereyra was referred to a surgeon who performed two surgical procedures to remove the tumor. Pereyra underwent a series of radiation treatments, which were supervised by Dr. Usas. A CT scan revealed that the cancer had spread to his lungs. Dr. Usas and other consulting physicians recommended that chemotherapy be considered following the course of radiation treatments. Pereyra was advised that his chance of survival following chemotherapy was 50 percent or better. During the summer of 1987, Pereyra consulted with a number of physicians as to the best course of treatment. Pereyra continued to see Zabrecky throughout the summer and fall of 1987. Zabrecky recommended that Pereyra reject the chemotherapy treatments and undergo a course of treatment with neytumorin and neythymin (two compounds manufactured in Germany). The Food and Drug Administration had not approved either drug. Pereyra agreed to undergo the treatment. Zabrecky performed an initial enzyme study prior to treatment, but did not perform further tests after the course of treatment began. During the course of treatment, the cancer continued to spread. Additional radiation treatments were given. Pereyra's condition worsened, and he was admitted to the hospital. The physicians at the hospital had not been aware that Pereyra was injecting himself with drugs given to him by Zabrecky. Upon urging from his wife, Pereyra revealed this information to the physicians at the hospital. Pereyra died on December 17, 1987, approximately six weeks after he had begun treatment with neytumorin and neythymin. An autopsy revealed that Pereyra had died from necrosis of the liver caused by a toxic reaction to a foreign substance. Pereyra was taking only the drugs neytumorin and neythymin between July 1987 and his death. No cancer was found in the liver.

A lawsuit was filed against the defendants, seeking damages for negligent treatment. The alleged negligent acts included:

- Administering drugs statutorily prohibited for use

- Withholding information from treating physicians

- Failing to follow patient's blood work

- Advising the patient to use drugs that had expired

- Engaging in the unlicensed practice of medicine

- Inducing the patient to forgo appropriate therapy

The jury delivered a verdict for the plaintiff. The defendants appealed, claiming that the evidence introduced at trial did not support the jury's finding as to causation.

The appellate court held that Zabrecky's grossly negligent actions and the circumstantial evidence introduced supported the jury's finding of causation. Zabrecky violated a recognized standard of care by prescribing statutorily prohibited drugs. No evidence was presented that would have supported another cause of the patient's liver failure. Reports from treating physicians indicate that the plaintiff died of liver failure and not from cancer. The defendant's expert testified that necrosis of the liver can be caused by the injection of foreign substances. He also testified that the normal reaction time of the human liver to a foreign protein is, on average, six weeks. "One of the ways to establish the causal relationship between particular conduct of a defendant and a plaintiff's injury is the expert's deduction, by the process of eliminating causes other than the conduct, that the conduct was the cause of injury. . . . The submitted reports indicate that each physician deduced that the German drugs were the most probable cause of Pereyra's liver failure, even without analysis of the drugs."[28]

Foreseeability

Foreseeability is the reasonable anticipation that harm or injury is likely to result from an act or an omission to act. The test for foreseeability is whether a person of ordinary prudence and intelligence should have anticipated the danger to others caused by a negligent act. "The test is not what the wrongdoer believed would occur; it is whether he or she ought reasonably to have foreseen that the event in question, or some similar event, would occur."[29]

When a defendant's actions fail to meet the standard of care, negligence has occurred and the jury must make two determinations. First, was it foreseeable that harm would occur from the failure to meet the standard of care? Second, was the carelessness or negligence the proximate or immediate cause of the harm or injury to the plaintiff? "The broad test of negligence is what a reasonably prudent person would foresee and would do in the light of this foresight under the circumstances."[30]

There is no expectation that the actor can guard against events that cannot reasonably be foreseen or that are so unlikely to occur that they would be disregarded. For example, in *Haynes v. Hoffman,*[31] the plaintiff brought a medical malpractice action against the defendant physician for his alleged negligence in prescribing a medication to which the plaintiff suffered an allergic reaction. The trial court returned a verdict in favor of the defendant, and the plaintiff appealed. The evidence at trial revealed that the plaintiff had not disclosed her history of allergies to the physician. The physician testified that, at the time of the physical examination of the plaintiff, she denied having any allergies. The physician testified that he would not have prescribed the drug had he known the plaintiff's complete history. By failing to disclose her allergies to the physician, the plaintiff was contributorily negligent. Foreseeability involves guarding against that which is probable and likely to happen, not against that which is only remotely and slightly possible.

The question of foreseeability was an issue in *Ferguson v. Dr. McCarthy's Rest Home.*[32] In this case, the plaintiff, a resident in the defendant's nursing facility, suffered from paralysis of the left side but was able to roll toward the left side in bed. The defendant had knowledge of this ability. A radiator, which was approximately the same height as the bed, was next to the plaintiff's bed on the left side. During the night, the plaintiff's left foot came in contact with the radiator and she suffered third-degree burns. The court held that this type of accident was foreseeable with respect to a person in the plaintiff's condition, particularly because the defendant had knowledge of the plaintiff's condition. The defendant should have shielded the radiator or not placed the plaintiff next to it.

Generally, the issue of foreseeability is for the trial court to decide. A duty to prevent a wrongful act by a third party will be imposed only where those wrongful acts can be reasonably anticipated.

SUMMARY CASE

All the elements necessary to establish negligence were well established in *Niles v. City of San Rafael*.[33] On June 26, 1973, at approximately 3:30 P.M., Kelly Niles, a young boy, got into an argument with another boy on a ball field and he was hit on the right side of his head. He rode home on his bicycle and waited for his father, who was to pick him up for the weekend. At approximately 5:00 P.M., his father arrived to pick him up. By the time they arrived in San Francisco, Kelly appeared to be in a great deal of pain. His father then decided to take him to Mount Zion Hospital, which was a short distance away. He arrived at the hospital emergency department at approximately 5:45 P.M. On admission to the emergency department, Kelly was taken to a treatment room by a registered nurse. The nurse obtained a history of the injury and took Kelly's pulse and blood pressure. During his stay in the emergency department, he was irritable, vomited several times, and complained that his head hurt. An intern who had seen Kelly wrote, "pale, diaphoretic, and groggy," on the patient's chart. Skull X-rays were ordered and found to be negative except for soft tissue swelling that was not noted until later. The intern then decided to admit the patient. A second-year resident was called, and he agreed with the intern's decision. An admitting clerk called the intern and indicated that the patient had to be admitted by an attending physician. The resident went as far as to write "admit" on the chart and later crossed it out. A pediatrician who was in the emergency department at the time was asked to look at Kelly. The pediatrician was also the paid director of the Mount Zion Pediatric Out-Patient Clinic. The pediatrician asked Kelly a few questions and then decided to send him home. The physician could not recall what instructions he gave the patient's father, but he did give the father his business card.

The pediatrician could not recall giving the father a copy of the emergency department's head injury instructions, an information sheet that had been prepared for distribution to patients with head injuries. The sheet explained that an individual should be returned to the emergency department should any of the following signs appear: a large, soft lump on the head; unusual drowsiness (cannot be awakened); forceful or repeated vomiting; a fit or convulsion (jerking or spells); clumsy walking; bad headache; and/or one pupil larger than the other.

Kelly was taken back to his father's apartment at about 7:00 P.M. A psychiatrist friend stopped by at approximately 8:45 P.M. He examined Kelly and noted that one pupil was larger than the other. Because the pediatrician could not be reached, the patient was taken back to the emergency department. A physician on duty noted an epidural hematoma during his examination and ordered that a neurosurgeon be called.

Today, Kelly can move only his eyes and neck. A lawsuit against Mount Zion and the pediatrician for $5 million was instituted. The city of San Rafael and the public school district also were included in the lawsuit as defendants. Expert testimony by two neurosurgeons during the trial indicated that the patient's chances of recovery would have been very good if he had been admitted promptly. This testimony placed the proximate cause of the injury with the hospital. The final judgment was $4 million against the medical defendants, $2.5 million for compensatory damages, and another $1.5 million for pain and suffering.

Case Lessons

Each case presented in this textbook illustrates actual experiences of plaintiffs and defendants, enabling the reader to apply the lessons learned to real-life situations. The many lessons in *Niles v. City of San Rafael* include the following:

- An organization can improve the quality of patient care rendered in the facility by establishing and adhering to policies, procedures, and protocols that facilitate the delivery of quality care across all disciplines.

- The provision of quality health care requires collaboration across disciplines.

- A physician must conduct a thorough and responsible examination and order the appropriate tests for each patient, evaluating the results of those tests, and providing appropriate treatment prior to discharging the patient.

- A patient's vital signs must be monitored closely and documented in the medical record.

- Corrective measures must be taken when a patient's medical condition signals a medical problem.

- A complete review of a patient's medical record must be accomplished before discharging a patient. Review of the record must include review of test results, nurses' notes, residents' and interns' notes, and the notes of any other physician or consultant who may have attended the patient.

- An erroneous diagnosis leading to the premature dismissal of a case can result in liability for both the organization and physician.

FAILURE TO ADMINISTER PROPER NOURISHMENT

Citation: *Caruso v. Pine Manor Nursing Ctr.*, 538 N.E.2d 722 (Ill. App. Ct. 1989)

Facts

In Illinois, a nursing facility by statute has a duty to provide its residents with proper nutrition. Under the Nursing Home Care Reform Act, the owner and licensee of a nursing home are liable to a resident for any intentional or negligent act or omission of their agents or employees that injures a resident. The act defines *neglect* as a failure in a facility to provide adequate medical or personal care or maintenance, when failure results in physical or mental injury to a resident or in the deterioration of the resident's condition. Personal care and maintenance include providing food, water, and assistance with meals necessary to sustain a healthy life.

The nursing facility in this case maintained no records of the resident's fluid intake and output. A nurse testified that such a record was a required nursing facility procedure that should have been followed for a person in the resident's condition but was not. The resident's condition deteriorated after staying six and a half days at the facility. Upon leaving the facility and entering a hospital emergency department, the resident was diagnosed by the treating physician as suffering from severe dehydration caused by an inadequate intake of fluids. The nursing facility offered no alternative explanation for the resident's dehydrated condition. As a result of the facility's failure to maintain adequate records, the resident suffered severe dehydration that required hospital treatment.

The evidence demonstrated that the proximate cause of the resident's dehydration was the nursing facility's failure to administer proper nourishment.

The trial court found that the record supported a finding that the resident had suffered from dehydration as a result of the nursing facility's negligence. The defendant appealed the jury verdict.

Issue

Did the nursing facility resident suffer harm as a result of the facility's negligence?

Holding

The Illinois Appellate Court upheld the trial court's finding that the resident suffered dehydration due to the nursing facility's negligence.

Reason

The evidence demonstrated that the proximate cause of the resident's dehydration was the nursing facility's failure to administer proper nourishment. The jury reasonably concluded that the resident suffered dehydration and that the nursing facility's treatment caused the dehydration.

Discussion

1. Discuss the element of foreseeability as applied in this case.
2. Discuss the importance of timely nutritional screenings and assessments.
3. What is the mechanism for screening and assessing the nutritional needs of patients in your organization?

INTENTIONAL TORTS

There are two main differences between intentional and negligent wrongs. The first is intent, which is present in intentional but not in negligent wrongs. For a tort to be considered intentional, the act must be committed intentionally, and the wrongdoer must realize to a substantial certainty that harm would result. The second difference is less obvious. While a negligent wrong may simply be the failure to act when there is a legal duty to act, an intentional wrong always involves a willful act that violates another's interests. Intentional wrongs include such acts as assault, battery, false imprisonment, defamation of char-acter, fraud, invasion of privacy, and infliction of emotional distress.

Assault and Battery

It has long been recognized by law that a person possesses a right to be free from aggression and the threat of actual aggression against one's person. The right to expect others to respect the integrity of one's body has roots in both common and statutory law. The distinguishing feature between assault and battery is that assault effectuates an infringement on the mental security or tranquility of another whereas battery constitutes a violation of another's physical integrity.

Assault

An *assault* is defined as the deliberate threat, coupled with the apparent present ability, to do physical harm to another. No actual contact is necessary. To commit the tort of assault, two conditions must exist: First, the person attempting to touch another unlawfully must possess the apparent present ability to commit the battery; second, the person threatened must be aware of or have actual knowledge of and fear of an immediate threat of a battery.

Battery

Battery is the intentional touching of another's person in a socially impermissible manner, without that person's consent. The law provides a remedy if consent to a touching has not been obtained or if the act goes beyond the consent given. Therefore, the injured person may initiate a lawsuit against the wrongdoer for damages suffered. In *Peete v. Blackwell,*[34] punitive damages in the amount of $10,000 were awarded to a nurse in her action against a physician for assault and battery. Evidence showed that the physician struck the assisting nurse on the arm and cursed at her when the physician ordered her to turn on the suction. Although there were no injuries, $1 in compensatory damages and $10,000 in punitive damages were awarded by the jury.

In the health care context, the principle of law concerning battery and the requirement of consent to medical and surgical procedures is critically important. Liability of organizations and health care professionals for acts of battery is most common in situations involving lack of patient consent to medical and surgical procedures.

It is of no legal importance that a procedure constituting a battery has improved a patient's health. If the patient did not consent to the touching, the patient may be entitled to such damages as can be proved to have resulted from commission of the battery. In *Perna v. Pirozzi,*[35] the New Jersey Supreme Court held that a patient who consents to surgery by one surgeon and is actually operated on by another has an action for medical malpractice or battery. Proof of unauthorized invasion of the plaintiff's person, even if harmless, entitles one to nominal damages.

Not only must individual staff members be aware of potential assault and battery hazards by fellow employees, as well as themselves, but they also must be alert to potential problems between patients (e.g., problems caused by smoking, racial or religious bias, and emotional conflicts). A health care facility has a particular duty to closely supervise those patients whose mental conditions make it probable that they will injure themselves or others.

False Imprisonment

False imprisonment is the unlawful restraint of an individual's personal liberty or the unlawful restraint or confinement of an individual. The personal right to move freely and without hindrance is basic to the legal system. Any intentional infringement on this right may constitute false imprisonment. Actual physical force is not necessary to constitute false imprisonment; false imprisonment may occur when an individual who is physically confined to a given area reasonably fears detainment or intimidation without legal justification. Both intimidation and forced detainment may be implied by words, threats, or gestures. Excessive force used to restrain a patient may produce liability for both false imprisonment and battery.

To recover for damages for false imprisonment, a plaintiff must be aware of the confinement and have no reasonable means of escape. Availability of a reasonable means of escape may bar recovery. To lock a door when another is reasonably available to pass through is not imprisonment. However, if the only other door provides a way of escape that is dangerous, the law may consider it an unreasonable way of escape and, therefore, false imprisonment may be a cause of action. Whether false imprisonment has taken place will be a matter for the courts to decide. No actual damage need be shown for liability to be imposed.

Where legal justification is absent and an arrest or imprisonment is false, the person denied free movement will be permitted to seek a remedy at law for any injury. Some occasions and circumstances allow for a person's confinement, such as when a person presents a self-danger or a danger to others. Criminals are incarcerated, as are sometimes the mentally ill who may present a danger to themselves or others. Long-term care residents are sometimes restrained to prevent falls. Children are retained after school for disciplinary reasons. In these examples, the right to move about freely has been violated, but the infringement occurs for reasons that are justifiable under the law.

False Arrest

In *Desai v. SSM Healthcare,*[36] Dr. Desai was walking across a hospital parking lot, a shortcut to the St. Louis University Medical School's Institute of Molecular Virology, where Desai worked as part of his graduate studies. Two security guards, Mr. Mealey and Mr. Windam, stopped Desai and asked him for identification. Desai said that he was a doctor and that he did not have his identification with him. Following an argument, the two security guards grabbed Desai's arms and Windam slammed Desai's head against the trunk of a car. After handcuffing him, the security guards escorted Desai back to the security office where they were joined by the security guards' supervisor. The handcuffs were eventually removed after the security guards received verification that Desai was affiliated with the institute and confirmation from a nurse supervisor that he was a physician. Shortly thereafter, the university campus police arrived. One of the officers asked Desai to apologize to Mealey. Desai refused and said that he wanted the St. Louis City police called, as he wanted to file an official complaint of assault. At the request of the security guards, Desai was rehandcuffed and arrested by the St. Louis police for trespassing. The security guards later admitted that they had Desai arrested to avoid trouble for themselves. Desai was not released from jail until noon the following day. While in jail, he suffered headaches and seizures. Desai brought suit against the hospital and security guards for false imprisonment, battery, and malicious prosecution.

The defendants moved to have the malicious prosecution count dismissed, and the motion was granted. The jury had returned a verdict totaling $75,000 in damages for the false imprisonment claim and found in favor of the defendants on the battery claim. The trial court sustained the defendants' motions for judgment notwithstanding the verdict and the plaintiff appealed.

Did the plaintiff meet his burden of establishing his case by substantial evidence? The Missouri Court of Appeals held that the evidence supported a finding that the security guards falsely imprisoned the physician, and that the physician was entitled to punitive damages on the false imprisonment claim. The defendants' testimony provided the jury with sufficient evidence to establish that the plaintiff had been held against his will. The testimony supported a finding that the arrest was self-serving and resulted in the false imprisonment. The trial court erred in dismissing the punitive damages as to the false imprisonment claim and, therefore, prevented its submission to the jury.

Physically Violent Persons

In *Celestine v. United States,*[37] the right to move about freely had been violated; however, the infringement was permissible for reasons justifiable under the law. In this case, the plaintiff had brought an action alleging battery and false imprisonment because security guards had placed him in restraints. The plaintiff-appellant sought psychiatric care at a veterans administration (VA) hospital. He became physically violent while waiting to be seen by a physician. The VA security guards placed him in restraints until a psychiatrist could examine him. The U.S. Court of Appeals for the Eighth Circuit held that the record supported a finding that the hospital was justified in placing the patient under restraint. Under Missouri law, no false imprisonment or battery occurred in view of the common-law principle that a person believed to be mentally ill could be restrained lawfully if such was considered necessary to prevent immediate injury to that person or others.

Contagious Diseases

Protocols should be instituted for handling patients diagnosed as having contracted a highly contagious disease. Detaining such patients, without statutory protection, constitutes false imprisonment. State health codes generally provide guidelines for caring for such patients. Statutes in many states allow mentally ill and intoxicated individuals to be detained if they are found to be dangerous to themselves or others. Those who are mentally ill, however, can be restrained only to the degree necessary to prevent them from harming themselves or others. If a mentally ill patient cannot be released, procedures should be followed to provide commitment to an appropriate institution for the patient's care.

Intoxicated Persons

The patient in *Davis v. Charter by the Sea*[38] was found not entitled to a directed verdict on a false-imprisonment claim. The claim arose from her overnight, involuntary detention at a hospital. Evidence that the patient was highly intoxicated, confused, incoherent, and experiencing a low diastolic blood pressure raised a jury question as to the existence of a medical emergency authorizing her detention.

Restraints

Restraints generally are used to control behavior when patients are disoriented or may cause harm to themselves (e.g., from falling, contaminating wounds, or pulling out intravenous lines) or to others. The use of restraints raises many questions of a patient's rights in the areas of autonomy, freedom of movement, and the accompanying health problems that can result from continued immobility. In general, a patient has a right to be free from any physical restraints imposed or psychoactive drugs administered for purposes of discipline or convenience and that are not required to treat a patient's medical symptoms.

Although the motivations for using restraints appear sound, there has been a tendency toward overuse. The fear of litigation over injuries sustained because of the failure to apply restraints further compounds the problem of overuse. As a result, regulations governing the use of restraints under the Omnibus Budget Reconciliation Act of 1987 make it clear that restraints are to be applied as a last resort rather than as a first option in the control of a resident's behavior.

Because prescription drugs are sometimes used to restrain behavior, the regulations represent the first time that prescription drugs must by law "be justified by indications documented in the medical chart."[39]

To avoid legal problems, health care organizations should implement policies aimed at eliminating or reducing the use of restraints. Programs for the effective use of restraints should include the following:

- Written policies that conform to federal and state guidelines (e.g., a policy prescribing that the least-restrictive device will be utilized to maintain the safety of the patient, a policy requiring the periodic review of patients under restraint, and a policy requiring physician orders for restraints)

- Procedures for implementing organizational policies (e.g., alternatives to follow before restraining a patient may include family counseling to encourage increased visitations, environmental change, activity therapies, and patient counseling)

- Periodic review of policies and procedures, with revision as necessary

- Education and orientation programs for the staff to be conducted inside and outside the organization

- Education programs for patients and their families

- A sound appraisal of each patient's needs

- Informed consent from the patient or legal guardian

- The application of the least-restrictive restraints

- Constant monitoring of the patient to determine the continuing need for restraints, injury to the patient, and complaints by the patient

- Documentation that includes:

  - the need for restraints—time-limited orders ("as needed" PRN orders are not acceptable)

  - consents for the application of restraints—patient monitoring—reappraisal of the continuing need for restraints

In *Big Town Nursing Home, Inc. v. Newman,*[40] the court held there was sufficient evidence to support a finding that a 67-year-old male resident had been falsely imprisoned in a facility against his will. He had attempted to leave the facility three days after he arrived at the facility but was caught by the facility's employees and forcibly returned. He was placed in a wing with persons who were addicted to drugs and alcohol and those who were mentally disturbed. He asked during the ensuing weeks that he be permitted to leave and attempted to leave five or six times. He was eventually confined to a restraint chair, his clothes taken, and he was not permitted to

use the telephone. The actions of the staff were described as being in utter disregard of the resident's legal rights. There was no court order for his commitment and the agreement for his admission stated that he was not to be kept against his will. The court stated that the staff acted recklessly, willfully, and maliciously by unlawfully detaining him.

Discharge Against Medical Advice

Patients who decide to leave a facility against medical advice should be requested to sign a discharge against advice form. Should a patient refuse to sign such a form, such refusal should be noted in the patient's record.

Defamation of Character

Another type of intentional tort comes in the form of defamation of character. *Defamation of character* is a communication to someone about another person that tends to hold that person's reputation up to scorn and ridicule. To be an actionable wrong, defamation must be communicated to a third person; defamatory statements communicated only to the injured party are not grounds for an action. *Libel* is the written form of defamation and may be presented in such forms as signs, photographs, letters, and cartoons. *Slander* is the verbal form of defamation and tends to form prejudices against a person in the eyes of third persons.

In a libel or slander *per se* (on its face) action, a court will presume that certain words and accusations cause injury to a person's reputation without proof of damages. Words or accusations that require no proof of actual harm to one's reputation are: (1) accusing someone of a crime, (2) accusing someone of having a loathsome disease, (3) using words that affect a person's profession or business, and (4) calling a woman unchaste. Health care professionals are, however, legally protected against libel when complying with a law that requires the reporting of venereal or other diseases. Damages typically consist of economic losses, such as loss of business or employment.

Libel

Performance Appraisals Not for General Publication. A statement in a hospital newsletter regarding the discharge of a nursing supervisor constituted libel per se in *Kraus v. Brandsletter.*[41] The newsletter indicated that the hospital's medical board had discharged the nursing supervisor after a unanimous vote of no confidence. Couching the board's determination in terms of a vote gave the impression that the board's determination had been based on facts that justified the board's opinion. The statement tended to injure the nurse's reputation as a professional because it did not refer to specifics of her performance but rather to her abilities as a professional in general. The reasonable interpretation of the statement in the newsletter was that the supervisor was incompetent in her professional capacity, thus giving rise to a cause of action for libel per se.

On the flip side in the same case, an alleged statement that a physician said, "You nurses will receive your Christmas bonus early, your boss is going to get fired," was not slander per se in that it did not injure the nurse in her professional capacity.[42] In addition, the statement that she was going to be fired was true.

Performance Appraisal Statements Not Libelous. In *Schauer v. Memorial Care System,*[43] the plaintiff applied for and was given a supervisory position at Memorial Hospital's new catheterization laboratory. In March 1989, she received an employment appraisal for the period June 1988 through December 1988. At that time, Schauer's supervisor rated her performance as "commendable" in two categories and "fair" in eight categories, with an overall rating of "fair." Although Schauer did not lose her job as a result of the appraisal, she brought an action against the hospital and her former supervisor for libel and emotional distress as a result of the appraisal. The hospital moved for summary judgment on the grounds that the employment appraisal was not defamatory as a matter of law, the hospital had qualified privilege to write the performance appraisal, and the claim for emotional distress did not reach the level of severity required for a claim for intentional infliction of emotional distress. The trial court granted the hospital's motion for summary judgment, and Schauer appealed.

The Texas Court of Appeals held that the statements contained in the performance appraisal were not libelous and that the appraisal was subject to qualified privilege. Moreover, the hospital's conduct and the statements contained in the appraisal did not support the claim for intentional infliction of emotional distress.

To sustain her claim of defamation, Schauer had to show that the hospital published her appraisal in a defamatory manner that injured her reputation in some way. A statement can be unpleasant and objectionable to the plaintiff without being defamatory. The hospital argued that the statements contained in the appraisal were truthful, permissible expressions of opinion and not capable of a defamatory meaning. Schauer's supervisor prepared the appraisal as part of her supervisory duties. The appraisal was not published outside the hospital and was prepared in compliance with the hospital policy for all employees. Schauer disputed her overall rating of "fair" as being libelous. "Clearly, this is a statement of her supervisor's opinion and is not defamatory as a matter of law."[44]

In her performance appraisal, Schauer objected to the statement, "Ms. Schauer was not sensitive to employee rela-

tions."[45] Schauer conceded in her deposition that there were a number of interpersonal problems in the catheterization laboratory and that she did not get along with everyone. The court found that given these admissions, the statement was not defamatory.

As to the plaintiff's claim of emotional distress, the plaintiff failed to show that the hospital acted intentionally and recklessly. The Restatement of Torts, Second, § 46 (1977) provides:

> Liability has been found only where the conduct has been so outrageous in character, and so extreme in degree, as to go beyond all possible bounds of decency, and to be regarded as atrocious, and utterly intolerable in a civilized community. . . . The liability clearly does not extend to mere insults, indignities, threats, annoyances, petty oppressions, or other trivialities. Complete emotional tranquility is seldom attainable in this world, and some degree of transient and trivial emotional distress is part of the price of living among people. The law intervenes only where the distress is so severe that no reasonable man could be expected to endure it.

Newspaper Articles. A libel suit was brought against the Miami Herald Publishing Company more than two years after its publication of an editorial cartoon depicting a nursing facility in a distasteful manner.[46] The cartoon was described in the following manner:

> On October 29, 1980, *The Herald* published an editorial cartoon which depicted three men in a dilapidated room. On the back wall was written "Krest View Nursing Home," and on the side wall there was a board which read "Closed by Order of the State of Florida." The room itself was in a state of total disrepair. There were holes in the floor and ceiling, leaking water pipes, and exposed wiring. The men in the room were dressed in outfits resembling those commonly appearing in caricatures of gangsters. Each man carried a sack with a dollar sign on it. One of the men was larger than the other two and was more in the forefront of the picture. One of the others addressed him. The caption read: "Don't Worry, Boss, We Can Always Reopen It As a Haunted House for the Kiddies."[47]

The court held that the newspaper's editorial cartoon depicting persons resembling gangsters in a dilapidated building, identified as a particular nursing facility that had been closed by state order, was an expression of pure opinion and was protected by the First Amendment against the libel suit alleging that the cartoon defamed the owner of the facility.

In another newspaper libel case, the court in *Wisconsin Association of Nursing Homes*[48] would not compel the newspapers to accept and print an advertisement in the exact form submitted by the Wisconsin Association of Nursing Homes and various individual homes.

Plaintiffs allege in their complaint that the defendants published a series of "investigative reports" in the *Milwaukee Journal* which dealt with the quality of care and services in several nursing homes. Plaintiffs further characterized the conclusions of the article as being false and erroneous. As a result, the plaintiffs prepared a full-page advertisement which purported to respond to and refute the allegations set out in the above mentioned "reports." The defendant newspaper refused to publish the advertisement in the form presented, and referred the question of possibly libelous matter to the attention of plaintiffs' attorneys.[49]

The court held that it was within the newspaper's journalistic discretion to reject the advertisement on the ground that it contained possibly libelous material. "[T]he clear weight of authority has not sanctioned any enforceable right of access to the press. In sum, a court can no more dictate what a privately owned newspaper can print than what it cannot print."[50]

Unlike broadcasting, the publication of a newspaper is not a government-conferred privilege. As we have said, the press and the government have had a history of disassociation. We can find nothing in the United States Constitution, any federal statute, or any controlling precedent that allows us to compel a private newspaper to publish advertisements without editorial control merely because such advertisements are not legally obscene or unlawful.[51]

In a very different suit, the appellee in *Stevens v. Morris Communications Corp.*[52] alleged that a newspaper article, which identified her as a representative of a convalescent center at a city council meeting, had defamed her. She claims that the article implies that she has responsibility for the convalescent center's problems of maintenance and disrepair. The court held that the appellee was not defamed by the article. Using the reasonable person test, the court found that it was highly unlikely that a reasonable person could have read the newspaper article as being defamatory.

Slander

Slander lawsuits are rare because of the difficulty in proving defamation, the small awards, and the high legal fees.

With slander, the person who brings suit generally must prove special damages; however, when any allegedly defamatory words refer to a person in a professional capacity, the professional need not show that the words caused damage. It is presumed that any slanderous reference to someone's professional capacity is damaging. The Georgia case of *Barry v. Baugh*,[53] however, presented a unique situation. The case involved a nurse who brought a defamation action, charging that a physician slandered her in the course of a consultation concerning the commitment of her husband to a mental institution. The nurse requested damages for mental pain, shock, fright, humiliation, and embarrassment. The nurse alleged that if the physician's statement were made known to the public, her job and reputation would be affected adversely. The court held that the physician's statement concerning the nurse did not constitute slander because the physician was not referring to the nurse in a professional capacity.[54] In this case, because the court held that the physician's statement did not refer to the nurse in her professional capacity, the plaintiff had to demonstrate damages in order to recover. The plaintiff was unable to show damages.

Professionals who are called incompetent in front of others have a right to sue to defend their reputation. However, it is difficult to prove that an individual comment was injurious. If the person making an injurious comment cannot prove that the comment is true, then that person can be held liable for damages.

ACCUSATORY STATEMENTS NOT DEFAMATORY

Citation: *Chowdhry v. North Las Vegas Hospital, Inc.*, 851 P.2d 459 (Nev. 1993)

Facts

On October 2, 1985, a young woman entered the emergency department of a hospital complaining of chest pain and shortness of breath. Dr. Lapica, the emergency physician on duty, saw her. Lapica diagnosed the patient as suffering from a possible pneumo-hemothorax, which required the placement of a chest tube to drain accumulated fluids. Lapica contacted Dr. Chowdhry, a physician who had recently performed surgery on the young woman and who was also the on-call thoracic surgeon at the hospital, and informed Chowdhry that his services were required at the hospital. The record revealed that Chowdhry refused to return to the hospital to treat the patient because he had recently left there and would treat her only if she were transferred to University Medical Center (UMC). Chowdhry testified that he could not return to the hospital because of a conflicting emergency at UMC.

Lapica then contacted the hospital's chief of staff, Dr. Wilchins, and told him that Chowdhry refused to come to the hospital and attend to the patient. Both physicians concluded that if the patient could be safely transported to UMC, the transfer should be affected so that Chowdhry could treat her.

The patient was ultimately transported to UMC where Lapica and Ms. Crow, the supervising nurse at the hospital, prepared incident reports detailing the events and submitted them to the hospital administrator, Mr. Moore.

On October 3, 1985, Moore informed Dr. Silver, UMC's chief of surgery, that Chowdhry had refused to come to the hospital emergency department to treat the patient. The matter was directed to the hospital's surgery committee, which recommended summary suspension of Chowdhry's staff privileges.

On November 1, 1985, in response to Chowdhry's request, a hearing was held before the medical executive committee. As a result of the hearing, Chowdhry's staff privileges were reinstated, but a reprimand was placed in his file for jeopardizing himself, the patient, and the hospital. The hospital denied Chowdhry's subsequent request to have the reprimand expunged from his record, thus prompting Chowdhry to file an action against the hospital, Silver, Moore, Wilchins, and Lapica.

Chowdhry's complaint alleged theories of liability based upon negligence, breach of contract, conspiracy, defamation, and negligent and intentional infliction of emotional distress. The district court concluded that Chowdhry had no reasonable basis for bringing the action and awarded attorneys' fees and costs to the hospital, Silver, Moore, Wilchins, and Lapica; Chowdhry appealed.

Issue

Did the district court err in dismissing the claims of defamation and infliction of emotional distress?

Holding

The Nevada Supreme Court held that the district court did not err in dismissing the claims of defamation and infliction of emotional distress.

Reason

Chowdhry's emotional distress claims are premised upon respondents' accusations of patient abandonment. Chowdhry testified that as a result, "he was very upset" and could not sleep. Insomnia and general physical or emotional discomfort are insufficient to satisfy the physical impact requirement for emotional distress. Thus, Chowdhry failed, as a matter of law, to present sufficient evidence to sustain verdicts for negligent or intentional infliction of emotional distress.

To establish a prima facie case of defamation, a plaintiff must prove: (1) a false and defamatory statement by defendant concerning the plaintiff, (2) an unprivileged publication to a third person, (3) fault amounting to at least negligence, and (4) actual or presumed damages. The actual statements made by the various respondents were not that Chowdhry "abandoned" his patient, but that he "failed to respond" or "would not come" to the hospital to treat his patient. The record reflected that the respondents made the statements to hospital personnel and other interested parties (e.g., the patient's mother) in the context of reporting what was reasonably perceived to be Chowdhry's refusal to treat the patient at the hospital. The statements attributable to the respondents, taken in context, are not reasonably capable of a defamatory construction.

Discussion

1. Explain what a plaintiff must prove in order to establish an action for defamation.
2. How does libel differ from slander?

Defenses to a Defamation Action

Essentially, the two defenses to a defamation action are truth and privilege. When a person has said something that is damaging to another person's reputation, the person making the statement will not be liable for defamation if it can be shown that the statement is true. A privileged communication differs from a defamatory statement in that the person making the communication has a responsibility to do so. For example, many states have statutes providing immunity to physicians and health care institutions in connection with peer review proceedings. The person making the communication must do so in good faith, on the proper occasion, in the proper manner, and to persons who have a legitimate reason to receive the information.

An administrator's statements made to a physician's supervisor regarding the physician's alleged professional misconduct is not grounds for a defamation action as long as the statements are made in good faith. A hospital administrator has a duty to report complaints about alleged professional misconduct of physicians working in the hospital. The administrator has qualified privilege to report such complaints to the physician's supervisor and other hospital officials as necessary.[55]

Two types of privilege may provide a defense to an action for defamation: absolute privilege and qualified privilege. *Absolute privilege* attaches to statements made during judicial and legislative proceedings as well as to confidential communications between spouses. *Qualified privilege* attaches to statements such as those made as a result of a legal or moral duty to speak in the interests of third persons and may provide a successful defense only when such statements are made in the absence of malice. If it can be shown that a speaker made a statement out of monetary gain, hatred, or ill will, the law will not permit the speaker to hide behind the shield of privilege to avoid liability for defamation.

The defense of privilege is illustrated in the case of *Judge v. Rockford Memorial Hospital,*[56] whereby a nurse brought an action for libel. The action was based on a letter written to a nurses' professional registry by the director of nurses at the hospital to which the nurse had been assigned by the registry. In the letter, the director of nurses stated that the hospital did not wish to have the nurse's services available to them because of certain losses of narcotics during times when this particular nurse was on duty. The court refused the nurse recovery. Because the director of nurses had a legal duty to make the communication in the interests of society, the director's letter constituted a privileged communication. Therefore, the court held that the letter did not constitute libel because it was privileged.

It is important to note that public figures have more difficulty in pursuing defamation litigation than the average individual. One who occupies a position of considerable public responsibility is considered a public figure for the purposes of the law of defamation and is generally more vulnerable to public scrutiny. Legal action against a public figure generally will be denied in the absence of any showing of actual malice in connection with alleged defamatory references to a plaintiff. Actual malice applies only in cases involving public figures and encompasses knowledge of falsity or recklessness as to truth.

The chairman of a publicly owned and operated county hospital in *Drew v. KATV Television*[57] brought a suit against a television station for defamation. The station reported during a news broadcast that the board chairman had been charged with a felony when he had been charged with two misdemeanor counts of solicitation to tamper with evidence (both of which were dismissed at trial). The second news report implied that the plaintiff was involved in a drug investigation being conducted at the hospital where he served as chairman of the board. The plaintiff occupied a position of considerable public responsibility, and he was considered a public figure for the purposes of the law of defamation. The circuit court dismissed the case on the defendant's motion for summary judgment, and the plaintiff appealed. The Arkansas Supreme Court held that the trial court properly ordered summary dismissal of the plaintiff's action against the television station in the absence of any showing of malice in connection with the allegedly defamatory references to the plaintiff during the news broadcasts.

Fraud

The intentional tort of *fraud* is defined as willful and intentional misrepresentation that could cause harm or loss to a person or property. Fraud includes any cunning, deception, or artifice used, in violation of legal or equitable duty, to circumvent, cheat, or deceive another. The forms it may assume and the means by which it may be practiced are as multifarious as human ingenuity can devise, and the courts consider it unwise or impossible to formulate an exact, definite, and all-inclusive definition of the action.

To prove fraud, the following facts must be shown:

- An untrue statement known to be untrue by the party making it and made with the intent to deceive

- Justifiable reliance by the victim on the truth of the statement

- Damages as a result of that reliance

Concealment of Information from Patient

The plaintiff in *Robinson v. Shah*[58] was a long-time patient of defendant, Dr. Shah, from 1975 to 1986. During that period of time, the defendant treated the plaintiff for various gynecological disorders. On November 9, 1983, the defendant performed a total abdominal hysterectomy and bilateral salpingo-oophorectomy on the plaintiff. Approximately one week following surgery, the plaintiff was discharged from the hospital and was assured that there were no complications or potential problems that might arise as a result of the surgery. On the day after the plaintiff was discharged from the hospital, she began to experience abdominal distress. She consulted the defendant about these symptoms, and the defendant ordered X-rays to be taken of the plaintiff's kidneys, ureter, and bladder in an effort to explain her discomfort.

The X-rays were taken at St. Joseph Memorial Hospital and were read and interpreted by Dr. Cavanaugh, presumably a radiologist associated with that facility. After reading the X-rays, Cavanaugh called the defendant and reported that the slides showed the presence of surgical sponges that had been left in the plaintiff's abdomen after surgery. Cavanaugh also sent the defendant a copy of a written report that reflected the findings.

The defendant fraudulently concealed from the plaintiff the findings of the X-rays. Instead of being truthful, the defendant intentionally lied to the plaintiff and told her the X-rays were negative and that there were no apparent or unusual complications from the recent abdominal surgery, and she assured the plaintiff that she did not require further treatment. At no time did the defendant reveal to the plaintiff the fact that she had left surgical sponges in the plaintiff's abdomen after the most recent surgery.

Over the next several years, the plaintiff continued to see the defendant for gynecological checkups. She continued to experience abdominal pain and discomfort. The defendant, however, continued to conceal from the plaintiff the existence of the surgical sponges left in the plaintiff's abdomen. The plaintiff ceased seeing the defendant as her physician in 1986. However, she consulted other physicians and continued to experience frequent pain and discomfort in her abdomen as well as intestinal, urological, and gynecological problems. Although the plaintiff brought her complaints to the attention of other physicians, no one was able to diagnose the source of her problems.

In 1993, one of the physicians attending to the plaintiff's problems diagnosed a pelvic mass, which he felt could be causing some discomfort. The plaintiff underwent pelvic sonograms and X-rays, which revealed the existence of retained surgical sponges. The plaintiff contended that the defendant, from and after November 18, 1983, had knowledge of the presence of retained surgical sponges in her abdomen and knew the potential of future complications that could arise from this condition. Despite this knowledge, the plaintiff contended, the defendant fraudulently concealed the existence of this condition from the plaintiff.

The trial court found that the plaintiff was unable to discover the fact that the defendant negligently left surgical sponges in her abdomen and that this fact was fraudulently concealed from the plaintiff, who did not discover the defendant's fraud until August 11, 1993.

The appeals court held that although the action in this case was filed more than ten years after the fraud was perpetrated, the statute of limitations was not tolled because of the defendant's fraudulent concealment of information from the patient. The court decided that a physician may not blunt a malpractice cause of action by misrepresenting facts to a patient. Allowing such misrepresentation would serve only to encourage such behavior.

Invasion of Privacy

The *right to privacy* is implied in the Constitution. It is recognized by the law as the right to be left alone—the right to be free from unwarranted publicity and exposure to public view, as well as the right to live one's life without having one's name, picture, or private affairs made public against one's will. Health care organizations and professionals may become liable for invasion of privacy if, for example, they divulge information from a patient's medical record to improper sources or if they commit unwarranted intrusions into a patient's personal affairs.

Patients have a right to personal privacy and a right to the confidentiality of their personal and clinical records. The information in a patient's medical record is confidential and should not be disclosed without the patient's permission, with the exception of occasions when there is a legal obligation or duty to disclose the information (i.e., reporting of communicable diseases, gunshot wounds, and child abuse). Those who come into possession of the most intimate personal information about patients have both a legal and an ethical duty not to reveal confidential communications.

Unfortunately, familiarity with an organization's health care environment tends to diminish the conscious concern personnel should have for the protection of patient privacy. The plaintiff, a former hospital employee, in *Vernuil v. Poirie*[59] was awarded $15,000 in a legal action against her supervisor and hospital for invasion of privacy. The plaintiff claimed that while she was a patient and in the postoperative recovery room, her supervisor lifted her sheet in an attempt to view her abdominal incision. The court of appeals held that evidence sustained a finding of invasion of privacy. Because the supervisor's conduct occurred during the time and place of his employment, the hospital was jointly liable for damages. "Ensuring a patient's well-being from all others, including staff, while the patient is helpless under the effects of anesthesia is part of its normal business."[60]

Intentional Infliction of Mental Distress

The intentional or reckless infliction of mental distress is characterized by conduct that is so outrageous that it goes beyond the bounds tolerated by a decent society. *Mental distress* includes mental suffering resulting from painful emotions such as grief, public humiliation, despair, shame, and wounded pride. Liability for the wrongful infliction of mental distress may be based on either intentional or negligent misconduct. A plaintiff may recover damages if he or she can show that the defendant intended to inflict mental distress and knew or should have known that his or her actions would give rise to it.

The mother of a premature infant who died shortly after birth went to her physician for a six week check-up. She noticed a report in her medical chart that stated that the child was past the fifth month in development and that hospital rules and state law prohibited disposal of the infant as a surgical specimen. The mother questioned her physician regarding the infant. The physician requested that his nurse take the mother to the hospital. An employee at the hospital took the mother to a freezer. The freezer was opened and the mother was handed a jar containing her premature infant. The circuit court found that the hospital, through its employees, committed intentional infliction of emotional distress. On appeal, the court of appeals held that the jury could find that the hospital's conduct in displaying the infant was outrageous conduct.[61]

In another mental distress case, an action in *Greer v. Medders*[62] was brought by a patient and his wife against a physician. The defendant physician had been covering for the attending physician who was on vacation. When the hospitalized plaintiff had not seen the covering physician for several days, he called the physician's office to complain. The physician later entered the patient's room in an agitated manner and became verbally abusive in the presence of the patient's wife and a nurse. He said to the patient, "Let me tell you one damn thing, don't nobody call over to my office raising hell with my secretary. . . . I don't have to be here every damn day checking on you because I check with physical therapy. . . . I don't have to be your damn doctor."[63] When the physician left the room, the plaintiff's wife began to cry, and the plaintiff experienced episodes of uncontrollable shaking for which he received psychiatric treatment. The superior court entered summary judgment for the physician, and the plaintiff appealed. The Georgia Court of Appeals held that the physician's abusive language willfully caused emotional upset and precluded summary judgment for the defendant.

STRICT/PRODUCTS LIABILITY

Strict liability is a legal doctrine that makes some persons or entity responsible for damages their actions or products cause, regardless of "fault" on their part. Strict liability often applies when people engage in inherently hazardous activities, such as blasting in a city. If the blasting injures a person, no matter how careful the blasting company was, it can be liable for any injuries suffered. Strict liability also applies in the case of manufactured products such as drugs. This section focuses on products liability.

Products liability is the accountability of a manufacturer, seller, or supplier of chattels to a buyer or other third party for injuries sustained because of a defect in a product. An injured party may proceed with a lawsuit against a seller, manufacturer, or supplier on three legal theories: (1) negligence, (2) breach of warranty (express or implied), and (3) strict liability. Many states have enacted comprehensive products liability statutes. These statutory provisions can be very diverse such that the United States Department of Commerce has promulgated a Model Uniform Products Liability Act (MUPLA) for voluntary use by the states. Three types of product defects that incur liability are design defects, manufacturing defects, and defects in marketing (e.g., providing improper instructions for the product's use).

Negligence

Negligence, as applied to products liability, requires the plaintiff to establish duty, breach, injury, and causation. The manufacturer of a product is not liable for injuries suffered by a patient if they are the result of negligent use by the user. Product users must conform to the safety standards provided by the manufacturers of supplies and equipment. Failure to follow proper safety instructions can prevent recovery in a negligence suit if injury results from improper use.

Because manufacturers are liable for injuries that result from unsafe product design, they generally provide detailed safety instructions to the users of their products. Failure to provide such instructions could be considered negligence on the part of the manufacturer.

An action in *Airco v. Simmons National Bank, Guardian, et al.*[64] was brought against a physician partnership that provided anesthesia services to the hospital and Airco, Inc., the manufacturer of an artificial breathing machine used in the administration of anesthesia. It was alleged that the patient suffered irreversible brain damage because of the negligent use of the equipment and its unsafe design. The machine had been marketed despite prior reports of a foreseeable danger of human error brought about by the presence of several identical black hoses and the necessity of connecting them correctly to three ports of identical size placed closely together. The machine lacked adequate labels and warnings, according to the reports. The jury awarded $1,070,000 in compensatory damages against the physician partnership and Airco, Inc. Punitive damages in the amount of $3 million were awarded against Airco, Inc. On appeal of the punitive damages award, the Arkansas Supreme Court held that the evidence for punitive damages was sufficient for the jury. The manufacturer acted in a persistent reckless disregard of the foreseeable dangers in the machine by continuing to sell it with the known hazardous design.

Negligence, as well as breach of warranty and strict liability, was not established in the well-publicized case of the 1980s involving a woman who died after ingesting Tylenol capsules tainted with potassium cyanide. The decedent's estate in *Elsroth v. Johnson & Johnson*[65] sued the manufacturer and the retail grocery store that sold the over-the-counter drug. The defendants moved for a summary judgment. The U.S. district court held that the retailer did not have a duty to protect the decedent from acts of tampering by an unknown third party. The manufacturer was not liable under an inadequate warning theory. Manufacturers are under a duty to warn of the dangers that may be associated with the normal and lawful use of their products, but they need not warn that their products may be susceptible to criminal misuse.

Negligent use of a product, however, may lead to liability. In *Monk v. Doctors Hospital,* the negligent use of a Bovie plate led to liability.[66] The patient was admitted to the hospital for abdominal surgery. Before surgery, the patient asked the surgeon also to remove three moles from the right arm and one from the right leg. The surgeon instructed a hospital nurse to prepare a Bovie machine, but was not present while the machine was set up. The nurse placed the contact plate of the Bovie machine under the patient's right calf in a negligent manner, and the patient suffered burns. Manufacturer instruction manuals supported the claim that the plate was placed improperly on the patient. These manuals were available to the hospital. The trial court directed a verdict in favor of the hospital and the physician. The appellate court found that there was sufficient evidence from which the jury could conclude that the Bovie plate was applied in a negligent manner. There also was sufficient evidence, including the manufacturer's manual and expert testimony, from which the jury could find that the physician was independently negligent.[67]

This case demonstrates the necessity for an organization to require conformity to the safety standards provided by the manufacturers of supplies and equipment. As evidenced in the previous case, such failure can cause an organization and its staff to be held liable for negligence. This case should alert manufacturers of the necessity to provide appropriate safety instructions to the users of their products. It can be assumed that failure to provide such instructions could be considered negligence on the part of the supplier.

Defective Packaging

Cotita, a registered nurse, was stuck by a syringe manufactured by the defendant-appellee, PharmaPlast. The syringe, although still in its sterile packaging, was missing the protective cap that normally covers the tip of the needle. This improper packaging allowed the needle to pierce its sterile plastic covering and penetrate the protective gloves Cotita was wearing. Because of the presence of the patient's blood on his gloves at the time of the needle stick, Cotita feared that he had been exposed to the human immunodeficiency virus (HIV). Subsequent tests revealed that Cotita was not HIV-positive; nevertheless, he sued PharmaPlast, seeking damages for mental anguish stemming from his fear of contracting AIDS.

PharmaPlast admitted defective packaging, and the district court granted summary judgment for the plaintiff on the issue of the defective state of the syringe. PharmaPlast asserted Cotita was negligent in his use of the syringe. Cotita objected to the introduction of evidence concerning his negligence.

The damage issue was tried before a jury that returned a verdict for $150,000 in Cotita's favor. This amount was reduced by 30 percent, a figure that the jury found reflected his negligence. Cotita maintained that the issue of his negligence should not have been considered by the jury, nor used to reduce the amount of his award.

The U.S. Court of Appeals found no error in the district court's application of comparative fault. PharmaPlast presented evidence that the procedures used by the nurse were in violation of the universal precautions and procedures that are standard in the health care field. The district court here was entitled to determine that the application of comparative fault would ultimately encourage workers in the health care field to follow the established procedures for handling syringes.[68]

Failure to Warn

Merck pulled Vioxx off pharmacy shelves, a drug it manufactures for the treatment of arthritis, after participants in a study experienced adverse cardiovascular events compared to those taking a placebo. Approximately 20 million people have used Vioxx. Since the recall of Vioxx, approximately 4,200 product liability lawsuits representing about 7,500 plaintiff groups have been filed against Merck. Lawsuits have already been filed in Texas, New Jersey, and California. Merck has vowed to fight each case.

The first Vioxx trial took place in Texas, where Mrs. Ernst claims that if her husband had known of the true risks of Vioxx, he would not have taken the drug. The plaintiff's lawyers argued that Merck was aware of the problems with Vioxx for several years, concealed the negative information, and continued to sell the drug to the public. On a jury verdict, Merck was held liable for the death in May 2001 of Mr. Ernst, a marathon runner, who died eight months after he started using Vioxx. He died of a heart attack and was taking Vioxx at the time of his death. The jury awarded the plaintiff $253 million in damages. Because of malpractice caps in Texas, Mrs. Ernst will receive a substantially lesser amount for damages. Nevertheless, the ultimate financial impact on

Merck is expected to be in the billions. Merck is expected to appeal the jury's decision claiming that Ernst's arrhythmia had not been linked to Vioxx in the studies conducted.

Breach of Warranty

A *warranty* is a particular type of guarantee (a pledge or assurance of something) concerning goods or services provided by a seller to a buyer. Nearly everything purchased is covered by a warranty. To recover under a cause of action based on a breach of warranty theory, the plaintiff must establish whether there was an express or implied warranty.

Express Warranty

An *express warranty* includes specific promises or affirmations made by the seller to the buyer, such as "X" drug is not subject to addiction. If the product fails to perform as advertised, it is a breach of express warranty. For example, in *Crocker v. Winthrop Laboratories,*[69] the patient, Mr. Crocker, was admitted to the hospital for a hernia operation. His physician prescribed both Demerol and Talwin for pain. After discharge from the hospital, Crocker developed an addiction to Talwin and was able to obtain prescriptions from several physicians to support a habit he developed. He was eventually admitted to the hospital for detoxification. After six days, Crocker walked out of the hospital and went home. He became agitated and abusive, threatening his wife, and she eventually called a physician at his request. The physician arrived and gave Crocker an injection of Demerol. Crocker then retired to bed and subsequently died. Action was brought against the drug company for the suffering and subsequent wrongful death that occurred as the proximate result of the decedent's addiction to Talwin.

The district court rendered a judgment for the plaintiff and the court of appeals reversed. On further appeal, the Texas Supreme Court held that when a drug company positively and specifically represents its product to be free and safe from all dangers of addiction and when the treating physician relies on such representation, the drug company is liable when the representation proves to be false and injury results.

Implied Warranty

An *implied warranty* is a guarantee of a product's quality that is not expressed in a purchase contract. An implied warranty assumes that the item sold can perform the function for which it is designed. Implied warranties are in effect when the law implies that one exists by operation of law as a matter of public policy for the protection of the public. *Jacob E. Decker & Sons v. Capps*[70] is a case involving the question of the liability of a manufacturer of food products to the consumer for damages sustained by ingestion of contaminated sausage. One member of a family died and others became seriously ill as a result of eating contaminated food. The jury found that the sausage had been contaminated before being packaged by the defendant and that it was unfit for human consumption. The Texas Supreme Court decided that the defendant was liable for the injuries sustained by the consumers of the contaminated food under an implied warranty. Liability in such a case is based neither on negligence nor on a breach of the usual implied contractual warranty. It is based on the broad principle of the public policy to protect human health and life.

The patient in *Perlmutter v. Beth David Hospital*[71] contracted serum hepatitis from a blood transfusion. She relied on an implied sales warranty as the basis of her suit. The court denied recovery, pointing out that even though a separate charge of $60 was made for the blood, the charge was incidental to the primary contract with the hospital for services. Because there was no claim of negligence, the court determined that blood provided by the hospital was a service, rather than a sale, and, therefore, barred recovery by the patient. The rationale of this case did not extend to relieve commercial blood banks from liability on the basis of strict liability warranty theories. Action could have been instituted against the hospital if it had been shown that the hospital was negligent in handling the blood.

Strict Liability

Strict liability refers to responsibility without fault and makes possible an award of damages without any proof of manufacturer negligence. The plaintiff needs only to show that he or she suffered injury while using the manufacturer's product in the prescribed way.

The following elements must be present for a plaintiff to proceed with a case on the basis of strict liability:

- The product must have been manufactured by the defendant.

- The product must have been defective at the time it left the hands of the manufacturer or seller. The defect in the product normally consists of a manufacturing defect, a design defect in the product, or an absence or inadequacy of warnings for the use of the product.

- The plaintiff must have been injured by the specific product.

- The defective product must have been the proximate cause of injury to the plaintiff.

In *Green v. Smith & Nephew AHP, Inc.,*[72] Green began her employment at St. Joseph's Hospital in Milwaukee, where she worked as a radiology technologist. Hospital rules required Green to wear protective gloves while attending patients. To comply with these rules, Green wore powdered latex gloves manufactured by Smith & Nephew AHP (S&N). Initially, Green used one or two pairs of gloves per shift. However, upon her promotion to the CT department, this use began increasing. Green's job required her to change up to approximately 40 pairs of gloves per shift. Green began suffering various health problems. Her hands became red, cracked, and sore and began peeling. In response to this condition, she applied hand lotion, changed the soap she used and the type of hand towels she used, and tried various other remedies. Green was eventually diagnosed with a latex allergy. Her symptoms grew increasingly severe, eventually culminating in an acute shortness of breath, coughing, tightening of the throat, and hospitalization on more than one occasion.

Green claimed that S&N should be held strictly liable for her injuries. She argued that although S&N could have significantly reduced the protein levels in and discontinued powdering of its gloves by adjusting its production process, S&N nonetheless utilized a production process that maintained these defects in the gloves. These defects, Green alleged, created the unreasonable danger that S&N's gloves would cause consumers to develop latex allergy and suffer allergy-related conditions. The primary cause of latex allergy is latex gloves and, for this reason, latex allergy disproportionately affects members of the health care profession. According to Green's medical experts, the vast majority of people with latex allergy—up to 90 percent—are health care workers. And although latex allergy is not common among the general population, Green's medical experts testified that it affects between 5 and 17 percent of all health care workers in the United States.

Although a manufacturer is not under a duty to manufacture a product that is absolutely free from all possible harm to every individual, it is the duty of the manufacturer not to place upon the market a defective product that is unreasonably dangerous to the ordinary consumer.

The jury returned a verdict in favor of Green, finding that S&N's gloves were defective and unreasonably dangerous and that they caused Green's injuries. The jury awarded Green $1 million in damages. The court of appeals affirmed the circuit court judgment. S&N then petitioned the supreme court of Wisconsin to review the court of appeals decision.

The Wisconsin Supreme Court affirmed the decision of the court of appeals. Strict products liability imposes liability without regard to negligence and its attendant factors of duty of care and foreseeability. Regardless of whether a manufacturer could foresee the potential risks of harm inherent in its defective and unreasonably dangerous product, strict products liability holds the manufacturer responsible for injuries caused by that product. When a manufacturer places a defective and unreasonably dangerous product into the stream of commerce, the manufacturer, not the injured consumer, should bear the costs of the risks posed by the product.

Negligent blood handling held a blood bank strictly liable in *Weber v. Charity Hospital of Louisiana at New Orleans,*[73] when a hospital patient developed hepatitis from a transfusion of defective blood during surgery. Evidence established that the blood bank collected, processed, and sold the blood to the hospital. Although the hospital administered the blood, absent any negligence in its handling or administration, it was not liable for the patient's injury. Many states have enacted statutes to exempt blood from the product category and thus remove blood products from the theory of strict liability.

Res Ipsa Loquitur

Liability also may be based on the concept of *res ipsa loquitur* (the thing speaks for itself) by showing all of the following:

- The product did not perform in the way intended.

- The product was not tampered with by the buyer or third party.

- The defect existed at the time it left the defendant manufacturer.

For example, a manufacturer mislabeled a box of Duragesic patches, a strong prescription medication for moderate-to-severe chronic pain, marking the box as containing 25 mcg patches. In actuality, the box contained 100 mcg patches. The patient placed a patch on her back to provide relief of severe back pain. Instead of receiving the 25 mcg dosage recommended by her physician, she received 100 mcg, four times the recommended dosage. The patient went into a coma and eventually died.

Products Liability Defenses

Defenses against recovery in a products liability case include:

- *Assumption of a risk* (e.g., voluntary exposure to such risks as radiation treatments and chemotherapy treatments)

- Intervening cause (e.g., an intravenous solution contaminated by the negligence of the product user, rather than that of the manufacturer)

- Contributory negligence (e.g., use of a product in a way that it was not intended to be used)

- Comparative fault (e.g., injury is the result of the concurrent negligence of both the manufacturer and the plaintiff)

- Disclaimers (e.g., manufacturers' inserts and warnings regarding usage and contraindications of their products)

Disclaimers and waivers of liability for products are often invalidated by courts as against public policy. Warranties are limited so that manufacturers and retailers are held responsible for personal injuries caused by the use of the product.

Successful products liability cases tend to have a negative impact on the development of new drugs. In addition, manufacturers tend to remove older technologies from the marketplace to decrease their exposure to liability and potential financial risks. On the positive side, the slipshod manufacture of products is discouraged. This is increasingly evident in the sale of food products where consumers are demanding full disclosure of the contents of packaged products.

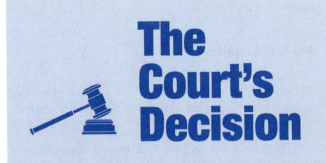

The Court's Decision

The Ohio Court of Appeals held that the delay in providing the plaintiff treatment fell below the medically acceptable standard of care. The court was appalled that the physician had characterized his evaluation as a medical examination or had implied that what he described as a "cursory breast examination" should be considered a medically sufficient breast examination. It seemed incredible to the court that a physician would deliberately choose not to take the additional few minutes or seconds to thoroughly palpitate the sides of the breasts, which is a standard minimally intrusive cancer detection technique. His admission that he merely "pressed" on the plaintiff's breasts, coupled with the additional admission that such acts would not necessarily disclose lumps in the breasts, constituted poor medical care.

It was probable that an earlier procedure would have safely and reliably conserved a large part of the plaintiff's right breast. Through inexcusable delays, the plaintiff lost this option and, instead, was medically required to have the entire breast removed. The court concluded that the defendant's negligence was the sole and proximate cause of the plaintiff's losses.

CHAPTER REVIEW

1. A *tort* is a civil wrong, not including breach of contract, that is committed against a person or property for which a court provides a remedy in the form of an action for damages. Three categories of torts are negligent torts, intentional torts, and torts where strict liability is assessed regardless of fault.
2. *Negligence* is a tort—a civil or personal wrong. It is the unintentional commission or omission of an act that a reasonably prudent person would or would not do under the same or similar circumstances.
3. *Negligence* has three basic forms:

   - *Malfeasance:* the execution of an unlawful or improper act

   - *Misfeasance:* the improper performance of an act that results in injury to another

   - *Nonfeasance:* a failure to act when there is a duty to do so
4. There are two degrees of negligence:

   - *Ordinary negligence* is the failure to do what a reasonably prudent person would do or doing what a reasonably prudent person would not do under the circumstances of the act or omission in question.

- Gross negligence is the intentional or wanton omission of care that should be provided or the performance of an improper act.

5. To recover damages caused by negligence, the following elements must be present:

   - *Duty to care:* exists when there is a legal obligation of care, performance, or observance imposed on one party to guard the rights of others

   - Breach of duty: failure to meet a prevailing standard of care

   - Injury: without proof of harm or injury, a defendant cannot be found liable for negligence

   - Causation: the defendant's negligence must be a substantial factor in having caused an injury

6. *Foreseeability* is the reasonable anticipation that harm or injury will result from an act or a failure to act. The test for foreseeability is whether one should have reasonably anticipated that the event in question or a similar event would occur.

7. For liability to be established based on failure to follow a specified standard of care outlined by statute, three elements must be present:

   - The defendant must have been within the specified class of persons outlined in the statute.

   - The plaintiff must have been injured in a way that the statute was designed to prevent.

   - The plaintiff must show that the injury would not have occurred had the statute not been violated.

8. Intentional wrongdoing involves a willful act that violates another person's interests. Not only must the action be intentional, but also the perpetrator must realize that the action will result in harm.

9. *Assault* is the infringement on the mental security or tranquility of another person; *battery* is the violation of another person's physical integrity. No actual physical harm need have occurred for an individual to be guilty of assault.

10. *False imprisonment* is the unlawful restraint of an individual's personal liberty or the unlawful restraint or confinement of an individual. For a false imprisonment charge to warrant recovery, the plaintiff must be aware of the confinement and have no reasonable means of escape.

11. *Defamation of character* is a false oral or written communication to someone other than the individual defamed that subjects that individual's reputation to scorn and ridicule in the eyes of a substantial number of respectable people in the community. Two aspects of defamation of character are *libel,* which results from the written word, and *slander,* which results from the spoken word.

12. *Fraud* is a willful and intentional misrepresentation that could cause harm or loss to an individual or property. To prove fraud, the following three facts must be shown:

   - An untrue statement known to be untrue by the party making it and made with the intent to deceive

   - A justifiable reliance by the victim on the truth of that statement

   - Damages as a result of that reliance

13. *Invasion of privacy* is a wrong that interferes with the right of an individual to personal privacy.

14. The intentional or reckless infliction of *mental distress* is conduct so outrageous that it goes beyond the bounds tolerated by a decent society. Mental distress can include mental suffering from painful emotions such as grief, public humiliation, despair, shame, and wounded pride.

15. *Strict liability* refers to liability without fault and makes possible an award of damages without any proof of manufacturer negligence. The plaintiff needs only to show that he or she suffered injury while using the manufacturer's product in the prescribed way.

16. *Products liability* is the liability of a manufacturer, seller, or supplier of chattels to a buyer or other third party for injuries sustained because of a defect in a product. An injured party may proceed with a lawsuit against a seller, manufacturer, or supplier on three legal theories: (1) negligence, (2) breach of warranty (express or implied), and (3) strict liability.

17. Products liability defenses include *assumption of a risk; intervening cause; contributory negligence; comparative fault;* and *disclaimers.*

REVIEW QUESTIONS

1. Describe the objectives of tort law.
2. Discuss the distinctions among negligent torts, intentional torts, and strict liability.
3. What forms of negligence are described in this chapter?
4. How does one distinguish between negligence and malpractice?
5. What elements must be proven in order to be successful in a negligence suit? Illustrate your answer with a case (the facts of the case can be hypothetical).
6. Can a "duty to care" be established by statute or contract? Discuss your answer.
7. Describe the categories of intentional torts.
8. How does slander differ from libel? Give an example of each.
9. What is products liability? Describe what legal theories an injured party may use in proceeding with a lawsuit against a seller, manufacturer, or supplier of goods.
10. Describe the defenses often used in a products liability case.

NOTES

1. *Tomcik v. Ohio Dep't of Rehabilitation & Correction,* 598 N.E.2d 900 (Ohio Ct. App. 1991).
2. *Id.* at 904.
3. www.wrongdiagnosis.com/malpractice/malpractice.htm.
4. 11 A.2d 132 (N.Y. App. Div. 1960).
5. 498 So. 2d 713 (La. Ct. App. 1986).
6. 787 S.W.2d 494 (Tex. Ct. App. 1990).
7. *Id.* at 496.
8. 57A AM. JUR. 2D Torts § 148 (1989).
9. 343 N.E.3d 589 (Ill. 1976).
10. No. 2004-00863 (N.Y. App. Div. 2004).
11. 175 N.W.2d 588, 596 (Iowa 1970).
12. 349 A.2d 245 (Md. 1975).
13. *Greene v. Bowen,* 639 F. Supp. 544, 561 (E.D. Cal. 1986).
14. 706 P.2d 1383 (Nev. 1985). 19. 355 S.E.2d 104 (Ga. Ct. App. 1987).
15. 355 S.E.2d 104 (Ga. Ct. App. 1987).
16. 57A AM. JUR. 2D Torts § 26 (1989).
17. 498 So. 2d 713 (La. Ct. App. 1986).
18. 128 So. 2d 485 (Ala. 1961).
19. 483 So. 2d 634 (La. Ct. App. 1985).
20. 57A AM. JUR. 2D Torts § 78 (1989).
21. 384 S.E.2d 92 (Va. 1989).
22. *Id.*
23. 498 So. 2d 713 (La. Ct. App. 1986).
24. *Dic v. Brooklyn Hospital Center,* No. 2003-01976 (N.Y. App. Div. 2004).
25. 691 A.2d 1147 (D.C. App. 1997).
26. 57A AM. JUR. 2D Torts § 80 (1989).
27. 33. 654 A.2d 771 (Conn. App. 1995).
28. *Id.* at 777.
29. *Clark v. Wagoner,* 452 S.W.2d 437, 440 (Tex. 1970).
30. 57A AM. JUR. 2D Torts § 134 (1989).
31. 296 S.E.2d 216 (Ga. Ct. App. 1982).
32. 142 N.E.2d 337 (Mass. 1957).
33. 116 Cal. Rptr. 733 (Cal. Ct. App. 1974).
34. 504 So. 2d 22 (Ala. 1986).
35. 457 A.2d 431 (N.J. 1983).
36. 865 S.W.2d 833 (Mo. Ct. App. 1993).
37. 841 F.2d 851 (8th Cir. 1988).
38. 358 S.E.2d 865 (Ga. Ct. App. 1987).
39. Garrard, *Evaluation of Neuroleptic Drug Use by Nursing Home Elderly under Proposed Medicare and Medicaid Regulations,* 265(4) JAMA 463 (1991).
40. 461 S.W.2d 195 (Tex. Ct. App. 1970).
41. 562 N.Y.2d 127 (N.Y. App. Div. 1990).
42. *Id.* at 129.
43. 856 S.W.2d 437 (Tex. Ct. App. 1993).
44. *Id.* at 447.
45. *Id.*
46. *Keller v. Miami Herald Publishing Company,* 778 F.2d 711 (11th Cir. 1985).
47. *Id.* at 713.
48. 285 N.W.2d 891 (Wis. Ct. App. 1979).
49. *Id.* at 893.
50. *Id.* at 894.
51. *Associates and Aldrich Co. v. Times Mirror Co.,* 440 F.2d 133, 136 (9th Cir. 1971).
52. 317 S.E.2d 652 (Ga. Ct. App. 1984).
53. 143 S.E. 489 (Ga. Ct. App. 1965).
54. *Id.*
55. *Miller-Douglas v. Keller,* 579 So. 2d 491 (La. Ct. App. 1991).
56. 150 N.E.2d 202 (Ill. App. Ct. 1958).
57. 739 S.W.2d 680 (Ark. 1987).
58. 936 P.2d 784 (Kans. App. 1997).
59. 589 So. 2d 1202 (La. Ct. App. 1991).
60. *Id.* at 1204.
61. 527 S.W.2d 133 (Tenn. Ct. App. 1975).
62. 336 S.E.2d 329 (Ga. App. 1985).
63. *Id.*
64. 638 S.W.2d 660 (Ark. 1982).
65. 700 F. Supp. 151 (S.D.N.Y. 1988).
66. 403 F.2d 580 (D.C. Cir. 1968).
67. *Id.*
68. 974 F.2d 598 (5th Cir. 1992).
69. 514 S.W.2d 429 (Tex. 1974).
70. 164 S.W.2d 828 (Tex. 1942).
71. 123 N.E.2d 793 (N.Y. 1955).
72. 629 N.W.2d 727 (2001).
73. 487 So. 2d 148 (La. Ct. App. 1986).

Criminal Aspects of Health Care

It's Your Gavel ...

NURSE SENTENCED FOR DIABOLICAL ACTS

From 1993 to 1995, Majors worked as a licensed practical nurse (LPN) in the intensive care unit (ICU) of a county hospital. He may have been a competent nurse, but he had one problem: An incredibly high number of elderly patients died under his watch. By 1995, after rumors started to circulate that he was euthanizing patients, the hospital suspended him, and the state board of nursing suspended his license.

In 1994, 100 of the 351 people admitted to the hospital's four-bed ICU died. A large percentage of those who died were elderly. In comparison, during the previous four years, an average of only 27 patients per year passed away, out of an average of 354 admitted to the ICU each year.

Spurred on by her suspicions (and those of other nurses), Nurse Stirek conducted an analysis showing that Majors was present for more deaths than any other nurse, almost twice as many as the nearest contender. After Stirek showed her analysis to Ling, the hospital's president and chief executive officer, Ling suspended Majors from work, with pay. Later, Ling asked the police to investigate. Majors was subsequently prosecuted.[1]

WHAT IS YOUR VERDICT?

Laws are made to restrain and punish the wicked; the wise and good do not need them as a guide, but only as a shield against rapine and oppression; they can live civilly and orderly, though there were no law in the world.

John Milton (1608–1674)

In an effort to provide the reader with a review of criminal law as it applies to the health care industry, this chapter presents the procedural aspects of criminal law, as well as an overview of criminal cases that have occurred in health care facilities.

CRIMINAL LAW

Criminal law (also known as *penal law*) is the body of statutory and common law that deals with crime and the legal punishment of criminal offenses. Criminal law represents society's expression of the limits of acceptable human behavior. A crime is any social harm defined and made punishable by law.

Crimes are classified as misdemeanors or felonies, dependent upon the severity of the crime. A *misdemeanor* is an offense generally punishable by less than one year in jail and/or a fine (e.g., petty larceny). A *felony* is a much more serious crime (e.g., rape or murder) and is punishable by imprisonment in a state or federal penitentiary for more than one year.

Criminal law distinguishes crimes from civil wrongs such as tort or breach of contract. Criminal law has been seen as a system of regulating the behavior of individuals and groups in relation to societal norms at large whereas civil law is aimed primarily at the relationship between private individuals and their rights and obligations under the law.

The objectives of criminal law are to maintain public order and safety, to protect the individual, to use punishment as a deterrent to crime, and to rehabilitate the criminal for return to society.

Particular to health care organizations is the fact that patients are often helpless and at the mercy of others. Health care facilities are far too often places where the morally weak and mentally deficient prey on the physically and sometimes mentally helpless. The very institutions designed to make the public well and feel safe can sometimes provide the setting for criminal conduct. The U.S. Department of Justice and state prosecutors vigorously pursue and prosecute health care organizations and individuals for criminal conduct. Health care fraud, patient abuse, and other such crimes have caused law enforcement agencies to assume a zero-tolerance level for such acts.

CRIMINAL PROCEDURE

Criminal procedure regulates the process for addressing violations of criminal law. The process begins with an alleged crime. A complainant makes an accusation, which is investigated by the police who act as agents of the government. When necessary, detectives may be assigned to a case to gather evidence, interview crime suspects and witnesses, and assist in preparing a case for possible trial. When a misdemeanor or felony has been committed, evidence gathered, and a target defendant has been identified, an arrest by a police officer is made. Upon arrest, the defendant is taken to the appropriate law enforcement agency for processing, which includes paperwork and fingerprinting. The police prepare and file accusatory statements, such as misdemeanor or felony complaints with a court in the appropriate jurisdiction. After processing has been completed, the defendant is either detained or released on bond. If the alleged offense is classified as a felony, the U.S. Constitution requires that the case be referred to a grand jury for an indictment. An *indictment* is the official charging instrument accusing the defendant of criminal conduct.

A prosecuting attorney represents the interests of the state, while the interests of the defendant are represented by his or her defense attorney. Although the specific process varies according to the local law, in virtually every jurisdiction the process culminates with a trial, followed by appeals to higher courts.

Criminal statutes spell out the exact circumstances that constitute a crime. These circumstances are known as the *elements* of the offense. Unless all the elements are proven by the prosecuting authority, the defendant is not guilty of the offense. There are three kinds of elements: the act itself, the *actus reus,* guilty act; the requisite mental state, the *mens rea,* guilty mind; and the attendant circumstances.

Criminal cases are presented to a grand jury by a prosecutor. Once the grand jury is presented with the prosecution's evidence, it may indict the target if jurors find in the evidence reasonable cause to believe that all the elements of a particular crime are present. Before indictment, the grand jury may request that witnesses be subpoenaed to testify; a defendant may also choose to testify. Finally, actions of a grand jury are handed to a judge, after which the defendant will be notified to appear to be arraigned for the crimes charged in the indictment.

Arraignment

The *arraignment* is a formal reading of the *accusatory instrument* (a generic term that describes a variety of documents, each of which accuses a defendant of an offense) and includes the setting of bail. After the charges are read, the defendant pleads guilty or not guilty. On a plea of not guilty, the defense attorney and prosecutor make arguments regarding bail. After the defendant's arraignment, the judge sets a date for the defendant to return to court. Between the time of arraignment and the next court date, the defense attorney and the prosecutor confer about the charges and evidence in the possession of the prosecutor. At that time, the defense will offer any mitigating circumstances it believes will convince the prosecutor to lessen or drop the charges.

Conference

If the defendant does not plead guilty, both felony and misdemeanor cases are taken to conference, and plea bargaining commences with the goal of an agreed-upon disposition. If no disposition can be reached, the case is adjourned, motions are made, and further plea bargaining takes place. After several adjournments, a case may be assigned to a trial court.

Criminal Trial

Most of the processes of a criminal trial are similar to that of a civil trial and include jury selection, opening statements, presentation of witnesses and other evidence, summations, instructions to the jury by the judge, jury deliberations, verdict, and opportunity for appeal to a higher court. In a criminal trial, the jury verdict must be unanimous, and the standard of proof must be beyond a reasonable doubt. Criminal trials involving health care professionals and organizations often involve health care fraud, falsification of records, misuse and theft of drugs, patient abuse, and murder. A variety of such cases are reviewed here.

FALSE CLAIMS

The False Claims Act of 1986 prohibits: knowingly presenting, or causing to be presented to the government a false claim for payment, knowingly making, using, or causing to be made or used, a false record or statement to get a false claim paid or approved by the government, conspiring to defraud the government by getting a false claim allowed or paid, and knowingly making, using, or causing to be made or used a false record to avoid, or decrease an obligation to pay or transmit property to the government.

As part of the effort to reduce fraud and abuse in federal health care programs, the Office of Inspector General (OIG) can impose monetary penalties, as well as exclude providers that violate the False Claims Act from participation in Medicare and other federal health care programs. Where the best interests of the programs are served by allowing continued participation by the provider, the OIG will often require that the provider adopt specific measures to better ensure its integrity. These measures are set forth in a corporate, institutional, or individual integrity agreement (collectively referred to as a corporate integrity agreement or CIA).

Consistent with the U.S. Sentencing Commission's *Federal Sentencing Guidelines Manual,* the CIA contains the following seven core elements of an effective compliance program.

1. leadership and structure, including a compliance officer and a corporate compliance counsel

2. written standards

3. education and training

4. internal lines of communication

5. auditing and monitoring

6. responding to potential violations

7. corrective action procedures

In addition to the abovementioned compliance elements, the provider may be required to submit periodic compliance reports. Inspector General June Gibbs Brown observed in her March 9, 2000, "Open Letter to Health Care Providers":

> The best evidence that a provider's compliance program is operating effectively occurs when the provider, through its compliance program, identifies problematic conduct, takes appropriate steps to remedy the conduct and prevent it from recurring, and makes a full and timely disclosure of the misconduct to appropriate authorities.[2]

KICKBACKS

The Medicare and Medicaid Patient Protection Act of 1987, as amended, 42 U.S.C. §1320a-7b (the "Antikickback Statute"), provides for criminal penalties for certain acts impacting Medicare and state health care (e.g., Medicaid) reimbursable services. The Anti-Kickback Statute, as amended, prohibits certain solicitations or receipt of remuneration. The statute penalizes anyone who knowingly and willfully solicits, receives, offers, or pays anything of value as an inducement in return for: referring an individual to a person for the furnishing or arranging for the furnishing of any item or service payable under the Medicare or Medicaid programs; and purchasing, leasing, or ordering or arranging for or recommending purchasing, leasing, or ordering any good, facility, service, or item payable under the Medicare or Medicaid programs.

The OIG investigates violations of the Medicare and Medicaid Anti-Kickback Statute. Violators are subject to criminal penalties or exclusion from participation in the Medicare and Medicaid programs. The OIG specifically targets four billing practices: claims for services not provided, claims for beneficiaries not homebound, claims for visits not made, and claims for visits not authorized by a physician.

Laboratory Kickback

In the case of *United States v. Katz,*[3] the owner of Tech Diagnostic Medical Lab agreed to kick back 50 percent of the Medicare payments received by Tech-Lab as a consequence of referrals from Total Health Care, a medical service company. Under the scheme, Total Health Care collected blood and urine samples from medical offices and clinics in southern California and sent them to Tech-Lab for testing. Tech-Lab billed Total Health Care, which in turn billed the private insurance carrier or the government-funded insurance programs Medi-Cal and Medicare for reimbursement.

Tech-Lab then kicked back half of its receipts to Total Health Care. The owners of Tech-Lab and Total Health Care arranged an identical scheme with a community medical clinic; Katz, the appellant, subsequently purchased a 25-percent interest in the clinic and began collecting payments under the scheme. Katz was convicted of conspiracy to commit Medicare fraud and of receipt of kickbacks in exchange for referral of Medicare patients. He appealed the decision. The court of appeals, however, affirmed the charges against him.

Architectural Contract Kickback

In *United States v. Thompson,*[4] three members of a county council, which served as the governing body of a county hospital, were convicted by a jury for soliciting and receiving $6,000 in kickbacks from architects. The architects testified that the appellants and others sought a one percent kickback on a hospital project, financed by federal funds, in return for being awarded the architectural contract. Mr. Galloway, of the architectural firm of Galloway and Guthrey, delivered the $6,000 to appellant Campbell at the Knoxville airport. The architects had informed the FBI, and an investigation was conducted. After the investigation, indictments, and trial by jury, the defendants were each sentenced to one year in prison. On appeal, the U.S. Court of Appeals for the Sixth Circuit held that the receipt of a kickback constituted an overt act in furtherance of a conspiracy to obstruct lawful government function and was a violation of the general conspiracy statute and a crime against the United States. It had been previously observed that "[t]o conspire to defraud the United States means primarily to cheat the government out of property or money, but it also means to interfere with or obstruct one of its lawful governmental functions by deceit, craft or trickery, or at least by means that are dishonest."[5] Proof that part of the architects' fee was reimbursed with federal funds was not necessary for a conviction. The criminal convictions were affirmed.

Ambulance Service Kickback

In *United States v. Bay State Ambulance and Hospital Rental Services,*[6] a city official was convicted in a federal district court for conspiring to commit Medicare fraud along with other defendants who were also convicted of making illegal payments. Bay State Ambulance and Hospital Rental Services, a privately owned ambulance company, gave cash and two automobiles to an official of a city-owned hospital. The gifts were given as an inducement to the city official for his recommendation that Bay State be awarded the Quincy City Hospital ambulance service contract, for which Bay State received some Medicare funds as reimbursement. The

defendants appealed, and the U.S. Court of Appeals for the First Circuit held that the evidence was sufficient to sustain a conviction.

HIPAA AND HEALTH CARE FRAUD

Congress passed, and President Clinton signed into law, the Health Insurance Portability and Accountability Act of 1996 (HIPAA). HIPAA provides new criminal and civil enforcement tools and funding dedicated to the fight against health care fraud. In addition, HIPAA requires the U.S. Attorney General and the U.S. Secretary of Department of Health and Human Services (DHHS), acting through the Office of Inspector General (OIG), to establish a coordinated national health care fraud and abuse control program. The program provides a coordinated national framework for federal, state, and local law enforcement agencies; the private sector; and the public to fight health care fraud. To combat fraud in home care settings, the DHHS announced Operation Restore Trust, an antifraud enforcement initiative targeted at home care agencies, nursing homes, and durable equipment suppliers. DHHS provided a toll-free telephone number (800-HHS-TIPS) to gather allegations of health care fraud from the public as well as from organizational whistle-blowers.

Medicare and Medicaid Fraud

The defendant physician in *United States v. Raithatha*[7] owned and operated two clinics. The defendant was convicted by a jury of making false statements and scheming to defraud. The defendant, sentenced to 27 months of imprisonment, appealed his conviction and sentence.

The indictment filed against the defendant included charges for instructing billing staff to raise the current procedural technology (CPT) codes on invoices when the physician reported a lower level of service; submit invoices to insurance companies for services performed by other physicians, as if the defendant had performed them; submit claims with a diagnosis listing an illness, when the patient did not have an illness; and, causing patients to present themselves for medically unnecessary visits by refusing to authorize refills on prescriptions and preventing employees from authorizing refills of prescriptions.

Charges also included making unannounced home visits to patients; approaching people on the street and ushering them into the clinic for unscheduled examinations; examining people who had come into the clinic for nonmedical reasons, such as to pay debts owed to the defendant; ordering medical tests not related to patients' conditions; falsely representing that other physician employees had specialties so that patients would be examined an additional time by a "specialist"; and refusing to give test results until an additional appointment was kept.

The defendant was also charged with defrauding Medicare/Medicaid by submitting a cost report for 1997 that included personal expenses unrelated to patient care. Included in those expenses was money that was actually spent to furnish and complete the defendant's home.

The defendant, on appeal, argued that there was insufficient evidence to sustain his conviction for defrauding or attempting to defraud. The defendant's staff members testified that the defendant instructed them to bill office visits covered by private insurance under CPT codes 99213 or 99203, regardless of the CPT code entered by the attending physician on the encounter form. Staff members were aware that this "up-coding" scheme resulted in higher reimbursement from private insurance companies.

In addition, staff members testified that the defendant routinely ordered tests unrelated to his patients' conditions and supported the tests with false diagnoses. Zeren, a nurse practitioner working at the McKee clinic, testified that after she performed sports physicals on children at local schools and found no indication of upper-respiratory infections, the defendant, who had not been present at the examinations, falsely diagnosed them as having upper respiratory infections.

A reasonable juror could have reasonably found the defendant physician guilty of defrauding or attempting to defraud Medicare/Medicaid. The conviction and sentence of the district court was affirmed.

False Medicaid Claims

In *United States v. Larm,*[8] a physician and his office manager were convicted on charges that they violated 42 U.S.C. § 139h(a)1 by submitting false Medicaid claims for medical services they never rendered to patients. Claims sometimes were submitted even when patients administered allergy injections themselves. In addition, sometimes more expensive serums were billed rather than those that were actually administered.

Fraudulent Billing for Laboratory Tests

The Court of Appeals of Georgia in *Culver v. State*[9] found that a reasonable fact-finder could conclude that the physician (Kell) maintained control over a laboratory and its Medicaid billings and received significant payments from the laboratory. The trier of fact could also find that although Medicaid paid the laboratory approximately $200 for each urine test conducted, the laboratory routinely charged self-pay patients $19.20 for what the laboratory employees described as the same test. Regulations prohibit providers from billing Medicaid for an amount greater than the lowest price routinely

offered to the general public for the same service or item on the same date of service.

Physician Bills for Services Not Rendered

A physician in *State v. Cargille*[10] was found to have submitted false information for the purpose of obtaining greater compensation than was otherwise permitted under the Medicaid program. Sufficient evidence was presented to sustain a conviction of Medicaid fraud. The physician argued that he felt justified for multiple billings for single office visits because of the actual amount of time that he saw a patient. He believed that his method of reimbursement was more equitable than Medicaid. The court disagreed with the physician's reasoning.

Pharmacist Submits False Drug Claims

The pharmacist in *State v. Heath*[11] submitted claims for reimbursement on brand-name medications rather than on the less-expensive generic drugs that were actually dispensed. A licensed pharmacist and former employee of the defendant contacted the Medicaid Fraud Unit of the Louisiana Attorney General's office and reported the defendant's conduct in substituting generic drugs for brand-name drugs. As a result of the complaint, the Medicaid Fraud Unit conducted a call-out, in which the unit sent letters to Medicaid recipients in the pharmacy's surrounding area:.

> In a recipient call out, the Medicaid Fraud Unit sends letters to Medicaid recipients in the general area of the pharmacy involved and asks them to bring all their prescription drugs to the welfare office on a specific date. The call out revealed that some of the prescription vials issued by the aforesaid pharmacies contained generic drugs while the labels indicated that they should contain brand name drugs.[12]

The pharmacist was convicted on three counts of Medicaid fraud.

Inaccurate Records and Controlled Drugs

The operator of a pharmacy, in a disciplinary proceeding before the California Board of Pharmacy, was found negligent because of inaccurate record keeping.[13] The pharmacist failed to keep accurate records of dangerous drugs, report thefts by employees, and report a burglary of pharmacy drugs. Such reporting is required by state statute.

Nursing Facility Stockholder Falsifies Records

The principal stockholder of a nursing home corporation in *Chapman v. United States, Department of Health and Human Services*[14] was convicted of making 19 false line item cost entries in reports to the Kansas Medicaid agency. The record shows that Chapman acted deliberately to submit false data to the Kansas Medicaid agency so that nursing homes owned by him would be reimbursed for goods and services they did not provide. When an audit was scheduled that threatened to reveal the false claims, Chapman prepared false invoices and had checks issued, but not signed, in an effort to cover up the discrepancies that the state audit would reveal.[15]

The U.S. Court of Appeals found that the DHHS did not act unreasonably when it imposed a $2,000 penalty for each of the false Medicaid claims and proposed an additional settlement of $118,136 even though the state already had recovered the $21,115 in excessive reimbursement by setoff. The court concluded that "the penalty reflects a fair amount of leniency on the part of the Inspector General and the Administrative Law Judge (ALJ)."[16]

Inflating Insurance Claims

The North Carolina Court of Appeals held that a chiropractor's license was properly suspended for six months in *Farlow v. North Carolina State Board of Chiropractic Examiners*[17] for inflating the insurance claims of victims of an automobile accident. Dr. Farlow prescribed a course of treatment for several patients that was not justified by the injuries they received. Instead, the treatment was prescribed to inflate insurance claims.

Fraud and Ethics

Behind every act of health care fraud lies a lapse in ethics. One particular type of fraud occurs when physicians refer their patients to hospitals and ancillary health care providers where the physician owns a financial interest in the provider to which the patient has been referred. The ethical risks inherent in physician self-referral were first noted in a 1986 Institute of Medicine study, and then again in a 1989 Health and Human Services inspector general study. The 1989 study concluded that physicians who owned or invested in independent clinical laboratories referred Medicare patients for 45 percent more laboratory services than did physicians without financial interests. It was in 1989 that the Ethics and Patient Referral Act was enacted, prohibiting unethical referrals, which were further defined in 1991, when the American Medical Association (AMA) Council on Ethical

and Judicial Affairs concluded that physicians should not refer patients to a health care facility in which they have a financial interest and they do not directly provide services. In the following year, the AMA House of Delegates voted to declare self-referral unethical in most instances.

The Omnibus Budget Reconciliation Act of 1989 (which took effect January 1, 1992) backed the AMA's position on self-referral, barring the referral of Medicare patients to clinical laboratories by physicians who have, or whose family members have, a financial interest in those laboratories. The scope of the ban on self-referral was expanded with the enactment of the Omnibus Reconciliation Act of 1993 (effective January 1, 1995), which added ten additional designated health services, including physical therapy; occupational therapy; radiology services; radiation therapy services and supplies; durable medical equipment and supplies; parenteral and enteral nutrients, equipment, and supplies; orthotics, prosthetics, and prosthetic devices and supplies; home health services; outpatient prescription drugs; and inpatient and outpatient hospital services. The 1993 law also expanded and clarified exceptions, and applied the referral limits to Medicaid.

While the antikickback law requires proof of "knowing" and "willful" illegal remuneration (i.e., bribes or rebates) for patient referrals and may result in criminal sanctions, self-referral laws usually are self-enforcing. If an improper financial relationship exists, a loss of Medicare payment or a civil fine may serve as punishment. Because of the law's preventative nature, it has been highly effective in protecting Medicare and Medicaid program integrity by motivating health care professionals to proactively comply with the law and to avoid financial arrangements that may unethically lead to substantial increases in use of service.

In *United States v. Greber*,[18] an osteopathic physician violated the Omnibus Budget Reconciliation when he unethically paid referring physicians after rendering services. The defendant, board certified in cardiology, was president of Cardio-Med, Inc., an organization that he formed. The company provided physicians with diagnostic services, one of which was Holter monitoring, a method of recording a patient's cardiac activity on tape, generally for a period of 24 hours. Cardio-Med billed Medicare for the monitoring service and, when payment was received, forwarded a portion to the referring physician. The government charged that the referral fee exceeded that permitted by Medicare and that there was evidence that physicians received interpretation fees even though the defendant actually evaluated the monitoring data. After a trial by jury, the physician was convicted on 20 of 23 counts in an indictment charging mail fraud, Medicare fraud, and false statement. On appeal the physician contended that the evidence was insufficient to support the guilty verdict. The court of appeals held that to the extent that payments made to a physician were made to induce referrals by that physician of Medicare patients to use payer laboratory services, Medicare fraud was established.

FALSIFICATION OF RECORDS

As with health care fraud, falsification of medical and business records is grounds for criminal prosecution. Anyone who suffers damage as a result of falsification of records may claim civil liability, which could result in the provider's loss of Medicare and Medicaid funding.

When a surgeon omitted a true entry in his operative report by not indicating that a nonphysician assisted in a patient's surgery, the surgeon was indicted for falsification of records. Two of the defendants, orthopedic surgeons Dr. Lipton and Dr. Massoff, in *People v. Smithtown General Hospital*[19] on the morning of July 3, 1975, performed an orthopedic procedure on a patient. The prosthesis used during surgery was supplied by a general sales manager, Mr. MacKay, who was present in the operating room during most of the operation, which began at 8 A.M. and ended at 11:30 A.M. After completion of the operation, an X-ray of the patient revealed that the "head of the femur popped out of the acetabulum."[20] At the request of Lipton, the salesman was located at a golf course and asked to return to the hospital. On arriving back in the operating room, he found Massoff reopening the surgical site. Massoff attempted to remove the prosthesis. MacKay offered his assistance and successfully removed the prosthesis. Massoff then returned to his office. With the consent of Lipton, MacKay removed the cement from the bone shaft and reinserted the prosthesis. An indictment charged Lipton with the intent to defraud and to conceal crimes of unauthorized practice of medicine and assault. A similar indictment was returned against a supervising nurse and the hospital for failure to make a true entry in the operating room register.

A motion to dismiss the indictments against the physicians and nurse charged with falsifying business records in the first degree was denied. A motion to dismiss the indictments for assault in the second degree was granted.

MISUSE AND THEFT OF DRUGS

Perhaps one of the most tempting and accessible crimes for a health care professional involves the misuse or theft of drugs. Drugs can offer significant financial gain when they fall into the hands of the wrong people. Such was the case in *United States v. Nelson,*[21] where a doctor cooperated in an Internet pharmacy and had the proceeds transferred to an offshore account for himself. Fuchs, an unindicted coconspirator, operated an Internet pharmacy called NationPharmacy.com, where customers could obtain prescription and nonprescription drugs. In accord with federal law, all requests for prescription drugs were first reviewed by a physician, defendant Nelson, who either approved or denied the request. Nelson, however, approved 90 to 95 percent of all prescription drug requests and did so without ever examining his purported patient. Customers who used Fuchs's Internet

pharmacy would have their orders routed through a brick-and-mortar pharmacy called Main Street Pharmacy. Nelson would physically visit Main Street Pharmacy to sign the prescription requests, and customers would receive prescriptions by mail and pay Fuchs directly. Nelson, the prescribing physician, was never paid by any customer. Instead, Nelson received a total of $175,000, which was wired directly from Fuchs into an offshore account.

Nelson was charged and convicted of both conspiracy to distribute controlled prescription drugs outside the usual course of professional practice, in violation of 21 U.S.C. § 846, and conspiracy to launder money, in violation of 18 U.S.C. § 1956(h). Nelson appealed his conviction, arguing that there was insufficient evidence to support a conviction because there was no evidence of a conspiracy.

The most significant evidence came from testimonies by Weeks, the person who set up the Web site; Shadid, the resident pharmacist at Main Street Pharmacy; Thompson, another pharmacist at Main Street Pharmacy; and Dupes, the office manager for Fuchs. Weeks's testimony described the general workings of the Fuchs Web site. He testified he established this Web site at Fuchs's behest as a means of providing prescription and nonprescription drugs over the Internet. Weeks testified that only those orders for prescription drugs that were specifically approved by Nelson were processed. He testified that he provided Nelson the means to review and approve prescription drug requests with a unique user name and password that enabled Nelson to access the medical history questionnaires required to be filled out by all customers who requested prescription drugs.

Shadid and Thompson testified at trial as to Nelson's personal participation in this scheme. Both men were pharmacists at Main Street Pharmacy, which processed all orders taken through NationPharmacy.com. Both testified that on numerous occasions, Nelson would personally come to Main Street Pharmacy to sign prescriptions and that Nelson signed "thousands" of prescriptions for NationPharmacy.com. Finally, Dupes testified that she transferred money, a total of $175,000, from an account controlled by Fuchs to an offshore account controlled by Nelson.

The evidence described a scheme that depended upon the participation of Nelson. Without his approval, requests for controlled prescription drugs taken on the Web site would not have been filled. Given the concert of action between Nelson and Fuchs in the common purpose of operating a Web site pharmacy, a reasonable jury could infer the existence of an agreement constituting a conspiracy to distribute prescription drugs outside the usual course of professional practice and to launder the proceeds of that distribution.

Physician Conspiracy to Distribute Dilaudid

The ophthalmologist in *Bouquett v. St. Elizabeth's Corp.*[22] brought an action to challenge suspension of his medical staff privileges after a felony conviction in a federal court for conspiracy to distribute Dilaudid. He later was sentenced to five years of incarceration. On appeal, the Ohio Supreme Court held that the conviction of the ophthalmologist justified summary suspension of his staff privileges pursuant to a hospital bylaw permitting summary suspension in the best interest of patient care in the hospital. The governing body of a private organization has broad discretion in determining who shall be granted medical staff privileges. Unless an organization has been arbitrary and capricious or has abused its discretion, the courts generally will not interfere with its decision to suspend physicians convicted on drug-related felony charges.

Pharmacist's Illegal Use and Sale of Marijuana

The pharmacist in *Brown v. Idaho State Board of Pharmacy*[23] admitted to using marijuana approximately twice a week. During a hearing by the Idaho State Board of Pharmacy, the hearing officer admitted into evidence a copy of a judgment of a conviction on Brown's plea of guilty to a criminal charge of possession of drug paraphernalia. The Idaho State Board of Pharmacy suspended Brown's license. On appeal, the Idaho Court of Appeals held that revocation of his license was supported by evidence that he engaged in the illegal use of marijuana and that he also had participated in the sale and delivery of a misbranded drug.

Theft of Drugs

The appellant, a licensed nurse, in *Chia v. Ohio Board of Nursing*,[24] took a patient's Percodan tablet for her own use. The appellant pled no contest and was found guilty of theft of drugs and a felony of the fourth degree. The licensing board mailed to the appellant a notice of immediate suspension and opportunity for hearing. In that notice, the board informed the appellant that her license was immediately suspended as a result of her felony drug abuse conviction. The notice also informed the appellant that the board proposed further sanctions to her license and that she was entitled to a hearing regarding those sanctions if she requested one within 30 days. The appellant did not respond to the notice.

Without having heard from the appellant, the board mailed her a letter informing her that it would consider sanctions to her license at its regularly scheduled meeting in May. At that meeting, the board permanently revoked the appellant's nursing license. The appellant appealed the board's decision to the court of common pleas. That court affirmed the board's decision, finding that it was supported by reliable, probative, and substantial evidence and was in accordance with law. The board's notice clearly informed the appellant that her license was immediately suspended due to her felony drug conviction.

The trial court did not abuse its discretion by finding that the board's decision to permanently revoke the appellant's license was supported by reliable, probative, and substantial evidence and was in accordance with law.

Fraudulent Billing

The physician in *Richstone v. Novello*[25] was found to have willfully filed false reports, practicing with negligence on more than one occasion, practicing fraudulently, failing to maintain adequate records, and performing unnecessary medical tests and treatment. The physician was found to be morally unfit to practice medicine as well as unsuitable for retraining or probation. A penalty was imposed by a hearing committee of the state to revoke the physician's license. The physician-petitioner challenged those determinations.

Given evidence that the physician was found to have been engaging in fraudulent billing, attempting to coerce a patient into dropping her complaint with the department of health, denying patients timely access to their records, performing substandard follow-up procedures, ordering excessive and medically unnecessary testing on patients, and falsifying his application for reappointment to the hospital's medical staff, the supreme court, appellate division declined to disturb the imposition of the penalty of revocation of the physician's license.

Distribution of Misbranded Drugs

Another such case occurred in *United States v. Milstein*,[26] in which the government established at trial that the defendant and others purchased Eldepryl, a medication used to treat Parkinson's disease, and the fertility drugs Pergonal and Metrodin, which were produced for distribution outside the United States, stripped them of their original factory packaging, and repackaged them with forged labels and packaging materials closely resembling those of drugs produced in accordance with FDA requirements for the U.S. market. They then fraudulently sold the drugs in the United States to doctors, pharmacists, and pharmaceutical wholesalers. The conviction for distributing the misbranded drugs in interstate commerce with fraudulent intent was appropriate.

PHYSICIANS CAN BE VICTIMS OF FRAUD

Physicians are not immune from being the victims of fraud. The detection, investigation, and prosecution of financial crimes against physicians are not uncommon occurrences. They involve such areas as computer billing crime, bookkeeper/office manager theft, insurance fraud, cash larceny, checkbook scams, and patient record tampering.

Physicians should be aware of how to analyze larcenous transactions, identify embezzled funds, and recognize the criminal employee. Physicians should be wary of bookkeepers who make themselves indispensable because of their perceived ability to operate the office computer system. To avoid being victimized by employee fraud, physicians should

- Familiarize themselves with patient-billing and record-keeping practices

- Avoid having one individual in charge of billing and collection procedures

- Arrange for an annual audit of office procedures and records by an outside auditor

PATIENT ABUSE

Gale . . . wasn't prepared for the rough treatment and cruel taunts she says her ailing mother suffered at the nursing home. She cried as a nurse's aide upbraided her mother for failing to straighten her arthritis-stricken legs. And she watched in disbelief as an assistant jerked her mother off her rubber bed pad and pushed her into the bed's metal rails.

All of these images were caught . . . by a "granny cam"—a camera hidden in her mother's room.

USA Today, September 14, 1999

Patient abuse is the mistreatment or neglect of individuals who are under the care of a health care organization. Abuse is not limited to an institutional setting and may occur in an individual's home as well as in an institution. Abuse can take many forms: physical, psychological, medical, and financial. To compound the issue, abuse is not always easy to identify because injuries often can be attributed to other causes, especially in elderly patients with their advanced age and failing health. In the hospital setting, patients are not generally as dependent upon the facility operator in the same manner as a resident in a nursing facility is. Persons are usually hospitalized for only brief periods of time, whereas nursing facility residents may be dependent upon the facility operator for a period of years. Thus, the potential for long-term abuse and neglect is far greater for nursing facility residents than hospital patients.

The abuse of the elderly is not a localized or isolated problem. Unfortunately, it permeates society. *Behind Closed Doors,* a landmark book on family violence, stated that the first national study of violence in American homes estimated that one in two homes are the scene of family violence at least once a year.[27]

We have always known that America is a violent society. . . . What is new and surprising is that the American family and the American home are perhaps as much or more violent than any other single institution or setting (with the exception of the military, and only then in the time of war). Americans run the greatest risk of assault, physical injury and even murder in their own homes by members of their own families.[28]

It is difficult to determine the extent of elder abuse because the abused elderly are reluctant to admit that their children or loved ones have assaulted them. According to a 2005 fact sheet by the Center on Elder Abuse, ". . . between 1 and 2 million Americans age 65 years of age or older have been injured, exploited, or otherwise been mistreated by someone on whom they depended for care and protection."[29]

The plaintiffs in *In re Estate of Smith v. O'Halloran*[30] instituted a lawsuit in an effort to improve deplorable conditions at many nursing homes. The court concluded that

The evidentiary record . . . supports a general finding that all is not well in the nation's nursing homes and that the enormous expenditures of public funds and the earnest efforts of public officials and public employees have not produced an equivalent return in benefits. That failure of expectations has produced frustration and anger among those who are aware of the realities of life in some nursing homes which provide so little service that they could be characterized as orphanages for the aged.[31]

Abuse of nursing facility residents gave impetus to the strengthening of resident rights under the Omnibus Budget Reconciliation Act of 1989. The Act provides that a "resident has the right to be free from verbal, sexual, physical, or mental abuse, corporal punishment, and involuntary seclusion."[32] Although resident rights have been significantly strengthened, resident abuse is often in the headlines. For example, the headline "Nurse's Aide Jailed for Punching Patient" topped a story about a nurse's aide who was jailed for punching a 91-year-old senile man in the nose.[33] The aide had been previously convicted of resident abuse.

Surveyors of health care organizations look for signs of patient abuse by watching for:

- Physician's orders for restraints

- Time-limited orders

- The number of patients who are physically restrained

- The type of restraints being used

- Whether the restraints are applied correctly

- The apparent physical and mental condition of the restrained patients

- Whether restraints are released as required by law and whether exercise is provided for the patient

- Whether the staff responds to requests for water, assistance to the bathroom, and so forth, from a patient who is restrained, and the interval of time between the request and the response

- How often restrained patients are observed by the staff

- The effect of restraints on patients and signs of overmedication

- The frequency of overmedication

- Signs of mental and physical abuse of patients

- Any signs of harassment, humiliation, or threats from staff or patients

- Whether patients are comfortable with the staff

- The numbers of patients with bruises or other injuries (because the skin of the elderly bruises easily, abuse or injury should not be assumed automatically)

- Patient-to-patient interactions and staff response to any physical or mental abuse of one patient by another

- Evidence of patient neglect or patients left in urine or feces without cleaning

Criminal Negligence

Criminal negligence is the reckless disregard for the safety of others. It is the willful indifference to an injury that could follow an act.

The defendants in *State v. Brenner*[34] were charged with cruelty to the infirm. The defendants brought a challenge stating that the criminal statutes under which they were charged were constitutionally vague. According to the court, Section 14.12 of Louisiana Revised Statutes defines criminal negligence as follows:

> Criminal negligence exists when, although neither specific nor general criminal intent is present, there is such disregard of the interest of others that the offender's conduct amounts to a gross deviation below the standard of care expected to be maintained by a reasonably careful man under like circumstances.[35]

Criminal negligence requires

> a gross deviation below the standard of care expected to be maintained by a reasonably careful man under like circumstances. It calls for substantially more than the ordinary lack of care which may be the basis of tort liability, and fur-

nishes a more explicit statement of that lack of care which has been variously characterized in criminal statutes as "gross negligence" and "recklessness."[36]

The state alleged that the administrator of the nursing facility neglected and mistreated residents by failing to ensure that the facility was maintained in a sanitary manner, necessary health services were performed, staff were properly trained, there were adequate medical supplies and sufficient staff, records were maintained properly, and the residents were adequately fed and cared for. In addition to allegations of neglect and mistreatment of residents, other allegations charged the director with failing to properly train the staff at the facility in correct nursing procedures. The controller was alleged to have failed to purchase adequate medical supplies for proper treatment. The admissions director allegedly failed to exercise proper judgment regarding admissions procedures, and the physical therapist allegedly failed to provide adequate physical therapy services. The defendants asserted that the term *neglect* was unconstitutionally vague. The Louisiana Supreme Court, on appeal by the defendants from two lower courts, held that the phrases "intentional or criminally negligent mistreatment or neglect" and "unjustifiable pain and suffering" were not vague and that they were sufficiently clear in meaning to afford a person of ordinary understanding fair notice of the conduct that was prohibited.[37]

Neglect of Residents

The defendant in *State v. Cunningham*[38] was the owner and administrator of a residential care facility that housed 30 to 37 mentally ill, mentally retarded, and elderly residents. The Iowa Department of Inspections and Appeals conducts routine inspections of health care facilities. All inspections are unannounced, and deficiency statements are sent to the administrator of the facility surveyed.

Various surveys were conducted at the defendant's facility between October 1989 and May 1990. All of the surveys except for one resulted in a $50 daily fine assessed against the defendant for violations of the regulations. On August 16, 1990, a grand jury filed an indictment charging the defendant with several counts of wanton neglect of a resident in violation of Iowa Code section 726.7 (1989), which provides: "A person commits wanton neglect of a resident of a health care facility when the person knowingly acts in a manner likely to be injurious to the physical, mental, or moral welfare of a resident of a health care facility. . . . Wanton neglect of a resident of a health care facility is a serious misdemeanor."

The district court held that the defendant had knowledge of the dangerous conditions that existed in the health care facility but willfully and consciously refused to provide or exercise adequate supervision to remedy or attempt to remedy the dangerous conditions. The residents were exposed to physical dangers, unhealthy and unsanitary physical conditions, and were grossly deprived of much-needed medical care and personal attention. The conditions were likely to and did cause injury to the physical and mental well-being of the facility's residents. The defendant was found guilty on five counts of wanton neglect. The district court sentenced the defendant to one year in jail for each of the five counts, to run concurrently. The district court suspended all but two days of the defendant's sentence and ordered him to pay $200 for each count, plus a surcharge and costs, and to perform community service. A motion for a new trial was denied, and the defendant appealed.

The Iowa Court of Appeals held that there was substantial evidence to support a finding that the defendant was responsible for not properly maintaining the nursing facility, which led to prosecution for wanton neglect of the facility's residents. *Substantial evidence* means evidence that would convince a rational fact finder that the defendant was guilty beyond a reasonable doubt. The defendant was found guilty of knowingly acting in a manner likely to be injurious to the physical or mental welfare of the facility's residents by creating, directing, or maintaining the following five hazardous conditions and unsafe practices:

1. There were fire hazards and circumstances that impeded safety from fire. For example, cigarette stubs were found in a cardboard box, and burn holes were found in patient clothing, on furniture, and in nonsmoking areas. Also, exposed electrical wiring was found, along with a bent and rusted fire door that could not close or latch.

2. The facility was not properly maintained, and demonstrated many health and safety violations, including broken glass in patients' rooms, excessively hot water in faucets, dried feces on public bathroom walls and grab bars, no soap in the kitchen, insufficient towels and linens, dead and live cockroaches and worms in the food preparation area, and debris, bugs, and grease throughout the facility.

3. Dietary facilities were unsanitary and inadequate to meet the dietary needs of the residents. In one particular case, an ordered "no concentrated sweets" diet for a diabetic patient was not followed, subjecting the patient to life-threatening blood sugar levels.

4. There were inadequate staffing patterns and supervision in the facility. No funds were spent on employee training, and the defendant did not spend the minimum amount of time at the facility, as required by administrative standards.

5. Improper dosages of medications were administered to the residents. For example, physicians distributed an ongoing overdose of heart medication to one resident while failing to administer medication to another (which resulted in a seizure).[39]

The defendant argued that he did not create the unsafe conditions at the facility. The court of appeals disagreed. The statute does not require that the defendant create the conditions at the facility to sustain a conviction. The defendant was the administrator of the facility and responsible for the conditions that existed.

Abuse and Revocation of License

The operator of a nursing facility appealed an order by the department of public welfare revoking his license because of resident abuse in *Nepa v. Commonwealth Department of Public Welfare*.[40] Substantial evidence supported the department's finding. Three former employees testified that the nursing facility operator had abused residents in the following incidents: he unbuckled the belt of one of the residents, causing his pants to drop, and then grabbed a second resident, forcing the two to kiss (petitioner's excuse for this behavior was to shame the resident because of his masturbating in public); on two occasions he forced a resident to remove toilet paper from a commode after she had urinated and defecated in it (denying that there was fecal matter in the commode, petitioner's excuse was that this was his way of trying to stop the resident from filling the commode with toilet paper); and he verbally abused a resident who was experiencing difficulty in breathing and accused him of being a fake as he attempted to feed him liquids.[41]

The nursing facility operator claimed that the findings of fact were not based on substantial evidence and that even if they were, the incidents did not amount to abuse under the code. The defendant attempted to discredit the witnesses with allegations from a resident and another employee that one of his former employees got into bed with a resident, and that another had taken a picture of a male resident while in the shower and had placed a baby bottle and a humiliating sign around the neck of another resident. The court was not impressed. Although these incidents, if true, were reprehensible, they were collateral matters that had no bearing on the witnesses' reputation for truthfulness and therefore could not be used for impeachment purposes. The court held that there was substantial evidence supporting the department's decision and that the activities committed by the operator were sufficient to support revocation of his license.

> We believe Petitioner's treatment of these residents as found by the hearing examiner to be truly disturbing. These residents were elderly and/or mentally incapacitated and wholly dependent on Petitioner while residing in his home. As residents, they are entitled to maintain their dignity and be cared for with respect, concern, and passion.

> Petitioner testified that he did not have adequate training to deal with the patients he received

who suffered from mental problems. Petitioner's lack of training in this area is absolutely no excuse for the reprehensible manner in which he treated various residents. Accordingly, DPW's order revoking Petitioner's license to operate a personal care home is affirmed.[42]

Abusive Search

A nurse in *People v. Coe*[43] was charged with a willful violation of the public health law in connection with an allegedly abusive search of an 86-year-old resident at a geriatric center and with the falsification of business records in the first degree. The resident, Mr. Gersh, had heart disease and difficulty in expressing himself verbally. Another resident claimed that two $5 bills were missing. Nurse Coe assumed that Gersh had taken them because he had been known to take things in the past. The nurse proceeded to search Gersh, who resisted. A security guard was summoned, and another search was undertaken. When Gersh again resisted, the security guard slammed a chair down in front of him and pinned his arms while the defendant nurse searched his pockets, failing to retrieve the two $5 bills. Five minutes later, Gersh collapsed, gasping for air, in a chair. Coe administered cardiopulmonary resuscitation but was unsuccessful, and Gersh died.

Coe was charged with violation of Section 175.10 of the New York Penal Law for falsifying records, because of the defendant's "omission" of the facts relating to the search of Gersh. These facts were considered relevant and should have been included in the nurse's notes regarding this incident. "The first sentence states, 'Observed resident was extremely confused and talks incoherently. Suddenly became unresponsive. . . .' This statement is simply false. It could only be true if some reference to the search and the loud noise was included."[44] A motion was made to dismiss the indictment at the end of the trial.

The court held that the search became an act of physical abuse and mistreatment, the evidence was sufficient to warrant a finding of guilt on both charges, and the fact that searches took place frequently did not excuse an otherwise illegal procedure.

It may well be that this incident reached the attention of the criminal justice system only because, in the end, a man had died. In those instances which are equally violative of residents' rights and equally contrary to standards of common decency but which do not result in visible harm to a patient, the acts are nevertheless illegal and subject to prosecution. A criminal act is not legitimized by the fact that others have, with impunity, engaged in that act.[45]

Physical Abuse

The revocation of a personal care home license was found to be proper in *Miller Home, Inc. v. Commonwealth, Department of Public Welfare*[46] because of repeated medication violations and resident abuse. Evidence was presented that the son of the personal care home's manager was hired as a staff member after having acted as a substitute, even though he had physical altercations with residents of the home. On one occasion, the manager's son punched a female resident, resulting in her hospitalization for broken bones around the eye, and on two prior occasions he had been involved in less-physical altercations that required police intervention.

A nursing facility orderly challenged a determination by the commissioner of the state department of health finding him guilty of resident abuse in *Reid v. Axelrod*.[47] The orderly maintained that the resident struck him with his cane, and that he merely pushed the cane away to avoid being struck a second time. A co-employee testified that the orderly struck the resident in the chest after being hit with the cane. The court held that the determination was supported by substantial evidence and that the three-year delay in conducting the hearing did not warrant dismissal of the petition charging the orderly with resident abuse. Public policy requires that residents must be protected from abusive health care workers.

The nursing facility resident in *Stiffelman v. Abrams*[48] died from:

". . . blows, kicks, kneeings, or bodily throwings intentionally, viciously, and murderously dealt him from among the facility's staff over a period of approximately two to three weeks prior to his death"; that the "beatings were repeated and were received by the decedent at ninety years of age and in a frail, defenseless, and dependent condition"; that the beatings so administered to the decedent were "physically and mentally torturous"; that he was caused by them to live out his final days in agony and terror; and that his physical injuries included thirteen fractures to his ribs, subpleural hemorrhaging, and marked lesions to his chest, flanks, abdomen, legs, arms, and hands; that during and following the period of the beatings the decedent lay at the facility for days unattended and unaided as to the deterioration and grave suffering he was undergoing.[49]

The executors of the estate had brought suit against the operator and individual and corporate owners of the facility for damages for personal injuries resulting in the death of the resident. The executors were requesting under Count I, $1.5 million in survival damages because of the physical and mental pain and suffering of the decedent, as well as $3 million for punitive damages, and under Count II, $1,504,084 in contractual breaches of the resident's admission contract with the facility. The executors claimed that certain standards of care and personal rights contained in the contract were violated. The trial court sustained the nursing facility's motion for dismissal of the case on the grounds that the plaintiffs failed to state a claim on which relief could be granted. On appeal, the judgment of the trial court was reversed with respect to Count I, and the dismissal of Count II was sustained. The case was remanded, requiring the executors to proceed under appropriate statutory authority and not under contract.

Forcible Administration of Medications

The medical employee in *In re Axelrod*[50] sought review of a determination by the commissioner of health that she was guilty of resident abuse. Evidence showed that the employee, after a resident refused medication, "held the patient's chin and poured the medication down her throat."[51] There was no indication or convincing evidence that an emergency existed that would have required the forced administration of the medication. The court held that substantial evidence supported the commissioner's finding that the employee had been guilty of resident abuse.

The commissioner properly found that the notation in the record that "staff are asked to, please, make every effort to make sure that she [the patient] takes them [her medication]"[52] does not authorize the forcible administration of medication. This is particularly so when a medical doctor did not make the notation authorized to prescribe medication and when the written policy of the facility was that the head nurse was to be notified if a patient refused medication.

ABUSE OF STROKE PATIENT

Citation: State v. Houle, 642 A.2d 1178 (Vt. 1994)

Facts

The defendant, an LPN, had criminal charges brought against her stemming from her treatment of a stroke patient. It was alleged that she had slapped the patient's legs repeatedly and shackled him to his bed at the wrists and ankles. By the time of trial, the patient had died of causes unrelated to the charged conduct. During the trial, the state pre-sented testimony of eyewitnesses, including the patient's wife, hospital employees, and an investigator from the office of the attorney general. The defendant did not deny that she had restrained the patient, but claimed that her actions were necessary for the patient's protection, as well as her own, and that her actions were neither assaultive nor cruel. The defendant claimed that the trial court improperly admitted evidence that the patient gave.

Issue

Was the evidence that the patient gave admissible in prosecution of the defendant?

Holding

The Vermont Supreme Court held that the evidence that the patient gave was relevant and admissible.

Reason

The patient's awareness of what happened to him was relevant to the state's case because the trial court, in its instruction to the jury, defined cruelty as "intentional and malicious infliction of physical or emotional pain or suffering upon a person." By showing that the patient was aware of what had happened to him, the state allowed the jury to infer that he had suffered physical or emotional pain. The state presented a witness who was present when the incident occurred and who was able to describe the acts of abuse in detail. The credibility of this eyewitness testimony, and not what the patient's testimony would have been, was the focus of the trial.

Discussion

1. Do you agree with the court's findings? Why?
2. At what point does the application of restraints become a cruelty?

MURDER

The tragedy of murder in institutions that are dedicated to the healing of the sick has been an all-too-frequent occurrence.

Fatal Injection of Pavulon

In a case involving Angelo, a registered nurse on the cardiac/intensive care unit at a Long Island hospital, the defendant was found guilty of second-degree murder for injecting two patients with the drug Pavulon. He was found guilty of the lesser charges of manslaughter and criminally negligent homicide in the deaths of two other patients. Angelo committed the murders in a bizarre scheme to revive the patients and be thought of as a hero.[53]

Fatal Injection of Lidocaine

In another case, *Hargrave v. Landon*,[54] the defendant, a nurse's aide, was convicted of murder in the first degree when he was found to have injected an elderly patient with a fatal dose of the drug Lidocaine. He was sentenced to life imprisonment by the circuit court. The defendant appealed the judgment of the circuit court, alleging that his due-process rights were violated during the trial, when the trial court failed to grant his motion for change of venue. Because of the carnival atmosphere surrounding the trial, he argued the trial court should have sequestered the jury. In addition, the defendant claimed the trial court improperly admitted evidence of other crimes. Finally, he asserted the evidence was insufficient as a matter of law to sustain the conviction.[55]

The U.S. district court held that the nurse's aide failed to establish that he was denied an impartial jury because of adverse pretrial publicity, especially because the tenor of newspaper articles before his trial was primarily informative and factual and the articles treated the story objectively. The evidence was found to have been sufficient to support the petitioner's conviction for murder.

Lethal Dose of Anesthesia

A licensed dentist and an oral surgeon in *People v. Protopappas*[56] were convicted in the superior court of second-degree murder for the deaths of three patients who died after receiving general anesthesia. The record revealed that the three patients received massive doses of drugs, which resulted in their deaths. The dosages had not been tailored to the patients' individual conditions. The dentist had also improperly instructed surrogate dentists, who were neither licensed nor qualified to administer general anesthesia, to administer preset dosages for an extended time with little or no personal supervision. In addition, the dentist had been habitually slow in reacting to resulting overdoses. In one case, the patient's general physician informed the defendant that the 24-year-old, 88-pound patient suffered from lupus, total kidney failure, high blood pressure, anemia, heart murmur, and chronic seizure disorder, and should not be placed under anesthesia even for a short time. The defendant consciously elected to ignore that medical opinion. On appeal, the court of appeals

found that there was sufficient evidence of implied malice to support the jury's findings that the dentist and the oral surgeon were guilty of second-degree murder.

> This is more than gross negligence. These are the acts of a person who knows that his conduct endangers the life of another and who acts with conscious disregard for life. . . . Many murders are committed to satisfy a feeling of a hatred or grudge, it is true, but this crime may be perpetrated without the slightest trace of personal ill-will.[57]

Not every charge of suspected murder ends in a conviction; however, there is a heavy price to be paid in the mental anguish suffered by those charged with the crime.

Lethal Dose of Codeine

Evidence supported a finding that a nurse killed the plaintiff's decedent in *Havrum v. United States*.[58] After a bench trial in an action brought under the Federal Tort Claims Act, the trial court concluded that Williams, a nurse at a VA hospital, killed veteran Elzie Havrum. On appeal, the government challenged the sufficiency of the evidence.

Ms. Havrum was required to show that the VA hospital had a duty to protect Mr. Havrum from injury and that its failure to perform that duty caused his death. The government did not challenge the trial court's conclusion that the hospital breached its duty to protect Havrum from the nurse, who presented a danger to patients. The government contends, however, that Havrum failed to establish causation because the evidence did not support the court's finding that the nurse killed Havrum.

The trial court found that Williams gave Havrum a lethal dose of codeine, and that even disregarding the evidence of codeine poisoning, the circumstantial evidence indicated that Williams killed Havrum. The trial court relied, in part, on a study by the hospital's epidemiologist, Dr. Christensen, who investigated a suspected link between Williams and an increase in deaths on the ward where Williams customarily worked. The study concluded that patients who were under Williams's care were nearly ten times more likely to die as were other patients. In addition, Williams was associated with many unexpected deaths that occurred in private rooms. Christensen also testified that he had never seen anything so unusual as the number of patients who died on the relevant ward from May through July 1992, between 1 A.M. and 3 A.M. (a period when fewer deaths generally occur). Williams was present for 11 of the 13 deaths in that interim, although he worked on only one third of the shifts.

Christensen concluded that there was only one chance in a million that the pattern of deaths on the ward was random, and that there was a compelling correlation between the deaths and Williams for which Christensen could find no benign explanation. Although the court agreed with the government, the statistical evidence alone does not establish that Williams caused Havrum's death; that evidence is nevertheless probative. It was, moreover, only one aspect of the circumstantial evidence upon which the trial court relied in finding causation.

With regard to Havrum specifically, the court noted that his death was among those that Christensen found highly unusual. Havrum died on the ward in question at 1:15 A.M. in a private room with Williams present. Havrum was not expected to die, and the government offered no evidence that he faced death as part of some short-term natural progression. Although Havrum suffered from a serious illness, the admitting physician did not place him in intensive care and did not believe that his death was imminent. Havrum actually reported feeling better while he was in the hospital, but 16 hours after his admission he was pronounced dead.

The trial court also referred to suspicious inconsistencies and alterations in the medical records. The court remarked that Williams first wrote a medical note indicating that he found Havrum in severe respiratory distress at about 1:15 A.M., the same time that the physician pronounced him dead. The time in the note was then changed to 1:10 A.M., a line was drawn through the note, and the note was marked "error R.W." Williams then wrote another medical note; this time he stated that he found Havrum in severe respiratory distress at about 1:10 A.M. and that the physician arrived at about 1:15 A.M., just as Havrum stopped breathing. Although the government suggests possible innocent explanations for the changed entries and omissions, the trial court, which noted that Williams had been fired by another hospital for inserting a false entry into a patient's chart, was free to draw its own less-innocent inferences from Havrum's hospital records. In addition, one permissible inference is that Williams's evident uncertainty about what to say and to note in the records indicates that there was, in fact, nothing particularly wrong with Havrum, and that Williams took his life. The appellate court concluded that, more likely than not, Williams did kill Havrum.

Removal of Life-Support Equipment

Although there may be a duty to provide life-sustaining equipment in the immediate aftermath of cardiopulmonary arrest, there is no duty to continue its use once it has become futile and ineffective to do so in the opinion of qualified medical personnel. Two physicians in *Barber v. Superior Court*[59] were charged with the crimes of murder and conspiracy to commit murder. The charges were based on their acceding to requests of the patient's family to discontinue life-support equipment and intravenous tubes. The patient suffered a cardiopulmonary arrest in the recovery room after surgery. A team of physicians and nurses revived the patient and placed him on life-support equipment. The patient suffered severe brain damage, which placed him in a comatose and vegetative state from which, according to tests and examinations by other specialists, he was unlikely to recover. On the written request

of the family, the patient was taken off life-support equipment. The family, his wife and eight children, made the decision together after consultation with the physicians. Evidence had been presented that the patient, before his incapacitation, had expressed to his wife that he would not want to be kept alive by a machine. There was no evidence indicating that the family was motivated in their decision by anything other than love and concern for the dignity of their loved one. The patient continued to breathe on his own. Showing no signs of improvement, the physicians again discussed the patient's poor prognosis with the family. The intravenous lines were removed, and the patient died sometime thereafter.

A complaint then was filed against the two physicians. The magistrate who heard the evidence determined that the physicians did not kill the deceased, because their conduct was not the proximate cause of the patient's death. On motion of the prosecution, the superior court determined as a matter of law that the evidence required the magistrate to hold the physicians to answer and ordered the complaint reinstated. The court of appeals held that the physicians' omission to continue treatment, although intentional and with knowledge that the patient would die, was not an unlawful failure to perform a legal duty. The evidence amply supported the magistrate's decision. The court of appeals determined that the superior court erred in determining that the evidence required the magistrate to hold the physicians to answer.

NURSE INJECTS PATIENTS WITH LIDOCAINE

Citation: *People v. Diaz,* 834 P.2d 1171 (Cal. 1992)

Facts

The defendant, a registered nurse, was working on the night shift at a community hospital. During a three-and-a-half-week period, 13 patients on the night shift had seizures, cardiac arrest, and respiratory arrest; nine died. The unit closed and the defendant went to work at another hospital. Within three days, a patient died after exhibiting the same symptoms as those in the previous hospital while the defendant was on duty. The defendant was arrested and tried for 12 counts of murder.

The testimony revealed that the defendant injected the patients with massive doses of Lidocaine (a rhythm-controlling drug). Evidence showed that the defendant assisted the patients before they exhibited seizures, providing opportunity for the nurse to administer the drug. She was observed acting strangely on the nights of the deaths and high concentrations of Lidocaine were found in the patients' syringes. Moreover, syringes containing the drug and Lidocaine vials were discovered in the defendant's home.

Pretrial investigation revealed that 26 other patients had died at the defendant's first hospital while under the nurse's care. All had the same symptoms. The defendant, who waived her right to trial by jury, was found guilty of the 12 counts of murder. The nurse appealed the judgment of death.

Issue

Did the expert testimony support the finding that an overdose of Lidocaine caused the patients' deaths? Did the evidence prove that the defendant had the opportunity to give patients overdoses of Lidocaine?

Holding

The California Supreme Court upheld the convictions.

Reason

The expert testimony about the levels of Lidocaine in the patients' tissue, coupled with the nurse's testimony concerning the symptoms prior to the deaths, confirmed that the patients died from overdoses given to them by the defendant. Testimony showed that the defendant was the only nurse on duty the night each patient was poisoned; other nurses were there on only some of the nights and only the defendant had the opportunity to administer the fatal doses.

Discussion

1. Examine how the evidence showed—when there were no eyewitnesses—that the defendant was the one who killed the 12 patients.

2. Discuss the processes hospitals should implement to prevent such occurrences (e.g., hiring practices and background checks).

PETTY THEFT

Health care organizations must be alert to the potential ongoing threat of theft by unscrupulous employees, physicians, patients, visitors, and trespassers. The theft of patient valuables, supplies, and equipment is substantial and costs health care organizations millions of dollars each year.

The evidence presented in *People v. Lancaster*[60] was found to have provided a probable cause foundation for information charging felony theft of nursing home residents' money by the office manager. Evidence showed that on repeated occasions the residents' income checks were cashed or cash was otherwise received on behalf of residents; that the defendant, by virtue of her office, had sole responsibility for maintaining the residents' ledger accounts; and that cash receipts frequently were never posted to the residents' accounts.

Nursing Facility Commingles Residents' Personal Funds

Criminal charges of theft were imposed because of misapplication of property in *State v. Pleasant Hill Health Facility*.[61] The facility commingled the residents' personal funds (Social Security checks and personal allowances) in a corporate account. There were times that the residents' funds remained in the corporate account for three to six months before being transferred to the residents' accounts, during which time the combined funds were used to pay corporate expenses. The facility described its relationship with the residents as debtor-creditor and not a trust relationship. The facility claimed that the funds were always available to residents, and they were never denied a request for their funds. The Maine Supreme Judicial Court held that the facility's handling of the residents' funds was not a debtor-creditor relationship but a trust relationship. Pleasant Hill's commingling of patients' personal need funds with corporate funds and use of the combined funds to pay corporate expenses constituted dealing with the money as its own and a violation of the corporation's trust agreement. The facility argued that it ultimately transferred all the residents' personal funds from a transfer account to the residents' accounts. The court concluded that a violation occurred at the moment the residents' personal funds were deposited without segregating them from the corporation's own funds.

SEXUAL ASSAULT

Sexual Assault of a Resident

An action was filed against a nursing home in *Dupree v. Plantation Pointe, L.P.*[62] after the plaintiff's mother was sexually assaulted at the nursing home by a dementia patient. A registered nurse testified that on the night of the incident, the nursing home was properly staffed and that no member of the nursing home staff did anything improper in the treatment of the assaulted resident. She stated measures were taken to protect residents from the dementia resident. Further, she testified that only a doctor had the power to restrain or transfer the patient and that the doctors did not do so. In addition, there was testimony that there was no penetration, that the resident suffered no physical injury, and that the she was not even aware of the assault. The trial court did not err in finding that the nursing home had not breached its duty of care.

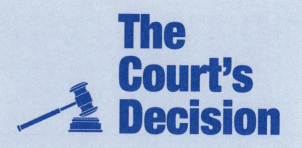

Majors was sentenced to spend the rest of his life in prison for murdering six elderly patients, a crime the judge referred to as a paragon of evil at its most wicked. Majors had been entrusted with these people's care. In response, he committed diabolical acts that extinguished the frail lives of six people.

CHAPTER REVIEW

1. The objectives of criminal law are to:
   - maintain public order and safety
   - protect individuals
   - use punishment as a deterrent to crime
   - rehabilitate criminals for return to society
2. A *crime*—a social harm defined and made punishable by law—is generally either a misdemeanor or a felony. A *misdemeanor* is an offense generally punishable by less than 1 year in jail and/or a fine. A *felony,* however, is punishable by imprisonment in a state or federal prison for a period of more than one year.
3. Criminal trials involving health care professionals and organizations often involve health care kickbacks, false claims, fraud, unethical referrals, falsification of records, misuse and theft of drugs, patient abuse, criminal negligence, murder, petty theft, and sexual abuse.
4. *Patient abuse* is the mistreatment or neglect of persons under the care of a health care organization. Abuse can occur in an institutional or home setting and can be in the form of physical, psychological, medical, financial, or other harm.
5. *Criminal negligence* is the reckless disregard for the safety of others and is the willful indifference to an injury that could result from an act. It differs from tort liability in that it provides for a more specific lack of care commonly characterized as gross negligence and recklessness.

REVIEW QUESTIONS

1. What are the objectives of criminal law?
2. Describe the difference between a misdemeanor and a felony. Give an example of each.

3. List the processes of a criminal trial.
4. Why has health care fraud been so costly to the nation?
5. Based on cases in the chapter, discuss why physicians historically have been reluctant to remove a patient's life-support systems.
6. Based on the cases reviewed in the chapter, discuss why you believe patients are sometimes reluctant to complain about their health care.

NOTES

1. *Majors v. Engelbrecht,* 149 F.3d 709 (1998).
2. http://oig.hhs.gov/fraud/cia/docs/assessment.htm.
3. 871 F.2d 105 (9th Cir. 1989).
4. 366 F.2d 167 (6th Cir. 1966).
5. 265 U.S. 182, 188 (1924).
6. 874 F.2d 20 (1st Cir. 1989).
7. 385 F.3d 1013 (C.A. 6, Ky. 2004).
8. 824 F.2d 780 (9th Cir. 1987).
9. 254 Ga. App. 297, 562 S.E.2d 201 (Ga. App. 2002).
10. 507 So. 2d 1254 (La. Ct. App. 1987).
11. 513 So. 2d 493 (La. Ct. App. 1987).
12. *Id.* at 495.
13. *Banks v. Board of Pharmacy,* 207 Cal. Rptr. 835 (Cal. Ct. App. 1984).
14. 821 F.2d 523 (10th Cir. 1987).
15. *Id.* at 529.
16. *Id.* at 530.
17. 322 S.E.2d 696 (N.C. Ct. App. 1985).
18. 760 F.2d 68 (3d Cir. 1985).
19. 402 N.Y.S.2d 318 (N.Y. Sup. Ct. 1978).
20. *Id.* at 320.
21. No. 02-6183 (C.A. 10, Okla. 2004).
22. 538 N.E.2d 113 (Ohio 1989).
23. 746 P.2d 1006 (Idaho Ct. App. 1987).
24. No. 04AP-143 (Ohio App. 2004).
25. 726 N.Y.S.2d 188 (2001).
26. 401 F.3d 53 (C.A. 2, N.Y. 2005).
27. RICHARD J. GELLES, MURRAY A. STRAUSS, & SUZABBE K. STEINMETZ, BEHIND CLOSED DOORS: VIOLENCE IN THE AMERICAN FAMILY (1981). Anchor Books, NY, New York.
28. *Id.*
29. www.elderabusecenter.org/default.cfm?p=statistics.cfm.
30. 557 F. Supp. 289 (D. Colo. 1983).
31. *Id.* at 293.
32. 42 C.F.R. § 483.13 (1989).
33. *Nurse's Aide Jailed for Punching Patient,* THE BALTIMORE SUN, June 29, 1990, §D, at 2.
34. 486 So. 2d 101 (La. 1986).
35. *Id.* at 103.
36. *Id.*
37. *Id.* at 101, 104.
38. *State v. Cunningham,* 493 N.W.2d 884 (Iowa Ct. App. 1992).
39. *Id.* at 887–888.
40. 551 A.2d 354 (Pa. Commw. Ct. 1988).
41. *Id.* at 355.
42. *Id.* at 357.
43. 501 N.Y.S.2d 997 (N.Y. Sup. Ct. 1986).
44. *Id.* at 1001.
45. *Id.*
46. 556 A.2d 1 (Pa. Commw. Ct. 1989).
47. 559 N.Y.S.2d 417 (N.Y. App. Div. 1990).
48. 655 S.W.2d 522 (Mo. 1983).
49. *Id.*
50. 560 N.Y.S.2d 573 (N.Y. App. Div. 1990).
51. *Id.*
52. *Id.* at 573–74.
53. Collwell, *The Verdict of Angelo,* 50(103) NEWSDAY 1989, at 3.
54. 584 F. Supp. 302 (E.D. Va. 1984).
55. *Id.* at 305.
56. 246 Cal. Rptr. 915 (Cal. Ct. App. 1988).
57. *Id.* at 927.
58. 204 F.3d 815 (8th Cir. 2000).
59. 195 Cal. Rptr. 484 (Cal. Ct. App. 1983).
60. 683 P.2d 1202 (Colo. 1984).
61. 496 A.2d 306 (Me. 1985).
62. No. 2002-CT-00556-SCT (Miss. 2004).

CHAPTER 5

Contracts and Antitrust

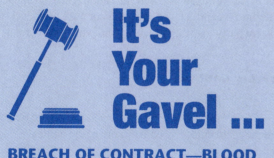

BREACH OF CONTRACT—BLOOD TRANSFUSION

Harvey was diagnosed with blockage in his carotid artery. Dr. Strickland recommended a surgical procedure. In anticipation of surgery, Harvey signed written forms entitled, "Refusal of Treatment/Release from Liability" and "Consent to Operation." The documents indicated that Harvey refused to have blood or blood products given to him and that he fully understood the attendant risks. The documents stated: "In all probability, my refusal for such treatment, medical intervention, and/or procedure (may)(will) seriously imperil my health or life." Hospital forms list Harvey's mother, Julia, as his emergency contact. The day before his surgery, Harvey signed another consent form indicating that he did "not give permission to the doctor to use blood or blood products if necessary."

Surgery was performed and appeared to have gone well. Harvey, however, developed a blood clot and had a stroke while in the recovery room. Because Harvey was unconscious, hospital personnel located his mother in the waiting room and obtained her permission to perform a CT scan and an arteriogram. A second surgery was performed and more blood clots were removed along the side of the carotid artery. Harvey was moved to the intensive care unit (ICU). He was intubated that evening by the on-call emergency room physician after the ICU nurse discovered Harvey was having trouble breathing. The next day, Harvey began bleeding from the surgical site at his neck. He had lost approximately 30 percent of his blood volume, and his heart rate was extremely high. Strickland was concerned that if they could not get the heart rate down, Harvey would have a heart attack and die. When his hemoglobin level reached 8, Strickland recommended a blood transfusion to Harvey's mother, Julia, who initially declined due to her son's faith as a Jehovah's Witness. Ultimately, Julia consented to giving Harvey two units of blood. Harvey recovered fully from the procedures. Harvey sued.[1]

WHAT IS YOUR VERDICT?

One of the many areas of law that affects health care providers is contracts. The intention here is to give the reader an introduction to contracts, focusing on providing a general understanding of their concepts, elements, and importance as they pertain to health care organizations and professionals.

PURPOSE OF A CONTRACT

A *contract* is a special kind of agreement, either written or oral, that involves legally binding obligations between two or more parties. A contract serves to provide one or more of the parties with a legal remedy if another of the parties does not perform his or her obligations pursuant to the terms of the contract. The major purpose of a contract is to specify, limit, and define the agreements that are legally enforceable. A contract forces the participants to be specific in their understandings and expectations of each other. Contracts, particularly those in writing, serve to minimize misunderstandings and offer a means for the parties of a contract to resolve any disputes that may arise.

TYPES OF CONTRACTS

The following is a general description of the various types of contracts and a brief definition of each. Health care professionals should be knowledgeable of each as they are commonly used in the health care setting.

Express Contract

An *express contract* is one in which the parties have an oral or written agreement.

Oral Contract. A court will not consider oral negotiations and agreements made before or at the same time a written contract is signed if the parties intended the document to be their complete and final agreement. Both written and oral contracts are generally recognized and are equally legal and binding.

Written Contract. It is always desirable to reduce any important contract to writing. In certain instances, the courts can enforce only written contracts.

Implied Contract

An *implied contract* is one that is inferred by law. It is based on the conduct of the parties, such as a handshake or similar conduct. Much of the litigation concerning excesses of corporate authority involves questions of whether a corporation has the implied authority—incidental to its express authority—to perform a questioned act. For example, even though its certificate of incorporation did not authorize such an act specifically, a hospital was permitted to construct a medical office building on land that had been donated for maintaining and carrying on a general hospital. The court, in recognizing a trend to encourage charitable hospitals to provide private offices for rental to staff members, held that such an act was within the implied powers of the hospital and that such offices aid in the work of a general hospital even though it went beyond the hospital corporation's express powers.[2]

Voidable Contract

A *voidable contract* is one in which one party, but not the other, has the right to escape from its legal obligations under the contract. It is considered a voidable contract at the option of that party. For example, a minor, not having the capacity to enter into a contract, can void the contract. However, the competent party to the contract may not void the contract.

Executory Contract

An *executory contract* is one in which something remains to be done (performed) by one or more of the parties.

Executed Contract

An *executed contract* is one in which all of the obligations of the parties have been performed fully.

Enforceable Contract

An *enforceable contract* is one that is a valid, legally binding agreement. If one party breaches it, the other will have an appropriate legal remedy.

Unenforceable Contract

An *unenforceable contract* is one in which, because of some defect, no legal remedy is available if breached by one of the parties to the contract.

Contracts for Realty, Goods, or Services

There are also contracts for *realty* (real estate or interests in real estate), *goods* (movable objects, with the exception of money and securities), and *services* (human energy).

ELEMENTS OF A CONTRACT

The law will enforce contracts only when they are executed between persons who are competent; that is, those with the legal and mental capacity to contract. Certain classes of persons, such as minors, the insane, and prisoners, traditionally have been considered unable to understand the consequences of their actions and have been deemed incompetent, or lacking in legal capacity, to make a binding contract. Whether contracts are executed in writing or agreed to orally, they must contain the following elements in order to be enforceable.

Offer/Communication

An *offer* is a promise by one party to do (or not to do) something if the other party agrees to do (or not do) something. Preliminary negotiations are not offers. An offer must be communicated to the other party so that it can be accepted or rejected.

Consideration

Each party to a contract must give up something of value in exchange for something of value. This is called *consideration*. No side can have a free way out or the ability to obtain something of value without providing something in exchange. Only when legal consideration has been given will a court treat the agreement as a contract. The adequacy or inadequacy of consideration, or the price paid, will not normally affect the formation of a contract.

Acceptance

Upon proper acceptance of an offer, a contract is formed. A valid acceptance requires the following:

Meeting of the Minds. Acceptance requires a *meeting of the minds* (mutual assent); in other words, the parties must understand and agree on the terms of the contract. This means that each side must be clear as to the details, rights, and obligations of the contract.

Definite and Complete. Acceptance requires mutual assent to be found between the parties. The terms must be so complete that both parties understand and agree to what has been proposed.

Duration. Generally, the *offeror* (the one who makes the offer) may revoke an offer at any time prior to a valid acceptance. When the offeror does revoke the proposal, the revocation is not effective until the *offeree* (the person to whom the offer is made) receives it. Once the

offeree has accepted the offer, any attempt to revoke the agreement is too late and is invalid.

Complete and Conforming. The acceptance must be a mirror image of the offer. In other words, the acceptance must comply with all the terms of the offer and not change or add any terms.

BREACH OF CONTRACT

A *breach of contract* occurs when there is a violation of one or more of the terms of the contract. The basic elements that a plaintiff must establish in order to be successful in a breach of contract lawsuit include the following:

- A valid contract was executed.

- The plaintiff performed as specified in the contract.

- The defendant failed to perform as specified in the contract.

- The plaintiff suffered an economic loss as a result of the defendant's breach of contract.

CORPORATE CONTRACTS

The ability of a corporation to enter into a contract is limited by its powers as contained in or inferred from its articles of incorporation (sometimes called a *charter*) or conferred upon it by general corporation law. Whenever a contract of any consequence is made with a corporation, appropriate corporate approval and authorization must be obtained. In the event that a contract is entered into with a corporation without the appropriate authority, the contract nevertheless may be ratified and made binding on the corporation by subsequent conduct or statements made on its behalf by its representatives.

When the chief executive officer (CEO) of an organization exceeds the limits of his or her authority, the question of whether the organization will be responsible for the CEO's acts may arise. If the actions of the governing body give rise to a third party's reasonable belief that the CEO acts with the authority of the organization, and such belief causes the third party to enter into an agreement with the CEO, expecting that the organization will be obligated under the contract, then the organization generally is responsible under the *concept of apparent authority* (the appearance of being the agent of another (employer or principal) with the power to act for the principal). However, if a third party deals with the CEO in the absence of indications of the CEO's authority created by the governing body and thereby unreasonably assumes that the CEO possesses the authority to bind the organization to a contract, then such third party deals with the CEO in an individual capacity and not as an agent of the organization. There are times when the CEO clearly may exceed the limitations of his or her authority, but the governing body subsequently may approve such actions through ratification by accepting any resulting responsibility as though it had been authorized previously.

If, for example, the governing body has imposed a limitation on equipment purchases that could be made without specific prior approval of the governing body, the price of the equipment would determine whether the governing body was bound under the contract. If the equipment was $26,000 and the limitation on purchases without specific governing body approval was $25,000, then the CEO would have no authority to bind the organization for the purchase of the equipment. The CEO generally would be liable to the supplier of the equipment.

PARTNERSHIPS

A *partnership* comprises two or more persons who agree to carry on a business for profit and to share profits and losses in some proportions. A partnership, unlike a corporation, can be created by the parties' actions without a written or oral agreement.

AGENTS

An *agent* is one who has the power to contract for and bind another person, who is known as the principal. Corporations can act only through agents (e.g., their officers).

Apparent Agent or Ostensible Agent

An *apparent* or *ostensible agent* is one who a third person believes is acting on behalf of the principal. If a hospital undertakes to provide physician services to a community, and the community reasonably believes that the physician is employed by the hospital to deliver services, then the hospital would generally be liable for the physician's negligent acts. For example, in *Jennison v. Providence St. Vincent Med. Ctr.,*[3] Jennison, having severe abdominal pain, was taken to the hospital emergency department. Unsure of the cause of Jennison's medical problems, Cook, Jennison's assigned physician, recommended surgery. Prior to surgery Cook asked Nunez, a member of an independent anesthesiology group at the hospital, to place a central venous catheter in Jennison.

Following surgery, at 1:10 P.M., Jennison was taken to the postanesthesia care unit (PACU) with the central line in place. Slater, a surgical resident who had assisted Cook during the surgery, wrote postoperative orders. These orders included a portable chest X-ray to be taken in the PACU.

The purpose of the chest X-ray was to check the placement of the central line. At approximately 4 P.M., Slater received a telephone call from the PACU nurse informing him that Jennison was still in a great deal of pain. Slater ordered more pain medication to be administered. Cook later called the PACU and was told about Jennison's pain problems. He then ordered the placement of an epidural line to treat Jennison's pain. Because Nunez was unavailable, Ing, an on-call anesthesiologist, placed the epidural line at 5:05 P.M. After a test dose was administered, Jennison's eyes rolled into the back of her head, her blood pressure fell dangerously low, and her heart rate rose. Ing decided to discontinue the epidural.

At approximately 5:30 P.M., Slater was called back to the PACU. He noticed that the central line placed during surgery earlier that day was not in use. He was unsure whether the X-ray, taken over four hours earlier, had been checked to confirm the correct placement of the central line. At that point Slater decided to check the X-ray himself. He discovered that the tip of the central line had gone into the pericardial sac of Jennison's heart. Slater went back to the PACU at approximately 5:45 P.M., and the central line was pulled back to its proper position. At some point before the central line had been properly positioned, fluids were infused through the central line and into the space between Jennison's heart and pericardial sac. The pressure of the fluid against her heart kept it from filling adequately, essentially crushing it. This in turn caused Jennison's blood pressure to drop, and eventually she went into cardiac arrest. The doctors attempted to remove the excess fluid. During the procedure, Jennison suffered a second cardiac arrest. The doctors were again able to resuscitate her. However, due to the lack of oxygen to her brain, Jennison suffered a severe brain injury.

The jury returned a multimillion dollar verdict in favor of the plaintiffs, finding the hospital 100 percent negligent, and the hospital appealed.

The record indicated that there was a written nursing policy pertaining to "nonurgent placement [of central venous lines] outside [the] surgical area." The hospital, however, had "no follow-up policy or procedure" describing what procedures were to be followed if the X-ray showed that the central line had been improperly placed. A procedure should have been established to notify the treating physicians that the central line had been dangerously misplaced.

The hospital argued that the trial court erroneously instructed the jury that it could find it liable for Jennison's injuries under an apparent agency theory if Jennison "reasonably believed" the nonemployee radiologists were employed by the hospital. The Court of Appeals of Oregon affirmed the findings of the trial court. The hospital presented itself as providing radiology services to the public. The public, looking to the hospital to provide such care, is unaware of and unconcerned with the technical complexities and nuances surrounding the contractual and employment arrangements between the hospital and the various medical personnel operating therein. Public policy dictates that the public has every right to assume and expect that the hospital is the medical provider it purports to be.

INDEPENDENT CONTRACTOR

An *independent contractor* is an individual who agrees to undertake work without being under the direct control or direction of another. Independent contractors are personally responsible for their own negligent acts. Whether a physician is an employee or an independent contractor is of primary importance in determining liability for damages. Generally, a health care organization is not liable for injuries resulting from negligent acts or omissions of independent physicians. There is no liability on the *theory of respondeat superior,* whereby a physician is an independent contractor as long as the physician is not an employee of the organization, is not compensated, maintains a private practice, and is chosen directly by his or her patients. The mere existence of an independent contractual relationship, however, is not sufficient to remove an organization from liability for the acts of certain of its professional personnel for which the independent contractor status is not readily known to the injured party.

Hospital Liable for Physician's Negligence

A hospital can be liable for a physician's negligence, even if the physician is under contract to provide services to the hospital. The appellate division of the New York State Supreme Court in *Mduba v. Benedictine Hospital*[4] held that the hospital was liable for the emergency department physician's negligence whether the physician was an independent contractor or, even if under contract, the physician was considered to be an independent contractor. The court held that the patient had no way of knowing of the existence of a contract and relied on the relationship between the hospital and the physician in seeking treatment in the emergency department.

Agency Liable for Negligent Hiring

The employer, Patient Support Services, Inc. (PSS), in *Maristany v. Patient Support Services, Inc.,*[5] was found not liable for negligent hiring for injuries received by a patient under the care of one of its independent contractors. By contract dated January 29, 1994, the plaintiff retained the services of PSS to furnish an independent nurse, Terry, to care for her husband, Santiago, a postoperative brain surgery patient at defendant Presbyterian Hospital.

At approximately 10 P.M., Terry assisted a hospital nurse in placing Santiago into a Posey restraining vest. At approximately 3:30 A.M., Terry returned from a break to find Santiago extremely agitated. Terry sought assistance and tried to restrain the patient physically, but the patient escaped from the vest, climbed over the rails, and fell to the floor, sustaining serious injury.

The plaintiffs did not contest that Terry's status was that of an independent contractor, not an employee. Although an employer is generally not liable for the torts or negligent acts of an independent contractor under the doctrine of *respondeat superior,* the employer had a right to rely on the supposed qualifications and good character of the contractor and is not bound to anticipate misconduct on the contractor's part. The employer is not liable on the ground of its having employed an incompetent or otherwise unsuitable contractor unless it also appears that the employer either knew or, in the exercise of reasonable care, should have ascertained that the contractor was not properly qualified to undertake the work.

There was no competent proof that PSS had any reason to question Terry's qualifications. At the time of the incident, Terry had her qualifying certificate for more than 10 years. She had received training in the use of Posey restraints and had previously cared for patients whose condition required these restraints. Because Terry had previously worked for PSS and had not given any indication of incompetence, there was no viability to the claim that PSS was negligent in assigning her to the care of Santiago.

LEGALITY OF OBJECT

To be a valid contract, the purpose or object of the contract must not be against state or federal policy and must not violate any statute, rule, or regulation. If the subject or purpose of the contract becomes illegal by some statute, rule, or regulation before actual formation of the contract, the parties no longer can form the contract.

CONDITIONS

A *condition precedent* is an act or event that must happen or be performed by one party before the other party has any responsibility to perform under the contract. An express condition is formally written into the contract in specific terms. An implied condition is one in which, although the parties may not have specifically mentioned the condition, it can reasonably be assumed that the parties intended the condition to be enforced.

PERFORMANCE

Ordinarily, substantial performance by one party to a contract will obligate the other parties to perform their function.

Many performance problems can be avoided by adequate drafting of contract terms.

NONPERFORMANCE DEFENSES

Under some circumstances the law gives a person a right not to perform under a contract. Defenses permitting non-performance of a contract include fraud, mistakes, duress, illegal contract, impossibility, and statute of limitations.

Fraud

A victim of fraud will not have to perform under a contract. *Fraud* occurs when one party intentionally misrepresents a material fact or term of the contract and intends that the other party rely on that misrepresentation. The second party must rely on the misrepresentation and suffer some damage before it will be excused from performing.

Mistake of Fact

Mistakes occur in contracts just as they do in everything else. However, a party will be allowed to claim mistake as a defense in only certain instances. There are two types of mistakes: mistake of fact and mistake of law. A *mistake of fact* is an incorrect belief regarding a fact. Both parties must have made the mistake. If only one is in error (and it is not known to the other), mistake of fact is not a defense. *Mistake of law,* on the other hand, is an incorrect judgment of the legal consequences of known facts. If the parties to a suit make a mistake as to the law involved, they usually must accept their plight without any remedy.

Duress

Duress is the use of unlawful threats or pressure to force an individual to act against his or her will. An act performed under duress is not legally binding.

Illegal Contract

No individual can recover damages when a contract is formed for illegal purposes.

Impossibility

Contracts that are impossible to perform do not have to be carried out by the parties.

STATUTE OF LIMITATIONS

A party who does not, within a period of time known as the *statute of limitations,* take action to enforce contract rights by suing for damages caused by a breach of contract or taking other action can be barred from doing so.

REMEDIES

What can a party do when another has breached the contract and refuses to or cannot perform? The general rule is that legal redress will attempt to make the injured party whole again.

Specified Performance

When an aggrieved party has subsequently complied with his or her obligations pursuant to the agreed-upon terms of a contract, that party might seek specific performance as a remedy rather than monetary remuneration. The most satisfactory remedy available to an injured party may be to require specific performance by the other party to the contract.

Monetary Damages

Money damages, sometimes called *compensatory damages,* are awarded in an attempt to restore to the aggrieved party the money that it would have had if the other party had not breached the contract. This can include the cost of making a substitute contract with another party and the expense of delays caused by the breach.

General and Consequential Damages

General damages are those that can be expected to arise from a breach of a contract. They are foreseeable and common in the circumstances. *Consequential damages* are those that occur because of some unexpected, unusual, or strange development involved in the particular contract in dispute. The distinction between the two types is one of foreseeability. If it is found that the party who breached the contract could have foreseen the damages that followed, that person could be liable for consequential as well as general damages.

Duty to Mitigate Damages

Once someone has breached a contract, the other party cannot stand idly by and let damages build indefinitely. Every injured party has a duty to mitigate (lessen) damages caused by the breach of another person or entity. Failure to do so will prevent the aggrieved party's full recovery of damages that could have been mitigated.

Arbitration

Under the modern view of contract law, agreements in contracts to arbitrate subsequent disputes are valid.

EMPLOYMENT CONTRACTS

An *employment contract* is an agreement between an employee and employer that specifies the terms of employment. The conditions of employment including wages, hours, and type of work are generally described in an employment contract. Depending on the level of employment and the responsibility of the new employee, the conditions of employment should include the terms of employment; the duties and responsibilities of the employee; compensation; confidentiality requirements (e.g., trade secrets and proprietary information); a noncompete clause; and provisions for termination of the agreement (e.g., an inability to perform one's duties and responsibilities).

A contract may be express or implied. Most employees work under employment contracts. For example, if an employee signs a document promising to abide by company policy and procedures, it likely constitutes an employment contract. Certain categories of employees (e.g., radiologists) often have the ability to negotiate their employment contracts. An employer's right to terminate an employee can be limited by express agreement with the employee or through a collective bargaining agreement to which the employee is a beneficiary.

The rights of employees have been expanding through judicial decisions in the different states. Court decisions have been based on verbal promises, historical practices of the employer, and documents such as employee handbooks and administrative policy and procedure manuals that describe employee rights.

Nurse Breaches Contract: Repayment of Tuition Required

The registered nurse in *Sweetwater Hosp. Ass'n v. Carpenter*[6] was found to have breached her contract with the hospital under which the hospital agreed to pay for her schooling as a nurse anesthetist in exchange for her agreeing to work for the hospital for five years following completion of her studies. The nurse agreed that if she failed to work at the hospital following completion of her studies, she would be responsible for cash advances by the hospital plus interest. Upon completion of her studies, the nurse sought employment elsewhere because it appeared to her that there were no nurse anesthetist positions available at the hospital.

The contract provided that one of the considerations for the loan was that the defendant agree to become or remain an employee of the hospital. The contract did not state in what capacity the defendant would become or remain an employee. There was nothing in the language of the contract stating that the hospital had an obligation to offer the defendant a nurse anesthetist position.

In this case, there was no proof by the defendant that the hospital breached the contract. The defendant breached her own contract by taking a job elsewhere without specifically getting proof that she was not going to be offered a job by the hospital. The defendant did not present herself for employment at the hospital after graduation. She accepted a position elsewhere. Because she did not become employed at the hospital, she was not entitled to rely upon the forgiveness provisions contained in the contract. She was, therefore, obligated to repay the hospital.

Geographic Practice Limitations Valid

The provisions of a covenant prohibiting the plaintiff in *Thompson v. Nason Hosp.,* a pediatrician, for a period of two years from practicing pediatric medicine within a 10-mile radius of the defendant's office, and prohibiting her for a period of one year from soliciting patients of the defendant, were found to be reasonable as to both duration and geographic area. When the plaintiff entered into the employment contract, she agreed to be bound by the restrictive covenants in the event that her employment should end. The defendant had the right to terminate the plaintiff's employment for any reason whatsoever or for no reason, upon 60 days' written notice to the plaintiff.[7]

No Express Agreement: Right to Terminate

No express agreement was found to exist in *O'Connor v. Eastman Kodak Co.,*[8] in which the court held that an employer had a right to terminate an employee at will at any time and for any reason or no reason. The plaintiff did not rely on any specific representation made to him during the course of his employment interviews nor did he rely on any documentation in the employee handbook, which would have limited the defendant's common-law right to discharge at will. The employee had relied on a popular perception of Kodak as a "womb-to-tomb" employer.

BREACH OF EMPLOYMENT CONTRACT

Citation: *Dutta v. St. Francis Reg'l Med. Ctr.,* 850 P.2d 928 (Kan. Ct. App. 1993)

Facts

On July 1, 1987, Dr. Dutta, a radiologist, began working in the radiology department of the hospital as an employee of Dr. Krause, the medical director of the hospital's radiology department. On August 5, 1988, the hospital terminated Krause's employment as medical director. On August 8, 1988, Dutta and the hospital entered into a written employment contract with a primary term of 90 days. The contract provided that if a new medical director had not been hired by the hospital within the 90-day period, the agreement was to be automatically extended for a second 90-day period.

Following a period of recruitment and interviews, the hospital offered Dr. Tan the position. Tan and the hospital executed a contract making him the medical director of the radiology department. The contract granted Tan the right "to provide radiation oncology services on an exclusive basis subject to the exception of allowing Dutta to continue her practice of radiation oncology at the hospital." On April 24, 1989, the hospital notified Dutta that the 90-day contract had expired and that Tan was appointed as the new medical director. The letter provided in part:

> It is our intent at this time to establish an exclusive contract with Dr. Donald C-S Tan for medical direction and radiation therapy at SFRMC. Your medical staff privileges to practice radiation therapy at SFRMC will not be affected by this action. You will be allowed to maintain your current office space for radiation oncology activities; however, you should make alternative arrangements for your billing and collection activities. *Id.* at 931.

Dutta and Tan then practiced independently of each other in the same facility. On October 13, 1989, Tan became unhappy with this arrangement and requested exclusive privileges, stating he could not continue as medical director without exclusivity. On February 2, 1990, an exclusive contract was authorized by the hospital. Dutta was notified that she would no longer be permitted to provide radiation therapy services at the hospital after May 1, 1990. By letter, Dutta twice requested a hearing on the hospital's decision to revoke her right to use hospital facilities. Both requests were denied.

Dutta sued the hospital for breach of employment contract after the hospital entered into an exclusive agreement with Tan, thereby denying Dutta the use of the hospital's radiology department and equipment. Dutta presented evidence about the purpose of the requirement in her contract with the hospital that provided that the new medical director be mutually acceptable to both parties. A hospital administrator testified that the hospital and Dutta included the phrase "mutually acceptable" in the contract because "[w]e both agreed that we wanted the person being recruited to be compatible with Dutta." *Id.* at 932.

Issue

Was the language, "mutually acceptable," ambiguous in the employment contract between the hospital and Dutta?

Holding

The Kansas Court of Appeals held that substantial evidence supported the jury's verdict that the hospital breached its written employment contract with Dutta by hiring a medical director who was not mutually acceptable to both the hospital and Dutta.

Reason

The language in the contract is ambiguous if the words in the contract are subject to two or more possible meanings. The determination of whether a contract is ambiguous is a question of law. Paragraphs four and five of the hospital's employment agreement with Dutta, dated August 8, 1988, read as follows:

4. During the term of this Agreement the Medical Center shall be actively recruiting for a full-time Medical Director for the Radiation Therapy department. . . . Dr. Dutta shall be involved in the interviewing process. The person selected for either of the above positions shall be mutually acceptable to the Medical Center and Dr. Dutta. Dr. Dutta may discuss potential business arrangements with each individual interviewed.

5. Once the full-time Medical Director or part-time radiation therapist is selected, Dr. Dutta will, in good faith, attempt to reach a satisfactory business arrangement with the selected individual. *Id.* at 936.

The testimony of Dutta, the hospital administrator, and the attorney who represented Dutta in contract negotiations, provides a factual basis for the jury to find that the phrase, "mutually acceptable," in the contract was intended by Dutta to ensure that the hospital would select a medical director who indicated a willingness to form a partnership or otherwise acceptable business relationship.

Discussion

1. What protective elements should each party to an employment contract negotiate?

2. What are the elements necessary to make a contract valid?

Restrictive Covenant Enforceable

The plaintiff-hospital, in *Sarah Bush Lincoln Health Ctr. v. Perket,*[9] sued its former director of physical medicine and rehabilitation to enforce a restrictive covenant in the employment contract precluding the director from accepting similar employment in the same county within one year of termination of employment. The parties to the complaint entered into a contract whereby the defendant was employed as the plaintiff's director of physical medicine. The contract provided that during the director's employment and for a period of one year thereafter, the director would not, directly or indirectly, invest in, own, manage, operate, control, be employed by, participate in, or be connected in any manner with the ownership, management, operation, or control of any person, firm, or corporation engaged in competition with the hospital in providing health services or facilities within Coles County, including the provision of services in a private office, without prior written consent of the hospital. Following the termination, the defendant engaged in the business of providing physical medicine and rehabilitation services in Coles County. The plaintiff argued that unless the defendant was enjoined, the hospital would suffer irreparable injury. The circuit court granted the hospital's motion for preliminary injunction. On appeal, the Illinois Appellate Court held that the grant of the preliminary injunction was proper and that the defendant was engaging in the business of providing physical medicine and rehabilitation services in Coles County. By hiring the defendant, the hospital was thereby bringing him in contact with a clientele that the hospital had established over a period of years. The hospital was naturally interested in protecting its clients from being taken over by the defendant as a result of these contacts.

Restrictive Covenant Not Enforceable

Not every restrictive covenant is enforceable; for example, the restrictive covenant in *Comprehensive Psychology System P.C. v. Prince*[10] limiting the ability of a psychologist from practicing his profession within 10 miles of his former employer's facility and from soliciting any of his patients was determined not to be enforceable. The nature of the practice of psychology and the uniquely personal patient-psychologist relationship forbid restrictions that might interfere with an ongoing course of treatment. A psychologist who changes his office location, voluntarily or involuntarily, has a duty to inform patients of the change and the new location and phone number. To do otherwise may be akin to abandonment. Before unilaterally withdrawing from treating a patient, a doctor must provide reasonable notice of withdrawal to enable the patient to obtain substitute care. The limitations plaintiff seeks to enforce against defendant interfere with a critical patient-psychologist relationship and with the right of the patient to continued treatment from that psychologist.

In another case, a restrictive covenant in an employment contract between a hospital and neurosurgeon was found to be geographically too restrictive whereby the neurosurgeon was not to practice within a 30-mile radius of the hospital. This restriction was determined to be excessive. Such a restriction was considered to be detrimental to public interest in that the restricted area was plagued with a shortage of neurosurgeons.[11]

The reader should understand that employment contracts that contain a restrictive covenant between a physician and a hospital, although not favored, are not per se unreasonable and unenforceable. The trial court must determine whether the restrictive covenant protects the legitimate interests of the employer, imposes no undue hardship on the employee, and is not adverse to the public interest.[12]

Employee Handbook: Considered a Contract

In order for an employee handbook to constitute a contract, thereby giving enforceable rights to the employee, the following elements must be present:

1. A policy statement that clearly sets forth a promise that the employee can construe to be an offer.

2. The policy statement must be distributed to the employee, making him or her aware of the offer.

3. After learning about the offer and policy statement, the employee must "begin" or "continue" to work.

The plaintiff-employee in *Weiner v. McGraw-Hill*[13] brought suit against his employer for wrongful termination. The plaintiff allegedly was discharged without the just-and-sufficient cause or the rehabilitative efforts specified in the defendant's handbook and allegedly promised at the time the plaintiff accepted employment. Further, on several occasions when the plaintiff recommended that certain of his subordinates be dismissed, he allegedly was instructed to proceed in strict compliance with the handbook and policy manuals. The court held that although the defendant did not engage the plaintiff for a fixed term of employment, the plaintiff pleaded a good cause of action for breach of contract. Even the employment application that the plaintiff signed at the time of employment stated that he would be subject to the provisions of McGraw-Hill's *Handbook on Personnel Policies and Procedures*.

In *Watson v. Idaho Falls Consolidated Hospitals, Inc.*[14] a nurse's aide was awarded $20,000 for damages when the hospital, as employer, violated the provisions of its employee handbook in the manner in which it terminated her employment. Although the nurse's aide had no formal written contract, the employee handbook and the hospital policies and procedures manual constituted a contract in view of evidence to the effect that these documents had been intended to be enforced and complied with by both employees and management. Employees read and relied on the handbook as creating terms of an employment contract. They were required to sign for the handbook to establish receipt of a revised handbook that explained hospital policy, discipline, counseling, and termination. A policy-and-procedure manual placed on each floor of the hospital also outlined termination procedures.

Employee Handbook: Not a Contract Due to Disclaimer

The employee handbook in *Churchill v. Waters*[15] was not a contract because of a disclaimer in the handbook. A nurse brought a civil rights action against the hospital and hospital officials after her discharge. The federal district court held for the defendants, finding that the hospital employee handbook did not give the nurse a protected property interest in continued employment: "Absent proof that the handbook contained clear promises which indicated the intent to bind the parties, no contract was created."[16] The "handbook contained a disclaimer" expressly disavowing any attempt to be bound by it and stated that its contents were not to be considered conditions of employment. The handbook was presented as a matter of information only, and the language contained therein was not intended to constitute a contract between McDonough District Hospital and the employee. Although an employee handbook may delineate specific disciplinary procedures, that fact does not in and of itself constitute an enforceable contract.[17]

Termination of Contract: Insubordination

The physician in *Trieger v. Montefiore Med. Ctr.*[18] circulated a memorandum to department chairs at the hospital strongly criticizing management and urging his cochairs "to set things right and reclaim their prerogatives and responsibilities." The appellate court found that the trial court correctly determined that the memorandum was insubordinate and that it gave just cause for termination of the physician's employment contract. In addition, the physician's age discrimination claim was dismissed for lack of evidence sufficient to raise an issue of fact as to whether the hospital's reason for the doctor's dismissal, circulation of the insubordinate memorandum, was a pretext for discrimination. The doctor was terminated immediately after circulating the insubordinate memorandum, and there was no other evidence in the record to support the claim that the hospital's actions were pretextual.

MEDICAL STAFF BYLAWS: A CONTRACT

Medical staff bylaws can be considered a contract. The plaintiff, Dr. Bass, in *Bass v. Ambrosius,*[19] alleged that the hospital's termination of his staff privileges violated its own bylaws. The hospital contended that its bylaws did not constitute a contract between itself and Bass, and, therefore, any violation of those bylaws would not support a breach-of-contract claim. The general rule that hospital bylaws can constitute a contract between the hospital and its staff is consistent with Wisconsin law that an employee handbook written and disseminated by the employer, and whose terms the employee has accepted, constitutes a contract between the employer and the employee. For instance, in *Ferraro v. Koelsch,*[20] an employee handbook was management's statement of what the company offered its employees and what it expected from its employees in return. It thus contained the essential elements of a binding contract: the promise of employment on stated terms and conditions by the employer and the promise by the employee to continue employment under those conditions. The court noted that a promise for a promise, or the exchange of promises, constitutes consideration to support any contract of this bilateral nature.

The bylaws at issue in *Bass v. Ambrosius,* required by Wis. Admin. Code § HSS 124.12(5) and approved by the hospital's board of directors, have the same contractual elements as did the handbook in Ferraro. First, the bylaws state that they provide the rules that govern the physicians and dentists practicing at the hospital. Second, members of the hospital's medical-dental staff must continuously meet the qualifications, standards, and requirements set forth in the bylaws. Third, an appointment to the medical-dental staff confers only those privileges provided by the letter of appointment and the bylaws. Fourth, all applicants for appointment to the medical-dental staff must submit a signed application acknowledging the requirement to familiarize themselves with the bylaws. Each applicant for appointment to the medical-dental staff must submit a signed application attesting that he or she has read and agreed to accept and abide by the provisions and directives in the bylaws. Thus, Bass's application to the medical-dental staff acknowledged by his signature that he would conduct his professional activities according to the bylaws and rules and regulations of both the hospital and the medical-dental staff of the hospital. In a separate letter, part of the application process, Bass agreed to conduct his activities according to the bylaws of the hospital, as well as the bylaws and rules and regulations of the hospital's medical-dental staff. For its part, the hospital promised that the medical-dental staff would be guided and governed by rules and regulations consistent with the bylaws, and it promised that any adverse action against a member of the medical-dental staff would comply with various procedural safeguards. The bylaws constituted a contract between Bass and the hospital. Accordingly, Bass was entitled to an order holding that the hospital had to comply with its bylaws before it could terminate his staff privileges.

In *Sadler v. Dimensions Health Corporation,*[21] Sadler, an obstetrician and gynecologist (OB/GYN), applied for medical staff privileges in the hospital's OB/GYN department. She was granted temporary privileges pending receipt of further information on her application. While practicing at the hospital, three incident reports concerning Sadler were filed. They involved her failure to respond to calls and initiate timely treatment, a broken humerus and permanent nerve injury following a birth, and a retained surgical sponge. The patient care committee (PCC) of the OB/GYN department reviewed the reports and concluded that continued observation of Sadler was warranted. The PCC met with Sadler to review five cases. Three involved nonindicated or precipitous cesarean sections and two involved delayed responses to calls from the hospital staff. Following review, the PCC recommended that Sadler consult with more senior practitioners for second opinions before performing Caesarean sections.

Two physician consultants were eventually retained by the OB/GYN department of the hospital to review charts of a variety of Sadler's cases. Random charts of other members of the OB/GYN department of the hospital were also reviewed. Following review, the consultants recommended in their report that Sadler be subjected to case-by-case premonitoring for surgical indications. The hospital's medical executive committee (MEC) reviewed the documentation regarding Sadler's performance. Based upon that review, the MEC voted not to extend provisional privileges and to impose monitoring of Sadler until her provisional privileges expired. Sadler was notified by letter of the MEC decision not to extend her provisional privileges. She was advised that she had a right to request a hearing pursuant to the provisions of the bylaws. Sadler exercised that right, and an ad hoc committee (a hearing committee) was formed pursuant to the bylaws. The committee concluded that there was compelling evidence that the physician consistently disregarded hospital policies, was unprofessional in her dealings with staff, and deviated from acceptable standards in her hospital record keeping and clinical practice. In addition, she ignored efforts by the hospital to bring her into compliance.

The parties agreed that the bylaws of the medical staff of the hospital to which Sadler subscribed when she applied for privileges at the hospital constitute an enforceable contract between her and the hospital. Those bylaws provide a process by which Sadler could challenge her termination of clinical privileges. Sadler fully pursued the prescribed process. Represented by counsel, she appeared before a panel of members of the medical staff who had no involvement with her case. She cross-examined witnesses under oath, called her own witnesses, offered evidence, and presented oral argument and posthearing written memoranda to the hearing committee. When the hearing committee agreed with the recommendation of the MEC that her privileges at the hospital should be terminated, she exercised her right under the bylaws to have that decision reviewed by the appellate review committee of the board of directors.

The court of appeals held that there was substantial evidence to support the conclusions of the hearing committee and the board of directors that the imposition of proctoring and monitoring upon Sadler and the termination of her hospital privileges were reasonable and proper.

Right to Hearing

A physician whose privileges are either suspended or terminated must exhaust all remedies provided in a facility's bylaws, rules, and regulations before commencing a court action. The U.S. Court of Appeals in *Northeast Georgia Radiological Associates v. Tidwell*[22] held that a contract with the hospital's radiologists, which incorporated the medical staff bylaws, sustained the plaintiffs' claim to a protected property interest entitling them to a hearing before the medical staff and the hospital authority.

EXCLUSIVE CONTRACTS

An organization often enters into an exclusive contract with physicians or medical groups for the purpose of providing a specific service to the organization. Exclusive contracts generally occur within the organization's ancillary service departments (e.g., radiology, anesthesiology, and pathology). Physicians who seek to practice at organizations in these ancillary areas but who are not part of the exclusive group have attempted to invoke the federal antitrust laws to challenge these exclusive contracts. These challenges generally have been unsuccessful.

In *Jefferson Parish Hospital v. Hyde,*[23] the defendant hospital had a contract with a firm of anesthesiologists that required all anesthesia services for the hospital's patients be performed by that firm. Because of this contract, the plaintiff anesthesiologist's application for admission to the hospital's medical staff was denied. Dr. Hyde commenced an action in the federal district court, claiming the exclusive contract violated Section 1 of the Sherman Antitrust Act. The district court rejected the plaintiff's complaint, but the U.S. Court of Appeals for the Fifth Circuit reversed, finding the contract illegal per se. The Supreme Court reversed the Fifth Circuit, holding that the exclusive contract in question does not violate Section 1 of the Sherman Antitrust Act. The Supreme Court's holding was based on the fact that the defendant hospital did not possess "market power," and therefore patients were free to enter a competing hospital and to use another anesthesiologist instead of the firm. Thus, the court concluded that the evidence was insufficient to provide a basis for finding that the contract, as it actually operates in the market, had unreasonably restrained competition.

Similarly, the anesthesiologists in *Belmar v. Cipolla*[24] brought an action challenging a hospital's exclusive contract with a different group of anesthesiologists. The New Jersey Supreme Court held that under state law the hospital's exclusive contract was reasonable and did not violate public policy.

COMPETITION CLAUSE NOT OVERLY RESTRICTIVE

Citation: *Dominy v. National Emergency Servs.,* 451 S.E.2d 472 (Ga. App. 1994)

Facts

The appellee, National Emergency Services (NES), assigned appellant, Dr. Dominy, to the emergency department at Memorial Hospital and Manor (MHM) in Bainbridge, Georgia, where he was working in 1987 when that hospital terminated its contract with NES and contracted with another provider, Coastal Emergency Services, for emergency department physicians. Dominy continued to perform emergency medical services at MHM under contract with Coastal until 1989.

The contract provided: "The period of this Agreement shall be for one (1) year from the date hereof, automatically renewable for a like period upon each expiration thereof. . . ." The only reasonable construction of this provision was that the parties intended to contract for Dominy's employment for automatically renewable 1-year terms upon the mutual assent of the parties. The fact that the agreement did not set out the mechanics by which mutual assent may be communicated did not invalidate the contract.

Dominy challenged the contract's noncompetition clause as overly restrictive. The covenant in this case provides, in pertinent part: "for a period of two (2) years after the termination of this agreement . . . Physician shall not directly or indirectly solicit a contract to perform nor have any ownership or financial interest in any corporation, partnership, or other entity soliciting or contracting to perform emergency medical service for any medical institution at which Physician has performed the same or similar services under this Agreement or any prior Agreement between Physician and Corporation." *Id.* at 474.

Issue

Was the contract's noncompetition clause overly restrictive?

Holding

The court of appeals held that the noncompetition clause was not overly restrictive.

Reason

The record reveals no attempt by either party to terminate the contract, and it is undisputed that Dominy received payment for his services at MHM and other benefits from NES consistent with the agreement until the hospital terminated its contract with NES. By their conduct, the parties assented to each of the contract's yearly renewals. Accordingly, the trial court properly granted summary judgment to NES.

As to the contract's noncompetition clause, this restriction prohibits Dominy from performing emergency medical services in only MHM in Bainbridge, Georgia, where he worked pursuant to a contract with NES, and from having an ownership or financial interest in an entity contracting to provide emergency medical services to that one hospital. He is not precluded from all practice of medicine, with staff privileges at MHM, nor is he prohibited from providing emergency medical services, directly or under contract to a provider of such services, to other hospitals in the immediate vicinity. The court found that such a restriction is reasonably limited in duration and territorial effect while it protects NES's interest in preventing Dominy from becoming its competitor immediately after termination of its contract with MHM.

Discussion

1. Discuss why hospitals place noncompetitive clauses in their contracts.
2. Discuss why the contract's noncompetitive clause was not overly restrictive.

Nurse Practitioner and Noncompetition Clause

The respondent-hospital in *Washington County Memorial Hospital v. Sidebottom*[25] employed the appellant-nurse practitioner from October 1993 through April 1998. Prior to beginning her employment, the nurse entered into an employment agreement with the hospital. The agreement included a noncompetition clause providing in part that the nurse during the term of the agreement and for a period of one year after the termination of her employment would not within a 50-mile radius directly or indirectly engage in the practice of nursing without the express direction or consent of the hospital. In February 1994, the nurse requested the hospital's permission to work for the Washington County Health Department doing prenatal nursing care. Because the hospital was not then

doing prenatal care, the hospital gave her permission to accept that employment but reserved the ability to withdraw the permission if the services the nurse was providing later came to be provided by the hospital. In January 1996, the nurse and the hospital entered into a second employment agreement that continued the parties' employment relationship through January 9, 1998. This agreement included a noncompetition clause identical to the 1993 employment agreement. It also provided for automatic renewal for an additional two years unless either party gave written termination notice no less than 90 days prior to the expiration of the agreement.

On March 11, 1998, the nurse gave the hospital written notice of her resignation effective April 15. On April 16, the nurse began working as a nurse practitioner with Dr. Mullen at his office. The office was located within 50 miles of the hospital. The nurse stopped working with Mullen on May 11 due to a temporary restraining order issued by the Washington County Circuit Court. The court granted a preliminary injunction on June 1. On October 16, the court entered a permanent injunction and final judgment and order prohibiting the nurse from practicing nursing within a 50-mile radius of the hospital for a period of one year from April 15. The nurse contended that the circuit court erred by enforcing the noncompetition clause contained in the nurse's employment agreement because there was no threat of significant patient loss to the hospital from the nurse's employment in the noncompete region, saying that the hospital is located in a medically underserved area and the nurse had agreed not to treat any of the hospital's patients.

The burden of demonstrating the covenant's validity is on the party seeking to enforce it. First, the covenant must be reasonable in scope as to geography and time. The nurse does not debate this aspect of the noncompetition clause in her employment agreement. Second, the covenant must be reasonably necessary to protect certain narrowly defined and well-recognized employer interests.

The hospital's interest lies in protecting its patient base, as a primary source of revenue. The specific enforcement of the nurse's noncompetition clause is reasonably necessary to protect the hospital's interest. Actual damage need not be proven to enforce a covenant not to compete. Rather, the employee's opportunity to influence customers justifies enforcement of the covenant. Thus, the quality, frequency, and duration of an employee's exposure to an employer's customers are crucial in determining the covenant's reasonableness. The nurse had opportunity to influence the hospital's patients. Prior to her employment with the hospital, the nurse never worked in Washington County, nor did she have a patient base there. The nurse helped to establish two rural health care clinics for the hospital, one of which she managed for her first year of employment. During her nearly five years of employment with the hospital, the nurse saw more than 3000 patients. Further, during her employment, the hospital promoted her as a nurse practitioner in the community by paying for advertisements with her picture and telephone number in the newspaper. In general, the nurse had a good rapport with her patients, and she had patients who requested her for medical services.

During the period that the nurse worked with Mullen, she actually saw at least six of the hospital's patients. Although the hospital is located in a medically underserved area, its patient base was affected nonetheless by the nurse's violation of the noncompetition clause. The nurse's violation of the noncompetition clause occurred because of her work as a nurse practitioner, not because of work as a nurse in general. The reasonableness of the noncompetition clause is unaffected by the nurse's offer to refrain from treating any patients treated by her during her employment with the hospital during the terms of the noncompetition clause. By the time the nurse made this offer, her violation of the clause already had occurred. The nurse already had treated some of the hospital's patients. Her opportunity to influence the hospital's patients already had occurred. In fact, prior to leaving the hospital, the nurse told several patients where she was going.

The noncompetition clause in the nurse's employment agreement was clear and unambiguous. The nurse obtained legal advice before signing her original employment agreement and before resigning. The hospital notified the nurse before her last day that the noncompetition clause would be enforced. The judgment of the circuit court was affirmed.

RESTRAINT OF TRADE

The increasing number of alternative delivery systems and resultant competition has created the potential for illegal activities to restrain trade. The emphasis on free enterprise and a competitive marketplace has resulted in careful scrutiny by the Federal Trade Commission (FTC), the federal agency responsible for monitoring the marketplace and enforcing federal antitrust laws.

The Antitrust Division of the U.S. Department of Justice has primary responsibility for enforcing federal antitrust laws, which includes investigation of possible violations of both the criminal and the civil provisions of the Sherman, Clayton, and Robinson-Patman Acts.

FEDERAL TRADE COMMISSION

The FTC is authorized to enforce Section 5 of the FTC Act, which prohibits unfair methods of competition and unfair or deceptive acts or practices. Together with the department of justice, the FTC also enforces the Clayton Act sections that prohibit discrimination (e.g., in price), exclusive dealings and similar arrangements, certain corporate acquisitions of stock or assets, and interlocking directorates.

SHERMAN ANTITRUST ACT

The primary federal law that comes into play in health care is the Sherman Antitrust Act. The Sherman Act proscribes the following:

Section 1. Every contract, combination in the form of trust or otherwise, or conspiracy, in restraint of trade or commerce among the several states . . . is declared to be illegal.

Section 2. Every person who shall monopolize, or attempt to monopolize, or combine or conspire with any other person or persons, to monopolize any part of the trade or commerce among the several states . . . shall be deemed . . . guilty of a felony. . . .[26]

Areas of concern for health care organizations include reduced market competition, price fixing, actions that bar or limit new entrants to the field, preferred provider arrangements, and exclusive contracts.

For example, a health care organization must be cognizant of the potential problems that may exist when limiting the number of physicians it will admit to its medical staff. Because closed staff determinations can effectively limit competition from other physicians, the governing body must ensure that the decision-making process in granting privileges is based on legislative, objective criteria and is not dominated by those who have the most to gain competitively by denying privileges.

Physicians have attempted to use state and federal antitrust laws to challenge determinations denying or limiting medical staff privileges. Generally, these actions claim that the organization conspired with other physicians to ensure that the complaining physician would not get privileges in order to reduce competition among physicians.

Conspiracy to Terminate Physician's Privileges

In *Patrick v. Burget,*[27] the U.S. Supreme Court upheld a $2 million jury verdict in favor of a surgeon practicing in Oregon who claimed that other physicians conspired to terminate his staff privileges at the only hospital in town and thus drove him out of practice. The defendant physicians argued that their conduct should be immune from liability under the state action doctrine because Oregon, like many states, has state agencies that regulate the procedures that hospitals may use to grant or deny staff privileges. The Supreme Court rejected this state action defense in the light of the egregious facts of the case (the defendant physicians were also participants in the state processes) and the fact that Oregon's statutory scheme did not actively supervise medical staff determinations.[28]

Claim of Group Boycott Denied

On February 29, 1984, the defendant hospital in *Cogan v. Harford Memorial Hospital,*[29] owned by Upper Chesapeake Health Systems, Inc. (UCHS), contracted with Dr. Cogan to act as the chief of radiology for five years. In 1988, the hospital and Cogan renegotiated the contract. Cogan's compensation was increased, and the contract extended until May 25, 1993, subject to termination by either party providing a 120-day written notice. During the renegotiation, Cogan sought compensation on a fee-for-service basis, but the hospital was uncomfortable with such an arrangement.

In December 1990, Cogan began discussing with NMR of America the possibility of opening a radiology clinic to provide testing with magnetic resonance imaging (MRI) separate from the hospital. The hospital expressed opposition to such an arrangement. In response, Cogan tied discussions of a new MRI clinic to renegotiation of his contract on a fee-for-service arrangement. The hospital agreed to discuss a fee-for-service contract. Under the proposed contract, Cogan's radiology group would not maintain any financial or professional interest with any competing medical facility within 20 miles of a hospital owned by UCHS. The parties failed to reach an agreement.

On March 1, 1991, the hospital informed Cogan of its intention to terminate his employment contract as of June 28, 1991. In October 1991, Cogan formed Cogan & Smith, a partnership with Dr. Smith, his former associate at the hospital.

In November 1991, Cogan & Smith signed a contract in which it agreed to act as the managing director of a radiology clinic. The clinic had a lower volume of business than anticipated, and Cogan filed suit against UCHS. He contended that the hospital's policy against sending patients to facilities not accredited by the Joint Commission on Accreditation of Healthcare Organizations impeded the clinic's business. The hospital claimed that the policy affected no more than seven patients. Cogan contended it affected 15,000 patients. He characterized this policy as a group boycott against the clinic. Under the Sherman Antitrust Act, group boycotts may be considered anticompetitive.

Cogan contended that the defendants violated the Sherman Act, breached the contract between himself and UCHS, interfered with his contractual relations, wrongfully discharged him, and deprived him of his constitutional rights in violation of 42 U.S.C. § 1983, as amended, 15 U.S.C.A. §§ 1, 2.

The U.S. District Court held that the harm suffered by Cogan because he was unable to continue working at the hospital was not compensable under the Sherman Act. The court found no evidence showing that competition in any relevant market had been harmed, reduced, or impacted by the termination of Cogan's contract or the alleged group boycott of the MRI clinic by the implementation of the hospital's policy. The only harm asserted was Cogan's inability to continue working at the hospital. The injury he incurred as a competitor of the hospital was not the "type the antitrust laws were intended to prevent."[30]

Physician Agreement for Professional Services/ Too Restrictive

In *Emergicare Systems Corporation v. Bourdon,*[31] Emergicare Systems Corporation (ESC) contracted to provide emergency department physicians to the Longview Regional Hospital for several years; Dr. Bourdon was one of those physicians. On October 23, 1991, ESC sent a letter to Bourdon confirming that its contract with Longview Regional Hospital would terminate on November 8, 1991, and that pursuant to his agreement for professional services with ESC, his agreement with ESC would also terminate. Bourdon talked to the hospital administrator and to Metroplex Emergency Physicians, PA. Arrangements were made for him to continue his work at the emergency department as an employee of Metroplex.

ESC sued Bourdon and Metroplex. ESC alleged that Bourdon breached a covenant not to compete and that Metroplex interfered with its contractual agreement with Bourdon. Following a nonjury trial, judgment was rendered on February 15, 1996, that ESC take nothing from the defendants. ESC appealed. The covenant purports to restrict the physician from working within five miles of any clinic operated by ESC, whether the physician ever worked in that clinic or not. Also, the covenant purports to restrict the physician from working in any emergency department where ESC provides emergency department physicians for one year following termination of such contract. This could be at some indefinite future date, more than one year following the physician's termination of employment by ESC.

The trial court was correct in rendering the take-nothing judgment on the appellant's claims against Metroplex. The appeals court held that covenants not to compete that are unreasonable restraints of trade, and being unenforceable on grounds of public policy cannot form the basis of an action for tortious interference.

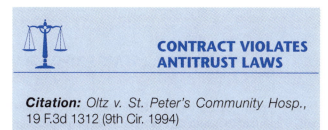

CONTRACT VIOLATES ANTITRUST LAWS

Citation: *Oltz v. St. Peter's Community Hosp.,* 19 F.3d 1312 (9th Cir. 1994)

Facts

Oltz, a nurse anesthetist, brought an antitrust action against physician anesthesiologists and

St. Peter's Community Hospital after he was terminated. Oltz had a billing agreement with the hospital, which provided 84 percent of the surgical services in the rural community that it served. The anesthesiologists did not like competing with the nurse anesthetist's lower fees and, as a result, entered into an exclusive contract with the hospital on April 29, 1980, in order to squeeze the nurse anesthetist out of the market. This resulted in cancellation of the nurse anesthetist's contract with the hospital. Oltz filed a suit against the anesthesiologists and hospital for violation of the Sherman Antitrust Act, 15 U.S.C. § 1. The anesthesiologists settled for $462,500 before trial.

The case against the hospital proceeded to trial. The jury found that the hospital conspired with the anesthesiologists and awarded the plaintiff $212,182 in lost income and $209,649 in future damages. The trial judge considered the damage award to be excessive and ordered a new trial.

The hospital motioned the court to exclude all damages after June 26, 1982, which was the date that the hospital renegotiated its exclusive contract with the anesthesiology group. The court decided that Oltz failed to prove that the renegotiated contract also violated antitrust laws, thus ruling that Oltz was not entitled to damages after June 26, 1982. Because Oltz conceded that he could not prove damages greater than those offset by his settlement with the physicians, his claim for damages against the hospital was disposed of by summary judgment.

The judge who presided over Oltz's request for attorneys' fees restricted the amount that he could claim. Because Oltz had been denied damages from the hospital, the judge refused to award attorneys' fees or costs for work performed after the 1986 liability trial.

Issue

Was Oltz entitled to seek recovery for all damages resulting from destruction of his business after June 26, 1982?

Holding

The U.S. Court of Appeals for the Ninth Circuit held that Oltz was entitled to seek recovery for all damages.

Reason

Oltz introduced evidence that the initial exclusive contract violated antitrust laws and that such violation destroyed his practice. "Because the initial conspiracy destroyed his practice, Oltz is entitled to seek recovery for all damages resulting from the destruction of his business. . . . The legality of any subsequent agreements between the conspirators is irrelevant, because the April 29, 1980, contract severed the lifeline to Oltz's thriving practice. . . ." *Id.* at 1314.

Discussion

1. What should parties to a contract be aware of when negotiating exclusive contracts?
2. What remedies are available when one party breaches a contract by refusing to perform an agreed-upon service?

HOSPITAL STAFF PRIVILEGES

Staff privileges are both professionally and economically important to health care professionals in the practice of their chosen professions. Health care organizations must be selective in the granting of staff privileges to maintain quality standards but every effort must be made to prevent anticompetitive abuses. As competition increases between podiatrists and orthopedic surgeons, psychologists and psychiatrists, nurse midwives and obstetricians, nurse anesthetists and anesthesiologists, and so on, it must be understood that there is a clear difference in denying staff privileges to an individual on a quality basis and denying such privileges to an entire group of professionals; the latter will serve only to raise a red flag and increase the chances of scrutiny by the courts. Competition for patients increases the potential for denial of privileges to prevent competitors from effectively entering the marketplace and practicing their respective professions.

Restricting Privileges

Moratoriums and closed medical staffs, as used in the health care field, describe an organization's policy of prohibiting further appointments to its medical staff. Generally, a moratorium is for a specified period of time. It is lifted at such time as the purpose for which it was instituted no longer exists. An HAL *closed staff* is of a more permanent nature and relates to the mission of the institution, such as a commitment to teaching and research. Such institutions are very selective in their medical staff appointments. Generally, physicians who are appointed have both high academic interests and abilities as well as national recognition for expertise in their specialties.

Organizations have adopted a moratorium policy in certain instances because of a high inpatient census and the difficulties that would be encountered in accommodating new physicians. If left unchecked, the closing of an organization's medical staff eventually could have the effect of discouraging a competitive environment in the physician marketplace.

Governing bodies that adopt a closed-staff policy must do so on a rational basis and take the following into consideration before closing the medical staff to new applicants:

- Effect on the organization's census

- Organization and community needs for additional physicians in certain medical and surgical specialties and subspecialties

- Strain that additional staff will put on the organization's supporting departments (e.g., radiology and laboratory services)

- Effect of denying medical staff privileges to applicants who presently are located within the geographic area of the organization and serving community residents

- Effect on any contracts the organization may have with other health care delivery systems, such as health maintenance organizations

- Effect a moratorium will have on physician groups that may desire to add a partner

- Effect additional staff may have on the quality of care rendered in the organization

- Whether closing the staff will confine control of the organization's beds to the existing medical staff, allowing them to enhance their economic interests at the expense of their patients and other qualified physicians

- Effect of a limited moratorium by specialty as opposed to a comprehensive one involving all specialties (Indiscriminately closing a staff in all departments and sections without a review could be considered an action in restraint of trade.)

- Existence of a mechanism for periodic review of the need to continue a moratorium

- Effect that medical staff resignations during the moratorium may have on the organization's census

- Existence of a mechanism for notifying potential medical staff candidates at such time that the organization determines that there is a need for an expanded medical staff

- Characteristics of the medical staff (Is the staff aging and in need of new membership?)

- Potential for restraint of trade legal action under antitrust laws

- Effect on physicians without staff privileges whose patients are admitted to the hospital

- Formation of a committee composed of representatives from the governing body, medical staff, administration, and legal counsel to develop an appropriate moratorium policy

- Selection of a consultant to study the demographics marketplace, physician referral patterns, literature, and organization use; conduct a medical staff opinion poll; develop patient-physician population ratios; determine population shifts; develop a formula to determine optimal staffing levels by department and section; and provide this information to the governing body for use in determining the appropriateness of closing the staff in selected medical departments and/or sections

The continuing pressure of new technology, third-party payers, a growing body of regulations, malpractice insurance rates, and a shortage of physicians in a variety of specialties emphasize the need for organizations to consider how they can effectively compete in the marketplace. In light of this, the imposition of a moratorium or the closing of an organization's medical staff may prove to be counterproductive to the long-term survival of an organization.

The governing body must ensure that any proposed action to close an organization's medical staff is based on objective criteria. Unless an organization can show that its actions are based on legitimate patient-care concerns or concerns related to the objectives of the organization, physicians might be successful in using antitrust and tort law to challenge the organization's actions.

PATIENT TRANSFER AGREEMENT

Health care organizations should have a written transfer agreement in effect with other organizations to help ensure the smooth transfer of patients from one facility to another when such is determined appropriate by the attending physician. A *transfer agreement* is a written document that sets forth the terms and conditions under which a patient may be transferred to a facility that more appropriately provides the kind of care required by the patient. It also establishes procedures to admit patients of one facility to another when their condition warrants a transfer.

Transfer agreements should be written in compliance with and reflect the provisions of the many federal and state laws, regulations, and standards affecting health care organizations. The parties to a transfer agreement should be particularly aware of applicable federal and state regulations.

Agreements that will aid in bringing about the maximum use of the services of each organization and in ensuring the best possible care for patients should be established. The basic elements of a transfer agreement include:

Identification of each party to the agreement, including the name and location of each organization to the agreement

Purpose of the agreement

Policies and procedures for transfer of patients (Language in this section of the agreement should make it clear that the patient's physician makes the determination as to the patient's need for the facilities and services of the receiving organization. The receiving organization should agree that, subject to its admission requirements and availability of space, it will admit the patient from the transferring organization as promptly as possible.)

Organizational responsibilities for arranging and making the transfer (Generally, the transferring organization is responsible for making transfer arrangements. The agreement should specify who will bear the costs involved in the transfer.)

Exchange of information (The agreement must provide a mechanism for the interchange of medical and other information relevant to the patient.)

Retention of autonomy (The agreement should make clear that each organization retains its autonomy, and that the governing bodies of each facility will continue to exercise exclusive legal responsibility and control over the management, assets, and affairs of the respective facilities. It also should be stipulated that neither organization assumes any liability by virtue of the agreement for any debts or obligations of a financial or legal nature incurred by the other.)

Procedure for settling disputes (The agreement should include a method of settling disputes that might arise over some aspect of the patient transfer relationship.)

Procedure for modification or termination of the agreement (The agreement should provide that it can be modified or amended by mutual consent of the parties.

It also should provide for termination by either organization on notice within a specified time period.)

Sharing of services (Depending on the situation, cooperative use of facilities and services on an outpatient basis [e.g., laboratory and X-ray testing] may be an important element of the relationship between organizations. The method of payment for services rendered should be carefully described in the agreement.)

Publicity (The agreement should provide that neither organization will use the name of the other in any promotional or advertising material without prior approval of the other.)

Exclusive versus nonexclusive agreement (It is advisable for organizations—when and where possible—to have transfer agreements with more than one organization. The agreement may include language to the effect that either party has the right to enter into transfer agreements with other organizations.)

INAPPROPRIATE TRANSFER OF A PATIENT

Citation: *J.B. v. Sacred Heart Hosp. of Pensacola,* 635 So. 2d 945 (Fla. 1994)

Facts

The facts of this case reveal that the hospital on or about April 17, 1989, was requested by its medical staff to arrange transportation for the patient, diagnosed with AIDS, to another treatment facility in Alabama. The social services department, unable to arrange ambulance transport, asked the patient's brother to provide the transportation. J.B., having visited his brother at the hospital when he was first admitted, was under the impression that his brother's diagnosis was Lyme disease. He had not been notified that there was a change in diagnosis. The patient was released to his brother from the hospital with excessive fever and a heparin lock in his arm. During the trip, J.B.'s brother began to thrash about and accidentally dislodged the dressing to his heparin lock, causing J.B. to reach over while driving in an attempt to prevent the lock from coming out of his brother's arm. In doing so, J.B. came in contact with fluid around the lock site. J.B.'s hand had multiple nicks and cuts due to a recent fishing trip. *Id.* at 947.

The complaint, which was filed after the two-year statute of limitation had tolled, alleged that the hospital was negligent in arranging for J.B. to transport his brother in that it knew of the patient's condition, the level of care that would be required in transporting him, and the risk involved. J.B. alleged that because he contracted the AIDS virus, his wife was exposed to it through him and his children have suffered a loss of relationship with him.

The Florida District Court ruled that J.B.'s complaint stated a claim for medical malpractice and was thus subject to the presuit notice and screening procedures set out in Florida statutes. Because J.B. did not follow those procedures, the court dismissed the complaint. On appeal, the Florida Circuit Court declined to rule on J.B.'s claim, concluding that the issues were appropriate for resolution by the Florida Supreme Court.

Issue

Was the claim of the patient's brother a claim for medical malpractice, and therefore subject to a two-year statute of limitations?

Holding

The Florida Supreme Court answered that the claim was not a claim for medical malpractice for purposes of the two-year statute of limitations or presuit notice and screening requirements.

Reason

Florida Statutes sets a two-year limitation period for medical malpractice actions. J.B.'s injury arose solely through the hospital's use of him as a transporter. Accordingly, this suit is not a medical malpractice action, and the two-year statute of limitations is inapplicable. According to the allegations in J.B.'s complaint, the hospital was negligent in using J.B. as a transporter. The complaint does not allege that the hospital was negligent in any way in the rendering of, or the failure to render, medical care or services to J.B.

Discussion

1. Why was the plaintiff's not an action in malpractice?
2. Were the transfer arrangements for the patient appropriate?

INSURANCE CONTRACT

Insurance is a form of risk management used primarily to hedge against the risk of potential loss. In an insurance contract, the insurer has an obligation to indemnify the insured for losses caused by specified events. In return, the insured must pay a fixed premium during the policy period. As noted, the interpretation of an insurance contract can give rise to a legal action when the insurer refuses to indemnify the insured.

Coverage Denied

Truett, in *Truett v. Community Mut. Ins. Co.,*[32] brought an action against the insurer to recover medical expenses. In

June 1991, Truett was treated for migraine headaches. As of August 1, 1991, Truett was covered under an employee benefit plan through a group health insurance contract with Community Mutual Insurance Co. On August 29, 1991, Truett was hospitalized for dizziness, vomiting, and weakness on his left side. After extensive testing, Dr. Moorthy diagnosed Truett as suffering from a complicated migraine. Truett sought reimbursement for medical expenses he incurred during the course of his illness.

Community Mutual concluded on January 20, 1992, that Truett's medical expenses were not covered because the expenses were for the care of a preexisting condition. Under the insurance policy, conditions that existed prior to the effective date of the policy were not covered if health problems related to the conditions were manifested after the effective date. Truett challenged this assessment to a Community Mutual appeals board. Dr. Morrow was recruited by

Community Mutual to provide an expert assessment of Truett's case. The Community Mutual appeals board found that Truett's condition was preexisting because he had been treated in June 1991 for migraine headaches. Therefore, Community Mutual denied his coverage for his expenses.

On September 1, 1992, the Truetts filed a complaint against Community Mutual to recover Truett's medical expenses. The court of common pleas entered summary judgment for Community Mutual, and Truett appealed.

The Ohio Court of Appeals held that the insurer's denial of coverage was not arbitrary or capricious. The appeals board had all of Truett's medical records from before and after the incident in question. It obtained Morrow's expert opinion that the complicated migraine was a continuation from Truett's previous bouts with normal migraines. The appeals board and Morrow relied on medical evidence in making their decisions and neither overlooked nor ignored relevant information. Thus, the decision was not arbitrary or capricious.

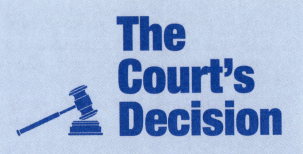

The Court's Decision

The trial court was found to have erred in granting a directed verdict to Strickland on Harvey's breach of contract claim. Harvey relied upon the documents he signed expressing his desire not to be administered blood. It was for the jury to determine whether an express contract was created. The trial court's grant of a directed verdict was reversed, and the matter was remanded for a new trial.

CHAPTER REVIEW

1. A *contract* is a written or oral agreement that involves legally binding obligations between two or more parties. The purpose of a contract is to provide legal recourse should one or more of the parties not perform its obligations as set forth under the contract.

2. Various types of contracts include:

   - *Express contracts* are those in which the parties have an oral agreement or have reduced agreements to writing. Written contracts are always the most desirable form. Although oral contracts are generally recognized, they cannot always be enforced by the courts.

   - *Implied contracts* are those that are inferred by law and are based on parties' conduct.

   - *Voidable contracts* allow one party, but not the other, to escape from legal obligations under the contract.

   - An *executory contract* is one in which something remains to be done (performed) by one or more of the parties.

   - *Executed contracts* are those in which obligations have been performed fully.

   - An *enforceable contract* is one that is a valid, legally binding agreement. If one party breaches it, the other will have an appropriate legal remedy.

   - An *unenforceable contract* is one in which, because of some defect, no legal remedy is available if breached by one of the parties to the contract.

   - There are also contracts for realty (real estate or interests in real estate), goods (movable objects, with the exception of money and securities), and services (human energy).

3. To be enforceable, contracts must contain an offer or *communication, consideration,* and *acceptance.* If one or more of the parties who have entered into the contract are not considered competent, the contract will not be enforceable. Examples of those often found incompetent include minors, the mentally insane, and prisoners.

4. In order to be successful in a breach of contract lawsuit, the following elements must be established:

   • A valid contract was executed.

   • The plaintiff performed as specified in the contract.

   • The defendant failed to perform as specified in the contract.

   • The plaintiff suffered an economic loss as a result of the defendant's breach of contract.

5. *Independent contractors* agree to perform work without being under the direct control or direction of another party. An employer is liable for the torts or negligence of an independent contractor in certain circumstances; these include negligence of the employer in selecting, instructing, or supervising the contractor.

6. Among the permissible defenses for not performing under a contract are *fraud, mistake of fact or law, duress, lack of legality of the contract, impossibility to perform the contract,* and expiration of the *statute of limitations.*

7. Forms of legal redress for breach of contract include specified performance of the duties set forth in the contract, the award of monetary (or compensatory) damages, and the award of general or consequential damages. General damages could be expected to result from the breach of the contract, while consequential damages are due to unforeseen damages.

8. The right of an employer to terminate an employee can be limited through an employment contract; an express agreement with the employee or a collective bargaining agreement to which the employee is the beneficiary.

9. Employee handbooks and medical staff bylaws can be viewed by a court as a binding contract between an employer and employee, unless such documents provide legally acceptable disclaimers.

10. *Exclusive contracts* allow organizations to contract with physicians and medical groups to provide specific services to the organization.

11. The Federal Trade Commission is a federal agency that monitors the marketplace and enforces federal antitrust laws with the goals of maintaining free enterprise and a competitive marketplace.

12. A *moratorium,* which prohibits further appointments to an organization's medical staff, must be applied with consistency and without discrimination. Although a moratorium is usually lifted at some point, a closed staff is more permanent in nature.

13. A *transfer agreement* is a written document that sets forth terms and conditions under which a patient may be transferred to an alternate facility for care.

14. In an insurance contract, the insurer has an obligation to indemnify the insured for losses caused by specified events. In return, the insured must pay a fixed premium during the policy period. The interpretation of an insurance contract can give rise to a legal action when the insurer refuses to indemnify the insured.

REVIEW QUESTIONS

1. What is a contract?
2. Describe the differences between an express and an implied contract.
3. What are the elements of a contract?
4. Discuss the remedies available for nonperformance of a contract.
5. Discuss the importance of disclaimers in employee handbooks.
6. Discuss why the courts often consider medical staff bylaws a contract.
7. Explain why exclusive contracts are so controversial.
8. Describe the advantages and disadvantages of closing a medical staff to new physicians.
9. What is an insurance contract?

NOTES

1. *Harvey v. Strickland,* 350 S.C. 303, 566 S.E.2d 529 (2002).

2. *Hungerford Hosp. v. Mulvey,* 225 A.2d 495 (Conn. 1966).

3. 25 P.3d 358 (2001).

4. 384 N.Y.S.2d 527 (N.Y. App. Div. 1976).

5. 693 N.Y.S.2d 143 (N.Y. App. Div. 1999).

6. No. E2004-00207-COA-R3-CV (Tenn. App. 2005).

7. *Gazzola-Kraenzlin v. Westchester Medical Group, P.C.,* 782 N.Y.S.2d 115 (N.Y. App. Div. 2004).

8. 492 N.Y.S.2d 9 (N.Y. 1985).

9. 605 N.E.2d 613 (Ill. App. Ct. 1992).

10. 867 A.2d 1187 (N.J. App. 2005).

11. *Community Hosp. Group, Inc. v. More,* No. A-75 September Term 2003 (N.J. 2005).

12. *Pierson v. Medical Health Ctrs.,* 869 A.2d 901 (N.J. 2005).

13. 457 N.Y.S.2d 193 (N.Y. 1982).

14. 720 P.2d 632 (Idaho 1986).

15. 731 F. Supp. 311 (D. Ill. 1990).

16. *Id.* at 321–322.

17. *Chesnick v. Saint Mary of Nazareth Hosp.,* 570 N.E.2d 545 (Ill. App. Ct. 1991).

18. 789 N.Y.S.2d 42 (N.Y. App. Div. 2005).

19. 520 N.W.2d 625 (Wis. App. 1994).

20. 368 N.W.2d 666, 668, 674 (1985).

21. 141 Md. App. 715 (2001).

22. 670 F.2d 507 (5th Cir. 1982).

23. 466 U.S. 2 (1984).

24. 475 A.2d 533 (N.J. 1984).

25. 7 S.W.3d 542 (Mo. App. 1999).

26. 15 U.S.C. § 1 (1982).

27. 108 S. CT. 1658 (1988).

28. 42 U.S.C.A. §§ 11101–11152 (1986).

29. 843 F. Supp. 1013 (D. Md. 1994).

30. *Id.* at 1018.

31. 942 S.W.2d 201 (Tex. App. 1997).

32. 633 N.E.2d 617 (Ohio Ct. App. 1993).

CHAPTER 6

Civil Procedure and Trial Practice

It's Your Gavel ...

CONFLICTING EVIDENCE

Gwendolyn was in Mississippi, when she felt light-headed and as though her heart was racing. Gwendolyn's sister brought her to the BCH hospital. Dr. Dorrough diagnosed Gwendolyn as suffering from supraventricular tachycardia. As Gwendolyn was discharged, she was told to follow up with her physician and to return to the emergency room if she experienced any further problems. Although Gwendolyn experienced more problems, she returned to Georgia and was admitted to a medical center. She complained of dizziness, shortness of breath, and chest tightness, and stayed at the medical center for over five hours. She was later transferred to St. Francis Hospital with a suspected diagnosis of acute pulmonary embolus. At St. Francis, Gwendolyn underwent emergency surgery. The surgery was unsuccessful, and Gwendolyn died of a pulmonary embolus.

The plaintiffs filed a complaint against Dorrough and BCH. The complaint alleged that Dorrough and BCH breached their duty to provide proper care to Gwendolyn. The plaintiffs had two expert witnesses, Dr. Vance and Dr. Falk. Dorrough had one expert witness, Dr. Dupuis. The jury heard conflicting testimony from the expert witnesses concerning the events leading up to Gwendolyn's death.

Vance testified that Dorrough did not meet the minimum standard of care based on the fact that there was a sustained rapid heart rate and abnormal laboratory findings. He stated that Gwendolyn suffered from sinus tachycardia and not supraventricular tachycardia. He defined *sinus tachycardia* as an increase in pulse rate in response to an underlying disease state. He testified that the two terms are not the same.

Falk testified that, in his opinion, Dorrough misdiagnosed Gwendolyn. He also believed that she suffered from sinus tachycardia, not supraventricular tachycardia, testifying that the two terms are not the same. Falk stated that, in his opinion, if Gwendolyn had been diagnosed and given the drug heparin then, she would not have embolized and would have survived. Further, he stated that most *emboli* (clots) come from the lower extremities and pelvis region.

Dupuis testified that Dorrough did not fall below the standard of care. He testified that Gwendolyn had a rare condition in that the clot that ultimately killed her was in the heart and did not come from the legs. Dupuis stated that Gwendolyn's death was unavoidable despite the best of care.

The jury returned a verdict in favor of the plaintiffs and assessed damages in the amount of $1.5 million against Dorrough. He appealed, asserting that the verdict of the jury was not supported by credible or sufficient evidence.[1]

WHAT IS YOUR VERDICT?

For many students and health care practitioners, this book will be their only formal introduction to the legal aspects of health care. This chapter in particular is valuable to readers in understanding the law and its application in the courtroom. Although many of the procedures leading up to and followed during a trial are discussed in this chapter, civil procedure and trial practice are governed by each state's statutory requirements. Cases on a federal level are governed by federal statutory requirements.

PLEADINGS

The pleadings of a case are the written statements of fact and law filed with a court by the parties to a lawsuit. Pleadings generally include such papers as a complaint, demurrer, answer, and bill of particulars. A *complaint* is the first pleading filed by a plaintiff that initiates a lawsuit. It sets forth the relevant allegations of fact that give rise to one or more legal causes of action along with the damages requested. A *demurrer* is a pleading filed by a defendant challenging the legal sufficiency of a complaint. An *answer* to a complaint is a pleading which admits or denies the specific allegations set forth in a complaint and constitutes a general appearance by a defendant. A *bill of particulars* is a request for a written itemization of the claims which a defendant can demand from the plaintiff to determine what the details of a claim are. A defendant may also file a cross-complaint and bring other parties into a lawsuit by the process. If only questions of law are at issue, the judge will decide the case based on the pleadings alone. If questions of fact are involved, a trial is conducted to determine those facts.

Summons and Complaint

The parties to a controversy are the plaintiff and the defendant. The *plaintiff* is the person who initiates an action by filing a complaint; the *defendant* is the person against whom a suit is brought. Many cases have multiple plaintiffs and defendants.

Although the procedures for beginning an action vary according to jurisdiction, there are procedural common denominators. All jurisdictions require service of process on the defendant (usually through a summons) and a return to the court of that process by the person who served it. Where a summons is not required to be issued directly by a court, an attorney, as an officer of the court, may prepare and cause a summons to be served without direct notice to or approval of a court.

The first pleading filed with the court in a negligence action is the complaint. The complaint identifies the parties to a suit, states a cause of action, and includes a demand for damages. It is filed by the plaintiff and is the first statement of a case by the plaintiff against the defendant. In some jurisdictions, a complaint must accompany a *summons* (an announcement to the defendant that a case has been commenced). The essential elements contained in a complaint are:

1. a short statement of the grounds on which the court's jurisdiction depends (the court's authority to hear the case)

2. a statement of the claim demonstrating that the pleader is entitled to relief

3. a demand for judgment for the relief to which the plaintiff deems him- or herself entitled

All these elements apply to any counterclaim, cross claim, or third-party claim.

The complaint can be served on the defendant either with the summons or within a prescribed time after the summons has been served. Specific formalities must be observed in the service of a summons so that appropriate jurisdiction over a defendant is obtained. Such formalities dictate the manner in which a summons is to be delivered, the time period within which service must be effected, and the geographic limitations within which service must be made. For example, a summons to commence an action in a local municipal court generally would require service within the particular municipality in order for the court to obtain jurisdiction. Where such service is not possible, the action may have to be brought in a different court.

In the preliminary motions, the defendant cites possible errors that would defeat the plaintiff's case. For example, the defendant may object that a summons or a complaint was served improperly, that the action was brought in the wrong jurisdiction, or that there was something technically incorrect about the complaint.

IMPROPER SERVICE OF A SUMMONS

Citation: *Collins v. Park,* 621 A.2d 996 (Pa. Super. Ct. 1993)

Facts

In this medical malpractice action, the trial court dismissed a complaint against Dr. Park because of improper service upon him. The plaintiff, Collins, appealed.

On March 14, 1989, the sheriff attempted to serve the writ on Park by leaving a copy with the receptionist at the hospital. Park had terminated his relationship with the hospital on February 22, 1988, and he did not thereafter maintain an office or place of business at the hospital.

Issue

Was the sheriff's attempt defective when he served the writ of summons upon Park in a medical malpractice action by leaving a copy with the receptionist at the hospital?

Holding

The Pennsylvania Superior Court held that the sheriff's attempt to serve the writ of summons upon the physician by leaving a copy with the receptionist at the hospital was defective, because Park did not have a proprietary interest in the hospital and, at the time of service, was no longer affiliated with the hospital. The service of a complaint by leaving a copy with the nurse at the intensive care unit was inadequate to confer jurisdiction over him.

Reason

The plaintiff's attempted service of the writ of summons was defective. Because Park was not affiliated with the hospital at which service was attempted, it seems clear that the hospital cannot be deemed his office or usual place of business. A copy of the complaint was left with a nurse at the intensive care unit of the hospital where Park was then a patient. The intensive care unit of a hospital, however, cannot be deemed the patient's place of residence, nor can it be said that the patient resides there.

Discussion

1. What is the difference between a summons and a complaint?
2. Why was the service of the summons determined to be improper?

Demurrer

On receiving a copy of the plaintiff's complaint, the defendant can file preliminary objections before answering the complaint. A *demurrer* is a formal objection by one of the parties to a lawsuit that the evidence presented by the other party is insufficient to sustain an issue or case.

Answer

After service of a complaint, a response is required from the defendant in a document called the *answer.* In the answer, the defendant responds to each of the allegations contained in the complaint by stating his or her defenses and by admitting to or denying each of the plaintiff's allegations. If the defendant fails to answer the complaint within the prescribed time, the plaintiff can seek judgment by default against the defendant. However, in certain instances, a default judgment will be vacated if the defendant can demonstrate an acceptable excuse for failing to answer. Even if a plaintiff has been granted judgment by default, he or she could be required to present the basis for damages at a hearing before a court. A defaulting defendant may be entitled to oppose the evidence presented by the plaintiff at such a hearing.

Personal appearance of the defendant to respond to a complaint is not necessary. To prevent default, the defendant's attorney responds to the complaint with an answer. The defense attorney attempts to show through evidence that the defendant is not responsible for the negligent act claimed by the plaintiff to have occurred. The answer generally consists of a denial of the charges made and specifies a defense or argument justifying the position taken. The defense may show that the claim is unfounded because: (1) the period within which a suit must be instituted has run out, (2) there is contributory negligence on the part of the plaintiff, (3) any obligation has been paid, (4) a general release was presented to the defendant, or (5) the contract was illegal and therefore canceled by mutual agreement. The original answer to the complaint is filed with the court having jurisdiction over the case, and a copy of the answer is forwarded to the plaintiff's attorney.

Counterclaim

In some cases, the defendant may file a counterclaim. For example, the plaintiff may have sued an organization for personal injuries and property damage caused by the negligent operation of an organization's ambulance. The organization may file a counterclaim on grounds that its driver was careful and that it was the plaintiff who was negligent and is liable to the organization for damage to the ambulance.

Bill of Particulars

The defense attorney may request a bill of particulars, seeking more specific and detailed information than is provided in the complaint. If a counterclaim has been filed, the plaintiff's attorney may request a bill of particulars from the defense attorney. More specifically, a bill of particulars for a malpractice suit may request, for example, from the plaintiff's attorney:

- the date and time of day when the alleged malpractice occurred

- if the claim involves

  - misdiagnosis or failure to diagnose correctly

  - failure to perform a test or diagnostic procedure

  - failure to medicate, treat, or operate

  - a contraindicated test given or a contraindicated test or surgical procedure performed

  - administration of a medicine or treatment or performance of a test or surgical procedure in a manner contrary to accepted standards of medical practice

- where the alleged malpractice occurred

- the commissions and/or omissions constituting the malpractice that is alleged to have occurred

- how the alleged malpractice occurred

- a listing of injuries claimed to have been caused by the defendant's alleged malpractice

- a listing of any witnesses to the alleged malpractice

- the length of time the plaintiff was confined to bed

- the weekly earnings of the plaintiff

- the name and address of the employer

A death action rider also may be attached if the malpractice allegedly caused death. The rider may request such information as the length of time the decedent experienced pain; the date, time, and place of death; and a statement setting forth the cause of death.

DISCOVERY AND EXAMINATION BEFORE TRIAL

Discovery is the process of investigating the facts of a case before trial. The objectives of discovery are to: (1) obtain evidence that might not be obtainable at the time of trial; (2) isolate and narrow the issues for trial; (3) gather knowledge of the existence of additional evidence that may be admissible at trial; and (4) obtain leads to enable the discovering party to gather further evidence.

The discovery process is available to promote more just trials by preventing unfair surprise. "Discovery rules were promulgated to prevent trial by ambush. To deny a party the right to know absolutely at some meaningful time before trial the names and addresses of all witnesses the opposing side proposes to call in its case-in-chief is an insult to this principle."[2]

Discovery may be obtained on any matter that is not privileged and that is relevant to the subject matter involved in the pending action. The parties to a lawsuit have the right to discovery and to examine witnesses before trial. Examination before trial (EBT) is one of several discovery techniques used to enable the parties of a lawsuit to learn more regarding the nature and substance of each other's case. An EBT consists of oral testimony under oath and includes cross examination. A deposition, taken at an EBT, is the testimony of a witness that has been recorded in a written format. Testimony given at a deposition becomes part of the permanent record of the case. Each question and answer is transcribed by a court stenographer and may be used at the subsequent trial. Truthfulness and consistency are important because answers from an EBT that differ from those given at trial will be used to attack the credibility of the witness.

ATTORNEY-CLIENT PRIVILEGE

Confidential communications made by a client and an attorney to one another are protected by attorney-client privilege. There are three elements required to successfully assert attorney-client privilege:

1. Both parties must agree that the attorney-client relationship does or will exist.

2. The client must seek advice from that attorney in his or her capacity as a legal advisor.

3. Communication between the attorney and client must be identified to be confidential.

INCIDENT AND INVESTIGATIVE REPORTS

Hospital incident and investigation reports are generally not protected from discovery. The burden rests upon the hospital to demonstrate that incident and investigation reports are protected from discovery under *attorney-client privilege* and *work product doctrine.* Attorney-client privilege is intended to ensure that a client remains free from apprehension that consultations with a legal advisor will be disclosed. Such privilege further encourages a client to talk freely with his or her attorney so that he or she may receive quality advice. Likewise, with regard to the work-product doctrine, not even the most liberal of discovery theories can justify unwarranted inquiries into the files and the mental impressions of an attorney. Courts are required to protect the integrity and fairness of the fact-finding process by requiring full disclosure of all relevant facts connected with the impending litigation while, at the same time, promoting full and frank consultation between a client and a legal advisor by removing the fear of compelled disclosure of information.

If in connection with an accident or an event, a business entity, in the ordinary course of business, conducts an investigation for its own purposes, the resulting investigative report is producible in civil pretrial discovery. The distinction between whether a defendant's in-house report was prepared in the ordinary course of business or was work product in anticipation of litigation is an important one. The fact that a defendant anticipates the contingency of litigation resulting from an accident or event does not automatically qualify an in-house report as work product. *A document that is not privileged does not become privileged by the mere act of sending it to an attorney.*

Incident Report Not Privileged

A hospital document, in *In re Bridges*,[3] entitled "Risk Management Variance Report August 2002," appeared to be an incident report generated in the regular course of business and did not fall within the privilege where the testimony of the hospital's risk manager indicated that such reports only go to risk management, which was not a hospital committee.

Statistical Data Are Not Necessarily Privileged

Statistical data collected are not necessarily protected from discovery during court proceedings. For example, the patient Braverman, in *Braverman v. Columbia Hospital, Inc.*,[4]

underwent surgery and was subsequently diagnosed with a nosocomial infection (hospital-acquired infection). She was rehospitalized several times for treatment of the infection.

Braverman filed a lawsuit and sought a variety of documents from the hospital. The hospital objected on the grounds that some of the information sought by Braverman was a record of its review and evaluation procedures under Wis. Stat. § 146.38 and therefore was privileged. In its written decision, the trial court found that the infection control materials, including meeting minutes, infection rates, and the results of any investigations conducted by quality assurance/peer review committees, were privileged. Braverman appealed.

As mandated by Wis. Admin. Code § HFS 124.08, the hospital maintains an infection control committee (ICC). Its purpose is to influence and improve the quality of health care through the practice of infection control. The ICC recommends practices to reduce the risk of infection to patients, visitors, and health care workers. The hospital infection control practitioners compile infection statistics. The ICC conducts an investigation or study of any postoperative infection for purposes of quality assurance. The ICC coordinates its infection control processes in compliance with the by-laws and rules of the medical staff in order to reduce the risk of hospital-acquired infections.

Braverman argued that this kind of statistical data is not covered by Wis. Stat. §146.38. The appeals court concluded that such information is exempt from the privilege pursuant to para. (3)(d), which reads:

> (3) Information acquired in connection with the review and evaluation of health care services shall be disclosed and records of such review and evaluation shall be released, with the identity of any patient whose treatment is reviewed being withheld unless the patient has granted permission to disclose identity, in the following circumstances:
>
> •   •   •   •
>
> (d) In a report in statistical form. The report may identify any provider or facility to which the statistics relate[.]

The court concluded that Braverman was entitled to discover the statistical data.

PREPARATION OF WITNESSES

The manner in which a witness handles questioning at a deposition or trial is often as important as the facts of the case. Each witness should be well prepared before testifying. Preparation should include a review of all pertinent records.

Helpful guidelines for witnesses undergoing examination in a trial or a court hearing include the following:

- Review the records (e.g., medical records and other business records) on which you might be questioned.

- Do not be antagonistic in answering the questions. The jury may already be somewhat sympathetic toward a particular party to the lawsuit; antagonism may only serve to reinforce such an impression.

- Be organized in your thinking and recollection of the facts regarding the incident.

- Answer only the questions asked.

- Explain your testimony in simple, succinct terminology.

- Do not overdramatize the facts you are relating.

- Do not allow yourself to become overpowered by the cross-examiner.

- Be polite, sincere, and courteous at all times.

- Dress appropriately and be neatly groomed.

- Pay close attention to any objections your attorney may have as to the line of questioning being conducted by the opposing counsel.

- Be sure to have reviewed any oral deposition in which you may have participated during EBT.

- Be straightforward with the examiner. Any answers designed to cover up or cloud an issue or fact will, if discovered, serve only to discredit any previous testimony that you may have given.

- Do not show any visible signs of displeasure regarding any testimony with which you are in disagreement.

- Be sure to have questions that you did not hear repeated and questions that you did not understand rephrased.

- If you are not sure of an answer, indicate that you are not sure or that you just do not know the answer.

MOTIONS

The procedural steps that occur before trial are specifically classified as pretrial proceedings. After the pleadings have been completed, many states permit either party to move for a judgment on the pleadings. When this motion is made, the court will examine the entire case and decide whether to enter judgment according to the merits of the case as indicated in the pleadings. In some states, the moving party is permitted to introduce sworn statements showing that a claim or defense is false or a sham. This procedure cannot be used when there is substantial dispute concerning the facts presented by the affidavits.

PRETRIAL CONFERENCE

In many states, a pretrial conference will be ordered at the judge's initiative or on the request of one of the parties to the lawsuit. The *pretrial conference* is an informal discussion during which the judge and the attorneys eliminate matters not in dispute, agree on the issues, and settle procedural matters relating to the trial. Although it is not the purpose of the pretrial conference to compel the parties to settle the case, it often happens that cases are settled at this point.

MOTION TO DISMISS

A defendant may make a motion to dismiss a case, alleging that the plaintiff's complaint, even if believed, does not set forth a claim or cause of action recognized by law. A motion to dismiss can be made before, during, or after a trial. Motions made before a trial may be made on the basis that the court lacks jurisdiction, that the case is barred by the statute of limitations, that another case is pending involving the same issues, and other similar matters. A motion during trial may be made after the plaintiff has presented his or her case, on the grounds that the court has heard the plaintiff's case and the defendant is entitled to a favorable judgment as a matter of law. In the case of a motion made by the defendant at the close of the plaintiff's case, the defendant normally will claim that the plaintiff has failed to present a prima facie case (i.e., that the plaintiff has failed to establish the minimum elements necessary to justify a verdict even if no contrary evidence is presented by the defendant). After a trial has been completed, either party may move for a directed verdict on the grounds that he or she is entitled to such verdict as a matter of law.

Case Dismissed

Mrs. Stewart was admitted to the hospital with inflammation of the gallbladder and the surgeon began antibiotics. Stewart, however, died early the next morning. The county medical examiner stated that the cause of death was due to a blood-borne infection. The plaintiff's nurse expert testified in a deposition that a registered nurse at the hospital failed to meet the nursing standard of care in treating the patient. A chart was produced identifying 11 instances in which the hospital nurse allegedly failed to meet the nursing standard of care, including failure to assess the need for oxygen therapy, failure to note abnormal breath sounds and severity or location of pain, failure to assess urinary retention, and failure to assess vital signs and nausea. The plaintiff, Stewart's husband, contended that the evidence established that the defendants violated the nursing standard of care and that their failures were the proximate cause of his wife's death. The defendants moved for dismissal and the superior court granted the motion. The Court of Appeals of Washington, Division Three in *Stewart v. Newbold*[5] found that the patient—Stewart's husband—failed to establish any genuine issue on the question of proximate causation. The trial court properly dismissed the claims against the nurse and hospital.

SUMMARY JUDGMENT

Either party to a suit may believe that there are no triable issues of fact and only issues of law to be decided. In such event, either party may make a motion for summary judgment. This motion asks the court to rule that there are no facts in dispute and that the rights of the parties can be determined as a matter of law, on the basis of submitted documents, without the need for a trial. Although the courts are reluctant to look favorably on motions for summary judgment, they will grant them if the circumstances of a particular case warrant it.

The plaintiff, in *Thomas v. New York University Med. Ctr.*,[6] while under general anesthesia, slid off the operating table during a surgical procedure. The plaintiff's head was pulled out of a head-stabilizing device, causing his head to be lacerated by one of the pins. The plaintiff suffered trauma to his neck and required mechanical assistance to breathe for six days following the accident. The Supreme Court, Appellate Division, on motion by the plaintiff, determined that summary judgment on the issue of liability was warranted. It could easily be reasoned that anesthetized patients do not fall from operating tables in the absence of negligence. The defendants, who were in joint and exclusive control of plaintiff, failed to explain their conduct in the operating room, and their failure to do so mandated summary judgment.

Tara and Donnie Reese, in *Reese v. Fort Worth Osteopathic Hospital, Inc.*,[7] are the biological parents of Clarence, a viable fetus who died in utero on May 12, 1998. Smith, Culton, and Beals were the treating physicians at the medical center where Tara sought treatment for a rapid heartbeat and dizziness prior to Clarence's death. The Reeses brought suit against the physicians on the grounds that their negligence caused Clarence's death. The physicians filed summary judgment motions contending that, as a matter of law, the parents may not recover for injury to or the death of a fetus. The trial court granted the physician's motions for summary judgment. On appeal, the appellants-parents contended the right of parents to bring a wrongful death claim for the in utero death of their viable fetus and the existence of a survival cause of action in favor of the fetus are guaranteed by the equal protection clauses of the Texas and U.S. Constitutions.

The Texas Court of Appeals found that the law permitted Tara to maintain a cause of action for medical negligence because she was the patient and was able to produce evidence of damages sufficient to defeat the appellees' summary judgment motion. Summary judgment on this issue was reversed, and the case was remanded for further proceedings. The Reeses' evidence included an affidavit by Halbridge, a board-certified specialist in obstetrics and gynecology, who stated that the physicians' failure to perform standard fetal diagnostic tests and the hospital nursing staff's failure to maintain continuous fetal rate heart monitoring proximately caused injuries to Tara. According to Halbridge, a timely Caesarean section delivery would have produced a viable child, thus avoiding what Tara described as a long and painful delivery process that produced her stillborn child.

NOTICE OF TRIAL

The examination before trial may reveal sufficient facts that would discourage the plaintiff from continuing the case or it may encourage one or both parties to settle out of court. Once a decision to go forward is reached, the case is placed on the court calendar. Postponement of the trial may be secured with the consent of both parties and the consent of the court. A case may not be postponed indefinitely without being dismissed by the court. If one party is ready to proceed and another party seeks a postponement, a valid excuse must be shown. Should a defendant fail to appear at trial, the judge can pass judgment against the defendant by default. A case also can be dismissed if the plaintiff fails to appear at trial.

MEMORANDUM OF LAW

A *memorandum of law* (or *trial brief*) presents to the court the nature of the case, cites case decisions to substantiate arguments, and aids the court regarding points of law. Trial briefs are prepared by both the plaintiff's and the defendant's attorneys. A trial brief is not required, but it is a recommended strategy. It provides the court with a basic understanding of the position of the party submitting the brief before the commencement of the trial. It also focuses the court's attention on specific legal points that may influence the court in ruling on objections and on the admissibility of evidence in the course of the trial.

THE COURT

A case is heard in the court that has jurisdiction over the subject of controversy. The judge decides questions of law and is responsible for ensuring that a trial is conducted properly in an impartial atmosphere and that it is fair to both parties of a lawsuit. He or she determines what constitutes the general standard of conduct required for the exercise of due care. The judge informs the jury of what the defendant's conduct should have been, thereby making a determination of the existence of a legal duty.

The judge decides whether evidence is admissible, charges the jury (defines the jurors' responsibility in relation to existing law), and may take a case away from the jury (by directed verdict or make a judgment notwithstanding the verdict) when he or she believes that there are no issues for the jury to consider or that the jury has erred in its decision. This right of the judge with respect to the role of the jury narrows the jury's responsibility with regard to the facts of the case. The judge maintains order throughout the suit, determines issues of procedure, and is generally responsible for the conduct of the trial.

THE JURY

The right to a trial by jury is a constitutional right, but an individual may waive the right to a jury trial. If this right is waived, the judge acts as judge and jury, becoming the trier of facts and deciding issues of law.

Members of the jury are selected from a jury list. They are summoned to court by a paper known as the *jury process.* Impartiality is a prerequisite of all jurors. The number of jurors who sit at trial is 12 in common law. If there are fewer than 12, the number must be established by statute.

Counsel for both parties of a lawsuit question each prospective jury member for impartiality, bias, and prejudicial thinking. This process is referred to as the *voir dire,* the examination of jurors. Once members of the jury are selected, they are sworn in to try the case.

The jury makes a determination of the facts that occurred, evaluating whether the plaintiff's damages were caused by the defendant's negligence and whether the defendant exercised due care. The jury makes a determination of the particular standard of conduct required in all cases in which the judgment of reasonable people might differ. The jury must pay close attention to the evidence presented by both sides to a suit in order to render a fair and impartial verdict. Jurors who fall asleep during the trial can be replaced with an alternate juror, as was the case in *Richbow v. District of Columbia.*[8]

The jury also determines the extent of damages, if any, and the degree to which the plaintiff's conduct may have contributed to his or her injury, thereby mitigating the responsibility of the defendant (contributory negligence).

A Jury Decision

A New York City jury awarded $26 million to a boy injured during surgery. What was it that so disturbed the jury that caused it to grant such a huge award? According to an article written by an alternate juror, who invited the jurors to his home three weeks after the trial:

> The defense lawyers were on their feet objecting they didn't want the jury to see Stephen. But that just raised a question for us: If his injuries were as slight as the defense had been insisting, why the resistance? The judge agreed that it was proper for Stephen to appear at his own trial, and the rear doors to the courtroom were opened.

> Most of the jurors had begun to cry. But we were also angry. The defense lawyers it seemed, had been trying to put one over on us, claiming that Stephen was a normal teenage boy with a few minor handicaps.

> For seven weeks, the jury had sat in that courtroom listening to the defense lawyers belittle Stephen's problems. We saw the doctors refuse to acknowledge Stephen's handicaps or to accept responsibility for them. To the jury at least, it seemed that the doctors had made mistakes, refused to admit them, and then tried to cover them up.[9]

SUBPOENAS

A *subpoena* is a legal order requiring the appearance of a person and/or the presentation of documents to a court or administrative body. Attorneys, judges, and certain law enforcement and administrative officials, depending on the jurisdiction, may issue subpoenas. Subpoenas generally include

- reference number
- names of plaintiff and defendant
- date, time, and place to appear
- name, address, and telephone number of opposing attorney
- documents requested if a subpoena is for records

Some jurisdictions require the service of a subpoena at a specified time in advance of the requested appearance (e.g., 24 hours). In other jurisdictions, no such time limitation exists. A court clerk, sheriff, attorney, process server, or other person as provided by state statute can serve a subpoena.

A *subpoena ad testificandum* orders the appearance of a person at a trial or other investigative proceeding to give testimony. Witnesses have a duty to appear and may suffer a penalty for contempt of court should they fail to appear.

They may not deny knowledge of a subpoena if they simply refused to accept it. The court may issue a bench warrant, ordering the appearance of a witness in court, if a witness fails to answer a subpoena. Failure to appear may be excused if extenuating circumstances exist.

A subpoena for records, known as a *subpoena duces tecum,* is a written command to bring records, documents, or other evidence described in the subpoena to a trial or other investigative proceeding. The subpoena is served on one able to produce such records. Disobedience in answering a *subpoena duces tecum* is considered contempt of court and carries a penalty of a fine or imprisonment.

BURDEN OF PROOF

The burden of proof in a criminal case requires that the evidence presented against the defendant must be beyond a reasonable doubt. Note the terminology: reasonable doubt—not all doubt. The burden of proof in a criminal case lies with the prosecution. In a civil suit, the evidence presented need only tip the scales of justice.

The burden of proof in a civil lawsuit is the obligation of the plaintiff to persuade the jury regarding the truth of his or her case. A preponderance of the credible evidence must be presented in order for a plaintiff to recover damages. *Credible evidence* is evidence that in the light of reason and common sense is worthy of belief. A preponderance of credible evidence requires that the prevailing side of the case carry more weight than the evidence on the opposing side.

The burden of proof requires that the plaintiff's attorney show that the defendant violated a legal duty by not following an acceptable standard of care and that the plaintiff suffered injury because of the defendant's breach. If the evidence presented does not support the allegations made, the case is dismissed. Where a plaintiff, who has the burden of proof, fails to sustain such burden, the case may be dismissed despite the failure of the defendant to present any evidence to the contrary on his or her behalf. The burden of proof in some states shifts from the plaintiff to the defendant when it is obvious that the injury would not have occurred unless there was negligence.

STATUTORY VIOLATION

Violation of a statute may constitute direct evidence of negligence, or it simply may voice a duty that is owed to a particular class of persons who are protected by the statute or regulation. For example, assume a regulation specifies a nurse-patient ratio of no less than one registered nurse for two patients on intensive care units. This regulation is an expression of the duty imposed on the facility to provide adequate nursing care to patients. Patients are, therefore, a class of persons identified within the regulation who are to have the benefits of the protection to be gained by having a predetermined minimum standard nurse-patient ratio.

POLICY AND PROCEDURE VIOLATIONS

Policies and procedures of a health care organization are established for the day-to-day operations. If a violation of a facility's policy and procedures cause injury to one whom the policy or procedure is designed to protect, such violation can give rise to evidence for negligent conduct.

RES IPSA LOQUITUR

Res ipsa loquitur ("the thing speaks for itself" or "circumstances speak for themselves") is the legal doctrine that shifts the burden of proof from the plaintiff to the defendant. It is an evidentiary device that allows the plaintiff to make a case legally adequate to go to the jury on the basis of well-defined circumstantial evidence even though direct evidence is lacking. This does not mean that the plaintiff has proven fully the defendant's negligence. It merely shifts the burden of going forward to the defendant who must argue to dismiss the circumstantial evidence presented as "speaking for itself."

An inference of negligence is permitted from the mere occurrence of an injury when the defendant owed a duty and possessed the sole power of preventing the injury by exercise of reasonable care. For example, the presence of severe burns on a patient's body after being bathed by an employee raises the question of negligence without the need for expert testimony. Negligence is considered so obvious that expert testimony is not necessary. It lies within a layperson's realm of knowledge that people generally do not suffer burns from a bath. That alone is sufficient to require a defendant to come forward with a rebuttal. The three elements necessary to shift the burden of proof from the plaintiff to the defendant under the doctrine of res ipsa loquitur are as follows:

1. The event would not normally have occurred in the absence of negligence.

2. The defendant must have had exclusive control over the instrumentality that caused the injury.

3. The plaintiff must not have contributed to the injury.

An action was brought against the nursing facility in *Franklin v. Collins Chapel Correctional Hospital*[10] to recover damages for the wrongful death of an 82-year-old resident. Extensive thermal burns were discovered soon after an attendant bathed the resident. The complaint sought to invoke the doctrine of res ipsa loquitur because the injuries suffered by the resident do not occur in the absence of negligence, and the deceased was in the defendant's sole care, custody, and control.

The trial court entered a judgment for the nursing facility pursuant to a jury verdict, and the administrators of the estate appealed. The appeals court held that proof that the nursing facility had exclusive control over the bath wherein burns were allegedly suffered and that the burns normally would not occur absent negligence entitled the administrators to a jury instruction on the doctrine of res ipsa loquitur. The case was reversed and remanded for a new trial.

The general rule for all cases of circumstantial evidence, both ordinary negligence cases and res ipsa loquitur cases, is that, to make his or her case, the plaintiff does not have to eliminate all other possible causes or inferences other than that of the defendant's negligence, and it is enough for him or her if the evidence makes such negligence more probable than any other cause.[11]

The patient in *Mack v. Lydia E. Hall Hospital*[12] was properly permitted to invoke the doctrine of res ipsa loquitur in her suit to recover damages for a third-degree burn on the side of her left thigh caused by an electro-coagulator used during surgery. The prerequisites for application of the doctrine were satisfied by evidence that the injury was unusual, the surgeon had exclusive control over the electro-coagulator, and the patient could not have contributed to the injury.

The oxygen mask discussed in *Gold v. Ishak*[13] caught fire during surgery. In performing surgery, the physician used an electrocautery unit provided by the hospital. At some point during surgery the oxygen mask caught on fire and the patient was injured. A claim of negligent treatment was presented to a medical review panel, which concluded that the medical providers had complied with the requisite standard of care. The plaintiff then filed a complaint against the medical providers for medical malpractice. The trial court refused to apply the doctrine of res ipsa loquitur.

On appeal, the trial court was found to have erred by refusing to apply the doctrine of res ipsa loquitur. The evidence presented at trial, as described here, clearly shows that the elements necessary for the inference of res ipsa loquitur had been established

1. The injuring instrumentality was under the management or exclusive control of the medical providers.

2. A fire under these circumstances is such that in the ordinary course of things would not have occurred if the medical providers had used proper care in relation to the electrocautery unit and oxygen mask.

3. Expert testimony is not required because a fire occurring during surgery where an instrument that emits a spark is used near a source of oxygen is not beyond the realm of the layperson to understand. It is easily understandable to the common person that careless use of the two could cause a fire and result in bodily injury.

RES IPSA LOQUITUR AND EXCLUSIVE CONTROL

Citation: *Seavers v. Methodist Medical Center of Oak Ridge*, 9 S.W.3d 86 (Tenn. 1999)

Facts

While in the intensive care unit (ICU), a nurse's note indicated that the grip in appellant-Seavers's right hand was weaker than that in her left hand. Both of her hands had been placed in wrist restraints, fastened to bed rails, to prevent her from pulling out her endotracheal tube. When the endotracheal tube was removed and the appellant could speak, she complained that her right arm was numb; Seavers had suffered severe damage to her right ulnar nerve. The appellant and her husband filed suit against the medical center, alleging that the injury was the result of the nurses negligently restraining her arm. She later amended her complaint to include the theory of res ipsa loquitur.

The medical center filed a motion for summary judgment, supported by the affidavits of two experts. Both experts opined that the nerve damage in appellant's right arm was "of unknown etiology" and that the injury could have developed during her stay in the ICU without any deviation from standards of professional care.

The appellant opposed the medical center's motion for summary judgment, arguing that there were genuine issues of material fact. The appellant's response was supported by the deposition of Natelson, a neurosurgeon, and the affidavits of both Natelson and Woodworth, a registered nurse who worked in the ICU. Both Natelson and Woodworth opined that the appellant was under the exclusive control and care of the medical center's nursing staff when the nerve injury occurred. Natelson and Woodworth stated that when treating ICU patients who are unconscious or under heavy sedation or restraint, the standard of professional care requires the protection of the patients' extremities so that injuries to the ulnar nerves do not occur. Based upon their independent review of the appellant's medical records and EMG results, they opined that the injury was the type that would not have occurred if the nursing staff had upheld the standard of care.

Finding no genuine issues of material fact, the trial court granted the medical center's motion for summary judgment. A majority of the court of appeals affirmed the trial court's order granting summary judgment for the medical center. The court of appeals held that res ipsa loquitur did not apply because the appellant's injury was not within the common knowledge of laypersons.

Issue

Does the doctrine of res ipsa loquitur apply in this case?

Holding

The doctrine of res ipsa loquitur may be applied in this case.

Reason

The parties agreed that the appellant was under the exclusive control and care of the medical center when the nerve injury occurred. The record further shows that the appellant's right arm and hand were fully functional when she entered the medical center's ICU and that no problem was detected until the ICU nurses noticed that the grip in her right hand was not as strong as the grip in her left hand. During that time, the appellant was heavily sedated, restrained, and under the complete care of the ICU nurses. Based upon EMG results, the appellant has shown that the dysfunction in her right arm resulted from damage to her right ulnar nerve. According to Natelson, this injury was likely caused by prolonged pressure on the nerve from a hard object such as a bed rail. This theory was corroborated by evidence that the appellant's arms were strapped to the hospital bed during her stay in the ICU. The appellant satisfied the res ipsa requirements under Tennessee code and raised a genuine issue of material fact on the allegation of negligence. Summary judgment in favor of the medical center was improper in this case.

Discussion

1. Was the appellant's injury within the common knowledge of laypersons? Discuss your answer.
2. What procedures should the medical center implement to reduce the likelihood of similar occurrences?

OPENING STATEMENTS

During the opening statement, the plaintiff's attorney attempts to prove the wrongdoing of the defendant by presenting credible evidence favorable to his or her client. The *opening statement* by the plaintiff's attorney provides, in capsule form, the facts of the case, what he or she intends to prove by means of a summary of the evidence to be presented, and a description of the damages to his or her client. Opening statements are prepared so that each jury member can sympathize with the plaintiff, relate to the injustice, and then see it happening to themselves. The opening statement must be concise and to the point.

The defense attorney makes his or her opening statement indicating the position of the defendant and the points of the plaintiff's case he or she intends to refute. The defense attorney explains the facts as they apply to the case for the defendant.

EXAMINATION OF WITNESSES

After conclusion of the opening statements, the judge calls for the plaintiff's witnesses. An officer of the court administers an oath to each witness, and direct examination begins. The attorney obtains information from each witness in the form of questions. On cross-examination by the defense, an attempt is made to challenge or discredit the plaintiff's witness. Redirect examination by the plaintiff's attorney can follow the cross-examination, if so desired. The plaintiff's attorney may at this time wish to have his or her witness review an important point that the jury may have forgotten during cross-examination. The plaintiff's attorney may ask the same witness more questions in an effort to overcome the effect of the cross-examination. Recross-examination may take place, if necessary, for the defense of the defendant.

A sampling of preliminary questions that a physician might expect to be asked on a personal injury case, for example, may take the following form:

- Please state your name, residence, and any prior residences.

- Where did you attend medical school?

- Are you licensed in this state?

- Where did you serve your internship?

- Where did you serve your residency?

- Is your practice general or special?

- Are you board certified in one or more specialties?

- How does a physician obtain board certification?

- Are you presently practicing medicine?

- How long have you been in practice?

- During your _____ years of practice, have you had occasion to treat a good number of personal injury cases?

- On or about _____ did you have occasion to see the patient on a professional basis?

- Where? Describe the patient's condition at the time.

- What, if anything, did you do on that occasion?

- Have you been the attending physician since that date?

- Describe the nature of the examination that you made on the patient and any others from time to time since then.

- Did you see the patient daily, several times a day at first?

- Did you continue to see the patient? How often?

- Of what, generally, did your treatment consist?

- From your examination and treatment of the patient, did you determine what injuries were sustained?

- As a result of your examination, did you find it necessary to seek consultation from another physician or specialist?

- Did there come a time when you found it necessary to transfer the patient to another health care facility?

The credibility of a witness may be impeached if prior statements are inconsistent with later statements or if there is bias in favor of a party or prejudice against a party to a lawsuit. Either attorney to a lawsuit may ask the judge for permission to recall a witness.

After all the witnesses of the plaintiff have testified, the defense may call its witnesses, and the process of direct, cross, redirect, and recross-examination is repeated until the defense rests.

EVIDENCE

Evidence consists of the facts proved or disproved during a lawsuit. The law of evidence is a body of rules under which facts are proved. The rules of evidence govern the admission of items of proof in a lawsuit. A fact can be proven by either circumstantial or direct evidence. Evidence must be competent, relevant, and material to be admitted at trial.

Direct Evidence

Direct evidence is proof offered through direct testimony. It is the jury's function to receive testimony presented by witnesses and to draw conclusions in the determination of the facts of a case.

Demonstrative Evidence

Demonstrative (*real*) *evidence* is proof furnished by things themselves. It is considered the most trustworthy and preferred type of evidence. It consists of tangible objects to which testimony refers (e.g., medical instruments and broken infusion needles) that can be requested by a jury. Demonstrative evidence is admissible in court if it is relevant, has probative value, and serves the interest of justice. It is not admissible if it will prejudice, mislead, confuse, offend, inflame, or arouse the sympathy or passion of the jury. Other forms of demonstrative evidence include photographs, motion pictures, X-ray films, drawings, human bodies as exhibits, pathology slides, fetal monitoring strips, safety committee minutes, infection committee reports, medical staff bylaws, rules and regulations, nursing policy and procedure manuals, census data, and staffing patterns. The plaintiff's attorney uses all pertinent evidence to reconstruct chronologically the care and treatment rendered.

When presenting photographs as a form of evidence, the photographer or a reliable witness who is familiar with the object photographed must testify that the picture is an accurate representation and a fair likeness of the object portrayed. The photograph must not exaggerate a client's physical condition. Such exaggeration could unfairly prejudice a jury. Photographs can be valuable legal evidence when they illustrate graphically the nature and extent of a medical injury. Motion pictures also are valuable evidence. The same principles that apply to photographs apply to motion pictures. Motion pictures must be accurately portrayed. The cutting and/or splicing of videos are suspect and may have no probative value. Videotape is admissible in court, assuming the matter being taped, the time of the taping, and the manner in which such taping took place can be authenticated.

Imaging films are considered pictures of the interior of the object portrayed and are admissible under the same requirements as photographs and motion pictures. Competent evidence must be offered to show that the films are those of the patient, the object, or body part under consideration; that the films were made in a recognized manner, taken by a competent technician; and that they were interpreted by a competent physician trained to read the films. The value of films is that they illustrate fractures, foreign objects, and so forth.

Where an issue as to personal injuries is involved, an injured person may be permitted to exhibit to the jury the wound or injury, or the member or portion of his body upon which such wound or injury was inflicted, and if relevant, the exhibition is allowable in the discretion of the court where there is no reason to expect that the sympathy of the jury will be excited. The human body is considered the best evidence as to the nature and extent of the alleged injury/injuries. If there is no controversy about either the nature or the extent of an injury, presenting such evidence could be considered prejudicial, and an objection can be made as to its presentation to a jury.

Demonstrations are permitted in some instances to illustrate the extent of injuries. The resident in *Hendricks v. Sanford*[14] developed serious bed sores on her back. The defendant objected to the offer of the plaintiff to display her back to the jury. The court found that the plaintiff's injuries, which had healed, were completely relevant as evidence. Even though the injuries had healed and a skin graft had been performed, a declivity of about three and a half inches in diameter and about the depth of a shallow ashtray was still discernible on the plaintiff's back.

Documentary Evidence

Documentary evidence is written information capable of making a truthful statement (e.g., drug manufacturer inserts, autopsy reports, birth certificates, and medical records). Documentary evidence must satisfy the jury as to authenticity. Proof of authenticity is not necessary if the opposing party accepts its genuineness. In some instances (e.g., wills), witnesses are necessary. In the case of documentation, the original of a document must be produced unless it can be demonstrated that the original has been lost or destroyed, in which case a properly authenticated copy may be substituted.

A sampling of preliminary questions that a witness might be asked on entering a medical record into evidence includes the following:

- Please state your name.
- Where are you employed?
- What is your position?
- What is your official title?
- Did you receive a subpoena for certain records?
- Did you bring those records with you?
- Can you identify these records?
- Did you retrieve the records yourself?
- Are these the complete records?
- Are these the original records or copies of the originals?
- How were these records prepared?
- Are these records maintained under your care, custody, and control?
- Were these records made in the regular course of business?
- Was the record made at the time the act, condition, or event occurred or transpired?
- Is this record regularly kept or maintained?

A manufacturer's drug insert or manual describing the proper use of medical equipment is generally admissible in court as evidence. In *Mueller v. Mueller,*[15] a physician was sued by a patient who charged that she had suffered a deterioration of bone structure and ultimately a collapsed hip as a result of the administration of cortisone over an extended period of time. The jury decided that the physician's prolonged use of cortisone was negligent, and the physician appealed. The appeals court held that the manufacturer's recommendations are not only admissible but also essential in determining a physician's possible lack of proper care.

In another case, *Mulligan v. Lederle Laboratories,*[16] the plaintiff, a medical laboratory technician, brought an action against the drug manufacturer as the result of the side effects of the drug Varidase. The plaintiff developed several chronic health problems including mouth sores, microscopic hematuria, and red cell cast, indicating kidney disease. The trial court awarded $50,000 in compensatory damages and $100,000 in punitive damages for the drug manufacturer's failure to warn of the side effects of Varidase. On appeal by the manufacturer, the appeals court held that the products liability action was not barred by a three-year statute of limitations contained in an Arkansas products-liability act and that the evidence was sufficient to award punitive damages. Evidence presented at trial indicated that several side effects were associated with the drug.

Judicial Notice Rule

The judicial notice rule prescribes that well-known facts (e.g., that fractures need prompt attention and that two X-rays of the same patient may show different results) need not be proven, but, rather, they are recognized by the court as fact. If a fact can be disputed, the rule does not apply.

The use of X-rays as a diagnostic aid in cases of fracture can be considered a matter of common knowledge to which a court, in the absence of expert testimony, can take judicial notice. Should a patient have a serious fall and a fracture is indicated, under the foregoing rule, it is a matter of common knowledge that the ordinary physician in good standing, in the exercise of ordinary care and diligence, would have ordered X-rays.

The patient-plaintiff in *Arthur v. St. Peter's Hospital*[17] sought treatment in the emergency department of St. Peter's Hospital after an injury to his left wrist. After being examined, he was sent to the radiology department for X-rays of his wrist. He later was released after being advised that there were no fractures. Due to continued swelling and pain, the plaintiff decided to seek care from another physician, who subsequently diagnosed a fracture of the navicular bone. The plaintiff sued and the hospital motioned for summary judgment, stating that the physicians were independent contractors and not employees of the hospital.

Copies of the emergency department record, X-ray report, and billing record contained the logo of the hospital. There was nothing on the records to identify the physicians as being independent contractors. The court took judicial notice, finding that people who seek medical help through emergency departments of hospitals are unaware of the status of the different professionals working there. Unless a patient had been put, in some manner, on notice that those physicians with whom he might come into contact during the course of his treatment were independent contractors, it would be natural to assume that they were employees of the hospital.

Hearsay Evidence

Hearsay evidence is based on what another has said or done and is not the result of the personal knowledge of the witness. *Hearsay* consists of written and oral statements. When a witness testifies to the utterance of a statement made outside court and the statement is offered in court for the truth of the facts that are contained in the statement, this is hearsay and therefore objectionable.

The court in *Costal Health Services, Inc. v. Rozier*[18] held that a written report by an ombudsman (who did not testify at trial) concerning injuries and treatment of an 85-year-old patient was inadmissible as evidence. It contained hearsay accounts of conversations as well as impressions, opinions, and conclusions regarding the nursing facility's negligence when a patient wandered into another patient's room and was injured by that resident. However, the court found that the testimony about one patient's own account of his violent past, made to the nursing home personnel upon his admission, was admissible as original evidence, not as proof of the

actual prior incidents, but to show the defendant's notice of the possibility of violent behavior on the part of that patient.

If a statement is offered not as proof of the facts asserted in the statement but rather only to show that the statement was made, the statement can come into evidence. For example, if it is relevant that a conversation took place, the testimony relating to the conversation may be entered as evidence. The purpose of that testimony would be to establish that a conversation took place and not to prove what was said during the course of the conversation. If testimony is based on personal knowledge, it would be admissible as evidence.

Because of the ability to challenge hearsay evidence successfully, which rests on the credibility of the witness as well as on the competency and veracity of other persons not before the court, it is admitted as evidence in a trial under very strict rules.

There are many exceptions to the hearsay rule that allow testimony that ordinarily would not be admitted. Included in the list of exceptions are admissions made by one of the parties to the action, threats made by a victim, dying declarations, statements to refresh a witness's recollection if he or she is unable to remember the facts known earlier, business records, medical records, and other official records (e.g., certified copies of birth and death records). "Where hearsay evidence is admitted without objection, its probative value is for the jury to determine."[19] This list of exceptions to hearsay evidence is by no means all-inclusive, and therefore state statutes should be consulted.

A police officer's testimony that he overheard a drug dealer tell an informant, who was wearing a concealed transmitter, that he could obtain drugs for the informant from a pharmacist friend was properly admitted in a disciplinary proceeding in *Brown v. Idaho State Board of Pharmacy.*[20] The testimony was presented before the Idaho State Board of Pharmacy for proving a dealer's state of mind and explaining his subsequent visit to the pharmacy. The testimony was not subject to hearsay objection.

⚖ **HEARSAY AND LOST CHANCE OF SURVIVAL**

Citation: *Stroud v. Golson,* 741 So. 2d 182 (La. App. 2d Cir. June 16, 1999)

Facts

Dr. Mikey examined Stroud. After viewing X-rays, Mikey told Stroud that she might have lung cancer and referred her to Dr. Gullatt for follow-up care. A

CT scan was performed at St. Francis Medical Center and the findings were interpreted by a radiologist, Dr. Golson, who interpreted Stroud's CT scan as negative for lung cancer.

Approximately one year later, Stroud was hospitalized at St. Francis for a cerebral hemorrhage. X-rays and CT scans revealed inoperative cancer in Stroud's left lung.

Stroud was discharged from St. Francis and later died as a result of the cancer. The decedent's husband and sons filed a suit seeking damages arising from Golson's failure to properly interpret Stroud's CT scan. Before trial, the plaintiffs settled with Golson and his insurer.

On February 23, 1998, a trial by jury commenced against the Patients' Compensation Fund (PCF), which admitted medical negligence but claimed that Stroud would have died from the fast-acting cancer even if it had been diagnosed earlier. The jury returned a verdict finding that Stroud lost a less-than-even chance of survival because of Golson's negligence.

Issue

Did the trial judge err when overruled the hearsay objection regarding Stroud's testimony?

Holding

The appeals court found no abuse of discretion by the trial court.

Reason

Stroud suffered a great deal of mental anguish from the hopeless condition she faced, knowing that earlier detection was lost because her CT scan was not properly read. Her decision not to undergo the painful and debilitating chemotherapy, when the odds were so stacked against her recovery, was justified. It is a reasonable conclusion that Stroud would have, in all likelihood, opted for the treatment had the cancer been properly diagnosed earlier.

The defendant argued that the trial judge erred when he overruled the hearsay objection regarding Mr. Stroud's testimony concerning his wife's rea-

sons for declining treatment after her cancer was diagnosed. The testimony at issue centered around the following:

Mr. Thomas: Now, did your wife discuss—you—you and your wife discuss whether or not she should have treatment for her cancer?

Mr. Stroud: Yes, we did.

Mr. Thomas: And were you a part in making a decision with her with why she did not agree to have treatment?

Mr. Stroud: Yes.

Mr. Thomas: Share with the jury what she said about that.

Mr. Stroud: She, ah,—

Mr. Anzelmo: Your Honor, I object to hearsay.

The Court: I understand. But, I think it—It is hearsay but it's reliable. I'll allow it.

Mr. Thomas: Go ahead.

Mr. Stroud: Ah, I had a—My sister passed away in November '94 with lung cancer, and she found out in July of '94 that she had lung cancer. So she went and took the radium treatments, and she weighed 125 pounds and was eating and doing all right until she started taking the radium treatments, and by the end of the radium treatments she could hardly get about, and actually she just laid down and starved herself to death. She weighed 65 pounds when she passed away, and was bedridden all that time. And the wife felt that it was too far gone in her for any treatments to do any good, plus what few days she had left she didn't want to be like my sister.

Stroud's testimony regarding statements his wife made were statements of her then-existing state of mind. The testimony showed the motive behind Stroud's decision not to receive treatment; namely, her belief that the treatments would not be effective, as well as her desire to avoid the severe pain and discomfort that can accompany chemotherapy.

Discussion

1. Discuss how the court viewed hearsay evidence in this case.
2. Discuss under what circumstances the courts sustain objection to the entry of hearsay into evidence.

Medical Books as Hearsay Evidence

Medical books are considered hearsay because the authors are not generally available for cross-examination. Although medical books are not admissible as evidence, a physician may testify as to how he or she formed an opinion and what part textbooks played in forming that opinion. During cross-examination, medical experts may be asked to comment on statements from medical books that contradict their testimony.

EXPERT TESTIMONY

It is the jury's function to receive testimony presented by witnesses and draw conclusions in the determination of facts. The law recognizes that a jury is composed of ordinary men and women and that some fact-finding will involve subjects beyond their knowledge. When a jury cannot otherwise obtain sufficient facts from which to draw conclusions, an expert witness who has special knowledge, skill, experience, or training can be called on to submit an opinion. The expert witness assists the jury when the issues to be resolved in the case are outside the experience of the average juror.

Laypeople are quite able to render opinions about a great variety of general subjects, but for technical questions the opinion of an expert is necessary. At the time of testifying, each expert's training, experience, and special qualifications will be explained to the jury. The experts will be asked to give an opinion concerning hypothetical questions based on the facts of the case. Should the testimony of two experts conflict, the jury will determine which expert opinion to accept. Expert witnesses may be used to assist a plaintiff in proving the wrongful act of a defendant or to assist a defendant in refuting such evidence. In addition, expert testimony may be used to show the extent of the plaintiff's damages or to show the lack of such damages. To qualify as an expert witness in a specified area, that person must have the appropriate training, experience, and qualifications necessary to explain and/or answer questions based on the facts of a particular case.

Pharmacist Not Always Qualified as an Expert

The pharmacist in *Nail v. Laros*[21] was found not competent to render an expert opinion regarding the proper standard of care required of a physician practicing a medical specialty. The patient, Mrs. Nail, developed a staphylococcal infection following spinal surgery. The orthopedic surgeon, Dr. Laros, treated the patient with the antibiotic Ansef for six days. The patient was released from the hospital without any sign of an infection. The patient, while under the treatment of an orthopedic surgeon (Hanley), was discovered through blood tests to have contracted a staphylococcal infection at the operative site. The patient eventually developed osteomyelitis. She brought a lawsuit against Laros for negligence in diagnosing and treating her infection. Nail obtained an affidavit from a pharmacist (Neff) who stated an opinion that Laros should have treated the patient for a longer period of time on Ansef and that his failure to do so was the proximate cause of Nail's staph infection found by Hanley. The court reasoned that there was nothing in the record to support the pharmacist's claim of being an expert in this case. Neither his education nor his training qualified him to be an expert on equal footing with a board-certified orthopedic surgeon in diagnosing and treating infections associated with surgical implants. The court of appeals took judicial notice by ruling that the pharmacist cannot legally prescribe medication, and is even prohibited from dispensing a dangerous drug, which by definition includes Ansef, without a valid prescription from a practitioner.

Expert Testimony Not Necessary

Not all negligence cases require testimony from an expert witness. Citing *Donovan v. State,* "If a doctor operates on the wrong limb or amputates the wrong limb, a plaintiff would not have to introduce expert testimony to establish that the doctor was negligent. On the other hand, highly technical questions of diagnoses and causation which lie beyond the understanding of a layperson require introduction of expert testimony."[22]

Surgical Sponge Left in Patient

Expert testimony was not required in *Powell v. Mullins,*[23] in which a surgical lap sponge was left in the abdomen of a patient during the performance of a cesarean section. Testimony of an expert witness generally is not required when an understanding of the physician's alleged lack of skill or due care requires only common knowledge or experience. The Alabama Supreme Court held that it was the physician's responsibility to remove all sponges from inside the patient before closing the incision.

Patient Falls

In medical malpractice cases where lack of care or want of skill is so gross as to be apparent, or the alleged breach relates to noncomplex matters of diagnosis and treatment within the understanding of lay jurors by resort to common knowledge and experience, failure to present expert testimony on the accepted standard of care and degree of skill under such circumstances is not fatal to a plaintiff's prima facie case showing of negligence. The court in *McGraw v. St. Joseph's Hospital*[24] reviewed cases addressing hospital fall incidents and found that a majority of jurisdictions do not require expert testimony in such cases where for example, a

- bed rail is left down contrary to the physician's order and the patient falls and is injured

- patient is known to be in weakened condition and is left alone in a shower and falls

- nurse fails to respond to a sedated patient's call and the patient gets out of bed and falls

A hospital owes the patient a duty to exercise reasonable care in rendering care and, in the performance of such duty, due regard must be given to the mental and physical condition of the patient of which the hospital, in the exercise of reasonable care, should have knowledge. If a patient requires professional care, then expert testimony as to the standard of care is necessary. The standard of nonmedical, administrative, ministerial, or routine care in a hospital need not be established by expert testimony. A jury is competent from its own experience to determine and apply a reasonable-care standard.

Negligent Insertion of an IV

The patient, Ms. Welte, in *Welte v. Bello,*[25] was admitted to the hospital for surgery. Approximately three hours prior to surgery, Welte conferred with her surgeon about the procedure. She then conferred with her anesthesiologist, Dr. Bello, who informed her that he would be administering sodium pentothal through an IV inserted into a vein in her arm. He told her about the potential risks associated with general anesthesia. Welte read and signed a consent form for surgery, administration of anesthetics, and the rendering of other medical services. Both Welte and Bello signed the consent form. Prior to surgery, a nurse inserted a catheter into the vein of Welte's right arm. Welte complained of pain after the IV was inserted. The nurse checked the IV and concluded that it was properly positioned. Bello began injecting drugs through a port in the IV. Bello then rechecked the site of the IV and noticed swelling on Welte's arm near the point at which the IV had been inserted. As a consequence of the sodium pentothal infiltration of the tissues surrounding the vein, Welte sustained first-, second-, and third-degree burns, resulting in a large, permanent scar.

Welte and her husband commenced two separate malpractice actions, one against the hospital and another against Bello. The separate suits were consolidated for trial. Prior to trial, Bello filed a motion for summary judgment, claiming that Welte failed to retain a qualified expert to testify against him and, therefore, they would be precluded from offering any expert testimony at trial. Welte argued that the tort claim of failure to obtain an informed consent did not require expert testimony. The trial court concluded that any alleged negligence of the anesthesiologist was not so obvious as to be within the comprehension of a layperson.

On appeal, the Iowa Supreme Court held that expert testimony was not required to establish a claim against Bello. The chemical burn to Welte's arm was caused by sodium pentothal that the anesthesiologist injected into the patient's vein, which then infiltrated or escaped from the vein into the surrounding tissues. The insertion of a needle into a vein is a common medical procedure, one that has become so common that laypersons know certain occurrences would not take place if ordinary care were used. Even Bello's expert testified in his deposition that in the usual course of events, an IV inserted for the purpose of anesthesia does not infiltrate surrounding tissue.

DEFENSES AGAINST PLAINTIFF'S ALLEGATIONS

Once a plaintiff's case has been established, the defendant may put forward a defense against the claim for damages. The defendant's case is presented to discredit the plaintiff's cause of action and prevent recovery of damages. This section covers the defenses available to defendants in a negligence suit. These are principles of law that may relieve a defendant from liability.

Ignorance of Fact and Unintentional Wrongs

Ignorance of the law excuses no man; not that all men know the law, but because it is an excuse every man will plead, and no man can tell how to confute him.

John Selden (1584–1654)

Ignorance of the law is not a defense otherwise an individual would be rewarded by pleading ignorance. Arguing that a negligent act is unintentional is no defense. If such a defense were acceptable, all defendants would use it.

Assumption of the Risk

Assumption of the risk is knowing that a danger exists and voluntarily accepting the risk by exposing oneself to it, aware that harm might occur. Assumption of the risk may be implicitly assumed, as in alcohol consumption, or expressly assumed, as in relation to warnings found on cigarette packaging.

This defense provides that the plaintiff expressly has given consent in advance, relieving the defendant of an obligation of conduct toward the plaintiff and taking the chances of injury from a known risk arising from the defendant's conduct. For example, one who agrees to care for a patient with a communicable disease and then contracts the disease would not be entitled to recover from the patient for damages suffered. In taking the job, the individual agreed to assume the risk of infection, thereby releasing the patient from all legal obligations.

The following two requirements must be established in order for a defendant to be successful in an assumption of the risk defense:

1. the plaintiff must know and understand the risk that is being incurred

2. the choice to incur the risk must be free and voluntary

The patient in *Faile v. Bycura*[26] was awarded $75,000 in damages on her allegations that a podiatrist used inappropriate techniques during an unsuccessful attempt to treat her heel spurs. On appeal, it was held that the trial court erred in striking the podiatrist's defense of assumption of the risk. Evidence established that the patient signed consent forms that indicated the risks of treatment as well as alternative treatment modalities.

Contributory Negligence

A person is contributorily negligent when that person does not exercise reasonable care for his or her own safety. As a general proposition, if a person has knowledge of a dangerous situation and disregards the danger, then the person is contributorily negligent. Actual knowledge of the danger of injury is not necessary for a person to be contributorily negligent. It is sufficient if a reasonable person should have been aware of the possibility of the danger.

In some jurisdictions, contributory negligence, no matter how slight, is sufficient to defeat a plaintiff's claim. Generally, the defense of contributory negligence has been recognized in a medical malpractice action when the patient has: (1) failed to follow a medical instruction, (2) refused or neglected prescribed treatment, or (3) intentionally given erroneous, incomplete, or misleading information that is the basis for medical care or treatment of the patient.

The elements necessary to establish contributory negligence are: (1) the plaintiff's conduct fell below the required standard of personal care, and (2) there is a causal connection between the plaintiff's careless conduct and the plaintiff's injury. Thus, the defendant contends that some, if not all, liability is attributable to the plaintiff's own actions. To establish a defense of contributory negligence, the defendant must show that the plaintiff's negligence was an active and efficient contributing cause of the injury. This was not the case in *Bird v. Pritchard*,[27] in which the plaintiff, on July 3, 1970, slipped and fell, cutting her right hand on a mayonnaise jar and thus injuring the ulnar nerve. She was taken to Hocking Valley Memorial Hospital where she requested the services of Dr. Najm, a board-certified general surgeon. However, he was not available. The defendant, an osteopathic surgeon, was available, and he treated the patient's wound. The patient complained that the fourth and fifth fingers of her right hand were numb. The defendant cleaned the wound and advised the patient to see him on Monday, July 7. The patient did not return to the osteopathic surgeon but went to see Najm that same Monday. A suit was filed, the court of common pleas rendered a judgment for the defendant, and the plaintiff appealed. The court of appeals held that the patient could not be found to have been contributorily negligent or to have assumed the risk. By the time of her scheduled visit, it was impossible to perform primary or secondary repair of the injured nerves that had not been treated on the initial visit when she had first complained of numbness. For contributory negligence to defeat the claim of the plaintiff, there must not only be negligent conduct by the plaintiff but also a direct and proximate causal relationship between the negligent act and the injury the plaintiff received.

The Delaware Supreme Court affirmed a lower court's dismissal of a wrongful death action against a medical center's emergency department personnel in *Rochester v. Katalan*.[28] The decedent, Rochester, and a friend had been brought to the emergency department at approximately 6:30 P.M. under the custody of two police officers.

Rochester and his friend, claiming to be heroin addicts suffering withdrawal symptoms, requested some form of medication. Rochester stated that he had a habit requiring four to five bags of heroin a day. His actions were symptomatic of withdrawal. He and his friend were loud, abusive, and uncooperative. Rochester complained of abdominal pains, his eyes appeared glassy, and his body was shaking, among other symptoms that he exhibited. The physician on duty in the emergency department asked whether Rochester had ever participated in a methadone clinic program. Rochester indicated that he had, but that he had dropped out of it because he found a new supply source for heroin. The physician then ordered the administration of 40 mg of methadone. Rochester began beating his head against a wall claiming that he was still sick and needed more methadone. The plea was granted, and the physician ordered a second dose of 40 mg of methadone. After eventually calming down, Rochester was taken to a cell by police officers. The following morning it was impossible to awaken him, and he was later pronounced dead. It was discovered that he had never been an addict or on a methadone program. Rather, the previous night he had been drinking beer and taking Librium. He had not told this to hospital authorities. Rochester's estate sued the physician, and the trial court dismissed the suit. The appellate court affirmed, saying that by Rochester's failure to provide the physician accurate information, he had contributed to his own death. On appeal, the plaintiff argued that the physician and staff could have done more to determine the truth of Rochester's assertions that he was a drug addict. The Delaware Supreme Court held that it already had assumed negligence in that respect. Rochester contributed to his own death by failing to provide a true account of the facts to the emergency department staff. He was guilty of negligent conduct, more accurately "willful" or "intentional" conduct, which was the proximate cause of his death, resulting from multiple drug intoxication. His estate was barred from recovering any monetary damages.

The patient, Cammatte, in *Jenkins v. Bogalusa Community Medical Center,*[29] was admitted to Bogalusa Community Medical Center on September 11 for the treatment of a severe gouty arthritic condition. He had been advised not to get out of bed without first ringing for assistance. On the morning of September 16, he got out of bed without ringing for assistance and went to a bathroom across the hall. As he returned to his room, he fell and fractured his hip. Cammatte was transferred to Touro Infirmary in New Orleans where he underwent hip surgery and died on October 5, during recuperation, caused by an apparent pulmonary embolism. The trial court entered judgment for the defendants, and the plaintiffs appealed. The appeals court found that the patient was in full possession of his faculties at the time he fell and fractured his hip. The accident was the result of the patient's knowing failure to follow instructions not to get out of bed without ringing for assistance. The injury in this case was not the result of any breach of the institution's duty to exercise due care.

The rationale for contributory negligence is based on the principle that all persons must be both careful and responsible for their acts. A plaintiff is required to conform to the broad standard of conduct of the reasonable person. The plaintiff's negligence will be determined and governed by the same tests and rules as the negligence of the defendant. A person incurs the risk of injury if he knew of a danger, understood the risk involved, and voluntarily exposed himself to such danger.

Good Samaritan Statutes

Various states have enacted Good Samaritan laws, which relieve physicians, nurses, dentists, and other health care professionals, and, in some instances, laypersons, from lia-

bility in certain emergency situations. Good Samaritan legislation encourages health care professionals to render assistance at the scene of emergencies. The language that grants immunity also supports the conclusion that the physician, nurse, or layperson who is covered by the act will be protected from liability for ordinary negligence in rendering assistance in an emergency.

Under most statutes, immunity is granted only during an emergency or when rendering emergency care. The concept of *emergency* usually refers to a combination of unforeseen circumstances that require spontaneous action to avoid impending danger. Some states have sought to be more precise regarding what constitutes an emergency or accident. According to the Alaska statute 09.65.090(a), the emergency circumstances must suggest that the giving of aid is the only alternative to death or serious bodily injury.

Apparently, this provision was inserted to emphasize that the actions of a Good Samaritan must be voluntary. To be legally immune under the Good Samaritan laws, a physician or nurse must render help voluntarily and without expectation of later pay.

⚖️ **GOOD SAMARITAN STATUTE: NOT APPLICABLE IF THERE IS A PREEXISTING DUTY TO CARE**

Citation: *Deal v. Kearney,* 851 P.2d 1353 (Alaska 1993)

Facts

The plaintiff, Kearney, suffered a life-threatening injury and was taken by ambulance to the emergency department of Kodiak Island Hospital (KIH). Kearney was examined by the on-call emergency department physician, a family practitioner. It was determined that a surgical consultation was necessary and Deal, a surgeon with staff privileges at the hospital, was called. After ordering certain tests, Deal was of the opinion that Kearney could not survive a transfer to Anchorage. Deal then performed emergency surgery that lasted over nine hours, ending the following morning.

The plaintiff was eventually transferred to Anchorage. His condition worsened, and he suffered loss of circulation and tissue death in both legs. The plaintiff alleged that the KIH was negligent in failing to properly evacuate him to Anchorage. Kearney reached a settlement totaling $510,000. He also brought an action against Deal for negligent acts. Deal moved for summary judgment claiming to be immune from suit under the Good Samaritan statute.

The trial court denied Deal's motion for summary judgment, ruling that the Good Samaritan statute was not applicable to Deal because he was acting under a preexisting duty to render emergency care to Kearney. Deal petitioned for review, and his petition was granted.

The superior court held that the immunity provided by the Good Samaritan statute is unavailable to physicians with a preexisting duty to respond to emergency situations. The court concluded that Deal was under a preexisting duty in the instant case by virtue of his contract with KIH, the duty being part of the consideration that Deal gave to KIH in exchange for staff privileges at the hospital. The court further found that the Good Samaritan statute did not apply to Deal in any event, because the actions allegedly constituting malpractice occurred during the follow-up care and treatment given Kearney after surgery. By then, the court reasoned, Deal had become Kearney's treating physician, and was no longer responding to an emergency situation. Deal appealed to the Alaska Supreme Court.

Issue

Does the Good Samaritan statute extend immunity to physicians who have a preexisting duty to render emergency care?

Holding

The Alaska Supreme Court held that the Good Samaritan statute does not extend immunity to physicians who have preexisting duty to render emergency care.

Reason

Alaska Statute 09.65.090(a) states:

A person at a hospital or any other location who renders emergency care or emergency counseling to an injured, ill, or emotionally distraught person who reasonably appears to be in immediate need of emergency aid in order to avoid serious harm or death is not liable for civil damages as a result of an act or omission in rendering emergency aid.

The legislature clearly intended this provision to encourage health care providers, including medical professionals, to administer emergency medical care, whether in a hospital or not, to persons who are not their patients, by immunizing them from civil liability. The clear inference of this recommendation is that the statute would not cover those with a preexisting duty to care.

Discussion

1. Do you agree with the court's interpretation of the Alaska Statute 09.65.090(a)? Explain.
2. Discuss the legal implications if the court had ruled that the Alaska statute could be interpreted as extending immunity to physicians who have a preexisting duty to render emergency care.

Emergency Assistance

A physician who responds to an emergency call by a surgeon to assist in the completion of a tubal ligation, for example, most likely will be immune from a negligence claim under the state's Good Samaritan law if he or she had a good-faith belief that the patient was in a life-threatening situation. Such was the case in *Pemberton v. Dharmani*,[30] where the court of appeals held that the Michigan Good Samaritan statute merely requires a good-faith belief by health care personnel that they are attending a life-threatening emergency in order to be cloaked with the immunity provided by the statute, regardless of whether a life-threatening emergency actually exists. To construe the statute otherwise would controvert the purpose of the statute and render it meaningless. Health care personnel would be discouraged from giving treatment in emergency situations if an actual life-threatening situation were required to exist before they would be cloaked with immunity. Treatment may be even delayed in a given case, worsening the condition of the patient by waiting until the patient is in an obviously life-threatening situation before rendering treatment.[31]

Borrowed Servant Doctrine

The borrowed servant doctrine is a special application of the doctrine of respondeat superior and applies when an employer lends an employee to another for a particular employment. Although an employee remains the servant of the employer, under the borrowed servant doctrine, the employer is not liable for injury negligently caused by the servant while in the special service of another. For example, in certain situations, a nurse employed by a hospital may be considered the employee of the physician. In these situations, the physician is the special or temporary employer and is liable for the negligence of the nurse. To determine whether a physician is liable for the negligence of a nurse, it must be established that the physician had the right to control and direct the nurse at the time of the negligent act. If the physician is found to be in exclusive control and if the nurse is deemed to be the physician's temporary special employee, the hospital is not generally liable for the nurse's negligent acts.

Hospital Responsible for Resident's Negligence

The hospital in *Brickner v. Osteopathic Hospital*[32] was held vicariously liable for a surgical resident's failure to diagnose testicular cancer during exploratory surgery performed under the supervision of a staff physician. The hospital was not insulated from liability under the borrowed servant doctrine even though the supervising surgeon had authority over the resident during the operation. The hospital never relinquished control over the resident, who was required under the hospital's training program to assist in diagnosis and who could have taken a biopsy without express instructions of the operating surgeon. Liability was not precluded because of the hospital's lack of actual control over the resident's medical decision not to perform a biopsy. The resident was performing a service for which he had been employed.

Physician Not Liable for Technician's Negligence

Oberzan brought a medical malpractice action against a hospital radiologist, Dr. Smith, for injuries allegedly incurred because of an X-ray technician's negligence in performing a barium enema.[33] The plaintiff alleged that Smith or Davis, the X-ray technician, perforated his rectum during a barium enema procedure. Davis inserted the enema tip into the rectum of the plaintiff for the barium enema before Smith entered the X-ray room for the procedure. After Smith entered the room, the exam began. Immediately after Davis began injecting the barium, she noticed bleeding at the tip of the rectum.

Oberzan claimed the physician was vicariously liable for the employee's negligent conduct. The Kansas Supreme Court held that the respondeat superior doctrine did not apply to the relationship between the technician employed by the hospital and the radiologist so as to impose vicarious liability on the radiologist.

Davis was not an employee of Smith. She was not under his direct supervision and control at the time the injury occurred. Smith did not select Davis to perform the insertion of the enema tip; she was assigned by the hospital. A master-servant relationship was not established because Smith was not exercising personal control or supervision over Davis.

Oberzan argued that Kansas law K.A.R. 28-34-86(a) ("the radiology department and all patient services rendered therein shall be under the supervision of a designated medical staff physician; wherever possible, this physician shall be attending or consulting radiologist") imposes a duty on radiologists to supervise patient services rendered in a hospital radiology department. However, none of the statute's subsections require that the preparation of a patient for a barium enema be performed under a physician's direct supervision. The purpose of K.A.R. 28-34-12(c) is to establish an administrative head for the radiology department. Oberzan cited no authority in support of his position that the Kansas statute created a legal duty for a designated medical staff physician to personally control and supervise all activities that occur in a radiology department. Such an interpretation of the statute would create physician liability extending far beyond the intent of the regulation.

Captain of the Ship Doctrine

In the context of the operating room, the application of the borrowed servant doctrine generally is referred to as the *captain of the ship doctrine.* Historically, under this doctrine, the surgeon was viewed as being the one in command in the operating room. The rationale for this concept was provided in the Minnesota case of *St. Paul-Mercury Indemnity Co. v. St. Joseph Hospital,* when the court stated:

> [t]he desirability of the rule is obvious. The patient is completely at the mercy of the surgeon and relies upon him to see that all the acts relative to the operation are performed in a careful manner. It is the surgeon's duty to guard against any and all avoidable acts that may result in injury to his patient. In the operating room, the surgeon must be master. He cannot tolerate any other voice in the control of his assistants. In the case at bar, the evidence is clear that the doctor had exclusive control over the acts in question, and therefore the hospital cannot be said to have been a "joint master" or "comaster," even though the nurses were in its general employ and paid by it.[34]

In *Krane v. Saint Anthony Hospital Systems,*[35] the factual question that had to be determined was whether, at the time of the alleged negligent act, the operating surgeon had assumed control of a surgical nurse. If so, the responsibility of the surgeon supersedes that of the hospital. Because it was uncontradicted that the alleged negligent act of the surgical nurse took place over two and a half hours into surgery, there could be no factual dispute that the surgeon had assumed control over the nurse.

Several courts have developed a distinction between a nurse's clerical or administrative acts and those involving professional skill and judgment, which are considered medical acts. Some courts use this distinction in allocating liability for the acts of a nurse as between the surgeon and the hospital. If the act is characterized as administrative or clerical, it is the hospital's responsibility; if the act is considered to be medical, it is the surgeon's responsibility. This rule was followed in the Minnesota case of *Swigerd v. City of Ortonville,*[36] in which the court found that the hospital is liable as an employer for the negligence of its nurses in performing acts that are basically administrative. Administrative acts, although constituting a component of a patient's prescribed medical treatment, do not require the application of specialized procedures and techniques or the understanding of a skilled physician or surgeon.

Today's courts recognize that surgeons do not always have the right to control all persons within the operating room. An assignment of liability based on the theory of who had actual control over the patient more realistically reflects the actual relationship that exists in a modern operating room. For example, summary dismissal in *Thomas v. Raleigh*[37] was properly ordered for those portions of a patient's medical malpractice action that sought to hold a surgeon vicariously liable for throat injuries suffered by his patient because of the negligent manner in which an endotracheal tube was inserted during the administration of anesthesia. The patient's allegations that the surgeon exercised control over the administration of anesthesia were rebutted by evidence to the contrary. Liability of the surgeon could not be premised on the captain of the ship doctrine because that doctrine would not be recognized in West Virginia, where the surgery took place.

Comparative Negligence

A defense of comparative negligence provides that the degree of negligence or carelessness of each party to a lawsuit must be established by the finder of fact and that each party then is responsible for his or her proportional share of any damages awarded. For example, when a plaintiff suffers injuries of $10,000 from an accident and when the plaintiff is found 20 percent negligent and the defendant 80 percent negligent, the defendant would be required to pay $8,000 to the plaintiff. Thus, with comparative negligence, the plaintiff can collect for 80 percent of the injuries, whereas an application of contributory negligence would deprive the plaintiff of any monetary judgment. This doctrine relieves the plaintiff from the hardship of losing an entire claim when a defendant has been successful in establishing that the plaintiff contributed to his or her own injuries. A defense that provides that the plaintiff will forfeit an entire claim if he or she has been contributorily negligent is considered too harsh a result in jurisdictions that recognize comparative negligence.

The plaintiff in *Quinones v. Public Administrator*[38] sought to recover damages for the alleged negligence of the defendant's physicians for their failure to treat a fractured ankle. The plaintiff claimed that there was a nonunion of the fracture and that he was advised to put weight on his leg. As a result of this advice, the plaintiff claimed that there was an exacerbation of the original injury requiring two operative procedures, which resulted in the fusion of his left ankle. The defendant claimed that if there was any subsequent injury, it was because of the failure of the plaintiff to return for care. The New York Supreme Court entered a judgment in favor of the defendant hospital, and the plaintiff appealed. The New York Supreme Court, Appellate Division, held that a patient's failure to follow instructions does not defeat an action for malpractice where the alleged improper professional treatment occurred before the patient's own negligence.[39] Damages would be reduced to the degree that the plaintiff's negligence increased the extent of the injury.

Statute of Limitations

The *statute of limitations* refers to legislatively imposed time constraints that restrict the period of time after the occurrence of an injury during which a legal action must be commenced. Should a cause of action be initiated later than the period of time prescribed, the case cannot proceed. Many technical rules are associated with statutes of limitations. Statutes in each state specify that malpractice suits and other personal injury suits must be brought within fixed periods of time. An injured person who is a minor or is otherwise under a legal disability may, in many states, extend the period within which an action for injury may be filed. Computation of the period when the statute begins to run in a particular state may be based on any of the following factors:

- the date that the physician terminated treatment

- the time of the wrongful act

- the time when the patient should have reasonably discovered the injury

- the date that the injury is discovered

- the date when the contract between the patient and the physician ended

The running of the statute will not begin if fraud (the deliberate concealment from a patient of facts that might present a cause of action for damages) is involved. The cause of action begins at the time fraud is discovered.

Malpractice actions must be filed in a timely manner. The action filed in *Russell v. Williford*[40] was not filed in a timely manner under the statute of limitations. Reasonable diligence should have led the plaintiff to seek a second opinion or additional treatment much sooner when the abnormal condition in his left leg persisted. This simple action, if taken within one to two years after surgery instead of 27 years after, might have made the true problem with the plaintiff's leg known a long time ago. The problem with his leg might have been discovered through reasonable diligence after or very soon after the surgery. Therefore, the plaintiff may not bring this action now, over a quarter of a century after the alleged act or omission. To allow the plaintiff to proceed under this set of facts on such an ancient claim would set a very dangerous precedent.

The statute of limitations does not generally begin to run in those cases where a patient is unaware that an act of malpractice has occurred. Such is the case when foreign objects are left in a patient during surgery. A New Hampshire patient in *Shillady v. Elliot Community Hospital*[41] sued the hospital for negligence in treatment that was administered 31 years earlier. A needle had been left in the patient's spine after a spinal tap in 1940. In 1970, an X-ray showed the needle. The patient had suffered severe pain immediately after the spinal tap, which had decreased over the intervening years to about three "spells" a year. The court held that the six-year statute of limitations does not begin "until the patient learns or in the exercise of reasonable care and diligence should have learned of its presence."[42] Therefore, the defendant's motion to dismiss the case on the grounds that the statute of limitations had run out was not granted.

Fraud prevents the tolling of the statute of limitations. In a 1949 Michigan case, *Buchanan v. Kull,*[43] a patient who had undergone a thyroidectomy suffered paralyzed vocal cords. The patient had been told that the injury was due to a lack of calcium. The patient later learned that the vocal cords had been cut. The statute of limitations normally would have run out in this case; however, the presence of fraud did not permit the statute to commence until the patient became aware of the fraud.

Sovereign Immunity

Sovereign immunity refers to the common-law doctrine by which federal and state governments historically have been immune from liability for harm suffered from the tortious conduct of employees. For the most part, both federal and state governments have abolished sovereign immunity. Congress enacted the Federal Tort Claims Act (FTCA) to provide redress for those who have been negligently injured by employees of the federal government acting within their scope of employment. In an action under the FTCA,[44] the Veterans Administration Hospital of Memphis, Tennessee, was held negligent for injuries sustained by an 83-year-old patient found lying in a hallway of the hospital. The patient suffered severe head injuries that required surgery. Damages in the amount of $80,000 were awarded the plaintiff. The court held that the evidence was sufficient to raise a duty on the part of hospital personnel attending the patient to use reasonable care to protect him from getting out of bed and injuring himself. This duty was breached, and the patient was injured. The proximate cause of the patient's injuries was related to the hospital's failure to put up the patient's bed rails and its failure to remind him to call a nurse if he needed help.

Action was brought on behalf of a minor in *Steele v. United States,*[45] who received treatment at a U.S. Army hospital and suffered injury because of the optometrist's failure to refer the child to an ophthalmologist for examination. The U.S. district court held that it was probable that an ophthalmologist would have diagnosed the child's problem and prevented the loss of his right eye. Recovery was permitted against the United States under the FTCA.

NURSE'S NEGLIGENCE: IMMUNITY DENIED

Citation: *Sullivan v. Sumrall by Ritchey,* 618 So. 2d 1274 (Miss. 1993)

Facts

In April 26, 1988, the patient was admitted to the hospital suffering from a severe headache. Her physician ordered a CT scan for the following morning and prescribed Demerol and Dramamine to alleviate pain. Referring to the patient's medical chart, the nurse stated in her deposition that the patient received injections of Demerol and Dramamine at 6:45 P.M. and 10:00 P.M. on April 26. The nurse checked on the patient at 11:00 P.M. The patient's temperature and blood pressure were taken at midnight. Her blood pressure was recorded at 90/60, down from 160/80 at 8:00 P.M. At 12:25 A.M., two hours and 25 minutes after her last medication, the nurse administered another injection of Demerol and Dramamine because the patient was still complaining of pain. Although hospital rules require consultation with a patient's admitting physician when there is a question regarding the administration of medication, the nurse stated that she did not call the physician before administering another injection.

At 4:00 A.M., when the nurse made an hourly check of the patient, she discovered that the patient was not breathing. She called a Code 99 (an emergency signal for a patient in acute distress). An emergency department physician responded and revived the patient. The patient was diagnosed as having suffered "respiratory arrest, with what appears to be hypoxic brain injury." CT scans revealed no bleeding, but other tests revealed a grossly abnormal EEG. The patient was transferred to a nursing facility where she remained in a coma at the time of trial.

The patient's daughter and husband filed a complaint against the hospital, alleging that the hospital had been negligent in monitoring and medicating the patient, in failing to notify a physician when her vital signs became irregular, in failing to properly assess her condition and intervene, and in failing to exercise reasonable care. Later, the complaint was amended to include the nurse.

The defendant nurse filed a motion for summary judgment. She asserted that, as a matter of law, she was shielded from liability under the qualified immunity afforded public officials. The circuit court denied the motion and the nurse appealed.

Reason

There is no qualified immunity for any public hospital employees making treatment decisions. Discretion exercised by medical personnel in making treatment decisions is not the sort of individual judgment sought to be protected by the qualified immunity bestowed upon public officials.

Issue

Is a nurse employed by a county hospital shielded by public official qualified immunity from a medical negligence action brought against her individually?

Holding

The Mississippi Supreme Court held that an employee of a county hospital enjoys no qualified immunity.

Discussion

1. Do you agree that the nurse should not be shielded from liability on the basis that she is a public official? Explain.
2. What assessment and reassessment issues do you see in this case?
3. Should the dramatic change in the patient's blood pressure have signaled a need to notify the attending physician of the patient's change in health status? Explain.
4. Was the nurse practicing medicine when she administered the second injection without contacting the attending physician?

Intervening Cause

Intervening cause arises when the act of a third party, independent of the defendant's original negligent conduct, is the proximate cause of an injury. If the negligent act of a third party is extraordinary under the circumstances and unforeseeable as a normal and probable consequence of the defendant's negligence, then the third party's negligence supersedes that of the defendant and relieves the defendant of liability.

For example, in *DePesa v. Westchester Square Medical Center*,[46] a 49-year-old woman experiencing severe pain in her abdomen entered the emergency department at Westchester Square Medical Center (W.S.M.C.). There, she was prescribed Mylanta and sent home with the advice that she should contact her personal physician if her condition worsened. She took the Mylanta, but her condition continued to deteriorate and, after 20 more days, she went to the emergency department at a second hospital. She was admitted and was operated on for a perforated bowel and peritonitis. Although the evidence indicated that the operation itself was successful, she died at the hospital on May 25. The autopsy report indicated the presence of yellow fluid in the pleural cavity and peritoneal cavity, and the cause of the death as status post-bowel resection, bronchopneumonia, and congestive heart failure.

The appellate court found that the trial court should have provided an instruction directing the jury to decide whether the postoperative care of the decedent by the second hospital, despite W.S.M.C.'s negligence in misdiagnosing the patient's condition, was the proximate and superseding cause of death. W.S.M.C.'s expert testified, based on the medical evidence, that while the decedent was recovering from surgery, employees at the second hospital administered almost double the amount of fluids that the decedent could output, resulting in congestive heart failure and her ultimate demise. W.S.M.C.'s theory at trial was that the perforation of the bowel occurred at the second hospital, where staff allegedly administered substantially more fluid to the patient than she could excrete, that these causes of death were independent of W.S.M.C.'s own negligence in failing to detect bowel conditions, and that such intervening cause would not have been foreseeable by a reasonably prudent person.

In *Cohran v. Harper,*[47] a patient sued a physician, charging him with malpractice for an alleged staphylococcus infection that she received from a hypodermic needle used by the physician's nurse. The nurse gave the patient an injection that resulted in osteomyelitis. The grounds of negligence included an allegation that the physician failed to properly sterilize the hypodermic needle that was used to administer penicillin. The evidence showed, without dispute, that a prepackaged sterilized needle and syringe were used in accordance with proper and accepted medical practice. The physician was not liable. There was inadequate proof that either the physician or his nurse was negligent. The court found that even if there was evidence that the needle was contaminated and that the patient's ailment was caused thereby, there was no evidence that either the physician, his nurse, or anyone in his office knew, or by the exercise of ordinary care could have discovered, that the prepackaged needle and syringe were so contaminated. The defense of intervening cause would have been an adequate defense against recovery of damages if it had been established that the needle was contaminated when packaged.

CLOSING STATEMENTS

After completion of the plaintiff's case and the defendant's defense, the judge calls for closing statements. The defense proceeds first, followed by the plaintiff. Closing statements provide attorneys with an opportunity to summarize for the jury and the court what they have proven. They may point out faults in their opponent's case and emphasize points they want the jury to remember.

If there appears to be only a question of law at the end of a case, a motion can be made for a directed verdict. The court will grant the motion if there is no question of fact to be decided by the jury. A directed verdict also may, for example, be made on the grounds that the plaintiff has failed to present sufficient facts to prove his or her case or that the evidence fails to establish a legal basis for a verdict in the plaintiff's favor.

JUDGE'S CHARGE TO THE JURY

After the attorneys' summations, the court charges the jury before the jurors recess to deliberate. Because the jury determines issues of fact, it is necessary for the court to instruct the jury with regard to applicable law. This is done by means of a charge. The charge defines the responsibility of the jury, describes the applicable law, and advises the jury of the alternatives available to it. As an example, statements from the trial judge's oral charge to the jurors in *Estes Health Care Centers v. Bannerman,*[48] in which a nursing facility resident died after transfer to a hospital after suffering burns in a bath, included

The complaint alleges the defendant Jackson Hospital undertook to provide hospital and nursing care to the deceased, and that the defendant negligently failed to provide proper hospital and nursing care to the plaintiff's intestate.

•   •   •   •

The defendants in response to these allegations . . . have each separately entered pleas of the general issue or general denial. Under the law, a plea of the general issue has the effect of placing the burden of proof on the plaintiffs to reasonably satisfy you from the evidence, the truth of those things claimed by them in the bill of the complaint. The defendants carry no burden of proof.

•   •   •   •

As to the defendant Jackson Hospital, the duty arises in that in rendering services to a patient, a hospital must use that degree of care, skill, and diligence used by hospitals generally in the community under similar circumstances.

•   •   •   •

Negligence is not actionable unless the negligence is the proximate cause of the injury. The law defines proximate cause as that cause which is the natural and probable sequence of events and without the intervention of any new or independent cause, produces the injury, and without which such injury would not have occurred. For an act to constitute actionable negligence, there must not only be some causal connection between the negligent act complained of and the injury suffered, but connection must be by natural and unbroken sequence, without intervening sufficient causes, so that but for the negligence of the defendant, the injury would not have occurred.

•   •   •   •

If one is guilty of negligence which concurs or combines with the negligence of another, and the two combine to produce injury, each negligent person is liable for the resulting injury. And the negligence of each will be deemed the proximate cause of the injury. Concurrent causes may be defined as two or more causes which run together and act contemporaneously to produce a given result or to inflict an injury. This does not mean that the causes of the acts producing the injury must necessarily occur simultaneously, but they must be active simultaneously to efficiently and proximately produce a result.

· · · · ·

In an action against two or more defendants for injury allegedly caused by combined or concurring negligence of the defendants, it is not necessary to show negligence of all the defendants in order for recovery to be had against one or more to be negligent. If you are reasonably satisfied from the evidence in this case that all the defendants are negligent and that their negligence concurred and combined to proximately cause the injury complained by the plaintiffs, then each defendant is liable to the plaintiffs.[49]

When a charge given by the court is not clear enough on a particular point, it is the obligation of the attorneys for both sides to request clarification of the charge. When the jury retires to deliberate, the members are reminded not to discuss the case except among themselves.

Jury instructions must be clear and accurate. The nursing assistant in *Myers v. Heritage Enterprises, Inc.*[50] was determined not to be in a professional position. The standard of care required by the nursing assistant was one of ordinary negligence. Therefore, the trial court should have instructed the jury that it had to decide how a reasonably prudent person would have acted under the circumstances. The trial court abused its discretion by instructing the jury on professional negligence rather than ordinary negligence. The instructions given misled the jury and resulted in prejudice to the plaintiff. The case was remanded for a new trial.

Jury Instructions: Surgery Sponge Count

The medical malpractice action in *Houserman v. Garrett*[51] was filed after a gauze pad was discovered in the patient approximately eight months after surgery. The trial court was found to have erred when it instructed the jury that the physician's conduct was negligent without any argument as to the surrounding circumstances (negligence per se). The physician alone was understood to be liable for failure to

remove the pad from the patient's body. Without clarification elsewhere in the charge, it was hard to determine what, if anything, a physician could do, to have defended himself.

It is undisputed that a nurse was responsible for counting the surgical sponges and surgical devices used in this procedure before and after the surgery and that she apparently did not include the pad in her presurgery count. In addition, she did not advise the physician, before the surgical site was closed, that a pad was unaccounted for.

The trial judge charged the jury that the nurse's count amounted only to an added precaution when, in fact, in light of the evidence, the jury was entitled to find that the nurse's count was valid evidence that the physician had satisfied one component of the standard of care. On appeal, the judgment was reversed, and the case was remanded to the trial court for further proceedings.

JURY DELIBERATION AND DETERMINATION

After the judge's charge, the jury retires to the jury room to deliberate and determine the defendant's liability. The jury members return to the courtroom upon reaching a verdict, and their determinations are presented to the court.

If a verdict is against the weight of the evidence, a judge may dismiss the case, order a new trial, or set his or her own verdict. At the time judgment is rendered, the losing party has an opportunity to motion for a new trial.

AWARDING DAMAGES

Monetary damages generally are awarded to individuals in cases of personal injury and wrongful death. Damages generally are fixed by the jury and are nominal, compensatory, hedonic, or punitive.

- *Nominal damages* are awarded as a mere token in recognition that wrong has been committed when the actual amount of compensation is insignificant.

- *Compensatory damages* are estimated reparation in money for detriment or injury sustained (including loss of earnings, medical costs, and loss of financial support).

- *Hedonic damages* are those damages awarded to compensate an individual for the loss of enjoyment of life. Such damages are awarded because of the failure of compensatory damages to compensate an individual adequately for the pain and suffering that he or she has endured as a result of a negligent wrong.

- *Punitive damages* are additional money awards authorized when an injury is caused by gross carelessness or disregard for the safety of others.

Plaintiff's Schedule of Damages

Plaintiffs seek recovery for a great variety of damages. The following are typical:

- personal injuries

- permanent physical disabilities

- permanent mental disabilities

- past and future physical and mental pain and suffering sustained and to be sustained

- loss of enjoyment of life

- loss of consortium where a spouse is injured in the accident

- loss of child's services where a minor child is injured in the accident

- medical and other health expenses reasonably paid or incurred, or reasonably certain to be incurred in the future

- past and future loss of earnings sustained and to be sustained

- permanent diminution in the plaintiff's earning capacity

The following cases illustrate the types of damages sought by plaintiffs.

Damages/Future Pain and Suffering

In *Luecke v. Bitterman,*[52] an award of $490,000 for future pain and suffering was found reasonable with respect to a 20-year-old patient who, as a result of a physician's negligent application of liquid nitrogen to remove a wart, suffered a 12- by 4-inch third-degree burn. The burn resulted in a scar on the right buttock extending to the back of the thigh. The plaintiff suffered excruciating pain and posttraumatic stress disorder.

Punitive Damages/Mighty Engine of Deterrence

Punitive damages are awarded over and above that which is intended to compensate the plaintiff for economic losses resulting from the injury. Punitive damages cover such items as physical disability, mental anguish, loss of a spouse's services, physical suffering, injury to one's reputation, and loss of companionship. Punitive damages were referred to as that mighty engine of deterrence in *Johnson v. Terry.*[53]

The court in *Henry v. Deen*[54] held that allegations of gross and wanton negligence incidental to wrongful death in the plaintiff's complaint gave sufficient notice of a claim against the treating physician and physician's assistant for punitive damages. The original complaint, which alleged

that the treating physician, the physician's assistant, and the consulting physician agreed to create and did create false and misleading entries in the patient's medical record, was sufficient to allege a civil conspiracy. The decision of the lower court was reversed, and the case was remanded for further proceedings.

In *Estes Health Care Centers v. Bannerman,* discussed earlier, the court stated:

> While human life is incapable of translation into a compensatory measurement, the amount of an award of punitive damages may be measured by the gravity of the wrong done, the punishment called for by the act of the wrongdoer, and the need to deter similar wrongs in order to preserve human life.[55]

In *Payton Health Care Facilities, Inc. v. Estate of Campbell,*[56] a punitive damage award in the amount of $1.7 million for the wrongful death of a patient from infected decubitus ulcers was found to be justified. The treating physician had agreed to a settlement prior to trial in the amount of $50,000. The deceased, a stroke victim, had been admitted to the Lakeland Health Care Center for nursing and medical care. While at the center, the patient developed several severe skin ulcers that eventually necessitated hospitalization in Lakeland General Hospital. The patient's condition deteriorated to such a state that further treatment was inadequate to prolong his life. Expert testimony had been presented that indicated that the standard of care received by the patient while at the nursing facility was an outrageous deviation from acceptable standards of care. There was sufficient evidence of the willful and wanton disregard for rights of others to permit an award of punitive damages against the companies who owned and managed the nursing facility. The cause of death was determined to be bacteremia with sepsis, because of extensive infected necrotic decubitus ulcers, that the patient developed at the nursing facility.

Punitive Damages for Failure to Diagnose Inappropriate

Punitive damages in *Brooking v. Polito*[57] were determined to be inappropriate in an action alleging failure to timely diagnose pancreatic cancer. It was undisputed that the defendants performed various tests on the decedent, which included blood tests, CAT scans, an MRI, and ultrasound. The tests had been analyzed and the patient was treated accordingly.

Damages/Surviving Spouse and Children

Damages may be awarded given evidence of a patient's pain and the mental anguish of the surviving husband and children. In *Jefferson Hospital Association v. Garrett,*[58] damages in the amount of $180,000 were found not to be excessive given evidence of the patient's pain and the mental suffering of the surviving spouse and children.

Damages/Emotional Distress

The court of appeals in *Haught v. Maceluch*[59] held that under Texas law the mother was entitled to recover for her emotional distress, even though she was not conscious at the time her child was born. The mother had brought a medical malpractice action, alleging that the physician was negligent in the delivery of her child, causing her daughter to suffer permanent brain injury. The district court entered judgment of $1,160,000 for the child's medical expenses and $175,000 for her lost future earnings. The court deleted a jury award of $118,000 for the mother's mental suffering over her daughter's impaired condition. On appeal, the court of appeals permitted recovery, under Texas law, for mental suffering. The mother was conscious for more than 11 hours of labor and was aware of the physician's negligent acts, his absence in a near-emergency situation, and the overadministration of the labor-inducing drug Pitocin.

Damages/Not Excessive

The plaintiff in *Burge v. Parker*[60] suffered a laceration of his right foot on April 2 and was taken to St. Margaret's Hospital. A physician in the emergency department cleaned and stitched the laceration and released the patient with instructions to keep the foot elevated. Even though reports prepared by the fire medic who arrived on the scene of the accident and by ambulance personnel indicated the chief complaint as being a fracture of the foot, no X-rays were ordered in the emergency department. The admitting clerk had typed a statement on the admission form indicating possible fracture of the right foot. However, a handwritten note stated the chief complaint as being a laceration of the right foot. The patient returned to the hospital later in the day with his mother, complaining of pain in the right foot. His mother asked if X-rays had been taken. The physician said that it was not necessary. The wound was redressed, and the patient was sent home again with instructions to keep the foot elevated. The pain continued to worsen, and the patient was taken to see another physician on April 5. X-rays were ordered, and an orthopedic surgeon called for a consultation diagnosed three fractures and a compartment syndrome, a swelling of tissue in the muscle compartments. The swelling increased pressure on the blood vessels, thus decreasing circulation, which tends to cause muscles to die.

Approximately one half pint of clotted blood was removed from the wound. By April 11, the big toe had to be surgically removed. It was alleged that the emergency department physician failed to obtain a full medical history, to order the necessary X-rays, and to diagnose and treat the fractures of the foot. As a result, the patient ultimately suffered loss of his big toe. The Macon County Circuit Court awarded damages totaling $450,000 for loss of a big toe, and the physician appealed. The Alabama Supreme Court found the damages not to have been excessive.

In *Tesauro v. Perrige,*[61] Mrs. Tesauro, the appellee, went to Dr. Perrige, the appellant, to have a lower left molar removed. A blood clot failed to form and the appellant administered an injection of alcohol near the affected area. The appellee began to experience pain, burning, and numbness on the left side of her face at the site of the injection. Several physicians diagnosed her as suffering from muscle spasms caused by a damaged trigeminal nerve. Over a five-year period, the appellee was treated by a variety of specialists. In 1989, the plaintiff underwent radical experimental surgery. The surgery corrected the plaintiff's most oppressive symptoms. Although the most painful symptoms had been eliminated, the appellee continued to suffer numbness and burning on the left side of her face. A dental malpractice lawsuit was filed against Dr. Perrige alleging that he was negligent in administering the alcohol injection so close to the trigeminal nerve. The jury returned a verdict in favor of the plaintiffs in the amounts of $2,747,000 to Mrs. Tesauro and $593,000 to Mr. Tesauro for loss of consortium. Perrige, the defendant/appellant, appealed for a new trial to be based on the excessiveness of the jury verdict.

The superior court held that the evidence supported the damage awards. The decision to grant or not to grant a new trial based on the excessiveness of a jury verdict is within the sound discretion of the trial court, and its decision will be upheld on appeal based on a gross abuse of that discretion. In determining excessiveness, a court should consider:

1. the severity of the injury

2. whether the injury is manifested by objective physical evidence or whether it is revealed only by the subjective testimony

3. whether the injury is permanent

4. whether the plaintiff can continue with his or her employment

5. the size of out-of-pocket expenses

6. the amount of compensation demanded in the original complaint

The superior court determined that the severity of the plaintiff's injury in itself would support the compensatory award. The plaintiff spent five years trying to find a cure for her pain. Although much recovered, the plaintiff continued to suffer from numbness and burning. Her experience clearly fell into the category of severe injury. The severity of the injury had a huge impact on the marital relationship. The compensation awarded to Mr. Tesauro was, therefore, fair and just.

A medical malpractice action was brought against the employer of a physician, alleging that the physician's failure to properly treat an abscess some three weeks after an infant received a live polio vaccine resulted in suppression of the infant's immune system and the infant's contraction of paralytic polio. The jury in the circuit court returned a $16 million verdict in favor of the plaintiffs, and the defendant appealed. The case was transferred from the court of appeals to the state supreme court.[62] Was the $16 million verdict excessive, and did the trial court err in denying a new trial based on the alleged excessive verdict?

The Missouri Supreme Court held that there was no basis for a new trial on the grounds of excessiveness of the $16 million verdict. There is no formula for determining the excessiveness of a verdict. Each case must be decided on its own facts to determine what is fair and reasonable. A jury is in the best position to make such a determination. The trial judge could have set aside the verdict if a determination was made that passion and prejudice brought about an excessive verdict. The size of the verdict alone does not establish passion and prejudice. The appellant failed to establish that the verdict was: (1) glaringly unwarranted and (2) based on prejudice and passion. Compensation of a plaintiff is based on such factors as the age of the patient, the nature and extent of injury, diminished earnings capacity, economic condition, and awards in comparable cases. A jury is entitled to consider such intangibles that do not lend themselves to precise calculation, such as past and future pain, suffering, effect on lifestyle, embarrassment, humiliation, and economic loss.

Damages Award Appropriate

An award of $350,000 for conscious pain and suffering arising from the death of an inmate from an overdose of medication during the inmate's 13-day hospitalization was determined appropriate in *Arias v. State*[63] where numerous invasive procedures (i.e., intubation, catheterizations, and tracheotomy) had been performed and where each of these was a source of discomfort. However, the inmate's mother failed to establish that there was a reasonable expectancy of financial support, gifts, or inheritance that would have caused injury to her had her son lived. She offered only her own testimony unsupported by any historical documentation in support of her claim. The record indicated that the inmate had a history of mental health problems, had been institutionalized periodically since the age of 12, and had a limited work history. The mother did establish her personal claim that the defendant was negligent by not notifying her of her son's admission to an outside hospital in violation of DOCS Directive 4451 and would be awarded $25,000 for her personal claim.

THE WRONG BLOOD

Citation: *Dodson v. Community Blood Ctr.,* 633 So. 2d 252 (La. Ct. App. 1993)

Facts

The patient was scheduled to undergo surgery at a medical center. In anticipation of the surgery and out of fear of contracting the acquired immune deficiency syndrome (AIDS) through blood transfusions from unknown donors, he arranged to have three known donors donate blood earmarked for his use should transfusion be required.

After surgery, the patient was transfused with two pints of blood. However, the blood used was not the blood obtained from the patient's voluntary donors. The blood had been taken from the hospital's general inventory, which had been obtained from the community blood center. The patient subsequently learned that as a result of the transfusions, he had been infected with hepatitis C.

Issue

Was the award of $325,000 in general damages to the patient excessive?

Holding

The Louisiana Court of Appeal held that the award of damages was not excessive.

Reason

In reasons for judgment, the trial court found that the patient was a credible witness. He did not exaggerate his symptoms, fears, or worries about his condition. The court believed the patient when he said he felt like a leper and feared infecting his wife, child, and friends with the disease. The trial court arrived at what it determined to be an appropriate award for general damages. After careful review of the record and in light of the vast discretion of the trial court to assess general damages, the court found that there was no abuse of discretion.

Discussion

1. Under what circumstances will an appellate court overturn the decision of a lower court?

2. Do you agree with the court's decision? Discuss your answer.

Damages Excessive

A jury verdict totaling $12,393,130 was considered an excessive award in *Merrill v. Albany Medical Center,*[64] in which damages were sought with respect to the severe brain damage sustained by a 22-month-old infant as the result of oxygen deprivation. This occurred when the infant went into cardiac arrest during surgery for removal of a suspected malignant tumor from her right lung. Reduction of the amount to $6,143,130 was considered appropriate.

Damages Capped

The trial court in *Judd v. Drezga*[65] was found to have properly limited a brain-damaged infant's recovery of quality-of-life damages to $250,000. The Idaho cap on damages was designed to reduce health care costs, increase the availability of medical malpractice insurance, and secure the continued availability of health care resources—all legitimate legislative goals given the clear social and economic evil of rising health care costs and a shortage of qualified health care professionals. In attempting to meet its goals, the legislature had not unreasonably or arbitrarily limited recovery. Rather, it had chosen to place a limit on the recovery of noneconomic quality-of-life damages—one area where legislation had been shown to actually and substantially further these goals. Applying each individual test, the open courts, uniform operation of laws, and due-process provisions of the constitution were not offended by the damage cap. Additionally, neither the right to a jury trial nor the constitutional guarantee of separation of powers were offended by the cap.

JOINT AND SEVERAL LIABILITY

The doctrine of joint and several liability permits the plaintiff to bring suit against all persons who share responsibility for his or her injury. The doctrine allows the plaintiff to recover monetary damages from any one of or all the defendants. Any one defendant, even though partially responsible for the plaintiff's injury, can be required to pay the full judgment awarded by the jury. Awards tend to fall in greater amounts on defendants with the better insurance. This is the deep-pockets concept: whoever has the most pays the greater percentage of the award.

APPEALS

An appellate court reviews a case on the basis of the trial record as well as written briefs and, if requested, concise oral arguments by the attorneys. A brief summarizes the facts of a case, testimony of the witnesses, laws affecting the case, and arguments of counsel. The party making the appeal is the *appellant.* The party answering the appeal is the *appellee.* After hearing oral arguments, the court takes the case under advisement until such time as the judges consider it and agree on a decision. An opinion then is prepared explaining the reasons for a decision.

Grounds for appeal may result from one or more of the following:

- The verdict was excessive or inadequate in the lower court.
- Evidence was rejected that should have been accepted.
- Inadmissible evidence was permitted.
- Testimony that should have been admissible was excluded.
- The verdict was contrary to the weight of the evidence.
- The court improperly charged the jury.
- The jury is confused by jury instructions.
- The jury verdict is the result of bias, prejudice, and/or passion.

Notice of appeal must be filed with the trial court, the appellate court, and the adverse party. The party wishing to prevent execution of an adverse judgment until such time as the case has been heard and decided by an appellate court also should file a stay of execution.

The appellate court may modify, affirm, or reverse the judgment or reorder a new trial on an appeal. The majority ruling of the judges in the appellate court is binding on the parties of a lawsuit. If the appellate court's decision is not unanimous, the minority may render a dissenting opinion. Further appeal may be made, as set by statute, to the highest court of appeals. If an appeal involves a constitutional question, it eventually may be appealed to the U.S. Supreme Court.

When the highest appellate court in a state decides a case, a final judgment results, and the matter is ended. The instances when one may appeal the ruling of a state court to the U.S. Supreme Court are rare. A federal question must be involved, and even then the Supreme Court must decide whether it will hear the case. A federal question is one involving the U.S. Constitution or a statute enacted by Congress, so it is unlikely that a negligence case arising in a state court would be reviewed and decided by the Supreme Court.

EXECUTION OF JUDGMENTS

Once the amount of damages has been established and all the appeals have been heard, the defendant must comply with the judgment. If he or she fails to do so, a court order may be executed requiring the sheriff or other judicial officer to sell as much of the defendant's property as necessary, within statutory limitations, to satisfy the plaintiff's judgment.

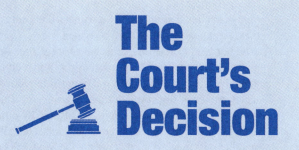

The Court's Decision

The Supreme Court of Mississippi found that Dorrough's arguments were without merit, holding that the verdict by the jury was supported by the weight of the evidence. When evidence is in conflict, the jury is the sole judge of both the credibility of a witness and the weight of his or her testimony. The jury was presented with conflicting testimony concerning the alleged negligence of Dorrough. The jury, being the sole judge of the weight and credibility of the witnesses, determined that Dorrough was liable for the death of Gwendolyn and awarded damages.[66]

CHAPTER REVIEW

1. The pleadings of a case are the written statements of fact and law filed with a court by the parties to a lawsuit. Pleadings generally include such papers as a complaint, demurrer, answer, and bill of particulars. In a case, if only questions of law are at issue, the judge will decide the case based on the pleadings. If there are questions of fact, a trial will be held to determine those facts. In a negligence action, the first pleading filed with the court is a complaint, which identifies the parties to a suit, the cause of action, and the demand for damages.

2. Once a defendant receives a copy of the *complaint,* the defendant can file a preliminary objection before submitting an answer, or response, to the complaint. A formal objection to the lawsuit is called a *demurrer,* and it holds that the evidence presented by the plaintiff is insufficient to sustain an issue or case. The defendant can file a counterclaim if he or she has a claim against the plaintiff.

3. Before the trial, facts are investigated in a process called *discovery.* The discovery process helps to prevent surprises during trial. *Examination before trial* is part of the discovery process and allows for witnesses to be examined before the trial. Generally, hospital incident and investigation reports are not protected from discovery. However, communications between client and attorney are protected under attorney-client privilege.

4. A *motion to dismiss* a case can be made before, during, or after the trial. The motion alleges that the plaintiff's complaint does not set forth a claim or cause of action that is recognized by law. If either party to a suit believes that there are no issues of fact in contention, only issues of law, they may make a motion for a summary judgment, in which the court is asked to rule without a trial.

5. The *jury* determines the facts in a case and makes a determination of the particular standards of conduct required in all cases in which the judgment of reasonable people might differ. The jury also determines the extent of damages and degree to which the plaintiff's conduct may have contributed to his or her injury.

6. A legal order requiring a person to appear in court or that documents be presented to a court or administrative body is called a *subpoena.* If a witness does not respond to a subpoena, then a bench warrant, which orders a witness to appear in court, may be issued.

7. The burden of proof in a criminal case requires that the evidence presented against the defendant must be *beyond a reasonable doubt.* The burden of proof in a civil lawsuit requires that a *preponderance of the credible evidence* must be presented in order for a plaintiff to recover damages.

8. Facts proved or disproved during a lawsuit constitute *evidence. Direct evidence* is proof that is offered via direct testimony. *Demonstrative evidence* is offered by objects themselves. Written evidence capable of making a truthful statement is considered *documentary evidence.* Written and oral statements that another has said or actions that another person has done that are not the result of personal knowledge of the witness are considered *hearsay evidence.*

9. When the issues to be resolved in the case are outside the understanding or experience of the average juror, an expert witness is allowed to offer testimony to assist in explanation of technical matters. The testimony of two experts may conflict, in which case the jury will determine which opinion to accept. An expert witness must have experience and training sufficient to explain the facts or answer the questions of a particular case.

10. After a plaintiff's case has been established, there are several defenses that may protect the defendant from recovery of damages:

    - *Assumption of a risk* is the knowledge that a danger exists and acceptance of the risk of exposing oneself to it knowing that to do so may result in harm.

    - The *borrowed servant doctrine* applies to cases in which an employee is lent to another for a particular employment. In such cases, the original employer is not responsible for injuries caused by the negligence of the temporary employer.

    - In cases of *comparative negligence,* a plaintiff found negligent and, therefore, partially responsible, is responsible for his or her proportional share of damages awarded.

    - When the defendant claims that the conduct of the plaintiff is below the standard of care that reasonably prudent persons would exercise for their own safety, the issue is one of *contributory negligence.* In such cases, the lack of ordinary care on the part of the plaintiff, combined with another's negligent act, caused the injury.

    - *Good Samaritan laws* encourage volunteer assistance in emergency situations and protect the volunteers from liability for ordinary negligence in rendering assistance in emergency situations.

    - When a third party is determined to be the proximate cause of death or injury, independent of the defendant's original negligence, there exists *intervening cause.*

    - If a cause of action is initiated beyond a prescribed period of time, the case cannot proceed according to the *statute of limitations.*

11. Damages, which are usually determined by the jury, come in four forms:

    - *Nominal damages* are a token in recognition that a wrong has been committed. In such cases, the amount of compensation is insignificant.

    - *Compensatory damages* are intended as reparation for detriment or injury sustained.

    - *Hedonic damages* are awarded to compensate the plaintiff for the loss of enjoyment of life. This is supplementary to the compensation offered by compensatory damages.

    - *Punitive damages* are additional monetary awards when an injury is caused by gross carelessness or disregard for others' safety.

REVIEW QUESTIONS

1. Describe the trial process, including pretrial motions and the functions of the judge, jury, and attorneys.
2. Describe the kinds of evidence that a plaintiff can present in order to establish a negligent act.

3. What defenses can a defendant present in order to refute a plaintiff's evidence?
4. Describe how statutes of limitations favor defendants in a lawsuit.
5. Describe the differences between nominal, compensatory, hedonic, and punitive damages.

NOTES

1. *Dorrough v. Wilkes,* 817 So. 2d 567 (2002).
2. *Kern v. Gulf Coast Nursing Home of Moss Point, Inc.,* 502 So. 2d 1198, 1202 (Miss. 1987).
3. No. 13-05-00062-CV (Tex. App. 2005).
4. 629 N.W.2d 66 (2001).
5. 112 Wash. App. 1027 (2002).
6. 725 N.Y.S.2d 35 (2001).
7. 87 S.W.3d 203 (Tex. App. 2002).
8. 600 A.2d 1063 (D.C. 1991).
9. STEVE COHEN, *Malpractice,* NEW YORKER MAGAZINE, Oct. 1, 1990, at 43, 47.
10. 696 S.W.2d 16 (Tenn. Ct. App. 1985).
11. *Roberts v. Ray,* 322 S.W.2d 435 (Tenn. Ct. App. 1958).
12. 503 N.Y.S.2d 131 (N.Y. App. Div. 1986).
13. 720 N.E.2d 1175 (Ind. App. 1999)
14. 337 P.2d 974 (Or. 1959).
15. 221 N.W.2d 39 (S.D. 1974).
16. 786 F.2d 859 (8th Cir. 1986).
17. 405 A.2d 443 (N.J. Sup. Ct. 1979).
18. 335 S.E.2d 712 (Ga. Ct. App. 1985).
19. *Spirito v. Temple Corp.,* 466 N.E.2d 491 (Ind. Ct. App. 1984).
20. 746 P.2d 1006 (Idaho Ct. App. 1987).
21. 854 S.W.2d 250 (Tex. Ct. App. 1993).
22. 445 N.W.2d 763 (Iowa 1989).
23. 479 So. 2d 1119 (Ala. 1985).
24. 488 S.E.2d 389 (W. Va. 1997).
25. 482 N.W.2d 437 (Iowa 1992).
26. 346 S.E.2d 528 (S.C. 1986).
27. 291 N.E.2d 769 (Ohio Ct. App. 1973).
28. 320 A.2d 704 (Del. 1974).
29. 340 So. 2d 1065 (La. Ct. App. 1976).
30. 469 N.W.2d 74 (Mich. Ct. App. 1991).
31. *Id.* at 76.
32. 746 S.W.2d 108 (Mo. Ct. App. 1988).
33. *Oberzan v. Smith,* 869 P.2d 682 (Kan. 1994).
34. 4 N.W.2d 637–639 (Minn. 1942).
35. 738 P.2d 75 (Colo. Ct. App. 1987).
36. 75 N.W.2d 217 (Minn. 1956).
37. 358 S.E.2d 222 (W. Va. 1987).
38. 373 N.Y.S.2d 224 (N.Y. App. Div. 1975).
39. 320 A.2d 704 (Del. 1974).
40. No. 2003-CA-01573-COA (Miss. Ct. App. 2004).
41. 320 A.2d 637 (N.H. 1974).
42. *Id.*
43. 25 N.W.2d 351 (Mich. 1949).
44. *Wooten v. United States,* 574 F. Supp. 200 (W.D. Tenn. 1982).
45. 463 F. Supp. 321 (D. Alaska 1978).
46. 657 N.Y.S.2d 419 (N.Y. App. Div. 1997).
47. 154 S.E.2d 461 (Ga. Ct. App. 1967).
48. 411 So. 2d 109 (Ala. 1982).
49. 657 N.Y.S.2d 419 (N.Y. App. Div. 1997).
50. 820 N.E.2d 604, 354 Ill. App.3d 241, 289 (Ill. App. Ct. 2004)
51. Nos. 1030587 & 1030789 (Ala. 2004).
52. 658 N.Y.S.2d 34 (N.Y. App. Div. 1997).
53. No. 537-907 (Wis. Cir. Ct. Mar. 18, 1983).
54. 310 S.E.2d 326 (N.C. 1984).
55. 411 So. 2d 109, 113 (Ala. 1982).
56. 497 So. 2d 1233 (Fla. Dist. Ct. App. 1986).
57. 16 A.D.3d 898, 791 N.Y.S.2d 686 (N.Y. App. Div. 2005).
58. 804 S.W.2d 711 (Ark. 1991).
59. 681 F.2d 291 (5th Cir. 1982).
60. 510 So. 2d 538 (Ala. 1987).
61. 650 A.2d 1079 (Pa. Super. 1994).
62. *Callahan v. Cardinal Glennon Hosp.,* 863 S.W.2d 852 (Mo. 1993).
63. No. 97942 (N.C.Ct.Cl. 2005).
64. 512 N.Y.S.2d 519 (N.Y. App. Div. 1987).
65. 103 P.3d 135, 2004 UT 91 (Utah, 2004).
66. *Roussel v. Robbins,* 688 So. 2d 714, 723–24 (Miss. 1996).

Corporate Structure and Liability

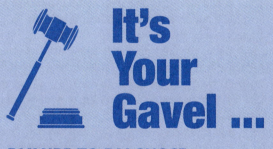

It's Your Gavel ...

FAILURE TO DIAGNOSE BREAST CANCER

The appellee, Condon, underwent a routine mammogram in July 1988. The mammogram revealed suspicious lesions in her right breast. Dr. Moore performed a biopsy at the AA Medical Center (AAMC). Dr. Williams, who was a pathologist working for Weisburger, MD, a pathology corporation providing contract pathology services to the hospital, performed an evaluation of the tissue. Williams reported noncancerous lesions in the right breast. Moore advised Condon that she did not have cancer but advised her to undergo frequent mammograms.

Condon, experiencing inflammation of her right breast, consulted with Moore in February 1990. Moore performed another biopsy. Condon was advised that the biopsy results indicated invasive carcinoma of the breast. As a result of the diagnosis, Condon underwent a bilateral modified radical mastectomy.

Condon brought a malpractice action against Williams and AAMC. The suit alleged malpractice on the part of Williams for failure to properly diagnose a biopsy as breast cancer. On the eve of the trial, Williams agreed to a $1 million settlement with the plaintiff. The circuit court entered judgment on a jury verdict in favor of the plaintiff. AAMC appealed, claiming that the release of the agent-Williams served to act as a release for AAMC.[1]

WHAT IS YOUR VERDICT?

This chapter introduces the health care professional to the responsibilities, as well as legal risks, of health care organizations and their governing bodies. Health care organizations are incorporated under state law as freestanding for-profit or not-for-profit corporations. Each corporation has a governing body (e.g., board of directors) that has ultimate responsibility for the operation of the organization. The existence of this authority creates certain duties and liabilities for governing boards and their individual members. The governing body is legally responsible for establishing and implementing policies regarding the management and operation of the organization. Responsibility for the day-to-day operations of an organization is generally accomplished by appointing a chief executive officer.

Not-for-profit health care organizations are usually exempt from federal taxation under Section 501(c)(3) of the

Internal Revenue Code of 1986, as amended. Such federal exemption usually entitles the organization to an automatic exemption from state taxes as well. Such tax exemption not only relieves the organization from the payment of income taxes and sales taxes, but also permits the organization to receive contributions from donors, who then may obtain charitable deductions on their personal income tax returns.

Although health care organizations may operate as sole proprietorships or partnerships, most function as corporations. Thus, an important source of law applicable to governing boards and to the duties and responsibilities of their members is found in state incorporation laws. These duties include holding meetings, establishing policies, being financially scrupulous, providing adequate insurance, and paying taxes.

AUTHORITY OF HEALTH CARE CORPORATIONS

Health care corporations—governmental, charitable, or proprietary—have certain powers expressly or implicitly granted to them by state statutes. Generally, the authority of a corporation is expressed in the law under which the corporation is chartered and in the corporation's articles of incorporation. The existence of this authority creates certain duties and liabilities for governing bodies and their individual members. Members of the governing body of an organization have both express and implied corporate authority.

Express Corporate Authority

Express corporate authority is the power specifically delegated by statute. A health care corporation derives its authority to act from the laws of the state in which it is incorporated. The articles of incorporation set forth the purpose(s) of the corporation's existence and the powers the corporation is authorized to exercise in order to carry out its purposes.

Implied Corporate Authority

Implied corporate authority is the right to perform any and all acts necessary to exercise a corporation's expressly conferred authority and to accomplish the purpose(s) for which it was created. Generally, implied corporate authority arises from situations in which such authority is required or suggested as a result of a need for corporate powers not specifically granted in the articles of incorporation. A governing body, at its own discretion, may enact new bylaws, rules, and regulations; purchase or mortgage property; borrow money; purchase equipment; select employees; adopt corporate resolutions that delineate decision-making responsibilities; and so

forth. These powers can be enumerated in the articles of incorporation and, in such cases, would be categorized as express rather than implied corporate authority.

Implied Duty: Select Competent Physicians

The Florida Supreme Court held in *Insinga v. LaBella*[2] that the *corporate negligence doctrine* imposes on hospitals an implied duty to patients to select competent physicians who, although they are independent practitioners, would be providing in-hospital care to their patients through staff privileges. Hospitals are in the best position to protect their patients and consequently have an independent duty to select competent independent physicians seeking staff privileges.

In this case, an action was brought against Canton (who was masquerading as a physician, Dr. LaBella), a hospital, and others for the wrongful death of a 68-year-old woman whom Canton had admitted. The patient died while she was in the hospital. Canton was found to be a fugitive from justice in Canada where he was under indictment for the manufacture and sale of illegal drugs. He fraudulently obtained a medical license from the state of Florida and staff privileges at the hospital by using the name of LaBella, a deceased physician. Canton was extradited to Canada without being served process.

The surgeon in *Purcell & Tucson General Hospital v. Zimbelman*[3] performed inappropriate surgery because of his misdiagnosis of the patient's ailment. Prior malpractice suits against the surgeon revealed that the hospital had reason to know or should have known that the surgeon apparently lacked the skill to treat the patient's condition. The court held that the hospital had a clear duty to select competent physicians; to regulate the privileges granted to staff physicians; to ensure that privileges are conferred only for those procedures for which the physician is trained and qualified; and to restrict, suspend, or require supervision when a physician has demonstrated an inability to perform certain procedures. The hospital assumed the duty of supervising the competence of its physicians. The department of surgery was acting for and on behalf of the hospital in fulfilling this duty. If the department was negligent in not taking action against the surgeon or recommending to the governing body that action be taken, the hospital would be negligent. The court noted that it is reasonable to conclude that if the hospital had taken some action against the surgeon, the patient would not have been injured.

Ultra Vires Acts

A governing body can be held liable for acting beyond its scope of authority, which is either expressed (e.g., in its articles of incorporation) or implied in law. Acts of this nature are referred to as *ultra vires acts.* The governing body acts in and on behalf of the corporation. If any action is in violation of a statute or regulation, it is illegal. An example of an illegal act would be the employment of an unlicensed person in a position that by law requires a license. The state, through its attorney general, has the power to prevent the performance of an ultra vires act by injunction. Governing bodies should have their corporate charters reviewed periodically by legal counsel to ensure that their express powers are consistent with the organization's mission, operations, and development plans.

In certain circumstances, members of an organization's governing body, as well as its corporate officers, may be individually responsible for ultra vires acts. This might be true, for example, if a member of a governing body or a corporate officer exceeded the powers of the corporation for individual benefit.

CORPORATE ORGANIZATION AND COMMITTEE STRUCTURE

Ultimate responsibility for the functioning of a health care corporation rests with the governing body. Ideally, the governing body includes representation from both the community and the organization's medical staff. The business of the governing body is generally conducted through a variety of committees. Some of those committees are described here.

Executive Committee

The executive committee is a working group of the governing body that has delegated authority to act on behalf of the full board. It must act within the scope and authority assigned by the governing body. The duties and responsibilities of the committee should be delineated in the corporate bylaws. The functions of the executive committee generally include acting as a liaison between management and the full board, reviewing and making recommendations on management proposals, and performing special assignments as may be delegated by the full board from time to time. Business transacted and actions taken by the executive committee should be reported at regular sessions of the governing body and ratified. The executive committee generally has all the powers of the governing body, except such powers as the governing body may be prohibited from delegating in accordance with applicable laws.

Bylaws Committee

The bylaws committee reviews and recommends bylaw changes to the governing body. Bylaws generally are amended or rescinded by a majority vote of the governing body.

Finance Committee

The finance committee is responsible for overseeing the financial affairs of the organization and making recommendations to the governing body. This committee is responsible for directing and reviewing the preparation of financial statements, operating budgets, major capital requests, and so on. The governing body must approve actions of the finance committee.

Joint Conference Committee

The joint conference committee is often a group consisting of an equal number of representatives from both the executive committees of the governing body and medical staff, along with representation from administration and nursing. The committee acts as a forum for discussion of matters of policy and practice pertaining to patient care. The committee generally meets quarterly and reports on its activities to the governing body.

Nominating Committee

The nominating committee is generally responsible for developing and recommending to the governing body criteria for governing body membership. The requirements for membership on a governing body generally include a willingness to devote the time and energy necessary to fulfill the commitment as a board member; residence in the community or an identifiable association with the community served; demonstration of a knowledge of local health care issues; possession of the traits of good moral character and maturity; and professional, as well as appropriate, life experiences necessary to make managerial decisions in the health care setting.

Planning Committee

The planning committee is responsible for recommending to the governing body the use and development of organizational resources as they relate to the mission and vision of the organization. The committee develops a plan and oversees its implementation throughout the organization. Major issues that the planning committee reviews include the organization's need to increase market share, expand services, downsize where appropriate, and integrate services across the entire continuum of care in a competitive marketplace. Specifically, the planning committee oversees:

- periodic review of the organization's mission and vision statements

- conducting of community health needs assessments
- development of strategic plans and ongoing monitoring
- development of short-term and long-range goals
- maintenance of the organization's physical facilities
- preparation of capital budgets
- oversight of expansion programs
- acquisition of major equipment
- addition of new services based on identified community need
- downsizing and closing services
- regular planning progress reports to the full board
- program development
- corporate development

The committee generally includes representation from the governing body, administration, medical staff, and nursing. When organizational planning affects the delivery of patient care services, a mechanism for obtaining community input is incorporated into the planning process.

Patient Care Committee

The patient care committee reviews the quality of patient care rendered in the organization and makes recommendations for the improvement of such care. The committee is generally responsible for developing a process to identify patient and family needs and expectations and to establish a process to continuously improve customer relations. This process often includes:

- development of a tool to identify patient and family needs and expectations
- methodology for reviewing data
- identification of patterns of concern
- mechanism for forwarding information to those responsible for implementing change in the organization
- continuing review, evaluation, and implementation of plans for improving organizational performance

Audit and Regulatory Compliance Committee

The audit and regulatory compliance committee is responsible for the assessment of various functions and control systems of the organization and for providing management with analysis and recommendations regarding activities

reviewed. Health care organizations must be vigilant in conducting their financial affairs. As the boards of several investment organizations have experienced in recent years, failure to do so can result in fines and imprisonment. An effective audit committee can be helpful in uncovering and thwarting poor or inept financial decision making. The committee should include members from the governing body and internal auditing staff. Responsibilities of the committee include:

- developing corporate auditing policies and procedures
- recommending independent auditors to the governing body
- reviewing the credentials of the independent auditors and facilitating change in auditors as may be deemed appropriate
- reviewing with independent auditors the proposed scope and general extent of their auditing duties and responsibilities
- reviewing the scope and results of the annual audit with the independent auditors and the organization's management staff
- setting, overseeing, reviewing, and acting on the recommendations of the internal audit staff
- reviewing the internal accounting practices of the corporation, including policies and procedures
- reviewing and evaluating financial statements (e.g., income statements, balance sheets, cash flow reports, investment accounts)
- promoting the prevention, detection, deterrence, and reporting of fraud
- reviewing the means for safeguarding assets, and, as appropriate, the existence of such assets
- ensuring that financial reporting functions are in keeping with generally accepted accounting principles
- reviewing the reliability and integrity of financial and operating information

Failure on the part of an audit committee to question management's representations may be the basis for committee malfeasance, because the committee and the governing body may be held liable for their failure to know what they were responsible for recognizing.

Safety Committee

The safety committee is generally charged with responsibility for overseeing the organization's safety management program. The committee reviews and acts on reports involving the organization's emergency preparedness, equipment management, and fire safety risk management and utilities management programs.

SARBANES-OXLEY ACT

The Sarbanes-Oxley Act of 2002, commonly called SOX or SARBOX, was enacted as a response to the misconduct committed by executives in companies such as Enron, World Com, and Tyco, resulting in investor losses exceeding a half a trillion dollars. To protect investors in public companies and improve the accuracy and reliability of corporate disclosures, SOX requires top executives of public corporations to vouch for the financial reports of their companies. The act encourages self-regulation and the need to promote due diligence; select a leader with morals and core values; examine incentives; constantly monitor the organization's culture; build a strong, knowledgeable governing body; continuously search for conflicts of interest in the organization; focus attention on processes and controls that support accurate financial reporting through documented policies and procedures; and establish strong standards of conduct and a code of ethics that encourages employees to report unethical or fraudulent behavior without fear of retribution.

The act covers issues such as establishing a public company accounting oversight board, auditor independence, corporate responsibility, and enhanced financial disclosure.

Major provisions of SOX include:

– Certification of financial reports by CEOs and CFOs

– Ban on personal loans to any executive officer and director

– Accelerated reporting of trades by insiders

– Prohibition on insider trades during pension fund blackout periods

– Public reporting of CEO and CFO compensation and profits

– Inside audit board independence

– Criminal and civil penalties for securities violations

– Obligation to have an internal audit function, which will need to be certified by external auditors

– Significantly longer jail sentences and larger fines for corporate executives who knowingly misstate financial statements

– Codes of ethics and standards of conduct for executive officers and board members. (Most companies have expanded their code of ethics to include all employees and attach the document to their public reports.)

Although not-for-profit organizations are not legally required to adopt SOX, the accountability and financial reporting requirements are being adopted by many hospitals.

DOCTRINE OF RESPONDEAT SUPERIOR

Respondeat superior (let the master respond) is a legal doctrine holding employers liable, in certain cases, for the wrongful acts of their agents (employees). This doctrine has also been referred to as *vicarious liability,* whereby an employer is answerable for the torts committed by employees. In the health care setting, an organization, for example, is liable for the negligent acts of its employees, even though there has been no wrongful conduct on the part of the organization. For liability to be imputed to the employer:

1. A master-servant relationship must exist between the employer and the employee; and

2. The wrongful act of the employee must have occurred within the scope of his or her employment.

The question of liability frequently rests on whether persons treating a patient are independent agents (responsible for their own acts) or employees of the organization. The answer to this depends on whether the organization can exercise control over the particular act that was the proximate cause of the injury. The basic rationale for imposing liability on an employer developed because of the employer's right to control the physical acts of its employees. It is not necessary that the employer actually exercise control, only that it possesses the right, power, or authority to do so.

When filing a lawsuit, the plaintiff's attorney generally names both the employer and employee. This occurs because the employer is generally in a better financial condition to cover the judgment. The employer is not without remedy if liability has been imposed against the organization due an employee's negligent act. The employer, if sued, may seek *indemnification* (i.e., compensation for the financial loss caused by the employee's negligent act) from the employee.

Hospitals can be vicariously liable for the negligent acts of independent contracted emergency department physicians. In *Schiavone v. Victory Mem. Hosp.,*[4] the decedent was transported to the hospital emergency department by ambulance. The patient sought emergency treatment from the hospital, not from any specific physician of the patient's own choosing. Thus, the hospital was vicariously liable for the alleged malpractice of the appellant even though he was an independent contractor with the hospital at the time of the occurrence.

INDEPENDENT CONTRACTOR: RESPONDEAT SUPERIOR NOT APPLICABLE

Citation: *Hoffman v. Moore Reg'l Hosp., Inc.,* 441 S.E.2d 567 (N.C. Ct. App. 1994)

Facts

Hoffman was admitted to the hospital with an order for a renal arteriogram. After her admission, Hoffman was presented with a consent form for the procedure. The consent listed five radiologists on the form but did not specify which radiologist would perform the procedure. The list of radiologists was composed of members of the Pinehurst radiology group. The group determined which radiologist would cover the hospital each day. Dr. Lina was assigned to perform Hoffman's procedure. Following the renal arteriogram, Lina determined that an angioplasty was necessary. Because of complications during the procedure, Hoffman had to be transferred to University Medical Center. Her condition deteriorated during the following year and she eventually died. Mr. Hoffman then sought to hold the hospital liable for the negligence of the radiologist under the theory of respondeat superior. The trial court dismissed the claim that the hospital was liable under the theory of respondeat superior.

Issue

Was the hospital liable for the malpractice of Lina under the theory of respondeat superior?

Holding

The North Carolina Court of Appeals held that the hospital was not liable for the negligence of Lina under the theory of respondeat superior.

Reason

The court of appeals held that Lina was not an employee of the hospital. He was not subject to supervision or control by the hospital. There was no evidence that Hoffman would have sought treatment elsewhere if she had known for a fact that Lina was not an employee.

Discussion

1. Under what conditions could the hospital have been liable for Lina's alleged negligence?
2. Can the patient recover damages from the radiologist who performed the radiologic procedure?
3. Can the patient recover damages from the Pinehurst radiology group?

Independent Contractor

An independent contractor relationship is established when the principal has no right of control over the manner in which the agent's work is to be performed. The independent contractor therefore is responsible for his or her own negligent acts. However, some cases indicate that an organization may be held liable for an independent contractor's negligence. For example, in *Mehlman v. Powell,*[5] the court held that a hospital may be found vicariously liable for the negligence of an emergency department physician who was not a hospital employee but who worked in the emergency department in the capacity of an independent contractor. The court reasoned that the hospital maintained control over billing procedures, maintained an emergency department in the main hospital, and represented to the patient that the members of the emergency department staff were its employees, which may have caused the patient to rely on the skill and competence of the staff.

The doctrine of respondeat superior may impose liability on an organization for a nurse's acts or omissions that result in injury to a patient. Whether such liability attaches depends on whether the conduct of the nurse was wrongful and whether the nurse was subject to the control of the organization at the time the act in question was performed. Determination of whether the nurse's conduct was wrongful in a given situation depends on the standard of conduct to which the nurse is expected to adhere. In liability deliberations, the nurse who is subject to the control of the organization at the time of the negligent conduct is considered an employee and is not a borrowed servant.

Corporate Officer/Director

An officer or a director of a corporation is not personally liable for the torts of corporate employees. To incur liability, the officer or the director ordinarily must be shown to have in some way authorized, directed, or participated in a tortious act. The administrator of the estate of the deceased in *Hunt v. Rabon*[6] brought a malpractice action against hospital trustees and others for the wrongful death of the decedent during an operation at the hospital. A contractor had incorrectly crossed the oxygen and nitrous oxide lines of a newly installed medical gas system leading to the operating room. The trustees filed a *demurrer*—a pleading claiming that the facts of the case were not sufficient for an action against them individually as trustees. The lower court sustained the demurrer, and the plaintiff appealed. On appeal, the South Carolina Supreme Court held that the allegations presented were insufficient to hold the trustees liable for the wrongs alleged.

CORPORATE NEGLIGENCE

There are duties that the corporation itself owes to the general public and to its patients. These duties arise from statutes, regulations, principles of law developed by the courts, and the internal operating rules of the organization. A corporation is treated no differently than an individual. If a corporation has a duty and fails in the exercise of that duty, it has the same liability to the injured party as an individual would have.

> Corporate negligence is a doctrine under which the hospital is liable if it fails to uphold the proper standard of care owed the patient, which is to ensure the patient's safety and well-being while at the hospital. This theory of liability creates a non-delegable duty which the hospital owes directly to a patient. Therefore, an injured party does not have to rely on and establish the negligence of a third party.[7]

Corporate negligence occurs when a health care corporation fails to perform those duties it owes directly to a patient or to anyone else to whom a duty may extend. If such a duty is breached and a patient is injured as a result of that breach, the organization can be held culpable under the theory of corporate negligence.

Hospitals once enjoyed complete tort immunity as charitable institutions. As hospitals evolved into more sophisticated corporate entities that expected fees for their services, their tort immunity receded. Courts first recognized that hospitals could be held liable for the negligence of their employees under the theory of respondeat superior. Liability later extended for nonemployees who acted as a hospital's ostensible agents. In *Thompson v. Nason Hospital,*[8] the evolution continued. The Pennsylvania court recognized that hospitals are more than mere conduits through which health care professionals are brought into contact with patients. Hospitals owe some nondelegable duties directly to their patients independent of the negligence of their employees or ostensible agents, such as a duty to:

- use reasonable care in the maintenance of safe facilities and equipment

- select and retain competent physicians

- oversee all persons who practice medicine within their walls

- formulate, adopt, and enforce rules and policies to ensure quality care

Darling—A Benchmark Case

The benchmark case in the health care field, which has had a major impact on the liability of health care organizations, was decided in 1965 in *Darling v. Charleston Community Memorial Hospital.*[9] The court enunciated a *corporate negligence doctrine* under which hospitals have a duty to provide an adequately trained medical and nursing staff. A hospital is responsible, in conjunction with its medical staff, for establishing policies and procedures for monitoring the quality of medicine practiced within the hospital.

The Darling case involved an 18-year-old college football player who was preparing for a career as a teacher and coach. The patient, a defensive halfback for his college football team, was injured during a play. He was rushed to the emergency department of a small, accredited community hospital where the only physician on emergency duty that day was Dr. Alexander, a general practitioner. Alexander had not treated a major leg fracture in three years.

The physician examined the patient and ordered an X-ray that revealed that the tibia and the fibula of the right leg had been fractured. The physician reduced the fracture and applied a plaster cast from a point three or four inches below the groin to the toes. Shortly after the cast had been applied, the patient began to complain continually of pain. The physician split the cast and continued to visit the patient frequently while the patient remained in the hospital. Not thinking it was necessary, the emergency department physician did not call in any specialist for consultation.

After two weeks, the student was transferred to a larger hospital and placed under the care of an orthopedic surgeon. The specialist found a considerable amount of dead tissue in the fractured leg. During a period of two months, the specialist removed increasing amounts of tissue in a futile attempt to save the leg until it became necessary to amputate the leg eight inches below the knee. The student's father did not agree to a settlement and filed suit against the emergency department physician and the hospital. Although the physician later settled out of court for $40,000, the case continued against the hospital.

The documentary evidence relied on to establish the standard of care included the rules and regulations of the Illinois Department of Public Health under the Hospital Licensing Act; the standards for hospital accreditation, today known as

The Joint Commission; and the bylaws, rules, and regulations of Charleston Hospital. These documents were admitted into evidence without objection. No specific evidence was offered that the hospital failed to conform to the usual and customary practices of hospitals in the community.

The trial court instructed the jury to consider those documents, along with all other evidence, in determining the hospital's liability. Under the circumstances in which the case reached the Illinois Supreme Court, it was held that the verdict against the hospital should be sustained if the evidence supported the verdict on any one or more of the 20 allegations of negligence. Allegations asserted that the hospital was negligent in its failure to: (1) provide a sufficient number of trained nurses for bedside care—in this case, nurses who were capable of recognizing the progressive gangrenous condition of the plaintiff's right leg; and (2) failure of its nurses to bring the patient's condition to the attention of the administration and staff so that adequate consultation could be secured.

Although these generalities provided the jury with no practical guidance for determining what constitutes reasonable care, they were considered relevant to aid the jury in deciding what was feasible and what the hospital knew or should have known concerning its responsibilities for patient care.

Evidence relating to the hospital's failure to review Alexander's work, to require consultation or examination by specialists, and to require proper nursing care was found to be sufficient to support a verdict for the patient. Judgment was eventually returned against the hospital in the amount of $100,000. The Illinois Supreme Court held that the hospital could not limit its liability as a charitable corporation to the amount of its liability insurance.

> [T]he doctrine of charitable immunity can no longer stand . . . a doctrine which limits the liability of charitable corporations to the amount of liability insurance that they see fit to carry permits them to determine whether or not they will be liable for their torts and the amount of that liability, if any.[10]

In effect, the hospital was liable as a corporate entity for the negligent acts of its employees and physicians. Among other things, the Darling case indicates the importance of instituting effective credentialing and continuing medical evaluation and review programs for all members of a professional staff.

Corporate Responsibility and Physician Competency

Health care organizations have a responsibility to ensure the competency of their medical staffs and to evaluate the quality of medical treatment rendered on their premises. A court of appeals in *Elam v. College Park Hospital*[11] held that a hospital is liable to a patient under the doctrine of corporate negligence for the negligent conduct of independent physicians and surgeons who are neither employees nor agents of the hospital.

In *Dykema v. Carolina Emergency Physicians, P.C.,*[12] Dykema began having respiratory symptoms, cough, and shortness of breath for which he was seen by Dr. King, his family physician. He sought a second opinion from the Center for Family Medicine (center), part of the Greenville Hospital System. Dykema went to the center with complaints of cough, shortness of breath, and tightness in the chest. He was seen that day by a third-year medical student, Dr. Gemas, and Dr. Pearman, an attending faculty member. Pearman prescribed antibiotics for persistent bronchitis and told Dykema to return in one week or sooner if his condition worsened. Early Sunday morning, February 6, Mrs. Dykema called the center concerning her husband's worsening condition and was advised to take him to the hospital the next day. She brought him to the hospital at approximately 1:00 P.M. on February 6, and he was seen by Dr. Connell, a medical resident and employee of Greenville Hospital System. Connell diagnosed viral bronchitis and advised Dykema to continue his antibiotics and keep his follow-up appointment at the center on February 8. The next morning, February 7, Mrs. Dykema called the center and spoke with a receptionist and requested that her husband be seen immediately due to his worsening condition. She was told there were no earlier appointments available and that she should keep the appointment on February 8. Dykema died on the morning of February 8, prior to his scheduled appointment. The cause of death was a progressive showering of pulmonary emboli, pieces of which moved to his lungs and caused a fatal blockage. The defendant hospital was found liable for the full $2 million in actual damages.

Joint Liability

Joint liability is based on the concept that all joint or concurrent tort-feasors are actually independently at fault for their own wrongful acts. Both a hospital and its physicians can be held jointly liable for damages suffered by patients. In *Gonzales v. Nork & Mercy Hospital,*[13] the hospital was found negligent for failing to protect the patient, a 27-year-old man, from acts of malpractice by an independent, privately retained physician. The patient had been injured in an automobile accident and was operated on by Dr. Nork, an orthopedic surgeon. The plaintiff's life expectancy was reduced as a result of an unsuccessful and allegedly unnecessary laminectomy. It was found that the hospital knew or should have known of the surgeon's incompetence because the surgeon previously had performed many operations either unnecessarily or negligently. In such cases the defendant produced false and inadequate findings as well as false-positive myelograms. He deceived his patients with this information and caused them to undergo surgery. Evidence was presented showing that the surgeon had performed more than three dozen similar operations unnecessarily or in a negligent manner. Even if the hospital was not aware of the surgeon's acts of negligence, an effective monitoring system should have been in place for monitoring his abilities. Consequently, the surgeon and hospital were jointly liable for damages suffered.

An organization owes its patients a duty of care, and this duty includes the obligation to protect them from negligent and fraudulent acts of those physicians with a propensity to commit malpractice. The courts will not permit organizations to hide behind a cloak of ignorance in this responsibility.

DUTIES OF HEALTH CARE CORPORATIONS

Governing body members are considered by law to have the highest measure of accountability. They have a fiduciary duty that requires acting primarily for the benefit of the corporation. The general duties of a governing body are both implied and express. The duty to supervise and manage is applicable to the trustees just as it is to the managers of any other business corporation. In both instances, there is a duty to act as a reasonably prudent person would act under similar circumstances.

Appoint a CEO

The governing body is responsible for appointing a CEO to act as an agent in the management of the organization. The individual selected as CEO must possess the competence and the character necessary to maintain satisfactory standards of patient care within the organization. The responsibilities and authority of the CEO should be expressed in an appropriate job description, as well as in any formal agreement or contract that the organization has with the CEO. Some state health codes describe the responsibilities of administrators in broad terms. They generally provide that the CEO/administrator shall be responsible for the overall management of the organization; enforcement of any applicable federal, state, and local regulations, as well as the organization's bylaws, policies, and procedures; appointment of, with the approval of the governing body, a qualified medical director; liaison between the governing body and staff (including both employed and appointed members of the professional staff); and appointment of an administrative person to act during the CEO's absence from the organization.

The general duty of a governing body is to exercise due care and diligence in supervising and managing the organization. This duty does not cease with the selection of a CEO.

A governing body can be liable if the level of patient care becomes inadequate because of the governing body's failure to supervise properly the management of the organization. CEOs, as is the case with board members, can be personally liable for their own acts of negligence that injure others.

Administrator Licensure

To comply with federal requirements, the various states have incorporated licensing requirements in their regulations. Administrators are licensed under the laws of their individual states. Statutes generally provide that the administrator of a nursing facility be licensed in accordance with state law.

States that require administrators to be licensed provide penalties ranging from fines to imprisonment for those administrators functioning without a license. A $5,000 fine was imposed on a nursing facility for operating without a licensed administrator for 54 days in *Magnolias Nursing and Convalescent Center v. Department of Health and Rehabilitation Services.*[14] The statute prohibiting operation of a nursing home without a licensed administrator was not considered vague, ambiguous, or unconstitutional.

Comply with the Law

The governing body in general and its agents (assigned representatives) in particular are responsible for compliance with federal, state, and local laws regarding the operation of the organization. Depending on the scope of the wrong committed and the intent of the governing body, failure to comply could subject board members and/or their agents to civil liability and, in some instances, to criminal prosecution.

Failure to comply with applicable statutory regulations can be costly. This was the case in *People v. Casa Blanca Convalescent Homes,*[15] in which there was evidence of numerous and prolonged deficiencies in resident care. The nursing home's practice of providing insufficient personnel constituted not only illegal practice but also unfair business practice in violation of Section 17200 of the California Business and Professions Code. The trial court was found to have properly assessed a fine of $2,500 for each of 67 violations, totaling $167,500, where the evidence showed that the operator of the nursing home had the financial ability to pay that amount.

Comply with Joint Commission Standards

The governing body, if accredited by the Joint Commission, is responsible for compliance with applicable standards promulgated by the Joint Commission. Noncompliance could cause an organization to lose accreditation, which in turn would provide grounds for third-party reimbursement agencies (e.g., Medicare) to refuse payment for treatment rendered to patients.

Provide Timely Treatment

Health care organizations can be held liable for delays in treatment that result in injuries to their patients. For example, the patient in *Heddinger v. Ashford Memorial Community Hospital*[16] filed a malpractice action against a hospital and its insurer, alleging that a delay in treating her left hand resulted in the loss of her little finger. Medical testimony presented at trial indicated that if proper and timely treatment had been rendered, the finger would have been saved. The U.S. District Court entered judgment on a jury verdict for the plaintiff in the amount of $175,000. The hospital appealed, and the U.S. Court of Appeals held that even if the physicians who attended the patient were not employees of the hospital but were independent contractors, the risk of negligent treatment was clearly foreseeable by the hospital.

Avoid Self-Dealing and Conflicts of Interest

Governing body members must refrain from self-dealing and avoid conflict-of-interest situations. Each board member should submit in writing all outstanding voting shares (where applicable) or any relationships or transactions in which the director might or could have a conflict of interest. Membership on the governing body or its committees should not be used for private gain. Board members are expected to disclose potential conflict-of-interest situations and withdraw from the boardroom at the time of voting on such issues. Board members who suspect a conflict-of-interest situation have a right and a duty to raise pertinent questions regarding any potential conflict. Conflict of interest is presumed to exist when a board member or a firm with which he or she is associated may benefit or lose from the passage of a proposed action.

Membership on the governing body of a nonprofit organization is deemed a public service. Neither the court nor the community expects or desires such public service to be turned to private gain. Thus, the standards imposed on board members regarding the investment of trust funds, self-dealing transactions, or personal compensation may be stricter than those for directors of business corporations. The essential rules regarding self-dealing are clear. Generally, a contract between the organization and a trustee financially interested in the transaction is voidable by the organization in the event that the interested trustee spoke or voted in favor of the arrangement or did not disclose fully the material facts regarding his or her interest. This resolution of the self-dealing problem is based on the belief that if an interested board member does not participate in the gov-

erning body's action and does make full disclosure of his or her interest, the disinterested remaining members of the governing body are able to protect the organization's interests. Statutory provisions in some states specifically forbid self-dealing transactions altogether, irrespective of disclosure or the fairness of the deal.

Provide Adequate Staff

Staffing shortages for both hospitals and nursing homes continue to plague the health care industry. Because the quality of care provided by nursing homes is the subject of much scrutiny, American families face difficult decisions about whether to move a loved one into such a setting.

Under federal law, nursing facilities must have sufficient nursing staff to provide nursing and related services adequate to attain and maintain the highest practicable physical, mental, and psychosocial well-being of each resident, as determined by resident assessments and individual plans of care. As nursing facilities are increasingly filled with older, disabled residents with ever-increasing complex care needs, the demands for highly educated and trained nursing personnel continue to grow.[17] Organizations that fail to meet federal standards can lose certification as a provider of patient care. This can in turn lead to the denial of reimbursement under federal entitlement programs.

"Federal health officials have concluded that most nursing homes are understaffed to the point that patients may be endangered. For the first time, the government is recommending strict new rules that would require thousands of the homes to hire more nurses and health aides."[18] A report released by Rep. Ciro Rodriguez and Rep. Gene Green in 2002 found that the vast majority of Texas nursing homes are understaffed and fail to comply with federal standards.[19] The continuing problems of nursing facility staffing prompted Rep. Waxman to introduce the Nursing Home Staffing Act of 2005 to establish minimum staff requirements for nursing homes receiving payments under the Medicare or Medicaid Program.

> Many medical and regulatory investigators who work in nursing homes every day characterize the number of wrongful deaths in terms such as "massive" and "pervasive," based on their daily experience. Most of the deaths can be traced to an inadequate number of nurses and aides to provide life-sustaining care. The U.S. Department of Health and Human Services reported to Congress this year that nine out of 10 nursing homes have staffing levels too low to provide adequate care.[20]

The answer to staffing requires a continuing emphasis on recruitment and education, development of career ladders, respect for caregivers, salaries commensurate with the requirements of the job, and severe prosecution of those who seek financial gain by purposely understaffing their facilities.

Deficient Nursing Care

The nursing facility in *Our Lady of the Woods v. Commonwealth of Kentucky Health Facilities*[21] was closed because of deficiencies found during an inspection of the facility, the most serious of which was the lack of continuous nursing care on all shifts. The court held that evidence that the nursing facility lacked continuous services required by regulation was sufficient to sustain an order to close the facility. The appellants in this case had been notified of the deficiencies and were ordered to correct them. Many witnesses testified concerning the deficiencies, and even the administrator admitted to the most serious violation—lack of continuous nursing services. The hearing officer, although noting that the quality of care provided to the facility's residents was satisfactory, concluded:

> The facts clearly reveal that the respondent has long violated one of the "essential functions of a nursing home" by not providing continuous graduate nursing supervision. To contend that such supervision can be provided from afar (by an "on-call" nurse) is to contend that a resident will never be confronted with a medical problem of such immediacy that his health or even his life would not be endangered while awaiting the arrival of the "on-call" professional. Such contention is unacceptable; the facility violated on a protracted basis one of its most substantive mandates. Absent proof that an adequate nursing staff could not be obtained (there is no such proof herein), it must be concluded that there is no justification for this violation.[22]

The court held that "deference is given to the trier of the fact, and agency determinations are to be upheld if the decision is supported by substantial, reliable, and probative evidence in the record as a whole."[23]

Timely Response to Patient Calls

Health care organizations must provide for adequate staffing. The court of appeal in *Leavitt v. St. Tammany Parish Hospital*[24] held that the hospital owed a duty to respond promptly to patient calls for help. The hospital breached its duty by having less-than-adequate staff on hand and by failing to at least verbally answer an assistance light to inquire what the patient needed.

Postoperative Care

The patient in *Czubinsky v. Doctors Hospital,*[25] recovering from anesthesia, went into cardiac arrest and sustained permanent damages. The court of appeals held that the injuries sustained by the patient were the direct result of the hospital's failure to properly monitor and render aid when needed in the immediate postoperative period. The registered nurse assigned to the patient had a duty to remain with her until the patient was transferred to the recovery room. The nurse's absence was the proximate cause of the patient's injuries. Failure of the hospital to provide adequate staff to assist the patient in the immediate postoperative period was an act in dereliction of duty—a failure that resulted in readily foreseeable permanent damages.

Nursing Facility Staffing

Residents in nursing facilities must be under the care and supervision of a physician. Provision should be made by the facility to obtain the services of at least one physician to oversee the quality of medical care.

States are more exacting than Medicare regulations in expressing nurse-resident ratios. In *Koelbl v. Whalen,*[26] regulations requiring the employment of sufficient personnel to provide for resident needs in nursing or convalescent homes were found to be sufficiently clear to avoid their being held unconstitutionally vague. State regulations vary in the methods used to establish staffing requirements. State regulations are often developed to ensure that the resident receives treatment, therapies, medications, and nourishment as prescribed in the resident care plans; the resident is kept clean, comfortable, and well groomed; and the resident is protected from accident, infection, and so forth.

In addition to nurses and physicians, a variety of other health care workers in nursing facilities support the care and services provided to residents. They include dietitians, physical therapists, social workers, activity directors, and others. The members of this group have specialized training and usually are licensed or certified by the state to practice their specialties. They differ from the medical or nursing staff in that they may not be involved with all residents, but rather limit their activities to residents needing their special skills.

Deficient Care Given

In *Montgomery Health Care Facility v. Ballard,*[27] three nurses testified that the nursing facility was understaffed. One nurse testified that she asked her supervisor for more help but did not get it. The estate of a nursing home resident, who had expired as the result of multiple infected bedsores, brought a malpractice action against the nursing home. First American Health Care, Inc., is the parent corporation of the Montgomery Health Care Facility. The trial court entered a judgment on a jury verdict against the home, and an appeal was taken. The Alabama Supreme Court held that reports compiled by the Alabama Department of Public Health concerning deficiencies found in the nursing home were admissible as evidence. Evidence showed that the care given to the deceased was deficient in the same ways as noted in the survey and complaint reports, which indicated that deficiencies in the home included:

> [I]nadequate documentation of treatment given for decubitus ulcers; 23 patients found with decubitus ulcers, 10 of whom developed those ulcers in the facility; dressings on the sores were not changed as ordered; nursing progress notes did not describe patients' ongoing conditions, particularly with respect to descriptions of decubitus ulcers; ineffective policies and procedures with respect to sterile dressing supplies; lack of nursing assessments; incomplete patient care plans; inadequate documentation of doctor's visits, orders or progress notes; A.M. care not consistently documented; inadequate documentation of turning of patients; incomplete "activities of daily living" sheets; "range of motion" exercises not documented; patients found wet and soiled with dried fecal matter; lack of bowel and bladder retaining programs; incomplete documentation of ordered force fluids. . . .[28]

From a corporate standpoint, the parent corporation of the nursing facility could be held liable for the nursing facility's negligence, where the parent company controlled or retained the right to control the day-to-day operations of the home. The defendants argued that the punitive damage award of $2 million against the home was greater than what was necessary to meet society's goal of punishing them. The Alabama Supreme Court, however, found the award not to be excessive. "The trial court also found that because of the large number of nursing home residents vulnerable to the type of neglect found in Mrs. Stovall's case, the verdict would further the goal of discouraging others from similar conduct in the future."[29]

Provide Adequate Facilities and Equipment

Health care organizations are under a duty to exercise reasonable care to furnish adequate equipment, appliances, and supplies for use in the diagnosis or treatment of patients. Equipment furnished by an organization should be fit for the purposes and uses intended. Within its duty to provide adequate facilities and equipment, the governing body must exercise reasonable care and skill in supervising and managing facility property. This obligation includes protecting property from destruction and loss.

Health care organizations must be designed, constructed, equipped, and maintained to provide a safe, healthy, functional, sanitary, and comfortable environment for patients, employees, and the public. Buildings and equipment should be maintained and operated to prevent fire and other hazards to personal safety. Patient rooms should be designed and equipped for adequate nursing care, comfort, and privacy. Mechanical, electric, and patient care equipment should be maintained in a safe operating condition.

Driftwood Convalescent Hospital, operated by Western Medical Enterprises, Inc., in *Beach v. Western Medical Enterprises, Inc.,*[30] was fined $2,500 in civil penalties because of nonfunctioning hallway lights and the facility's failure to provide the required type and amount of decubitus preventive equipment necessary for resident care as required by the California Health and Safety Code. The regulations required that equipment necessary for care to patients, as ordered or indicated be provided.

> Though no evidence was introduced to show that the decubitus equipment had been ordered by a physician, the phrase "as indicated" supports an inference that when a patient's condition requires certain equipment, the fact that no physician has ordered that equipment does not relieve the hospital (nursing facility) of the responsibility for providing equipment necessary for patient care.[31]

Provide Adequate Insurance

One basic protection for tangible property is adequate insurance against fire and other risks. This duty extends to keeping the physical plant of the corporation in good repair and appropriating funds for such purpose when necessary.

The duty of the governing body is to purchase insurance against different risks. Organizations face as much risk of losing their tangible and intangible assets through judgments for negligence as they do through fires or other disasters. When this is true, the duty to insure against the risks of fire is as great as the duty to insure against the risks of negligent conduct.

Be Financially Scrupulous

Health care organizations searching for alternate sources of income must do so scrupulously and not find themselves in what could be construed as questionable corporate activities. *Smith v. van Gorkum*[32] involved a board of directors that authorized the sale of its company through a cash-out merger for a tendered price per share nearly 50 percent over the market price. Although that might sound like a good deal, the governing body did not make any inquiry to determine whether it was the best deal available. In fact, it made no decision during a hastily arranged, brief meeting in which it relied solely on the CEO's report regarding the desirability of the move. The Delaware Supreme Court held that the board's decision to approve a proposed cash-out merger was not a product of informed business judgment and that it acted in a grossly negligent manner in approving amendments to the merger proposal.

A triable claim of illegal fee splitting was stated in *Hauptman v. Grand Manor Health Related Facility, Inc.,*[33] by the allegations of a psychiatrist that a nursing home barred him from continuing to treat its residents unless he joined a professional corporation, the members of which included owners of the nursing home. Under the proposed agreement, the nursing home would retain 20 percent of the fees collected on his behalf. Although Section 6509 (a) of the New York Education Law does not prohibit members of a professional corporation from pooling fees, the statute did not apply to forced conscription into a corporation at the price of surrendering a portion of one's fees unwillingly. Likewise, Title 8, Section 29.1[b][4] of the New York Compilation of Codes and Rules expressly forbids a professional corporation from charging a fee for billing and office expenses based on a percentage of income from a practice. The psychiatrist's allegations also showed possible violation of New York Public Health Law § 2801(b), which prohibited exclusion of a practitioner on grounds not related to reasonable objectives of the organization.

In *Lynch v. Redfield Foundation,*[34] a California bank refused to honor corporate drafts unless all trustees concurred. They could not agree, and funds in a noninterest-bearing account continued to grow in principal from $4,900 to $47,000 over a five-year period. Although two trustees did try to carry on corporate functions despite a dissident trustee, their good faith did not protect them from liability in this case. The money could have been transferred to at least an interest-bearing account without the third trustee's signature. The trustees were held jointly liable to pay to the corporation the statutory rate of simple interest.

Require Competitive Bidding

Many states have developed regulations requiring competitive bidding for work or services commissioned by public organizations. The fundamental purpose of this requirement is to eliminate or at least reduce the possibility that such abuses as fraud, favoritism, improvidence, or extravagance will intrude into an organization's business practices. Contracts made in violation of a statute are considered illegal and could result in personal liability for board members, especially if the members become aware of a fraudulent activity

and allow it to continue. The mere appearance of favoritism toward one contractor over another could give rise to an unlawful action. For example, a board member's pressing the administrator to favor one ambulance transporter over others because of his or her social acquaintance with the owner is suspect. An organization's governing body should avoid even the appearance of wrongdoing by requiring competitive bidding.

Provide a Safe Environment

Each organization is responsible for providing a safe environment for patients, staff, and visitors. Responsibility for this function is often assigned to an organization's plant services/engineering department. Among other duties, the department is responsible for the provision of heat, water, electricity, and refrigeration and for maintenance of the organization's equipment and physical plant. The duties of the department may vary from one organization to the next, depending on the size of a particular organization's facilities.

It is essential that employers provide a safe environment for both patients and employees. Although one cannot guard against the unforeseeable, a health care organization is liable for injuries resulting from dangers that it knowingly failed to guard against or those that it should have known about and failed to guard against.

An organization can be subject to corporate liability if it fails to ensure a patient's safety and well-being. Health care corporations are liable for injuries to both patients and employees rising from environmental hazards. For example, the license of a nursing facility operator was revoked in *Erie Care Center, Inc. v. Ackerman*[35] on findings of uncleanliness, disrepair, inadequate record keeping, and nursing shortages. The court held that although violation of a single public health regulation may have been insufficient in and of itself to justify revocation of the nursing home's operating license, multiple violations, taken together, established the facility's practice and justified revocation.

Hospital Created Unsafe Conditions

The plaintiff in *Lutheran Hosp. of Ind. v. Blaser*[36] crossed the street one evening after visiting her husband in the hospital and was hit by a car as she was walking up the driveway to the hospital parking lot. She was struck from behind when the car was turning into the parking lot exit. The patient and her husband brought a negligence suit against the hospital as a result of the injuries she suffered.

Drivers in general could not determine that the driveway was not an exit until such time as they were alongside it or were in the process of turning into the driveway. Each night three or four cars mistakenly took the exit for an entrance. Outside visual cues actually drew pedestrians to cross the highway mid-block in order to enter the lot. Neither security guards nor the parking lot attendants had attempted to dissuade pedestrians from crossing the street mid-block. The superior court found that the funneling of pedestrians and vehicular traffic into the exit driveway created a dangerous condition that the hospital should have reasonably foreseen, and the court entered judgment for the plaintiffs. The hospital appealed, claiming that although it maintained the driveway, it did not have control over the driveway.

The Indiana Court of Appeals held that the accident was sufficiently foreseeable to require the hospital protect its invitees from such a mishap. The intervening act of the hit-and-run driver in and of itself does not relieve the hospital of its legal responsibility.

The hospital had a legal duty to exercise reasonable care for the plaintiff's protection. The hospital's failure to post adequate safeguards or warnings to pedestrians and automobiles against the use of the exit driveway as an entrance to the parking lot was the proximate cause of the injuries suffered by the plaintiff. Regardless of whether the hit-and-run driver was confused by inadequate signing or poor illumination, the accident was within the hospital's scope of foreseeability. The hospital was aware of how the driveway was used and yet failed to make any effort to correct the dangerous situation.

The hospital created an unsafe condition and risked a car hitting a pedestrian at the parking lot exit. This was exactly what occurred. Because the subsequent negligent act by the hit-and-run driver was foreseeable by the hospital, the original tort-feasor, the intervening act of the negligent driver does not in and of itself relieve the hospital of its legal responsibility.

Construction Hazards

The nursing facility's operating certificate in *Slocum v. Berman*[37] was revoked for violations of nursing home regulations relating to construction and safety standards. The most critical issues related to the facility's structure, which was neither protected wood frame nor fire resistive as required by regulation. This was a violation that adversely affected the health, safety, and welfare of the occupants. It was determined that the nursing home could not be made reasonably safe or functionally adequate for nursing home occupancy.

Fire Hazards

In *Stacy v. Truman Medical Center,*[38] the patients' families brought wrongful death actions against the medical center and one of its nurses. The wrongful death actions resulted from a fire in the decedents' room at the medical center. On the day of the fire, Ms. Stacy visited her brother, Stephen Stacy. When she arrived, Stephen, who suffered from head injuries and was not supposed to walk around, was sitting in a chair smoking a cigarette with the permission of one of the nurses. No one told Ms. Stacy not to allow her brother to smoke. Stacy also lit a cigarette and because she did not see an ashtray in the room, she used a juice cup and a plastic soup tray for her ashes.

At approximately 5:00 P.M., a nurse came in and restrained Stephen in his chair with ties to prevent him from sliding out of the chair. Before Stacy left, she lit a cigarette, held it to Stephen's mouth, and extinguished it in the soup tray. When Ms. Stacy left, she believed there were one or two cigarette butts in the soup container. Ms. Stacy testified that she did not think she dumped the soup tray into the wastebasket but that she could have.

Shortly after 5:00 P.M., a fire started in a wastebasket in the room. There was no smoke detector in the room. Another patient, Wheeler, was in the bed next to the windows. When Ms. Schreiner, the nurse in charge, discovered the fire, she did not think Wheeler was in immediate danger. She unsuccessfully tried to untie Stephen from his restraints. Then she attempted to put out the fire by smothering it with a sheet. When her attempts to extinguish the fire failed, she ran to the door of the room and yelled for help, which alerted Nurses Cominos and Rodriguez. After calling for help, Ms. Schreiner resumed her attempts to smother the flames with bed linens. Subsequently, she and others grabbed Stephen by the legs and pulled him and his chair toward the hallway. In the process, Stephen's restraints burned through, and he slid from the chair to the floor. Schreiner and her assistants pulled him the remaining few feet out of the room and into the hallway. Schreiner tried to get back into the room but was prevented by the intense smoke, flames, and heat.

After initially entering the room, both Rodriguez and Cominos returned to the nurse's station to sound alarms and to call security; neither attempted to remove Wheeler from the room. Both ran directly past a fire extinguisher, but neither grabbed it before returning to the room. After Stephen was removed from the room, Cominos entered the room with a fire extinguisher and tried to rescue Wheeler. Because of the intense smoke and heat, however, she was unable to reach Wheeler. Wheeler died in the room from smoke inhalation. Stephen survived for several weeks, and then died as a result of complications from infections secondary to burns.

The medical center's policy in case of fire provided for the removal of patients from the room and out of immediate danger first. In its fire-training programs, the medical center used the acronym of "RACE" to supply a chronology of steps to take in case of a fire.

R—Rescue or remove the patient first.

A—An alarm should be sounded second.

C—Contain the fire third.

E—Extinguish the fire last.

The medical center also had a training movie depicting a trash can fire started by smoking that showed how to pull a patient out of bed by the sheets and drag the patient across the floor at the first recognition of a fire.

The medical center's written smoking policy at the time of the fire stated: "No smoking shall be permitted in the Truman Medical Center Health Care Facility except in those areas specifically designated and posted as smoking areas." The patient's room was not posted as a designated smoking area on the date of the fire. The smoking policy further stated: "In the event violations of this policy are observed, the person violating the policy must be requested to discontinue such violation. This shall be the responsibility of all employees and particularly supervisory and security employees." Nurse Cominos admitted that she was a supervisor and that she violated this portion of the smoking policy on the date of the fire by observing smoking and the use of a juice cup for an ashtray.

On appeal, the Missouri Supreme Court held that a causal connection between the medical center's negligence and the patients' deaths was sufficiently established. The medical center owed a duty of reasonable care to all of its patients. The medical center argued that there was no evidence to causally link the alleged negligence in allowing smoking without an approved ashtray to the death of Wheeler. There was evidence that the fire started in the trash can from discarded smoking materials. The jury was free to believe from the evidence presented that if Ms. Stacy had been given a hospital-approved ashtray, she would have discarded her cigarette in a proper ashtray and the fire would not have occurred.

The individual in charge of fire-safety training at the medical center, Lieutenant Campbell, testified that the hospital's policy was to first remove a patient from the room and out of immediate danger in case of fire. Testimony was also offered that the particular training received by the medical center's nurses was below the standard of care and that attempting to put the fire out with linens would also be indicative of a lack of training. The medical center's expert, Fire Captain Gibson, testified that throwing dry sheets on the fire would have added to the problem by fueling the fire. The jury could have found that if the medical center's nurses would have been properly trained, they would have followed their training and prevented Wheeler's death by removing him from the room, in accordance with their training acronym "RACE."

Chemical Hazards

Employees should be warned of any unusual hazards related to their jobs. For example, pregnant employees may abort because of exposure to anesthetic gases in the operating or delivery room; the fetus of a pregnant employee may suffer cell damage because of exposure to chemotherapeutic agents and radioactive materials.

The proper test to determine whether a claimant's job caused his or her injury is set out in *Newman Brothers, Inc. v. McDowell.*[39] That test is:

> [i]f in the performance of his job he has to exert or strain himself or is exposed to conditions of risk or hazard and he would not have strained or exerted himself or been exposed to such conditions had he not been performing his job and the exertion or strain or the exposure to the conditions was, in fact, a contributing cause to his injury or death, the test whether the job caused the injury or death is satisfied.[40]

An employee's skin condition was found to be compensable in *Albertville Nursing Home v. Upton.*[41] The employee had developed a severe skin condition on his hands and feet as a result of daily exposure to various caustic cleaning solutions that he used while performing his duties in the nursing facility. The court held that the claimant was entitled to disability benefits for a period of 26 weeks.

A plan for the handling, storage, and disposal of hazardous materials to prevent user exposure should include:

- policies and procedures (e.g., receipt, storage, and disposal of hazardous materials)
- engineering controls (e.g., vertical laminar flow hood for the preparation of chemotherapeutic medications)
- personal protective clothing and equipment (e.g., masks, gowns, foot and head coverings, and gloves)
- work practices (who, where, when, and how hazardous materials are handled)
- medical surveillance of those who handle hazardous materials (e.g., hazardous materials handling history and exposure follow-up by employee)
- inventory of the location, use, and security of all hazardous materials
- orientation, education, training, annual updates, and meetings
- material safety data sheets readily available in appropriate locations for all staff

Refuse generated by health care facilities can be divided into five separate categories: (1) infectious; (2) biohazardous; (3) hazardous; (4) radioactive; and (5) general (solid) waste. Each category poses its own particular problems for receiving, storing, handling, and disposal.

Medical Equipment

Hospitals must have appropriate procedures in place for the proper selection, education, handling, storage, and maintenance of medical equipment.

Failure to Educate Staff

The plaintiff in *Parris v. Uni Med, Inc.*[42] was admitted to St. Francis Hospital with a decubitus ulcer. While there, he used a Mediscus bed, which was designed with air pockets to prevent decubitus ulcers. Upon discharge on May 31, 1987, the pressure ulcer was healing well. The plaintiff was readmitted on June 15th. At the time of the June admission, his pressure ulcer was healing. Four days later, a nurse noted that the ulcer condition had worsened and a new pressure ulcer had formed. The nurse noticed that the dressing on the first site was touching the metal frame on the bed, thus putting pressure on his sacral area. The nurse called Uni Med and a company employee made adjustments to the bed. In spite of observed improvement in the pressure ulcers at the time of discharge, the patient deteriorated and surgery was required. Evidence showed that the beds were not monitored regularly and that the nurses were not trained to turn the patients or adjust or regulate the beds.

The plaintiff, a 37-year-old paraplegic, brought an action against Uni Med, Inc., for pressure ulcers he sustained during his hospital stay. The jury found that the inadequate pressure setting on the bed was caused by its being improperly set up, thus causing worsening of the condition of the ulcers, necessitating surgery. An appellate court found that failure to set the bed up properly was the cause the patient's pressure ulcers and subsequent surgery. Evidence demonstrated that the bed had been set up hastily, that continuous pressure for two hours on one area of skin can cause pressure ulcers, and that the nurses had not been properly trained to use the bed.

Failure to Properly Maintain Equipment

The plaintiff, Thibodeaux, in *Thibodeaux v. Century Manufacturing Co.,*[43] a nurse's aide at the Rosewood nursing facility, sued Century Manufacturing Company after she was injured while operating a Saf-Kary chair lift, which was manufactured by Century. The plaintiff was injured when the chair fell and smashed her finger when the chair's lifting arm failed. The failure occurred when a patient was being lifted from a whirlpool bath. The plaintiff alleged that Century manufactured a defective chair lift that was the cause of her injuries.

Century argued that the chair lift was not defective in design and that the failure of the chair was caused by air in the Saf-Lift hydraulic system, resulting from the nursing facility's lack of maintenance. The plaintiff's expert witness testified that after inspecting the equipment he found that the accident was caused by the safety lock failing to prevent the chair from disconnecting from the lift. Century theorized that this lack of maintenance caused the whole lift apparatus, including the chair still connected to the lifting arm of the lift column, to rapidly descend on Irene's finger. Approximately four months before the accident, a Century-licensed service technician performed an inspection of the equipment. He found leaks of hydraulic fluid, deteriorating seals and rings, a corroded lift base, and an air-contaminated lifting column. He took the chair lift out of service and recommended that Rosewood not use it until repairs were made to restore it to safe operation. These findings were communicated to Rosewood in writing. Rosewood did not make the repairs. The court, on a jury verdict, found that the sole cause of the accident was due to poor maintenance on the part of the nursing facility. The plaintiff appealed.

The Louisiana Court of Appeal held that the evidence supported the conclusion that the accident was caused by the nursing facility's failure to properly maintain the equipment and that the injury was not the result of poor design. Virtually all products are subject to wear and tear and therefore need periodic maintenance. The nursing facility had been warned by the manufacturer of the need for repairs on the chair lift, but failed to heed that warning.

Contracted Preventative Maintenance

In *Palka v. Servicemaster Management Services,*[44] Servicemaster Management Services contracted with Ellis Hospital to develop and implement a maintenance program for the hospital. Servicemaster's duties included the training, management, and direction of support service employees, including the maintenance department. There had been preexisting wall-mounted fans that had been inspected for safety prior to Servicemaster taking over. The plaintiff, a registered nurse employed by the hospital, was injured when one of the fans fell from the wall onto her. She sued Servicemaster for negligence. The jury rendered a verdict for the plaintiff, and Servicemaster appealed, alleging that they had no duty to her. The appellate division reversed and dismissed the complaint. The nurse appealed.

The court of appeals reversed the decision of the appellate division and reinstated the jury verdict for the plaintiff. Servicemaster, by its contract with the hospital, assumed a duty to act. Although no specific mention of fan maintenance (including an inspection of them) was made in the contract, the director of operations for Servicemaster testified that part of their duties was to create a safe and clean environment for employees and patients, to reduce safety hazards, and to engage in preventative maintenance and casualty control or casualty prevention, which is defined as inspection and checking to see whether something needs to be repaired before it falls. He further testified that it was Servicemaster's responsibility to train hospital employees regarding how and when to perform maintenance on all electrical and mechanical equipment. The court found that all persons, including the nurse, who entered the hospital had a reasonable expectation that someone was in charge of maintenance and inspection of both the premises and the equipment. The contract between Servicemaster and the hospital clearly affected the safety of everyone who came onto the hospital premises. Servicemaster contracted with the hospital to perform certain services and performed those services negligently, which caused Palka's injury. Palka was part of a known and identifiable group of hospital employees, patients, and visitors who were to be protected by proper safety and maintenance protocols assumed exclusively by Servicemaster.

Duty to Prevent Falls

Falls are frequent occurrences in health care settings. They can occur anywhere from the time of arrival to the time of departure. The frequency of falls can be reduced by maintaining a safe environment, as well as, providing ongoing staff and patient education. The following cases describe some of the more common falls.

Parking Lot Safety

The plaintiff, Harkins, in *Harkins v. Natchitoches Parish Hospital*,[45] tripped on a piece of black vinyl garden border material, hidden in the grass, and seriously injured herself. Although the plaintiff had surgery, she never regained full use of her right shoulder. Prior to her fall, Harkins was completely independent and able to care for herself and her apartment. The loss of use was permanent, and the shoulder continued to be painful. The trial court awarded her $50,000.

On appeal, the court held that a hospital owes a duty to its visitors to exercise reasonable care commensurate with the particular circumstances. It must prove that it acted reasonably to discover and correct a dangerous condition reasonably anticipated in its business activity. The plaintiff was required to prove that she tripped and fell and was injured because of some defect at the hospital's premises, creating a presumption of negligence on the hospital's part.

Harkins established that she fell because she tripped on the black vinyl plastic gardening border, which was partially hidden by the grass. It was up to the hospital to exculpate itself from this presumption of liability. This it failed to do. It offered no proof to show that it acted with reasonable care under the circumstances, by having a hidden black vinyl gardening border in an area near its entrance that was regularly traversed by persons using the hospital's facilities. The hospital chose to defend itself by contending that Harkins made inconsistent statements about the location where she tripped.

The trial judge found that Harkins tripped on the gardening border on the grassy median. Given all of the evidence, this had a reasonable basis. On appeal, an appellate court

agreed with the trial judge that it was reasonable to believe that the groundskeeper knew the piece of vinyl border material was present and took no action to remove it or place warning signs that it existed. The failure to either remove the vinyl or place warning signs was a failure to exercise reasonable care.

Hospital Lobby Safety

The plaintiff in *Blitz v. Jefferson Parish Hospital Service District*[46] brought a slip-and-fall suit against a hospital, alleging that her fall was caused by loose vinyl stripping in the front entrance of the hospital. The plaintiff testified that as she walked across the lobby her foot got caught in vinyl stripping. She contends that the vinyl stripping was loose, so that the front of the sole of her shoe was caught between the vinyl stripping and the carpeting. She contended further that the vinyl stripping was defectively installed and maintained. An expert testified that there was an insufficient amount of vinyl adhesive on the underside of the vinyl trim stripping in contact with the top of the terrazzo floor.

The plaintiff filed suit against the hospital and was awarded $80,000 after a bench trial. The hospital appealed, contending that the finding of liability was erroneous and that the trial judge erred in refusing to accept several defense witnesses as experts. The appellate court held that the evidence supported a liability determination. The appellate court was reluctant to substitute its findings of fact for those of the trial judge.

Stretcher Safety

On June 14, 1986, Hussey, in *Hussey v. Montgomery Memorial Hospital*,[47] became ill and was taken to the Montgomery Memorial Hospital by his wife. Upon arrival, he was seated on a stretcher in the emergency department. The stretcher had no side rails. Hussey fell from the stretcher and suffered a severe head injury. After being treated by a physician, Mrs. Hussey was advised that her husband's condition was caused by swelling in the brain due to the head injury. Hussey was moved by ambulance to another hospital, where he was diagnosed with a dislocated clavicle, laceration of the skin, and two fractures of the lateral wall of the right orbit.

The plaintiffs alleged that on several occasions they questioned Dr. Andrews, the attending physician, as to whether there was any permanent brain damage. On each occasion, Andrews answered that there would not be any brain damage. Two months after the fall, the plaintiffs consulted with an attorney concerning a possible claim against the Montgomery Memorial Hospital, but decided not to pursue a lawsuit at that time because they feared doing so might impair the plaintiff husband's ability to receive medical treatment. For the next three and a half years, Hussey continued to see his medical providers. No physicians ever disclosed to the plaintiffs that Hussey may suffer permanent brain impairment.

By April 1990, Hussey's behavior became severely erratic and unpredictable to the point that Mrs. Hussey took him to Sandhills Center for Mental Health. Hussey was examined and transferred to the Dartmouth Clinic. A physician at the clinic informed the plaintiffs that test results indicated permanent and residual brain impairment. On June 12, 1990, the plaintiffs filed a complaint alleging negligence against the hospital. The hospital filed a motion to dismiss on the grounds that the action was barred by the three-year statute of limitations.

The trial judge granted the hospital's motion for summary judgment and the plaintiffs appealed. The appellate court held that the action was time barred.

The statute of limitations accrued on June 14, 1986, the date of Hussey's fall. The head injury was not latent. Hussey had a cause of action on the date he fell from the stretcher. Upon falling from the stretcher, he suffered a severe head injury and was rendered unconscious. A treating physician in the emergency department advised Hussey's wife that swelling in the brain caused her husband's condition. The probable cause of the accident was the hospital's negligence. On the date of the fall, it was apparent that there had been wrongdoing, most likely attributable to the hospital. The ultimate injuries sustained by Hussey were a direct result of the June 14, 1986, fall caused by the hospital's wrongdoing. Hussey's failure to pursue a cause of action on this date resulted in the tolling of the statute of limitations.

Safe Use of Restraints

Falls by patients often involve mixed allegations of a failure to restrain, supervise, assist, or attend the patient. Some plaintiffs have argued that, although restraints were applied, they were improperly applied. The plaintiff in *Smith v. Gravois Rest Haven, Inc.*[48] brought a lawsuit arising out of a fall and subsequent injuries suffered by his 78-year-old mother. The plaintiff's mother required use of a "posey" restraining device because of previous falls in the facility. There was sufficient evidence to establish that the restraints had been improperly applied. Evidence showed that the plaintiff was a frail, elderly woman who had a history of crippling arthritis, among other ailments, and who had been administered a sleeping pill one hour before her fall, making it highly unlikely that she could have untied properly installed restraints and gotten out of bed.

Window Safety

Health care organizations are required to exercise reasonable care and diligence in safeguarding a patient, measured by the capacity of the patient to provide for his or her own safety. The plaintiffs in *Horton v. Niagara Falls Memorial Medical Center*[49] sought recovery against the hospital for injuries sustained by the plaintiff-patient's fall from a second-story hospital window. The patient had been admitted to the hospital with a fever of unknown origin and was noted to be lacking in coordination and blurred vision. The patient had been placed in a private room with a single window that opened to a small balcony encircled by a two- to three-foot-high railing. Before the patient's fall, construction workers notified hospital personnel that the patient was standing on his balcony calling for a ladder. The patient had been confused and disoriented. On learning of the incident, the attending physician advised a nurse to keep the patient under restraint and to keep an eye on him. The patient's wife was called, and she indicated that her mother would come to the hospital in 10 to 15 minutes to watch her husband. The patient fell shortly before the mother's arrival. The Niagara Supreme Court entered judgment for the plaintiffs and the hospital appealed. The New York Supreme Court, Appellate Division, held that the hospital had a duty to supervise the patient and prevent him from injuring himself.

Slippery Floors

Slippery floors are often a major source of lawsuits. To reduce liability caused by falls, floors should be maintained properly. The following actions should be taken to reduce patient falls:

- Floors should not contain a dangerous amount of wax.

- Caution signs (e.g., slippery floors) should be used when and where appropriate.

- Floors should be cared for and maintained properly on rainy and/or snowy days.

- Broken floor tiles should be repaired promptly.

- Foreign matter should be quickly and completely wiped from the floor.

- Signs, ropes, and lights should be used where appropriate.

- Appropriate precautions should be taken for outdoor walkways to guard against dangers such as icy conditions and construction hazards.

The plaintiff in *Borota v. University Medical Center*,[50] a hospital visitor, brought an action against University Medical Center to recover for injuries she suffered as a result of slipping on a puddle of milk in the hospital corridor. The plaintiff claimed that the spill appeared fresh and that there were several spots of milk on the floor and on the walls. She also noted that the corridor was well lit. The trial court granted summary judgment for the hospital, and the plaintiff appealed.

The Arizona Court of Appeals held that the plaintiff did not establish constructive notice that would indicate that the hospital was aware of the spilled milk. Although it is the responsibility and duty of a hospital to keep its premises reasonably safe for invitees, the hospital does not ensure their safety. The hospital is not liable for the injuries sustained by the plaintiff unless she can establish that either (1) the hospital's employees caused the spill and failed to clean it on a timely basis or (2) the milk was there for a long period of time and the hospital had constructive notice that the spill was there, yet failed to clean it. The plaintiff failed to show evidence that the milk was spilled by a hospital employee. The plaintiff was unable to show that the hospital was aware of the spill.

Loading Dock Safety

In *Glowacki v. Underwood Memorial Hospital,*[51] a nurse, while employed as a pediatric transport nurse, was transporting a critically ill infant from the hospital. An isolette was needed for this purpose and the nurse was responsible for wheeling it to the ambulance. The ambulance arrived at the hospital and drove to the emergency department area where it backed up to a loading platform. The back of the ambulance made contact with hard rubbery pieces that jutted out from a wooden bumper. The bumper was separated from the concrete loading platform by intermittent rubber blocks, which left an open space of approximately three and one-half inches between the bumper and the dock. The nurse stepped from the ambulance directly onto the concrete platform. The nurse and the driver began the process of lifting the isolette up into the ambulance. The distance or height to the back of the ambulance appeared to have been approximately one foot. During this process, the nurse's foot became wedged into the space between the wooden bumper and the concrete platform. The nurse alleged that the space was as wide as her shoe.

A civil engineer testified at trial as an expert on behalf of the nurse that it was unsafe to have a hole or gap in the bumper system. The hospital produced a civil engineer who testified that there was no standard in the industry applicable to hospital bumpers. He admitted that any design should consider the nature of traffic going over it. It was his opinion that the system in the instant case did not create an unreasonable hazard of tripping or falling. The hospital's director of plant operations conceded that the hospital was aware of the spaces in the bumper system, but indicated there had never been a report of an incident since it was built.

The court charged the jury on principles of ordinary negligence and the liability of a property owner to business invitees for a dangerous condition on its property. The jury was also charged on contributory negligence. The jury returned a verdict finding that an unsafe condition existed on the hospital's platform, that the hospital was negligent, and that the negligence was a proximate cause of the nurse's accident. However, the court also found the nurse negligent and was found to be a proximate cause of the accident. The hospital was found 85 percent negligent and the nurse 15 percent negligent.

The defendant argued that the court erred in denying its motion for a new trial on damages because the verdict of $908,000 constituted a miscarriage of justice, was against the weight of the evidence, and was the result of passion, prejudice, sympathy, or mistake. The appeals court disagreed. The nurse's symptoms from the day following the accident to the date of trial eight years later never changed. The nurse's medical proofs were capable of supporting a jury finding that her back injury was one involving the spine and discs and not merely a low back sprain.

Duty to Safeguard Patient Valuables

Appropriate procedures should be developed for handling the personal property of patients. A health care facility can be held liable for the negligent handling of a patient's valuables. The following points should be remembered and followed when handling the personal belongings and valuables of patients:

- Send the belongings home when feasible.

- Deposit jewelry, wallets, and other appropriate items in the facility's safe.

- Select one department to handle valuables.

- Provide proper communication between the department handling lost-and-found articles and the department holding patient valuables for safekeeping.

- Encourage patients to keep with them as little money, jewelry, and other valuables as possible.

- Establish a valuables procedure for deceased patients, patients entering the emergency department, and patients scheduled for a surgical procedure or other diagnostic tests.

- Provide prenumbered envelopes that list those items placed in each valuables envelope. Verification of the contents should be made between the employee delivering an envelope and the employee accepting the envelope for safekeeping. A receipt should be given to the patient making a deposit. Strikeouts or corrections should not be permitted on the envelope; this will help prevent claims of mishandling.

CEO/ADMINISTRATOR'S ROLE AND RESPONSIBILITY

The CEO is responsible for the supervision of the administrative staff and managers who assist in the daily operations of the organization. The CEO derives authority from the owner or governing body. The CEO of an organization owned and operated by a governmental agency may be an appointed public official. CEOs, as is the case with governing body members, can be personally liable for their own acts of negligence that injure others.

The CEO must implement the policies of the governing body, as well as interpret policies. Appropriate action must be taken where noncompliance with rules and regulations occurs. The CEO is responsible for making periodic reports to the governing body regarding policy implementation.

There may be occasions when the CEO believes that following a direction of the governing body may create a danger to the patients or others. If the CEO knows or should have known, as a reasonably prudent CEO, of a danger or unreasonable risk or harm that will be created by certain directed activity but nevertheless proceeds as directed, he or she could become personally liable for any resulting injury. The CEO, therefore, must take appropriate steps to notify the governing body of any danger in carrying out policies that create dangers or unreasonable risks.

Although the CEO cannot assume the functions of the professional staff, he or she must ensure that proper admission and discharge policies and procedures are formulated and carried out. He or she must cooperate with the professional staff in maintaining satisfactory standards of medical care. The CEO must keep abreast of regulatory changes that affect organizational operations. Periodic meetings should be conducted to inform the staff of regulatory changes affecting their duties and responsibilities. The CEO should designate a representative for administrative coverage during those hours he or she is absent from the organization. This individual should be capable of dealing with administrative matters and be able to contact the CEO when major problems arise.

Tort Liability of the CEO

The wrongful injury to another by the CEO in the performance of his or her duties makes the CEO liable to the one injured. Because the CEO is subject to the control of the organization, the organization also may be liable for the torts of the CEO that occur within the scope of his or her employment. When performing the duties that he or she was hired to do, the CEO is working for the benefit of the organization and not as an individual. Because the organization gains from the work performed by its employees, the law renders the organization legally responsible for the acts of employees while performing the work of the organization.

CEO's Liability for the Acts of Others

The CEO is not liable for the negligent acts of other employees as long as he or she personally took no part in the commission of the negligent act and was not negligent in selecting or directing the person committing the injury. However, under the doctrine of respondeat superior, a health care facility can be liable for the employee's negligent acts.

Regulatory Agencies

The duties of the CEO include the correction of any deficiencies found during inspections by governmental agencies and nongovernmental agencies. The Joint Commission surveyors provide organizations with Requirements for Improvement (RFI) and consultative remarks. Consultative remarks are often given to highlight an area of concern that should be addressed by the organization. They should be regarded just as significant in identifying areas needing corrective action as written reports that may be given by the surveyor.

Case Overviews

Over the years, a fair number of cases have dealt with administrators and their management of health care organizations. In general, an administrator employed for the duration of satisfactory performance has no property right in the position, as was pointed out in *Bleeker v. Dukakis.*[52] The administrator of the Woodland Nursing Home had been hired through an oral agreement under which his continued employment was contingent upon satisfactory work performance. "The assistant commissioner determined that Woodland was being managed improperly and that the appellant should be replaced."[53] The administrator's appointment was considered to be at the will of the employers even though the nursing facility's policies provided a procedure for warning and an opportunity to correct work performance deficiencies.

Dealing with the legal system can be a harrowing experience, even in those instances where the administrator is eventually exonerated from either negligence or criminal activity. Presented here are a few agonizing moments in the lives of some boards and their administrators.

- An administrator's license was revoked for concealment of the identities of the facility's owners in *Loren v. Board of Examiners of Nursing Home Administrators.*[54] The court found that the record contained substantial evidence to support the board's finding. The administrator had actively participated in a scheme to divert checks belonging to the nursing home to undisclosed partners of the home. The crime of knowingly filing false statements as to the facility's ownership with the intent of defrauding the U.S. government and the state of New York involved moral turpitude and subjected the administrator to disciplinary action.

- An administrator's plea to misdemeanor counts for mismanagement was considered a proper basis for suspending his nursing home license for one year.[55]

- A nursing facility's exclusion from a Medicaid rate incentive program was considered rationally related to the encouragement of superior health care after the administrator was indicted for accepting excessive payments from the residents' relatives.[56]

- Although cases of alleged wrongdoing do not always end in a finding for the plaintiff, going through the ordeal is at best a most uncomfortable experience for the defendant. The court in *State v. Serebin*[57] held that the evidence of inadequate staffing and diet was found to be insufficient to support homicide charges against the administrator where the resident left the facility and died of exposure.

MEDICAL STAFF

The role of the governing body in setting policy and supervision of the medical staff is extremely important. The governing body should ensure that medical staff bylaws, rules, and regulations should include, for example, the following:

- application requirements for clinical privileges and admission to the medical staff
- a process for granting emergency staff privileges
- requirements for medical staff consultations
- a peer-review process
- a process auditing medical records
- a process for addressing disruptive physicians and substance abuse
- a process for instituting corrective action (disciplinary actions can take the form of a letter of reprimand, suspension, or termination of privileges)

CORPORATE REORGANIZATION

Traditionally, hospitals have functioned as independent, freestanding corporate entities or as units or divisions of multihospital systems. Until recently, a freestanding hospital functioned as a single corporate entity with most programs and activities carried out within such entity to meet increasing competition.

Dependence on government funding and related programs (e.g., Medicare, Medicaid, and Blue Cross) and the continuous shrinkage occurring in such revenues have forced hospitals to seek alternative sources of revenue. Greater competition from nonhospital sources also has contributed to this need to seek alternative revenue sources. It has become apparent that traditional corporate structures may no longer be appropriate to accommodate both normal hospital activities and those additional activities undertaken to provide alternative sources of revenue.

The typical hospital is incorporated under state law as a freestanding for-profit or not-for-profit corporation. The corporation has a governing body. Such governing body has an overall responsibility for the operation and management of the hospital with a necessary delegation of appropriate responsibility to administrative employees and the medical staff.

Not-for-profit hospitals are usually exempt from federal taxation under Section 501(c)(3) of the U.S. Internal Revenue Code of 1986 as amended. Such federal exemption usually entitles the organization to an automatic exemption from state taxes as well. Such tax exemption not only relieves the hospital from the payment of income taxes, sales taxes, and the like, but also permits the hospital to receive contributions from donors who then may obtain charitable deductions on their personal tax returns.

Given the need to obtain income and to meet competition, hospitals often consider establishing business enterprises. They also may consider other nonbusiness operations, such as the establishment of additional nonexempt undertakings (e.g., hospices and long-term care facilities). Because hospitals have resources including the physical plant, administrative talent, and technical expertise in areas that are potentially profitable, the first option usually considered is direct participation by the hospital in health-related business enterprises. There are, however, regulatory and legal pressures that present substantial impediments.

Taxation

Income earned by tax-exempt organizations from nonexempt activities is subject to unrelated business income taxes under the Internal Revenue Code. These taxes are similar to those paid by profit-making organizations. In addition, tax-exempt status may be lost if a substantial portion of the corporation's activities are related to nonexempt activities and/or if the benefits of the tax-exempt status accrue to individuals who control the entity either directly or indirectly (private inurement). Care also must be taken to avoid the use of facilities exempt from real estate taxation for nonexempt enterprises because this may lead to a partial or complete loss of such exemption.

Third-Party Reimbursement

Medicare, Medicaid, Blue Cross, and other third parties that reimburse hospitals directly for patient care require that no reimbursement be available for activities unrelated to the provision of such care. Thus, costs associated with unrelated activities must be deducted from costs submitted to third-party payers for reimbursement. The "carving out" of these costs can be detrimental to the hospital unless alternative revenues are found.

Certificate of Need

Generally, hospitals may not add additional programs or services nor may they expend monies for the acquisition of capital in excess of specified threshold limits without first obtaining approval from appropriate state regulatory agencies. The process by which this approval is granted generally is referred to as the *certificate of need (CON) process.*

The National Health Planning and Resources Development Act of 1974, Public Law No. 93-641, sought to encourage state review of all plans calling for the construction, expansion, or renovation of health facilities or services by conditioning receipt of certain federal funds on the establishment of an approved state CON program. Most states responded to this law by instituting state CON programs that complied with federal standards. Although the federal law is now history, CON programs remain in effect in a dwindling number of states. Some states continue to maintain control over Medicaid expenditures for hospital and nursing home care by controlling the number of beds through the CON process. This process can be lengthy and expensive. Further, it may not always result in approval of the request to offer the new program or service or to make the capital expenditure.

Health care providers have criticized CON requirements because they require review of those expenditures by or on behalf of a health care facility but may allow, for example, groups of physicians or independent laboratories to make large expenditures for equipment or services without triggering the state review mechanism.

Disapprovals of CONs often occur because they do not comply with state health plans that are designed to limit programs and services and prevent overbedding in predefined geographic areas. Some CON applicants have attempted to seek revisions in state health plans to obtain approval of their projects. *Nursing Home of Dothan v. Alabama State Health Planning & Development Agency*[58] was one such case. The nursing home filed a CON application with the state health planning agency (SHPA) to construct a 110-bed nursing home. SHPA informed Dothan that the state health plan failed to indicate a need for additional beds and advised Dothan to seek an amendment to the state health plan before proceeding with the CON process. The defendant filed the proposed amendment with the state health coordinating council, which approved the defendant's request for additional beds. The amendment, which required the governor's approval, was rejected. On appeal of the circuit court's finding for SHPA, denying Dothan's proposed amendment to the state health plan and subsequent denial of the CON application, the appeals court held that the governor properly disapproved the requested amendment.

Disapproval of a CON application also can be based on the financial feasibility of the project. A CON proposal to construct a long-term care nursing facility with 65 percent Medicaid beds was found to have been properly denied in *National Health Corp. v. South Carolina Department of Health & Environmental Control.*[59] The department of health and environmental control's decision was considered proper, reasonable, and consistent with applicable laws and regulations. The unsuccessful applicant, National Health Corporation (NHC), failed to establish its project's financial feasibility because of the unavailability of Medicaid funding. Discrepancies also existed between its budgets and its cost reports.

The record contains clear evidence that Medicaid funds would not be available for the NHC beds. The board also found that inconsistencies in four budgets submitted by NHC and the discrepancies between those budgets and the cost reports submitted by NHC to the state health and human services finance commission raised serious questions regarding the financial feasibility of the NHC project.[60]

The agency's competitor had shown the financial feasibility of its project and was, therefore, granted a CON.

There can be disagreement among justices within the same court as to whether an applicant has established the criteria for need within a specific geographic area. The record in *Heritage of Yankton, Inc. v. South Dakota Department of Health*[61] was found to have supported denial of a CON application for additional beds based on the argument that there was no need for additional beds in the service area. The department of health was found not to have acted arbitrarily and capriciously in denying the application. It provided valid reasons for rejecting new information submitted at a rehearing. The department of health rejected an argument that a bed shortage in the county demonstrated a need for more beds. The department argued that it had never considered county boundaries in determining bed need, and that the population of the facility's service area is the proper area for consideration. In view of its policy to maintain high occupancy rates in all facilities, the department also rejected Heritage's claim that the department's formula forces the elderly to be separated from their families and home communities.

Justice Henderson stated in a dissenting opinion:

> This health care facility submitted three items of new evidence which had not been previously considered. This consisted of population projections for the area and an in-and-out migration data with information pertaining to the existence of alternative services. The Department, summarily, expressed that it refused to consider this new evidence. Instead of opening its mind and then opening the door of reconsideration with relevant evidence, the Department of Health chose to be unyielding with its grip on the single formula and methodology it employed. If this health facility's evidence had been reconsidered, an open mind would see that there was an extensive need for beds existing in the city of Yankton and Yankton county.

• • • •

I cannot in good conscience, join the majority opinion which prevents elderly citizens from having a bed, with medical care and treatment, administered compassionately, in a community where their children and grandchildren reside. I would elevate reality over a single methodology and accordingly dissent.

"[T]herefore never send to know for whom the bell tolls; it tolls for thee." John Donne (1573–1631), Devotions upon Emergent Occasions, Meditation XVII. My mind drifts to Ernest Hemingway. And a clod of dirt. Chipped away at the shores of Europe by the sea. "If a clod be washed away by the sea, Europe is the less. . . ." Supra. All from whence Hemingway's great novel was born. And, yes, not a person is turned away from a bed of repose, in his older years, but South Dakota is lesser in spirit. A refrain also comes to my mind: "And crown thy good, with Brotherhood, from sea to shining sea."[62]

Financing

Even when a hospital has determined that it can and should add a program or service and when it is allowed to do so, it may lack the necessary capital financing. The hospital could join with private investors (who may, in fact, be members of the medical staff) to gain greater access to capital. Care must be taken, however, that no venture that includes physicians who refer to the hospital can be construed as providing an incentive or a reward for such referrals. Federal antifraud and abuse laws and regulations and similar state regulations impose severe penalties for such violations.

Recognizing the need to develop alternative sources of revenue, hospitals often establish an additional or restructured organization. Besides the need to develop alternative sources of capital, some restructurings come about simply because of the evolution of a multi-institutional system. Thus, when hospitals merge or consolidate, restructuring is virtually automatic. Also, when several hospitals fall under common ownership or when additional health enterprises are undertaken, restructuring usually evolves as more institutions are added to the system. In these instances, general legal principles applicable to corporations, as well as proper management considerations, will control the development of the appropriate corporate structure.

Corporate Restructuring

Assuming the existence of a single not-for-profit tax-exempt hospital, any restructuring undertaken normally involves the creation of at least one additional not-for-profit

tax-exempt entity. This entity may be referred to as a parent or holding company or a foundation. Its general function is to serve as the corporate vehicle to receive the ultimate benefits from the revenue-producing activities and to confer some or all of these benefits on the hospital. Under current rules regarding income taxation, income received directly (by providing goods or services) or indirectly (by means of dividends or other investment income) does not give rise to any tax obligation if the receiver of such benefit is exempt from taxation under any of several subsections of Section 501(c) of the Internal Revenue Code, provided that exempt activities are the organization's main source of income and expense.

Parent Holding Company Model

Under this model, a new not-for-profit corporation is formed in conformity with the laws of the state in which the hospital is located. This corporation then can seek to obtain a tax exemption under the Internal Revenue Code. The overall purposes of the corporation are general in nature but involve a promotion of the health and welfare of the public and also may directly involve benefit to a named hospital or hospitals. In some states, when one organization exists to benefit a licensed hospital, such organization must itself be approved through a CON or similar process. The government of the parent holding company usually is derived from the governing body of the hospital. Qualifications for certain categories of exempt status under the Internal Revenue Code may require overlapping governing bodies between the hospital and the new entity. Section 509(a) of the Internal Revenue Code deals with the qualification of a tax-exempt entity as a "private and/or non-private" foundation. Nonprivate is the preferred status, and the qualification for such status may depend in part on the relationship between the entity seeking tax exemption and the already exempt entity (i.e., the hospital).

Because there is no stock involved in a not-for-profit corporation (the ownership of which would confer control by one corporation over another), control of the not-for-profit hospital by the not-for-profit parent holding company generally arises when the parent holding company is the sole member of the hospital corporation. Membership carries with it the right to elect directors and thus creates the necessary linkage for the parent-subsidiary relationship.

As a tax-exempt entity, the parent holding company also may own one or more for-profit subsidiaries. Although such ownership cannot represent most activities of the parent holding company, the ownership of such entities would not in and of itself disqualify the parent holding company from achieving and maintaining a tax-exempt status. It is through the subsidiaries that for-profit activities are carried on. The for-profit ventures (which may be independent corporations, joint ventures with other investors, etc.) are tax-paying entities. The net revenues (after payment of taxes) are paid out as dividends to the entity owning the stock or other ownership interest (the parent holding company), which, being tax exempt, pays no taxes on the receipt of such dividends. The parent holding company may then, as a donation, confer benefits directly on the hospital or any other entity intended to benefit from the parent holding company. Again, it is important to monitor closely the activities of this corporation so that its participation in or ownership of for-profit entities does not destroy its tax-exempt status.

Controlled Foundation

An alternative structure to the parent holding company model is one in which the new, not-for-profit entity is controlled directly by the hospital. Instead of the parent holding company being a member of the hospital corporation, the reverse is true. The hospital is the member of the new entity. The structure described earlier to carry out for-profit activities would then fall under the controlled foundation. In many states, the regulators would view such a controlled foundation as nothing more than the alter ego of the hospital and therefore impose on this entity all regulatory restrictions, reimbursement restrictions, and the like.

Independent Foundation

The establishment of a separate not-for-profit corporation and the substructure for carrying out for-profit activities may be accomplished independent of the hospital. Even though members of the hospital's governing body are involved in the creation of the new not-for-profit entity, the two corporations themselves may not necessarily be linked. This "brother-sister" relationship frequently is found to be desirable when the governing body of a hospital does not favor the creation of a parent organization to control the hospital but nevertheless seeks to create a viable structure within which for-profit activities may be carried on outside the hospital. A concern frequently expressed in this brother-sister relationship is that the new entity, not being controlled directly by the hospital, or in the alternative, not controlling the hospital, may "run away" and not necessarily ultimately benefit the hospital as was originally intended. Whether such a concern will materialize is naturally dependent on the degree to which the governing bodies of the two organizations overlap and the degree to which each organization remains responsive to the other. The use of this model also may have certain reimbursement advantages regarding earnings on donated monies. If reimbursement regulations ever change to offset charitable gifts from reimbursable activities, an independent organization also may prove useful.

General Considerations

The organizational structures just described are not intended to alter the way a hospital is managed or the way care is delivered. The driving force behind the creation of alternative structures is the desire to develop alternative sources of revenue and/or to streamline management of multi-institutional systems. In many states, substantial changes in the governance of a hospital require regulatory approval. The establishment of the alternative structures previously described normally does not require such regulatory approval as long as the hospital continues to be governed by a governing body and continues to carry out its functions in accordance with applicable laws, rules, and regulations.

After restructuring has taken place, many additional entities will require legal and accounting attention. These entities (normally corporations) must maintain minutes, books, and records; file tax returns; and make other such filings as are required by state laws and by federal and state income tax laws and regulations. It is important that the structures be viewed as running independent of one another. This includes establishing separate bank accounts, holding regular meetings among officers and directors, and maintaining appropriate minutes. Too often the activities and records of one entity are difficult to discern from those of another, and then the benefits of the separate organizations may be lost. The concept of "piercing the corporate veil" may come into play when each corporate entity is not maintained separately and apart from every other entity. The corporate veil will be pierced when a court determines that the activities of the corporation are indistinguishable from the activities of either another corporation or the corporation's directors, officers, or members.

The parent corporation in *Boafo v. Hospital Corp. of America*[63] was held not liable for injuries sustained by a patient at a subsidiary hospital. Even though the parent corporation shared some officers with the subsidiary and furnished it with substantial administrative services, there was no basis for piercing the corporate veil of the parent, absent some showing that the subsidiary was a sham formed for the purpose of promoting fraud, defeating justice, concealing crime, or evading contractual or tort responsibility.

Although the hospital was a wholly owned subsidiary of a national management corporation, it was a fully capitalized corporate entity that was insured, owned the hospital property, autonomously managed and operated the hospital on a day-to-day basis, maintained its own payroll, and employed its own employees. Therefore, there was no basis for holding the parent corporation liable.

Medical Staff and Restructuring

Any discussion of corporate reorganization undertaken by a hospital must involve the medical staff. Although a reorganization may have little or no direct impact on the medical staff, the perception of major change requires, at the very least, a full explanation and involvement in the process.

Many hospitals have come to realize that the medical staff presents a fertile area for developing relationships and projects leading to additional revenues. Projects such as imaging centers, laboratories, durable medical equipment (DME) businesses, and the like may be organized in conjunction with one or more members of the medical staff. Other likely candidates to participate in joint ventures include existing laboratories, home care companies, DME companies, drug companies, surgical supply houses, and the like. As previously noted, ventures involving physicians are closely regulated. Laws and regulations have been designed to curb the practice of physicians and other professionals from referring patients to facilities or enterprises in which they have a financial interest.

Joint ventures with physician groups are not without risk, as was shown in *Arango v. Reyka,*[64] in which a hospital entered into a joint venture with an anesthesiology group and thus was vicariously liable for the malpractice of the members of that group. The hospital billed patients for anesthesiology services, retained 12 percent of all collections, owned and furnished anesthesiology equipment and medications used by the group, scheduled patients, and referred to the group as the hospital's department of anesthesiology. As a result, there existed a common purpose to provide anesthesiology services to hospital patients. Control was shared between the hospital and the group over the provision of anesthesia services, and there was a joint interest in the financial benefits and profits generated by the combination of their resources and services. The physicians had an obligation to maintain control over their medical judgment, but this did not prevent the creation of a joint venture contract.

Development of a business involving equity participation must be considered in the light of state and federal securities laws and other relevant laws, rules, and regulations to determine that there is full compliance. Shares of stock, shares in linked partnerships, and other similar equity participation interests may fall within the definition of a public offering of securities requiring filings and/or registrations under state and federal securities laws.

Fund-Raising

A not-for-profit hospital generally raises funds. Any new not-for-profit corporation formed as part of restructuring also may be able to engage in fund-raising if such entity obtains a tax exemption under the Internal Revenue Code.

Also, as part of a reorganization and despite the creation of a new entity as indicated, hospitals frequently determine that it is desirable to create an additional foundation, the sole purpose of which is fund-raising for the hospital. This, therefore, may lead to as many as three organizations with both the capability and the intent to engage in fund-raising to benefit the hospital. Obvious confusion may arise in the minds of the public being asked to give to these organizations. A coordinated approach to fund-raising is critical to avoid such confusion.

Any organization engaged in fund-raising may have local filing requirements at the state or other governmental level. Care must be taken that the public is informed completely as to the ultimate beneficiary of such fund-raising and the manner in which the monies raised will be spent. A donor to a charity may have a claim against that charity if the donor can show that he or she was misled regarding the ultimate beneficiary of the gift or the purposes for which the gift would be used. Members of the public may be reluctant to donate when capital is to be used to fund for-profit enterprises. The overall charitable purposes of the entity must be carried out, and the activities may not be so concentrated on the operation or participation in for-profit ventures that either the tax exemption is jeopardized or it is determined (usually by the state attorney general) that the funds have been raised improperly from the public.

Regulatory Authority Checklist

When considering restructuring, the following regulatory authority checklist may be helpful:

Not-for-profit corporations

- not-for-profit corporation law

- Internal Revenue Code (exemption and taxpayer identification number)

- state and local tax laws on exemptions (including real property)

- attorney general or similar charitable registration requirements

- bylaws, organization minutes, and minutes of first governing body meeting

- bank account

For-profit corporations

- business corporation law

- taxpayer identification number

- bylaws, organization minutes, minutes of first governing body meeting, and issuance of stock

- bank account

Hospitals

- reimbursement regulations

- CON regulations

– governing body bylaws and relationship to additional corporations

– fraud and abuse laws, rules, and regulations

Competition and Restructuring

Because an organization exerts a certain amount of influence and dominance over its patient population, the participation in for-profit enterprises to which an organization's patients are referred may give rise to anticompetitive activities and antitrust claims. Patients must be permitted free choice of goods and services. For example, if an organization (through its reorganized structure) participates in a DME business and seeks to recommend such business to its patients on discharge, these patients must be allowed to choose an alternate supplier. The patients must be advised that they are not required to use the vendor recommended by the organization. An organization should disclose its relationship to the DME company so that the patient knows the organization's involvement prior to making a choice.

Care must be taken that local vendors and merchants who have a traditional relationship with the organization or with the patients are not so affected by the proposed for-profit activity that ill will is generated within the community, leading to a potential legal claim regarding anticompetitive activity.

Restructuring requires a multidisciplinary approach. The issues to be considered include legal, financial, accounting, tax, regulatory, and reimbursement concerns. These disciplines must provide input on an ongoing basis, not merely at inception. Changing requirements and interpretations—especially in the areas of taxation and Medicare/Medicaid fraud and abuse regulations—mandate a continuous process of review and modification so that desired goals are not subverted by legal and financial problems.

> Nonetheless, a word of caution. Today's ventures require additional planning for the possibility that some, or part, of an enterprise might ultimately be found illegal. Therefore, potential buyers, and hopefully arrangements with them, as well as appropriate dissolution and unwinding provisions, now more than ever, need to be part of the fabric and documentation of any new joint venture. As well, the documentation of existing ventures must be reviewed in the light of current considerations and where necessary, needed revisions crafted.[65]

Restructuring and acquisitions can lead to collusive practices that are harmful to consumers. Such was the case when the FTC determined that the Hospital Corporation of America (HCA), a proprietary hospital chain, violated Section 7 of the Clayton Act, as amended, 15 U.S.C. § 18 (1982), by acquiring two hospital corporations in the Chattanooga area, Hospital Affiliates International, Inc., and Health Care Corporation, for $700 million. HCA already owned one hospital in the area. Hospital Affiliates International held management contracts with two other area hospitals.[66] This in effect gave HCA control of more than 5 of the 11 hospitals in the Chattanooga area. The management contract with one of the hospitals was canceled after the FTC began investigating HCA's acquisition of Hospital Affiliates. HCA sought judicial review by petitioning the court of appeals to set aside the decision of the FTC. The court of appeals held that there was substantial evidence to support the commission's determination that the acquisitions were likely to foster collusive practices harmful to consumers.

Restructuring is an undertaking that requires careful planning and legal and accounting advice, and should be undertaken not because it is "fashionable" but rather because it will provide the hospital with opportunities not available under its current structure.

Safe-Harbor Regulations

The safe-harbor regulations describe how health care providers should structure financial arrangements in order to be exempt from prosecution by the department of justice (DOJ) and the FTC. The safe-harbor regulation covers (1) investment interests, (2) space rentals, (3) equipment rentals, (4) personal services and mandatory contracts, (5) sales of practice, (6) referral services, (7) warranties, (8) discounts, (9) employees, (10) group purchasing organizations, and (11) waivers of beneficiary coinsurance and deductibles (for inpatient hospital services under a prospective payment system). "Under the rules, providers must be under no obligation to refer business to the venture. In addition, providers' financial return must be in proportion to the amount of their investment and not tied to their business referrals."[67]

The Medicare and Medicaid Patient and Program Protection Act specifically directed the secretary of the U.S. Department of Health and Human Services (DHHS), in consultation with the attorney general, to publish regulations specifying payment practices that would not be treated as a criminal offense under the antikickback provisions. Illegal remunerations (*kickbacks*) are a felony offense. The statute provides that once those rules have been promulgated, any payment practice specified in such regulations will not be considered illegal. Failure to fall squarely within a safe harbor, however, does not necessarily mean that the practice is illegal. It simply indicates that it is not automatically safe. Failure to comply with the regulations can result in civil or criminal sanctions, as well as exclusion from Medicare and Medicaid programs.

The regulations establishing safe harbors were published July 9, 1991, and became effective on that date.[68] The following briefly describes the safe harbors and some of the requirements that must be met in order to fall within the safe harbor:

- *Investments in large publicly traded entities:* No violation is inherent in a payment that is a return on an investment interest made to an investor as long as requirements, such as the following, are met: payment to an investor as return on investment must be directly proportional to the amount of that investor's capital investment.

- *Investments in smaller ventures:* No violation is inherent in a payment that is a return on an investment interest made to an investor.

- *Lease of space and equipment:* The OIG characterized as two different safe harbors two kinds of lease arrangements—those for space and those for equipment. Despite this characterization, however, the rules for the two safe harbors are very similar: rental payments made by lessees to lessors for use of space or equipment received are safe-harbor protected.

- *Personal services and management contracts:* Safe-harbor protection applies to payments made by a principal to an agent as compensation for the services of the agent.

- *Sale of practitioner practice:* Payments made to a practitioner by another practitioner in order to purchase a practice are protected.

- *Referral services:* Any payment or exchange of anything of value between a referral service and a referral service participant is protected.

- *Warranties:* This safe harbor covers warranties that meet the definition of that term in the Magnuson-Moss Warranty-Federal Trade Commission Improvement Act[69] as well as agreements by a manufacturer or supplier to replace another manufacturer's or supplier's defective item on terms equal to the agreement if replaced.

- *Standards for buyers:* Any payment or exchange of anything of value under a warranty provided by a manufacturer or supplier of an item to the buyer of the item receives safe-harbor protection.

- *Standards for manufacturers and suppliers:* To qualify for this safe-harbor protection, a manufacturer or supplier must meet certain requirements, such as reporting any price reduction that was obtained as part of the warranty.

- *Discounts:* Discounts are a reduction in the amount a seller charges a buyer (who buys either directly or through a wholesaler or a group purchasing organization) for a good or service based on an arm's-length transaction.[70] The term discount may include a rebate check or credit. It does not include any cash payment nor does it include furnishing one good or service without charge or at a reduced charge in exchange for any agreement to buy a different good or service.

- *Standards for buyers:* A hospital that receives a discount for a purchased good or service must comply with requirements, such as the discount being earned based on purchases of that same good or service bought within a single fiscal year.

- *Standards for sellers:* The person or entity that sells discounted goods or services to a hospital must comply with requirements, such as the seller must fully and accurately report such discount on the invoice or statement submitted to the buyer and inform the buyer of its obligations to report such discount.

- *Employees:* This safe harbor allows an employer to pay an employee, who has a bona fide employment relationship with the employer, for providing covered items or services.

- *Group purchasing organizations (GPOs):* A GPO is an entity authorized to act as a purchasing agent for a group of individuals or entities who are furnishing services for which payment may be made under Medicare or a state health care program, and who are neither wholly owned by the GPO nor subsidiaries of a parent corporation that wholly owns the GPO (either directly or through another wholly owned entity).

- *Waiver of beneficiary coinsurance and deductibles:* Hospitals may waive copayments or deductibles for inpatient hospital care for which Medicare pays under the prospective payment system.

- *Managed care:* Two additional safe harbors for managed care plans were published in the Federal Register on November 5, 1992. The safe harbors are intended to protect certain business and payment relationships between health care plans, providers, and enrollees that allow them to compete in the marketplace for managed care.

- *Coverage, cost-sharing, or premiums offered to enrollees:* Under this safe harbor, managed care plans may offer incentives to beneficiaries, including additional coverage of any item or service to an enrollee, reduction of some or all of the enrollee's obligations to pay the health plan or a contract health care provider for cost-sharing amounts (such as coinsurance, deductible, or copayment amounts), or reduction of the premium amounts attributable to items or services covered by the health plan, Medicare, or a state health plan.

- *Price reductions providers offer to health plans:* This safe harbor protects certain price-reduction agreements between health care plans and health care providers. Contract health care providers may offer a reduction in price to health plans as long as both the health plan and the contract health care provider comply with all of the applicable standards.

Antitrust Safety Zones

The DOJ and the FTC issued six policy statements that address the following antitrust safety zones[71]:

1. hospital mergers

2. hospital joint ventures involving high-technology or other expensive medical equipment

3. physicians' provision of information to purchasers of health care services

4. hospital participation in exchanges of price and cost information

5. joint purchasing arrangements among health care providers

6. physician network joint ventures

The policy statements are designed to provide education and instruction to the health care community on issues related to mergers and joint ventures. The policy statements give health care providers guidance in the form of antitrust safety zones, which describe the circumstances under which the agencies will not challenge conduct as violative of the antitrust law as a matter of prosecutorial discretion. The statements set forth in outline format the analysis the agencies will utilize to review conduct that falls outside the antitrust safety zones. The policy statements, for the first time, commit the agencies to responding to requests for business reviews or advisory opinions from the health care community no later than 90 days following the receipt of all information regarding any matters addressed in the statements, with the exception of requests regarding mergers falling outside the antitrust safety zone.[72]

Under HIPAA, DHHS is now required to provide formal guidance to individual parties with respect to the antikickback statute. DHHS, in collaboration with the DOJ, must issue written opinions relating to the following: what constitutes prohibited remuneration, whether an arrangement violates the antikickback and safe-harbors statutory scheme, what constitutes an inducement to limit or reduce services to Medicare and Medicaid beneficiaries in a managed care plan, and whether any activity exposes a provider to criminal or civil liability.

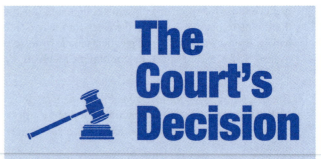

The court of special appeals held that, where the liability of AAMC was solely vicarious and based on the negligent conduct of the pathologist as its purported agent, AAMC and the pathologist were not joint tort-feasors. The patient's release of the pathologist acted as a release of AAMC as a matter of law.

CHAPTER REVIEW

1. The governing body of an organization oversees and controls the corporation's activities. This body is legally responsible for establishing and implementing policies for the management and operation of the organization.

2. *Articles of incorporation* detail the corporation's purpose and the powers it is authorized to exercise in order to carry out this purpose. *Express corporate authority* is delegated by a statute, while *implied corporate authority* is invoked in cases in which authority not specifically granted in the articles of incorporation is required to carry out its purpose. *Ultra vires acts* are those in which a governing body acts beyond its expressed or implied scope of authority.

3. Traditionally, a number of committees conduct the business of the governing body:

   - *Executive committee:* has the authority to act on behalf of the full board

   - *Bylaws committee:* reviews and recommends bylaws to the governing body

   - *Finance committee:* oversees financial affairs and makes recommendations to the governing body

   - *Joint conference committee:* acts as a forum for discussion of policy and practice matters

   - *Nominating committee:* develops and recommends criteria for governing body membership

- *Planning committee:* makes recommendations for the use and development of an organization's resources

- *Patient care committee:* reviews the quality of patient care and makes recommendations for its improvement

- *Audit and regulatory compliance committee:* assesses various functions and control systems of the organization and provides management with analysis and recommendations for activities reviewed

- *Safety committee:* oversees the organization's safety program

4. The *Sarbanes-Oxley Act of 2002* was enacted to protect investors by improving the accuracy and reliability of corporate disclosures. The act requires top executives of public corporations to vouch for the financial reports of their companies and encourages self-regulation.

5. An employer can be held responsible for the acts of its employees under the legal *doctrine of respondeat superior* or *vicarious liability.* The idea that all joint or concurrent tort-feasors are independently at fault for their own wrongful acts is called *joint liability.* An independent contractor relationship is one in which the principal has no right of control over the way in which the agent's work is to be performed. To be found liable for the torts of corporate employees, an officer or director of a corporation must have had direct involvement in the tortious act.

6. A corporation has a responsibility to ensure the patient's safety and well-being while at the hospital. If a corporation has a duty to fulfill and it fails to do so, it can be found guilty of corporate negligence. Under this doctrine, hospitals that fail to uphold proper standards of care are liable.

7. Corporations have certain duties specified by the corresponding state's corporation laws. These duties include holding meetings, establishing policies, being financially scrupulous, providing adequate insurance, and paying taxes.

8. The CEO, who is given authority by the owner or governing body, is charged with the supervision of the administrative staff and department heads. In addition, the CEO must implement the governing body's policies and interpret them to staff, and must notify the governing body of potential danger in carrying out policies that create unreasonable risks.

9. Dependence on government funding and related programs, the continuous shrinkage in such revenues, and increased competition from nonhospital sources have contributed to the need to seek alternative resources for revenue. The need to obtain income and meet competition has caused hospitals to consider establishing business enterprises.

10. A certificate of need (CON) is granted by a state regulatory agency and allows hospitals to add programs or services or expend monies for the acquisition of capital in excess of specified threshold limits. Health care providers have criticized CON requirements because they require the review of expenditures by or on behalf of a health care facility but may permit groups of physicians or independent laboratories to make large expenditures without triggering state review mechanisms.

11. Restructuring of a single not-for-profit tax-exempt hospital normally involves the formation of at least one additional not-for-profit tax-exempt entity, which may be referred to as a parent or holding company or foundation. This additional entity is created to serve as the corporate vehicle to receive the ultimate benefits for the revenue-producing activities and to confer some or all of those benefits to the hospital.

12. Patients must be allowed free choice of goods and services so that organizations can protect themselves from anticompetitive activities and antitrust claims. Patients must be advised that they are not required to use a vendor that an organization recommends and also should be informed of the organization's relationship to the company in advance of the patient's decision.

13. The regulations that describe how health care providers should structure financial arrangements in order to be exempt from prosecution by the department of justice and the FTC are called *safe-harbor regulations.*

14. The DOJ and the FTC have issued policy statements designed to educate and instruct health care community members on issues surrounding mergers and joint ventures. These statements outline the analysis the agencies will use to review conduct that falls outside antitrust safety zones.

REVIEW QUESTIONS

1. Describe the organization, responsibilities, duties, and legal risks of a governing body.
2. List some of the major provisions of the Sarbanes-Oxley Act, as presented in the text.
3. Describe the meaning of the legal doctrine respondeat superior.
4. Describe the term *corporate negligence.*

5. Why is the Darling case described as a benchmark case?
6. Does the legal doctrine respondeat superior apply to an independent contractor? Explain your answer.
7. What is meant by the parent holding company model?
8. What does the Safe Harbor Act regulate?

NOTES

1. *AA Medical Center v. Condon,* 649 A.2d 1189 (Md. App. 1994).

2. 543 So. 2d 209 (Fla. 1989).

3. 500 P.2d 335 (Ariz. Ct. App. 1972).

4. 738 N.Y.S.2d 87 (N.Y. App. Div. 2002).

5. 46 U.S.L.W. 2227 (Md. 1977).

6. 272 S.E.2d 643 (S.C. 1980).

7. *Thompson v. Nason Hosp.,* 591 A.2d 703, 707 (Pa. 1991).

8. *Id.*

9. 211 N.E.2d 253 (Ill. 1965).

10. *Id.* at 260.

11. 183 Cal. Rptr. 156 (Cal. Ct. App. 1982).

12. 348 S.C. 549, 560 S.E.2d 894 (2002).

13. No. 228566 (Cal. Super. Ct. Sacramento Co. 1976).

14. 438 So. 2d 412 (Fla. Dist. Ct. App. 1983).

15. 23. 206 Cal. Rptr. 164 (Cal. Ct. App. 1984). 24. 734 F.2d 81 (1st Cir. 1984).

16. 734 F.2d 81 (1st Cir. 1984).

17. *Educating and Licensing Nursing Home Administrators: Public Policy Issues,* 30 THE GERONTOLOGIST 582 (1990).

18. NEW YORK TIMES on Sun., July 23, 2000, available at www.massnurses.org/News/2000/000007/nursinghomes.htm

19. *Nursing Homes Conditions in Texas: Many Nursing Homes Fail to Meet Federal Standards for Adequate Care,* Minority Staff, Special Investigation Division, Committee on Government Reform, U.S. House of Representatives, October 20, 2002, www.democrats.reform.house.gov/story.asp?ID. Full report available at www.democrats.reform.house.gov/story.asp?ID=580.

20. *Nation's Nursing Homes Are Quietly Killing Thousands,* Andrew Schneider and Phillip O'Connor, St. Louis Post-Dispatch, October 12, 2002, www.stltoday.com/stltoday/news/special/neglected.nsf/0/D99DA8A06 D2CBA8C86256C500057AAC5?OpenDocument.

21. 655 S.W.2d 14 (Ky. Ct. App. 1982).

22. *Id.* at 26.

23. *Id.* at 26.

24. 396 So. 2d 406 (La. Ct. App. 1981).

25. 188 Cal. Rptr. 685 (Cal. Ct. App. 1983).

26. 406 N.Y.S.2d 621 (N.Y. App. Div. 1978).

27. 565 So. 2d 221, 224 (Ala. 1990).

28. *Id.* 223–224.

29. *Id.* at 226.

30. 171 Cal. Rptr. 846 (Cal. Ct. App. 1981).

31. *Id.* at 852.

32. 488 A.2d 858 (Del. 1985).

33. 502 N.Y.S.2d 1012 (N.Y. App. Div. 1986).

34. 88 Cal. Rptr. 86 (Cal. Ct. App. 1970).

35. 449 N.E.2d 486 (Ohio Ct. App. 1982).

36. 634 N.E.2d 864 (Ind. Ct. App. 1994).

37. 439 N.Y.S.2d 967 (N.Y. App. Div. 1981).

38. 836 S.W.2d 911 (Mo. 1992).

39. 354 So. 2d 1138 (Ala. Civ. App. 1987).

40. *Id.* at 1140.

41. 383 So. 2d 544 (Ala. Civ. App. 1980).

42. 861 S.W.2d 694 (Mo. Ct. App. 1993).

43. 625 So. 2d 351 (La. Ct. App. 1993).

44. 634 N.E.2d 189 (N.Y. 1994).

45. 696 So. 2d 19, 83–97 (La. App. 1997).

46. 636 So. 2d 1059 (La. Ct. App. 1994).

47. 441 S.E.2d 577 (N.C. Ct. App. 1994).

48. 662 S.W.2d 880 (Mo. Ct. App. 1983).

49. 380 N.Y.S.2d 116 (N.Y. App. Div. 1976).

50. 861 P.2d 679 (Ariz. Ct. App. 1993).

51. 636 A.2d 527 (N.J. Super. Ct. App. Div. 1994).

52. 665 F.2d 401 (1st Cir. 1981).

53. *Id.* at 402.

54. 430 N.Y.S.2d 402 (N.Y. App. Div. 1980).

55. *Feuereisen v. Axelrod,* 473 N.Y.S.2d 870 (N.Y. App. Div. 1984).

56. *Cliff House Nursing Home, Inc. v. Department of Pub. Health,* 463 N.E.2d 578 (Mass. App. Ct. 1984).

57. 338 N.W.2d 855 (Wis. Ct. App. 1983).

58. 542 So. 2d 935 (Ala. Civ. App. 1989).

59. 380 S.E.2d 841 (S.C. Ct. App. 1989).

60. *Id.* at 845.

61. 432 N.W.2d 68 (S.D. 1988).

62. *Id.* at 76–77.

63. 338 S.E.2d 477 (Ga. Ct. App. 1985).

64. 507 So. 2d 1211 (Fla. Dist. Ct. App. 1987).

65. WEISSBURG, *Joint Ventures: To Be or Not To Be,* FED'N OF AM. HEALTH SYS. REV., May–June 1989, at 50.

66. *Hospital Corp. of Am. v. Federal Trade Comm'n,* 807 F.2d 1381 (7th Cir. 1986).

67. 56 Fed. Reg. 35,952 (codified at 42 C.F.R. § 1001.951–953).

68. *HHS's Final "Safe-Harbor" Regulations Limit Referrals,* A.H.A. NEWS, July 29, 1991, at 1.

69. The term *written warranty* is defined as: (A) any written affirmation of fact or written promise made in connection with the sale of a consumer product by a supplier to a buyer that relates to the nature of the material or workmanship and affirms or promises that such material or workmanship is defect free or will meet a specified level of performance over a specified period of time, or (B) any undertaking in writing in connection with the sale by a supplier of a consumer product to refund, repair, replace, or take other remedial action with respect to such product in the event that product fails to meet the specifications set forth in the undertaking, which written affirmation, promise, or undertaking becomes part of the basis of the bargain between a supplier and a buyer for purposes other than resale of such product.

70. Safe Harbor, 42 C.F.R. § 1001.951–953.

71. 31. U.S. DEPT. OF JUSTICE AND FED. TRADE COMM'N, STATEMENTS OF ANTITRUST ENFORCEMENT POLICY IN THE HEALTH CARE AREA, Sept. 15, 1993, at 1.

72. *Id.* at 1–2.

Medical Staff

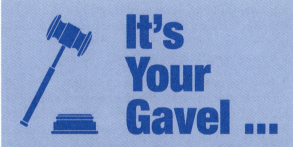

It's Your Gavel ...

RIGHT PATIENT, WRONG SURGERY

The plaintiff was diagnosed with a herniated disk at L4-L5. His surgeon performed a laminectomy. During a review of the plaintiff's postoperative X-rays, the surgeon noted that he had mistakenly removed the disk at L3-L4. The plaintiff testified that after the surgery his condition progressively worsened.

The plaintiff's expert testified that removal of the healthy disk caused the space between L3-L4 to collapse and the vertebrae to shift and settle. Even the defendant's expert witness testified that the removal of the healthy disk would increase the likelihood that the plaintiff would be more susceptible to future injuries.

The trial court directed a verdict against the defendant based on the defendant's own admission and that of his expert that he was negligent, and that his negligence caused at least some injury to the patient. The defendant appealed.[1]

WHAT IS YOUR VERDICT?

This chapter provides an overview of medical staff organization, the credentialing process, and a review of cases focused on the legal risks of physicians. The cases presented highlight those areas in which physicians tend to be most vulnerable to lawsuits.

MEDICAL STAFF ORGANIZATION

The medical staff is an integral part of a health care organization with defined responsibilities under its bylaws. The medical staff is formally organized with officers, com-

mittees, and bylaws. At regular intervals, the various committees of the medical staff review and analyze their responsibilities, clinical experiences, and opportunities for improvement. The responsibilities of a variety of medical staff committees are described here.

- **Executive Committee.** The executive committee oversees the activities of the medical staff. It is responsible for recommending to the governing body such things as medical staff structure, a process for reviewing credentials and appointing members to the medical staff, a process for delineating clinical privileges, a mechanism for the participation of the medical staff in performance improvement activities, a process for peer review, a mechanism by which medical staff membership may be terminated, and a mechanism for fair hearing procedures. The executive committee reviews and acts on the reports of medical staff departmental chairpersons and designated medical staff committees. Actions requiring approval of the governing body are forwarded to the governing body for approval. Membership on the executive committee generally includes the chief of staff as chairperson, medical staff officers, and departmental chairman. The chief executive and chief nursing officers are generally nonvoting members of the committee.

- **Bylaws Committee.** The functioning of the medical staff is described in its bylaws, rules, and regulations, which must be reviewed and approved by the organization's governing body. Bylaws must be kept current, and the governing body must approve recommended changes. The bylaws describe the various membership categories of the medical staff (e.g., active, courtesy, consultative, and allied professional staff) as well as the process for obtaining privileges.

- **Blood and Transfusion Committee.** The blood and transfusion committee develops blood usage policies and procedures. It is responsible for monitoring transfusion services and reviewing indications for transfusions, blood ordering practices, each transfusion episode, and transfusion reactions. The committee reports its findings and recommendations to the medical staff executive committee.

- **Credentials Committee.** The credentials committee oversees the application process for medical staff applicants, requests for clinical privileges, and reappointments to the medical staff. The committee makes its recommendations to the medical executive committee.

- **Infection Control Committee.** The infection control committee is generally responsible for the development of policies and procedures for investigating, controlling, and preventing infections.

- **Medical Records Committee.** The medical records committee develops policies and procedures as they pertain to the management of medical records, including release, security, and storage. The committee determines the format of complete medical records and reviews medical records for accuracy, completeness, legibility, and timely completion. Medical records are also reviewed for clinical pertinence. The committee ensures that medical records reflect the condition and progress of the patient, including the results of all tests and therapy given, and makes recommendations for disciplinary action as necessary.

- **Pharmacy and Therapeutics Committee.** The pharmacy and therapeutics committee is generally charged with developing policies and procedures relating to the selection, procurement, distribution, handling, use, and safe administration of drugs, biologicals, and diagnostic testing material. The committee oversees the development and maintenance of a drug formulary. The committee also evaluates and approves protocols for the use of investigational or experimental drugs. The committee oversees the tracking of medication errors and adverse drug reactions; the management, control, and effective and safe use of medications through monitoring and evaluation; the monitoring of problem-prone, high-risk, and high-volume medications utilizing parameters such as appropriateness, safety, effectiveness, medication errors, food-drug interactions, drug-drug interactions, drug-disease interactions, and adverse drug reactions; and performs other such activities that may be delegated to it by the medical executive committee.

- **Quality Improvement Council.** The quality improvement council functions as a patient care assessment and improvement committee. The council generally consists of representatives from the organization's administration, governing body, medical staff, and nursing.

- **Tissue Committee.** The tissue committee reviews all surgical procedures. Surgical case reviews address the justification and indications for surgical procedures. Representation on the tissue committee should include the departments of surgery, anesthesiology, pathology, nursing, risk management, and administration.

- **Utilization Review Committee.** The utilization review committee monitors and evaluates utilization issues such as medical necessity and appropriateness of admission and continued stay, as well as delay in the provision of diagnostic, therapeutic, and supportive services. The utilization review committee ensures that each patient is treated at an appropriate level of care. Objectives of the committee include timely transfer of patients requiring alternate levels of care; promotion of the efficient and effective use of the organization's resources; adherence to quality utilization standards of third-party payers; maintenance of high-quality, cost-effective care; and identification of opportunities for improvement

MEDICAL DIRECTOR

The medical director serves as a liaison between the medical staff and the organization's governing body and management. The medical director should have clearly written agreements with the organization, including duties, responsibilities, and compensation arrangements. State nursing home codes often provide for the designation of either a full-time or part-time physician to serve as medical director. The responsibilities of a medical director include enforcing the bylaws of the governing body and medical staff and monitoring the quality of medical care in the organization.

The medical director of an organization can be liable for failing to perform his or her duties and responsibilities. When a Texas nursing home was indicted by a grand jury in 1981 for the deaths of several residents, the medical director was also indicted.[2] His plea that he merely signed papers and attended meetings did not absolve him of the responsibility to ensure the adequacy and the appropriateness of medical services in the organization.

MEDICAL STAFF PRIVILEGES

Medical staff privileges are restricted to those professionals who fulfill the requirements as described in an organization's medical staff bylaws. Although cognizant of the importance of medical staff membership, the governing body must meet its obligation to maintain standards of good medical practice in dealing with matters of staff appointment, credentialing, and the disciplining of physicians for such things as disruptive behavior, incompetence, psychological problems, criminal actions, and substance abuse.

Appointment to the medical staff and medical staff privileges should be granted only after there has been a thorough investigation of the applicant. The delineation of clinical privileges should be discipline-specific and based on appropriate predetermined criteria that adhere to national standards.

Credentialing and Privileging Process

The purpose of the appointment process is to evaluate the competency of the applicant to determine whether he or she is qualified for appointment to the medical staff. The following sections describe the appointment process.

- **Application**

  The governing body should establish a policy of nondiscrimination on the basis of race, color, sex, religion, national origin, age, and physical disability. The medical staff application should provide pertinent information regarding the applicant's

  - residence
  - office location (Geographic requirements should not be unreasonably restrictive. If the applicant does not meet the organization's geographic requirements for residence and office location, provision should be available in the bylaws for exceptions that might be necessary to attract a distinguished consulting staff.)
  - medical school
  - internship

  - residency
  - license to practice medicine
  - board certification
  - fellowship
  - medical society membership (Board certification, fellowship, and medical society membership are not generally acceptable criteria for determining eligibility for medical staff appointment.)
  - malpractice coverage
  - special skills and talents
  - privileges requested and specialty
  - availability to provide on-call emergency department coverage where applicable
  - availability to serve on medical staff and/or organization committees
  - other medical staff appointments
  - previous disciplinary actions against the applicant
  - unexplained breaks in work history
  - voluntary and/or involuntary limitations or relinquishment of staff privileges

- **Medical Staff Bylaws.** Each staff member must adhere to the written bylaws governing the medical staff and care of patients. The bylaws should be approved by the medical executive committee and governing body. Each member of the organization's medical staff should be required to sign a statement attesting to the fact that the medical staff bylaws have been read and that the physician agrees to abide by the bylaws and other policies and procedures that may be adopted from time to time by the organization.

- **Physical and Mental Status.** Health care organizations must address issues regarding a physician's physical and mental capacity prior to the granting of medical staff privileges. Credentialed members of the medical staff should undergo a medical evaluation prior to reappointment to the medical staff.

- **Consent for Release of Information.** Consent for release of information from third parties should be obtained from the applicant.

- **Certificate of Insurance.** The applicant should provide evidence of professional liability insurance. The insurance policy should provide minimum levels of insurance coverage, with limits (e.g., $1 million to $3 million) determined by the organization.

- **State Licensure.** A physician's right to practice medicine is subject to the licensing laws contained in the statutes of the state in which the physician resides. The right to practice medicine is not a vested right, but is a condition of a right subordinate to the police power of the state to protect and preserve public health. Although a state has power to regulate the practice of medicine, for the benefit of the public health and welfare, this power is restricted. Regulations must be reasonably related to the public health and welfare and must not amount to arbitrary or unreasonable interference with the right to practice one's profession. Health professions commonly requiring licensure include chiropractors, dentists, nurses, pharmacists, physicians' assistants, optometrists, osteopaths, physicians, and podiatrists. A statute mandating that the Medical Board of California disclose to the public information regarding its licensees (Cal. Bus. & Prof. Code, § 803.1) and the statute mandating that the board post on the Internet information pertaining to its licensees (Section 2027), did not prohibit the board from posting on its Web site information regarding a licensee's completion of probation with a listing of the case number the case from which the probation arose.[3] Grounds for the revocation of a license to practice medicine include the following:

- a clear demonstration of the lack of good moral character

- deliberate falsification of a patient's medical record (to protect one's own interests at the expense of the patient)

- intentional fraudulent advertising

- gross incompetence

- sexual misconduct

- substance abuse

- performance of unnecessary medical procedures

- billing for services not performed

- disruptive behavior

• **National Practitioner Data Bank.** The National Practitioner Data Bank (NPDB) was created by Congress as a national repository of information with the primary purpose of facilitating a comprehensive review of physicians' and other health care practitioners' professional credentials (see Chapter 13). The National Practitioner Data Bank must be queried as to information in its files that may pertain to medical staff applicants. Health care organizations must query the data bank every two years on the renewal of clinical privileges of health care practitioners. The data bank serves as a flagging system whose principal purpose is to facilitate a more comprehensive review of professional credentials. As a nationwide flagging system, it is a resource to assist state licensing boards, hospitals, and other health care entities in conducting extensive independent reviews of the qualifications of health care practitioners they seek to license or hire or to whom they wish to grant clinical privileges.

• **References.** References should be checked thoroughly. Failure to do so can lead to corporate liability for a physician's negligent acts. Both written and oral references should be obtained from previous organizations with which the applicant has been affiliated. An action was brought against a hospital in *Rule v. Lutheran Hospitals & Homes Society of America*[4] for birth injuries sustained during an infant's breech delivery. The action was based on allegations that the hospital negligently failed to investigate the qualifications of the attending physician before granting him privileges. The jury's verdict of $650,000 was supported by evidence that the hospital failed to check with other hospitals where the physician had practiced. The physician's privileges at one hospital had been limited in that breech deliveries had to be performed under supervision.

• **Interview Process.** The preinterview and interview process should cover the following:

- Have all documents been received prior to the interview?

- Are there any unaccounted-for breaks or gaps in education or employment?

- Has any disciplinary action or misconduct investigation been initiated or are any pending against the applicant by any licensing body?

- Has the applicant's license to practice medicine in any state ever been denied, limited, suspended, or revoked?

- Have the applicant's medical staff privileges ever been suspended, diminished, revoked, or refused at any health care organization?

- Has the applicant ever withdrawn an application or resigned from any medical staff to avoid disciplinary action prior to a decision being rendered by an organization regarding application for membership?

- Has the applicant ever been named as a defendant in a lawsuit?

- Has the applicant ever been named as a defendant in a criminal proceeding?

- Is the applicant available for emergency on-call coverage?

- Does the applicant have back-up and cross-coverage?

- Does the applicant have any special skills or talents?

- Has the applicant reviewed medical staff bylaws, rules, and regulations, and, where applicable, departmental rules and regulations?

- Does the applicant agree to abide by the medical staff bylaws, rules, and regulations, and other policies and procedures set by the organization?

- Is the applicant a team player? Can he or she work well with others?

- Has the applicant ever been restricted from participating in any private or government (e.g., Medicare, Medicaid) health insurance program?

- Has the applicant's malpractice insurance coverage ever been terminated by action of an insurance carrier?

- Has the applicant ever been denied malpractice insurance coverage?

- Have there been any settlements and/or judgments against the applicant?

- Does the applicant have any physical or mental impairments that could affect his or her ability to practice the privileges requested?

- **Delineation of Clinical Privileges.** The delineation of clinical privileges is the process by which the medical staff determines precisely what procedures a physician is authorized to perform. This determination is based on predetermined criteria as to what credentials are necessary to competently perform the privileges requested.

- **Governing Body Responsibility.** The governing body has ultimate responsibility for the selection of the organization's professional staff and ensuring that applicants to the organization's medical staff are qualified to perform the clinical privileges requested. The duty to select members of the medical staff is legally vested in the governing body as the body charged with managing the organization. In light of the importance of staff appointments to physicians, the courts have prohibited an organization from acting unreasonably or capriciously in rejecting physicians for staff appointments or in limiting their privileges.

- **Appeal Process.** An appeal process should be described in the medical staff bylaws to cover issues such as the denial of professional staff privileges, grievances, and disciplinary actions. The governing body should reserve the right to hear any appeals and be the final decision maker within the organization. A physician whose privileges are either suspended or terminated must exhaust all remedies provided in a hospital's bylaws, rules, and regulations before commencing a court action. The physician in *Eidelson v. Archer*[5] failed to pursue the hospital's internal appeal procedure before bringing a suit. As a result, the Alaska Supreme Court reversed a superior court's judgment for the physician in his action for damages.

- **Reappointments.** Each physician's credentials and departmental evaluations should be reviewed at a minimum of every two years. The medical staff must provide effective mechanisms for monitoring and evaluating the quality of patient care and the clinical performance of physicians. For problematic physicians, consideration should be given to privileges with supervision, a reduction in privileges, suspension of privileges with purpose (e.g., suspension pending further training), or termination of privileges.

Screening for Competency

The governing body has a responsibility to appoint competent members to its professional staff. Failure to properly screen a medical staff applicant's credentials can lead to liability for injuries suffered by patients as a result of that omission. The patient in *Johnson v. Misericordia Community Hospital*[6] brought a malpractice action against the hospital and its liability insurer for alleged negligence in granting orthopedic privileges to a physician who performed an operation to remove a pin fragment from the patient's hip. The Wisconsin Court of Appeals found the hospital negligent for failing to scrutinize the physician's credentials before approving his application for orthopedic privileges. The hospital failed to adhere to procedures established under both its own bylaws and state statute. The measure of quality and the degree of quality control exercised in a hospital are the direct responsibilities of the medical staff. Hospital supervision of the manner of appointment of physicians to its staff is mandatory, not optional. On appeal by the hospital, the Wisconsin Supreme Court affirmed the appellate court's decision, finding that if the hospital had exercised ordinary care, it would not have appointed the physician to the medical staff.

HOSPITAL'S DUTY TO ENSURE COMPETENCY

Citation: *Candler Gen. Hosp., Inc. v. Persaud*, 442 S.E.2d 775 (Ga. Ct. App. 1994)

Facts

On or about February 15, 1990, the patient in this case was referred to Dr. Freeman for consultation and treatment of gallstones. Freeman recommended that the patient undergo a laparoscopic laser cholecystectomy procedure.

On February 16, 1990, Freeman requested and was granted temporary privileges to perform the procedure. The privileges were granted based on a certificate he had received after completing a laparoscopic laser cholecystectomy workshop, which he took on February 10, 1990. Freeman performed the cholecystectomy on February 20, 1990, with the assistance of Dr. Thomas.

A complaint by the administrator of the patient's estate, supported by an expert's affidavit, alleged that the cholecystectomy was negligently performed, and as a result the patient bled to death. The complaint charged the hospital with negligence in permitting Freeman to perform the procedure on the decedent without having instituted any standards, training requirements, "protocols," or otherwise instituted any method for judging the qualifications of a surgeon to perform the procedure. The complaint also alleged that the hospital knew or reasonably should have known that it did not have a credentialing process that could have assured the hospital of the physicians' education, training, and ability to perform the procedure.

The trial court denied the hospital's motion for summary judgment, finding that the plaintiffs' evidence was sufficient to raise a question of fact regarding whether surgical privileges should have been issued by the hospital to Freeman. The hospital appealed.

Issue

Was there a material issue of fact as to whether the hospital was negligent in granting the specific privileges requested by Freeman?

Holding

The Georgia Court of Appeals held that there was a material issue of fact as to whether the hospital was negligent in granting the specific privileges requested, thus precluding summary judgment.

Reason

The court found that a hospital has a direct and independent responsibility to its patients to take reasonable steps to ensure that physicians using hospital facilities are qualified for the privileges granted. The hospital owed a duty to the plaintiffs' decedent to act in good faith and with reasonable care to ensure that the surgeon was qualified to practice the procedure that he was granted privileges to perform.

Discussion

1. Describe the credentialing issues in this case.
2. Discuss what steps a hospital should take to help ensure that a physician is competent to perform the procedures he or she is requesting.

PHYSICIAN SUPERVISION AND MONITORING

The medical staff is responsible to the governing body for the quality of care rendered by members of the medical staff. The landmark decision in this area occurred in *Darling v. Charleston Community Memorial Hospital,*[7] in which it was decided that the hospital's governing body has a duty to establish a mechanism for the medical staff to evaluate, counsel, and, when necessary, take action against an unreasonable risk of harm to a patient arising from the patient's treatment by a physician. Physician monitoring is best accomplished through a system of peer review. Most states provide statutory protection from liability for peer-review activities when they are conducted in a reasonable manner and without malice.

DISRUPTIVE PHYSICIANS

Disruptive physicians can have a negative impact on an organization's staff and ultimately affect the quality of patient care. Having the right policies in place as they relate to conflict resolution is a must for an effective working environment. Criteria other than academic credentials (e.g., a physician's ability to work with others) should be considered before granting medical staff privileges. That factor was considered by the court in *Ladenheim v. Union County Hospital District,*[8] which held that the physician's inability to work with other members of the staff was sufficient grounds to deny him staff privileges. The physician's record was replete with evidence of his inability to work effectively with other members of the hospital staff. As stated in *Huffaker v. Bailey,*[9] most courts have found that the ability to work smoothly with others is reasonably related to the objective of ensuring patient welfare. The conclusion seems justified because health care professionals frequently are required to work together or in teams. A staff member who, because of personality characteristics or other problems, is incapable of getting along with others could severely hinder the effective treatment of patients.

The court, in *Pick v. Santa Ana-Tustin Community Hospital,*[10] held that the petitioner's demonstrated lack of ability to work with others in the hospital setting was sufficient to support the denial of his application for admission to the medical staff. There was evidence that the petitioner presented a real and substantial danger to patients treated by him and that the patients might receive other than a high quality of medical care.

PHYSICIAN NEGLIGENCE

Table 8-1, as reported by the National Practitioner Data Bank, describes the number of malpractice payment amounts by malpractice reason for physicians. The cases that follow illustrate of a variety of acts or failures to act that have led to lawsuits.

MISREPRESENTATION OF CREDENTIALS

There was reliable, probative, and substantial evidence in *Graor v. State Medical Board* to support the Ohio State Medical Board's decision to permanently revoke a physician's license for misrepresenting his credentials by claiming that he was board certified in internal medicine. The evidence submitted supported that, in many instances, the physician falsely indicated that he had American Board of Internal Medicine certification. The board contended that the hearing examiner addressed the physician's credibility and found many statements to support her conclusion that the physician intended to misrepresent his board status.[11]

LIMITATIONS ON REQUESTED PRIVILEGES

Dr. Warnick, a pediatrician, obtained associate staff privileges at the Natchez Community Hospital in 1997. She later applied for full privileges through the hospital's credentials committee. Concern was raised about her alleged difficulty with the intubation of children. As a result, action on Warnick's request for full privileges was deferred. In May of 1998, the credentials committee recommended full privileges with the exception of neonatal resuscitation. After several in-hospital appeals, Warnick filed a lawsuit. The court determined that there was substantial evidence to support

the hospital's suspension of Warnick's resuscitation privileges, and her right to due process was not violated.

Hospitals licensed in Mississippi pursuant to statute are authorized to suspend, deny, revoke, or limit the hospital privileges of any physician practicing or applying to practice therein, if the governing board of such hospital, after consultation with the medical staff, considers such physician to be unqualified because of any of the acts set forth in Miss. Code Ann. § 73-25-93 (1998); provided that the procedures for such actions comply with the hospital and/or medical staff bylaw requirements for due process. In this case, the hospital and medical staff abided by the bylaws and requirements for due process, as evidenced by two hearings afforded to Warnick. She did not complain that she was unable to present all relevant evidence. Her claims were heard in a timely and meaningful manner.[12]

MISDIAGNOSING UNCONSCIOUS ACCIDENT VICTIM

In *Ramberg v. Morgan,*[13] a police department physician, at the scene of an accident, examined an unconscious man who had been struck by an automobile. The physician concluded that the patient's insensibility was a result of alcohol intoxication, not the accident, and ordered the police to remove him to jail instead of the hospital. The man, to the physician's knowledge, remained semiconscious for several days and finally was taken from the cell to the hospital at the insistence of his family. The patient subsequently died, and the autopsy revealed massive skull fractures. The court found that any physician should reasonably anticipate the presence of head injuries when a person is struck by a car. Failure to refer an accident victim to another physician or a hospital is actionable neglect of the physician's duty. Although a physician does not ensure the correctness of the diagnosis or treatment, a patient is entitled to such thorough and careful examination as his or her condition and attending circumstances permit, with such diligence and methods of diagnosis as usually are approved and practiced by medical people of ordinary or average learning, judgment, and skill in the community or similar localities.

FAILURE TO RESPOND TO EMERGENCY CALL

Physicians on call in an emergency department are expected to respond to requests for emergency assistance when such is considered necessary. Failure to respond is grounds for negligence should a patient suffer injury as a result of a physician's failure to respond.

Issues of fact in *Dillon v. Silver*[14] precluded summary dismissal of an action charging that a woman's death from

TABLE 8-1 National Practitioner Data Bank, 2005 Annual Report

Mean and Median Medical Malpractice Payment Amounts by Malpractice Reason, 2005 and Cumulative Through 2005—Physicians*
National Practitioner Data Bank (September 1, 1990–December 31, 2005)

Malpractice Reason	2005 Only			Cumulative through 2005				
				Actual			Inflation-adjusted	
	Number of Payments	Mean Payment	Median Payment	Number of Payments	Mean Payment	Median Payment	Mean Payment	Median Payment
Anesthesia related	464	$357,673	$200,000	7,062	$271,465	$100,000	$318,926	$119,226
Behavioral health related**	47	$310,647	$120,000	90	$246,910	$100,000	$249,011	$101,241
Diagnosis related	4,542	$315,543	$200,000	76,133	$251,889	$140,912	$294,195	$163,751
Equipment or product related	76	$160,000	$66,875	853	$88,411	$25,000	$102,732	$28,975
IV or blood products related	26	$183,973	$131,250	811	$177,058	$75,000	$214,427	$92,900
Medication related	656	$245,034	$135,000	12,457	$171,424	$70,000	$203,042	$79,601
Monitoring related	456	$252,291	$146,341	3,093	$241,162	$100,000	$275,489	$125,000
Obstetrics related	1,258	$523,534	$300,000	19,304	$395,762	$200,000	$464,859	$250,000
Surgery related	3,670	$252,737	$150,000	60,812	$186,019	$95,000	$217,601	$107,606
Treatment related	2,610	$228,423	$112,101	39,785	$197,515	$92,500	$231,621	$105,777
Miscellaneous	229	$171,746	$70,000	3,097	$119,855	$30,000	$142,358	$37,160
All reasons	**14,034**	**$294,153**	**$174,569**	**223,497**	**$229,972**	**$100,000**	**$269,256**	**$128,764**

This table includes only disclosable reports in the NPDB as of the end of the current year. Voided reports have been excluded. Cumulative totals exclude 120 medical malpractice payment reports that are missing data necessary to calculate payment or malpractice reason.

*The "Physicians" category includes allopathic (M.D.) physicians, allopathic interns and residents, osteopathic (D.O.) physicians, and osteopathic interns and residents.

**The "Behavioral Health" category was added on January 31, 2004. Reports involving behavioral health issues filed before January 31, 2004 used other reporting categories. Cumulative data in this category includes only reports filed after January 31, 2004.

complications of an ectopic pregnancy occurred because of a gynecologist's refusal to treat her despite a request for aid by a hospital emergency department physician. Although the gynecologist contended that no physician-patient relationship had ever arisen, the hospital bylaws not only mandated that the physician accept all patients referred to him, but also stated that the emergency department physician had authority to decide which service physician should be called and required the service physician to respond to such a call.

DELAYING TREATMENT

A physician may be liable for failing to respond promptly if it can be established that such inaction caused a patient's death.[15] A patient afflicted with lung cancer was awarded damages in *Blackmon v. Langley* because of the failure of the examining physician to inform the patient in a timely manner that a chest X-ray showed a lesion in his lung.[16] The lesion eventually was diagnosed as cancerous. The physician contended that because the evidence showed the patient had less than a 50 percent chance of survival at the time of the alleged negligence, he could not be the proximate cause of injury. The Arkansas Supreme Court found that the jury was properly entitled to determine that the patient suffered and lost more than would have been the case had he been notified promptly of the lesion.

The Bureau of Professional Medical Conduct (BPMC), in *Bell v. New York State Department of Health*,[17] upon investigation of a complaint charged that the physician failed to properly treat and respond to his patient's evolving emergency cardiac condition despite symptoms and circumstances indicating the need for immediate hospitalization. The physician denied the allegations, and the state board for professional medical conduct (committee) conducted a hearing.

When the patient visited the physician in September 1994, he was suffering from high blood pressure and taking medication for that condition. From 1994 to 1996, the patient was treated by the physician for various medical conditions, including high cholesterol and hypertension. On May 29, 1997, the patient visited the physician complaining of chest pains, anxiety panic attacks, and shortness of breath. During that visit, the physician performed an EKG, ordered chest X-rays, and referred the patient to a cardiac specialist for consultation. The physician also ordered a test for cardiac enzymes; however, the results were not available for several days. The physician prescribed asthma medication and sent the patient home. The next day, the physician attempted to call the patient to inquire about his condition but was unable to reach him. Within less than a week, on June 2, 1997, the patient returned to the physician's office complaining of continued chest pain. At that time, the physician arranged a visit with the cardiologist for the same day. The cardiologist

reviewed the patient's medical history, performed an electro-cardiogram (EKG), reviewed the May 29, 1997, EKG, and concluded that the patient had a myocardial infarction followed by postinfarction angina. The patient was immediately sent to the hospital.

The physician was not present at the hearing and did not call any witnesses to rebut BPMC's expert witness. Expert opinion revealed that the physician's response to the patient's symptoms on May 29, 1997, and June 2, 1997, failed to meet medically acceptable standards of care. On February 21, 2001, the committee sustained the charge of negligence. The physician's license was suspended for two years; however, the suspension was stayed, and the physician was placed on probation.

On appeal, the Supreme Court of New York found that given the serious nature of the patient's complaints and symptoms and the potential consequences, the committee's conclusions were found by the court to be supported by substantial evidence. According to Greenburg, (one of the defendants in the case), the physician's course of conduct in performing an EKG, ordering a cardiac enzyme test, and referring the patient to a cardiologist demonstrated that the physician suspected that the patient was experiencing cardiac problems. However, given the patient's symptoms and history, it was Greenburg's opinion that the physician failed to adhere to medically acceptable standards of treatment by failing to obtain the results of the cardiac enzyme test expeditiously and not referring the patient to an emergency department immediately.

INADEQUATE HISTORY AND PHYSICAL EXAMINATIONS

Failure to obtain an adequate family history and perform an adequate physical examination violates a standard of care owed to the patient. In *Foley v. Bishop Clarkson Memorial Hospital*,[18] the spouse sued the hospital for the death of his wife. During her pregnancy, the patient was under the care of a private physician. She gave birth in the hospital on August 20, 1964, and died the following day. During July and August, her physician treated her for a sore throat. There was no evidence in the hospital record that the patient had complained about a sore throat while in the hospital. The hospital rules required a history and physical examination to be written promptly (within 24 hours of admission). No history had been taken, although the patient had been examined several times in regard to the progress of her labor. The trial judge directed a verdict in favor of the hospital. On appeal, the appellate court held that the case should have been submitted to the jury for determination. A jury might reasonably have inferred that if the patient's condition had been treated properly, the strep throat infection could have been combated successfully, and her life saved. It also reasonably might have been inferred that if a history had been taken promptly when she was admitted to the hospital, the sore throat would have been discovered and hospital personnel alerted to watch for possible complications of the nature that later developed. Quite possibly, this attention also would have helped in diagnosing the patient's condition, especially if it had been apparent that she had been exposed to a strep throat infection. The court held that a hospital must guard not only against known physical and mental conditions of patients, but also against conditions that reasonable care should have uncovered.

The physician in *Moheet v. State Board of Registration for the Healing Arts*[19] had adequate notice of the charges against him, in that he was fully aware of the link between his failure to obtain an adequate medical history and the possibility of harm to the patient. He had sufficient notice of the allegation of his failure to obtain an adequate patient history, and his own pleading showed that he knew the charges he would be defending against. The testimony of the expert witnesses, combined with the other evidence in the record, constituted competent and substantial evidence to support the commission's finding of conduct that might be harmful to a patient. There is ample evidence in the record to support a finding of gross negligence.

There was substantial evidence in *Solomon v. Connecticut Medical Examining Board*[20] to support disciplinary action against a physician where the record indicated that the physician failed to document adequately patient histories, perform adequate physical examinations, assess the patient's condition appropriately, or order appropriate laboratory tests or secure appropriate consultations. The Connecticut Medical Examining Board found that the physician had administered contraindicated medications to patients and did not practice medicine with reasonable skill and safety, and that his practice of medicine posed a threat to the health and safety of any person. The board concluded that there was a basis on which to subject the physician's license to disciplinary action.

CHOICE OF TREATMENT: TWO SCHOOLS OF THOUGHT

The potential for liability affects the choice of treatment a physician will follow with his or her patient. Use of unprecedented procedures that create an untoward result may cause a physician to be found negligent even though due care was followed. A physician will not be held liable for exercising his or her judgment in applying a course of treatment supported by a reputable and respected body of medical experts even if another body of expert medical opinion would favor a different course of treatment. The two schools of thought doctrine is only applicable in medical malpractice cases in which there is more than one method of accepted treatment for a patient's disease or injury. Under this doctrine, a physician will not be liable for medical malpractice if he or she follows a course of treatment supported by reputable, respected, and reasonable medical experts.

A physician's efforts do not constitute negligence simply because they were unsuccessful in a particular case. A physician cannot be required to guarantee the results of his or her treatment. The mere fact that an adverse result may occur following treatment is not in and of itself evidence of professional negligence.

FAILURE TO ORDER DIAGNOSTIC TESTS

A plaintiff who claims that a physician failed to order proper diagnostic tests must show the following:

- It is standard practice to use a certain diagnostic test under the circumstances of the case.

- The physician failed to use the test and therefore failed to diagnose the patient's illness.

- The patient suffered injury as a result.

Failure to order diagnostic tests resulted in the misdiagnosis of appendicitis in *Steeves v. United States*.[21] In this case, physicians failed to order the appropriate diagnostic tests for a child who was referred to a Navy hospital with a diagnosis of possible appendicitis. Judgment in this case was entered against the United States, on behalf of the U.S. Navy, for medical expenses and for pain and suffering. The child had been referred by an Air Force dispensary, where a test indicated a high white-blood cell count. A consultation sheet had been given to the mother, indicating the possible diagnosis. The physician who examined the child at the Navy hospital performed no tests, failed to diagnose the patient's condition, and sent him home at 5:02 P.M., some 32 minutes after his arrival on July 21. The child was returned to the emergency department on July 22, at about 2:30 A.M., only to be sent home again by an intern who diagnosed the boy's condition as gastroenteritis. Once again, no diagnostic tests were ordered. The boy was returned to the Navy hospital on July 23, at which time diagnostic tests were performed. The patient was subsequently operated on and found to have a ruptured appendix. Holding the Navy hospital liable for the negligence of the physicians who acted as its agents, the court pointed out that a wrong diagnosis will not in and of itself support a verdict of liability in a lawsuit. However, a physician must use ordinary care in making a diagnosis. Only where a patient is examined adequately is there no liability for an erroneous diagnosis. In this instance, the physicians' failure to perform further laboratory tests the first two times the child was brought to the emergency department was found to be a breach of good medical practice.

FAILURE TO PROMPTLY REVIEW TEST RESULTS

Can a physician's failure to promptly review test results be the proximate cause of a patient's injuries? The answer is yes; a physician's failure to promptly review test results can be the proximate cause of a patient's injuries. In *Smith v. U.S. Department of Veterans Affairs,*[22] the plaintiff, Smith, was first diagnosed as having schizophrenia in 1972. He had been admitted to the VA hospital psychiatric ward 15 times since 1972. His admissions grew longer and more frequent as time passed. On the occasion of his March 17, 1990, admission, he had been drinking in a bar, got into a fight, and was eventually taken to the VA hospital. Dr. Rizk was assigned as Smith's attending physician. Smith developed an acute problem with his respiration and level of consciousness. It was determined that his psychiatric medications were responsible for his condition. Some medications were discontinued and others reduced. An improvement in his condition was noted.

By March 23, Smith began to complain of pain in his shoulders and neck. He attributed the pain to more than 20 years of service as a letter carrier and to osteoarthritis. His medical record indicated that he had similar complaints in the past. A rheumatology consultation was requested and carried out on March 29. The rheumatology resident conducted an examination and noted that Smith reported bilateral shoulder pain increasing with activity as an ongoing problem since 1979. Various tests were ordered, including an erythrocyte sedimentation rate (ESR).

Smith was incontinent and complained of shoulder pain. By the afternoon, he was out of restraints, walked to the shower, and bathed himself. On returning to his room, he claimed that he could not get into bed. He was given a pillow and slept on the floor. By the morning of April 4, Smith was lying on the floor in urine and complaining of numbness. His failure to move was attributed to his psychosis. By evening it was noted that Smith could not lift himself and would not use his hands.

On April 5, a medical student noted that Smith was having difficulty breathing and called for a pulmonary consultation. By evening Smith was either unwilling or unable to grasp a nurse's hand and continued to complain that his legs would not hold him up.

On the morning of April 6, Smith was complaining that his neck and back hurt and that he had no feeling in his legs and feet. Later that day a medical student noted that the results of Smith's ESR was 110 (more than twice the normal rate for a man his age). His white blood count was 18.1, also well above the normal rate. A staff member noted on the medical record that Smith had been unable to move his extremities for about five days. A psychiatric resident noted that Smith had been incontinent for three days and had a fever of 101.1 degrees.

On the morning of April 7, Smith was taken to University Hospital for magnetic resonance imaging of his neck. Imaging revealed a mass subsequently identified as a spinal epidural abscess. By the time it was excised, it had been pressing on his spinal cord too long for any spinal function to remain below vertebrae four and five.

The plaintiff brought suit alleging that the physicians' failure to promptly review his test results was the proximate cause of his paralysis. Following a bench trial, the U.S. District Court agreed, holding that the negligent failure of physicians to promptly review laboratory test results was the proximate cause of the plaintiff's quadriplegia.

Of primary importance was the plaintiff's ESR of 110; the test results were available on the patient care unit by April 2 but were not seen, or at least not noted in the record, until April 6. Although witnesses for both sides disagree, there was little disagreement as to the nature and importance of this test. An elevated ESR generally accounts for one of three problems: infection, cancer, or a connective tissue disorder. Most experts agreed that at the very least a repeat ESR should have been ordered. The VA's care of the plaintiff fell below the reasonable standard of care in that no one read the laboratory results until April 6. The fact that the tests were ordered mandates the immediate review of the results. Although it cannot be known with certainty what would have occurred had the ESR been read and acted upon on April 2, it is certain that the plaintiff had a chance to fully recover from his infection. By April 6, that chance was gone.

In the absence of notes from Rizk in the plaintiff's chart, it is impossible to know whether Rizk was aware of the plaintiff's symptoms. However, it appears that the absence of notes by Rizk indicated Rizk's care of the plaintiff was negligent, and the failure to review the results of the plaintiff's ESR constituted negligence under the relevant standard of care. That led to the failure to make an early diagnosis of the plaintiff's epidural abscess and was the proximate cause of the patient's eventual paralysis. Given that a high ESR can manifest in a very serious illness, it was foreseeable that ignoring a high ESR could lead to serious injury.

A mechanism should be in place to expeditiously notify the patient's physician of abnormal test results (e.g., panic values from laboratory tests). Many hospitals use computer systems to help ensure that physicians are notified of critical data so that appropriate care decisions can be implemented.

EFFICACY OF TEST QUESTIONED

A medical malpractice action was brought against Mambu in *Sacks v. Mambu*[23] for failure to make a timely diagnosis of Sack's colon cancer. It was alleged that Mambu was negligent in that he failed to properly screen Sacks for fecal occult blood to determine whether there was blood in the colon.

Because of complaints of fatigue by the patient, Mambu ordered blood tests that revealed a normal hemoglobin, the results of which suggested that Sacks had not been losing blood. However, by late July 1984, Sacks experienced symptoms of jaundice. Mambu ordered an ultrasound test, and Sacks was subsequently diagnosed with a tumor of the liver. He was admitted to the hospital and diagnosed with having colon cancer. By the time the cancer was detected, it had invaded the wall of the bowel and had metastasized to the liver. Sacks died in March 1985. The trial court entered judgment on a jury verdict for Mambu and the plaintiff appealed.

The Pennsylvania Superior Court upheld the decision of the trial court. The jury determined that the physician's failure to administer the test had not increased the risk of harm by allowing the cancer to metastasize to the liver before discovery and, therefore, was not a substantial factor in causing the patient's death. Although the presence of blood in the stool may be suggestive of polyps, cancer, and a variety of other diseases, not all polyps and cancers bleed. Physicians are therefore in disagreement as to the efficacy of the test.

IMAGING STUDIES/RADIOLOGY

Misdiagnosis in general, and especially misdiagnosis related to medical imaging, represents a significant segment of malpractice litigation. Malpractice lawsuits generally involve allegations of misdiagnosis and can often be the result of the failure to order appropriate imaging tests; misinterpretation of an imaging study; failure to consult with a radiologist; failure to review imaging studies; delay in relaying test results; and failure to relay imaging results. Although the following cases describe many of these issues, they are not exhaustive of the problems that can arise in imaging-related lawsuits.

Failure to Order Appropriate X-Rays

The failure to order a proper set of X-rays is as legally risky as the failure to order X-rays. In *Betenbaugh v. Princeton Hospital,*[24] the plaintiff had been taken to the hospital because she injured the lower part of her back. One of the defendant physicians directed that an X-ray be taken of her sacrum. No evidence of a fracture was found. When the patient's pain did not subside, the family physician was consulted. He found that the films taken at the hospital did not include the entire lower portion of the spine and sent her to a radiologist for further study. On the basis of additional X-rays, a diagnosis of a fracture was made, and the patient was advised to wear a lumbosacral support. Two months later, the fracture was healed. The radiologist who had taken X-ray films on the second occasion testified that it was customary to take both an anterior-posterior and a lateral view when making an X-ray examination of the sacrum. In his opinion, the failure at the hospital to include the lower area of the sacrum was a failure to meet the standard required. The family physician testified that if the patient's fracture had been diagnosed at the hospital, then appropriate treatment could have been instituted earlier, and thus the patient would have suffered less pain and recovery time would have been reduced. The evidence was sufficient to support findings that the physicians and the hospital were negligent by not having taken adequate X-rays and that such negligence was the proximate cause of the patient's additional pain and delay in recovery.

X-Ray Misinterpretation Leads to Death

The deceased, Jane Fahr, in *Setterington v. Pontiac General Hospital,*[25] was concerned about a lump in her thigh. She had a CT scan taken at Pontiac General Hospital in August 1987. The radiologist, Dr. Mittner, did not mention that the lump could be cancerous. In reliance on the radiologist's report, Dr. Sanford, the plaintiff's treating physician, regarded the condition as a hematoma and believed that a biopsy was not warranted. In late January 1988, Fahr returned to Pontiac General Hospital for another CT scan because the lump seemed to be enlarging. The radiologist, Dr. Khalid, did not include the possibility of a malignant tumor in his report. As a result, Sanford continued to believe that Fahr had a hematoma. In early September 1988, Fahr returned to Sanford, who had another CT scan performed. Dr. Kayne, the radiologist, found an enlarged hematoma. In a follow-up discussion with Sanford, Kayne assured Sanford that the lump did not appear to be dangerous or invasive. As a result, Sanford concluded that Fahr had a hematoma with a leaking blood vessel. In October 1988, the tumor was biopsied and the cancer diagnosed. By December 1988, chest scans revealed metastasis. Fahr died on July 6, 1990, at the age of 32. Setterington, Fahr's personal representative, brought a malpractice action against Sanford and Pontiac General Hospital, alleging that they failed to timely diagnose and treat Fahr.

The jury found that the radiologists were agents of defendant Pontiac General Hospital and breached the standard of care. The jury also concluded that the breach was a proximate cause of Fahr's death. The jury returned a verdict for the plaintiff in the amount of just over $251,000. The trial court denied the plaintiff's motion for a new trial as to damages, as well as the defendant's motion for a new trial.

The court found that the evidence as to the malpractice of Khalid and Kayne supported the jury's finding that they were professionally negligent. Kayne failed to diagnose the cancer in September 1988. With a proper diagnosis, there could have been a full month or more of treatment before metastasis was visible in December. As to Khalid, whose malpractice was seven months earlier, the conclusion is even stronger.

The hospital provided the plaintiff with the radiologists. The evidence supports the jury's finding that an agency relationship existed between the radiologists and the hospital. Fahr did not have a patient-physician relationship with the radiologists independent of the hospital setting. Rather, the radiologists just happened to be on duty when Fahr arrived at the hospital. Moreover, the evidence showed that the radiology department is held out as part of the hospital, leading patients to understand that the services are being rendered by the hospital.

Failure to Consult with a Radiologist

The internist in *Lanzet v. Greenberg*[26] failed to consult with the radiologist after his conclusion that the patient suffered from congestive heart failure. This factor most likely contributed to the death of the patient while on the operating table.

Failure to Read X-Rays

The patient in *Tams v. Lotz*[27] had to undergo a second surgical procedure to remove a laparotomy pad that had been left in the patient during a previous surgical procedure. The trial court was found to have properly directed a verdict with respect to the patient's assertion that the surgeon who performed the first operation failed to read a postoperative X-ray report, which allegedly would have put him on notice both that the pad was present and that there was a need for emergency surgery to remove the pad, therefore averting the need to remove a portion of his intestine.

Delay in Conveying X-Ray Report

On April 20, 1995, Mr. Carrasco[28] was taken to the Tri City Community Hospital (Tri City) emergency department by ambulance, complaining of back pain. He was admitted for observation, then released on April 21. On April 22, Carrasco returned to Tri City complaining of continued back pain and the inability to stand. A chest X-ray taken on April 22 revealed a significantly widened mediastinum and an increase in the size of the cardiac silhouette. On April 24, a radiologist reported that the X-ray revealed that in the setting of back pain, consideration should be given for aortic dissection.

Sometime on April 24, Carrasco's condition deteriorated, and he was air lifted to Methodist Hospital in San Antonio. A CT scan revealed an aneurysm of the thoracic aorta. Carrasco underwent emergency surgery, and the surgeons found a ruptured aneurysm of the thoracic aorta. The following day, Carrasco suffered another pericardial effusion, had emergency surgery, coded, and died.

Tri City and the emergency department physician were sued. Tri City filed a motion for summary judgment, asserting that the plaintiffs failed to show it breached the standard of care owed to the patient. The trial court granted summary judgment on this ground.

In its motion for summary judgment, Tri City asserted that the plaintiffs failed to produce evidence of any actions causing Carrasco's death. The plaintiffs-appellants filed a response to two affidavits that were attached to the medical records from Tri City.

The affidavits of Dr. Youmans asserted that Carrasco's chance for survival would have been significantly better if the aneurysm was operated on an elective basis as opposed to a postrupture emergent basis. Although the X-ray report was not dictated until April 24, Tri City had the responsibility of seeing to it that the findings of the grossly abnormal chest X-rays were conveyed to the attending physician on an emergent basis.

Tri City stated that the affidavits did not suggest that the failure to properly diagnose the patient was the result of some failure to convey X-ray findings to the attending physician or that the physician would have made the correct diagnosis with the information.

The X-ray report stated that in the setting of back pain, consideration should be given for aortic dissection. Because the diagnosis that led to Carrasco's surgery was an aneurysm of the thoracic aorta, this is evidence that the X-ray reading would have led the attending physician to a correct diagnosis. Tri City failed to convey the X-ray reading on the day of admission. Youmans stated that "the correct diagnosis apparently was not suspected until the time the patient coded on April 24." This statement links Tri City's failure to convey the X-ray information with the misdiagnosis. At the very least, the evidence rises to a level that would enable reasonable and fair-minded people to conclude that the absence of the X-ray report caused the improper diagnosis.

Because Carrasco's condition did not deteriorate until April 24, an inference can be made that the rupture occurred sometime on April 24. If the X-ray results had been relayed on April 22, the second admission to Tri City, the surgery could have been elective instead of emergent. Youmans' affidavit provided evidence that Tri City's failure to ensure that the X-ray reading was promptly relayed to the attending physician was a proximate cause of the patient's death. The trial court's judgment was reversed, and the cause was remanded for trial.

Failure to Communicate X-Ray Results

The court of appeals in *Washington Healthcare Corp. v. Barrow*[29] held that evidence was sufficient to sustain a finding that the hospital was negligent in failing to provide a radiology report demonstrating pathology on patient Barrow's lung in a timely manner. An X-ray of the patient taken on April 4, 1982, disclosed a small nodular density in her right lung. Within a year, the cancerous nodule had grown to the size of a softball.

The most significant testimony at trial was that of Theresa James, a medical student who worked for Dr. Oweiss, the defendant, until April 23, 1982. James testified that her job entailed combing through Oweiss's mail and locating abnormal X-ray reports, which she then would bring to his attention. Emphasizing that she had come to know the patient personally, James said that she would have been upset if she had come across an abnormal report on the patient. James claimed that she received no such report while working for the physician, thus accounting for 19 days after the X-ray was taken. James stated that the X-ray reports were usually received within four or five days after being taken. Dr. Odenwald, who dictated the patient's report on April 4, 1982, gave testimony to corroborate her testimony. Odenwald, of Groover, Christie and Merritt, PC (GCM), who operated the radiology department at the Washington Hospital Center (WHC), stated that the X-ray reports usually were typed and mailed the same day that they were dictated. The jury could have determined that if the report did not reach Oweiss by April 23, 1982, then it did not reach him by May 3, 1982. The patient's record eventually was found; however, it was not in the patient's regular folder. One could infer that the record therefore was negligently filed.

Questions also arise as to why Oweiss did nothing to follow up on the matter in ensuing months. Oweiss testified that he did receive the report by May 3, 1982, and that he informed Mrs. Barrow of its contents. Barrow stated that although her folder was on the physician's desk at the time of her visit, he did not relay to her any information regarding an abnormal X-ray. Oweiss, however, was severely impeached at trial, and the jury chose not to believe him. Considering the entire record, there was reasonable probability that WHC was negligent and that Oweiss had not received the report. The plaintiff settled with Oweiss, the patient's personal physician, in the amount of $200,000 during pendency in the district court, and the action against him was dismissed with prejudice. The record did not support WHC's request of indemnification from Oweiss. The trial court directed a verdict in favor of GCM, leaving WHC as the sole defendant. The court of appeals remanded WHC's cross-claim for indemnification from GCM for further findings of fact and conclusions by the trial court.

FAILURE TO OBTAIN SECOND OPINION

Dr. Goodwich, an obstetrician and gynecologist, in *Goodwich v. Sinai Hospital,*[30] had clinical practice patterns that were subject to question by his peers on a wide variety of medical matters. Dr. Goldstein (chairman of the department of obstetrics and gynecology) met with him on several occasions in 1988 regarding those concerns. It was suggested to Goodwich that he obtain second opinions from board-certified OB/GYNs; he orally agreed to do so. This agreement was presented to Goodwich in writing on two

occasions in 1988. Goodwich failed to comply with the agreement, and Goldstein held a second meeting with him and his attorney in February 1990. Due to continued noncompliance, Goldstein asked the director of quality, risk, and utilization management to determine how often Goodwich failed to obtain a second opinion. The investigation uncovered several instances of noncompliance. Goldstein then met with Goodwich for a third time. Goodwich agreed that he would obtain a second opinion in high-risk obstetrical cases. Goldstein confirmed the agreement in writing on April 23, 1992.

Goldstein left the hospital in June 1992, and Dr. Taylor was appointed acting chief of obstetrics and gynecology. He asked for a recheck of Goodwich's compliance with the second-opinion agreement. By January, the hospital appointed Dr. Currie as the chief of obstetrics and gynecology. Because of Goodwich's continuing failure to obtain second opinions, Currie informed Goodwich in writing that pursuant to Article IV, Sec. 7C of the bylaws, rules, and regulations of the hospital's medical staff, his privileges were temporarily abridged. The letter also advised Goodwich that the MEC would consider a permanent abridgment of his privileges. The MEC met and abridged Goodwich's privileges for three months. The abridgement of Goodwich's privileges was reported to the Maryland State Board of Physician Quality Assurance and the National Practitioner Data Bank.

Goodwich appealed the MEC decision to two different physician panels and the hospital's governing board. Both physician panels and the governing board affirmed the MEC's decision to abridge Goodwich's privileges. Goodwich then sued the hospital for breach of contract, intentional interference with contractual relations, and tortious interference with prospective economic benefit after restrictions were placed on his practice privileges at the hospital. The circuit court entered summary judgment for the hospital on the grounds of statutory immunity. Goodwich appealed, and the court of special appeals held that the hospital acted reasonably, as required for immunity under the federal Health Care Quality Improvement Act of 1986. The record was replete with documentation of questionable patient management and continual failure to comply with second-opinion agreements.

FAILURE TO REFER

A physician has a duty to refer his or her patient whom he or she knows or should know needs referral to a physician familiar with and clinically capable of treating the patient's ailments. To recover damages, the plaintiff must show that the physician deviated from the standard of care and that the failure to refer resulted in injury.

The California Court of Appeals found that expert testimony is not necessary where good medical practice would require a general physician to suggest a specialist's consultation.[31] The court ruled that because specialists were called in after the patient's condition grew worse, it is reasonable to assume that they could have been called in sooner. The jury was instructed by the court that a general practitioner has a duty to suggest calling in a specialist if a reasonably prudent general practitioner would do so under similar circumstances.

A physician is in a position of trust, and it is his or her duty to act in good faith. If a preferred treatment in a given situation is outside a physician's field of expertise, it is his or her duty to advise the patient. Failure to do so could constitute a breach of duty. Today, with the rapid methods of transportation and easy means of communication, the duty of a physician is not fulfilled merely by using the means at hand in a particular area of practice.

In *Doan v. Griffith*,[32] an accident victim was admitted to the hospital with serious injuries, including multiple fractures of his facial bones. The patient contended that the physician was negligent in not advising him at the time of discharge that his facial bones needed to be realigned by a specialist before the bones became fused. As a result, his face became disfigured. Expert testimony demonstrated that the customary medical treatment for the patient's injuries would have been to realign his fractured bones surgically as soon as the swelling subsided and that such treatment would have restored the normal contour of his face. The appellate court held that the jury reasonably could have found that the physician failed to provide timely advice to the patient regarding his need for further medical treatment, and that such failure was the proximate cause of the patient's condition.

The convalescent home resident in *Stogsdill v. Manor Convalescent Home, Inc.*[33] brought an action against the physician, the home, and a coowner of the home for damages suffered when her leg was amputated as a proximate result of allegedly deficient medical and convalescent care. The resident had developed a decubitus ulcer on her left ankle, and gangrene developed sometime before November 7, 1972. Testimony by one of the nurses at the nursing facility stated that she noticed gangrene in August or September. The treating physician, Dr. Hiatt, prescribed certain medications but did not prescribe any antibiotics until November 6, 1972, at which time he prescribed Terramycin. Wet soaks, laboratory tests, and vascular studies also were not ordered. The treating physician did not request hospitalization or seek consultation from another physician. On November 7, 1972, the resident's son called another physician to see his mother. He diagnosed the resident's condition as a wet gangrene involving the entire outer surface of the ankle. The resident was taken to the hospital the same day. At the hospital, an orthopedic surgeon recommended amputation. After building up the patient for surgery with the use of intravenous fluids and feedings, her leg was amputated on November 10, 1972. Dr. Loutfy, a specialist in internal medicine, in response to a hypothetical question, was of the opinion, based on a reasonable degree of medical and surgical certainty, that with proper care and treatment the leg could have been saved. The defendant presented no witnesses at trial.

The trial court directed a verdict for the home and coowner, and it assessed damages against the physician in the amount of $40,000 for general damages and $80,000 for punitive damages. The defendant appealed. The appellate court affirmed the directed verdict for the home and coowner. Testimony was found sufficient to establish that the loss of the leg was proximately caused by Hiatt's negligence.

A directed verdict for the defendants in *Vito v. North Medical Family Physicians, P.C.*,[34] following the plaintiff's proof was found to be in error in an action alleging that the defendants were negligent in various aspects of their treatment of the plaintiff's lower back injury. The plaintiff established through expert testimony that the defendant physician failed to refer him to a specialist from 1996 to 2000 and that such failure was a departure from good medical practice and that the longer a herniation existed, the worse the prognosis. There is a rational process by which the jury could have found that Dr. Bonavita was negligent in failing to refer the plaintiff to a specialist to determine the cause of his pain. The physician allegedly failed to keep proper business records and continued to prescribe OxyContin to the plaintiff, and that negligence caused plaintiff's damages. The court denied the defendants' motion for a directed verdict, reinstated the complaint, and granted a new trial before a different justice.

PRACTICING OUTSIDE FIELD OF COMPETENCY

A physician should practice discretion when treating a patient outside his or her field of expertise or competence. The standard of care required in a malpractice case will be that of the specialty in which a physician is treating, whether or not he or she has been credentialed in that specialty.

In a California case, *Carrasco v. Bankoff*,[35] a small boy suffering third-degree burns over 18 percent of his body was admitted to a hospital. During his initial confinement, there was little done except to occasionally dress and redress the burned area. At the end of a 53-day confinement, the patient was suffering hypergranulation of the burned area and muscular-skeletal dysfunction. The surgeon treating him was not a board-certified plastic surgeon and apparently not properly trained in the management of burn cases. At trial, the patient's medical expert, a plastic surgeon who assumed responsibility for care after the first hospitalization, outlined the accepted medical practice in cases of this nature. The first surgeon acknowledged this accepted practice. The court held that there was substantial evidence to permit a finding of professional negligence because of the defendant surgeon's failure to perform to the accepted standard of care and that such failure resulted in the patient's injury.

TIMELY DIAGNOSIS

A physician can be liable for reducing a patient's chances for survival. The timely diagnosis of a patient's condition is as important as the need to accurately diagnose a patient's injury or disease. Failure to do so can constitute malpractice if a patient suffers injury as a result of such failure.

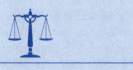

WRONGFUL DEATH

Citation: *Powell v. Margileth*, 524 S.E.2d 434 (Va. 2000)

Facts

On January 9, 1992, Dr. Massey, a specialist in otolaryngology, measured a node in Mr. Powell's neck as 4 cm × 3 cm and ordered a CT scan. The CT scan conducted January 11, 1992, indicated that the size of the left cervical mass was due to an enlarged internal jugular node, which most likely was an abscess. On January 14, 1992, Massey aspirated fluid from the enlarged node. Although he discussed the CT scan with Powell and ordered cultures, he did not suggest a need for an examination to rule out cancer. Because Powell told Massey that he had experienced some exposure to cats, Massey referred Powell to Dr. Margileth, an infectious disease specialist experienced in the diagnosis and treatment of cat scratch disease. On January 27, 1992, Margileth performed tests for tuberculosis and cat scratch disease and measured the swelling in the left anterior superior neck. He advised Powell that he had cat scratch disease and prescribed antibiotics. The results of the CT scan had been furnished to Margileth.

On February 18, 1992, Massey palpitated the nodule in Powell's neck which measured 4 cm × 2.8 cm. Massey performed another examination on April 7, 1992, during the course of which he suggested the possibility of cancer.

In June 1992, Powell discovered a second lump in his neck and in July went for help to the VA Medical Center Hospital. A needle aspiration of the two lumps resulted in the diagnosis of cancer, representing a progression from stage III in January 1992 when the CT scan was conducted to stage IV in July 1992. Powell underwent radiation therapy, surgery, and other treatment but died of cancer three years later at the age of 40.

The trial court held that there was not sufficient evidence that would allow a jury of reasonable persons to conclude that the defendant's breach of the standard of care: (1) proximately caused Powell's injuries; (2) adversely altered the required method of treatment; or (3) adversely affected Powell's rate of survival.

Issue

Did the trial court err in granting the defendant's motion to strike the plaintiff's evidence?

Holding

The appeals court ruled that there was adequate evidence that would allow a jury of reasonable persons to conclude that the defendant's breach of the standard of care proximately caused the decedent's injuries. The case was remanded for a new trial.

Reason

Dr. Holder, one of the plaintiff's expert witnesses, testified that the defendant's misdiagnosis of cat scratch disease caused his patient delay in diagnosis and treatment of his cancer from January until July, and that if Powell had been informed of the possibility of cancer in January, and options were offered in terms of biopsy for fine needle aspirations, then Powell would have had a diagnosis of cancer probably the first week of February. Asked whether the delay was a direct and proximate cause of the failure of Margileth to comply with the required standard of care, Holder answered, "Yes, it was."

Dr. Ali, who had treated Powell, said he would have had approximately a 75 percent chance of surviving five years compared with the 15 to 20 percent chance he had in July 1992. Dr. Tercilla, a professor at the Medical College of Virginia testified that, in his opinion, if Powell had been treated in January as opposed to July, he would have had a higher likelihood of being in control of this disease than he had when he presented at the VA hospital. Dr. Kipreos, a pathologist at the VA center, stated that in her opinion, that if Margileth would have requested a fine needle aspiration in January 1992, Powell's cancer would have been diagnosed at that time.

Discussion

1. Discuss how the outcome in this case might have been different if Massey had referred his patient to, for example, a family practitioner.
2. Discuss the role of expert testimony in this case.

MISDIAGNOSIS

Misdiagnosis is the most frequently cited injury event in malpractice suits against physicians. Although diagnosis is a medical art and not an exact science, early detection can be critical to a patient's recovery. Misdiagnosis may involve the diagnosis and treatment of a disease different from that which the patient actually suffers, or the diagnosis and treatment of a disease that the patient does not have. Misdiagnosis in and of itself will not necessarily impose liability on a physician, unless deviation from the accepted standard of care and injury can be established.

Mitral Valve Malfunction

In *Lauderdale v. United States,*[36] the federal government was held liable under the Federal Tort Claims Act for the death of a patient whose mitral valve malfunction was misdiagnosed at a military medical clinic. Under applicable Alabama law, the physician failed to conduct the necessary tests to determine the cause of a suspected heart problem. The physician never indicated to the patient that the problem was severe, that the treatment with digoxin was tentative, and that his well-being mandated that he return in a week. The patient subsequently died. He was found not to have been contributorily negligent by failing to return to the clinic. The patient had not been told sufficiently of the urgency of a return visit. This failure was considered the proximate cause of the patient's death because his illness might have been treated successfully.

FAILURE TO FORM A DIFFERENTIAL DIAGNOSIS

Citation: *Corley v. State Department of Health & Hospitals,* 749 So. 2d 926 (La. App. 1999)

Facts

Corley began experiencing low back pain on February 11, 1988. He sought medical treatment from Dr. Gremillion. Corley complained that he had been experiencing low back pain and abdominal discomfort for approximately four months. At Corley's request, Gremillion ordered X-rays of the lower spine, chest, kidneys, and gallbladder, as well as an upper GI series. Gremillion, feeling that a specialist should see Corley, then gave him a written referral to a medical center for an orthopedic evaluation.

On March 2, 1988, Corley went to the medical center's emergency department with his wife. The Corleys presented admitting personnel with Corley's records from Gremillion, including X-rays and other test reports. Dr. Fuller, an emergency department physician, took a history from Corley and reviewed Gremillion's notes and the X-ray reports. He also conducted a routine physical examination and had X-rays made of Corley's lower back. Fuller's impression was that Corley was suffering from low back pain. Fuller continued Corley on the medication prescribed by Gremillion and made an appointment for him with the orthopedic clinic on March 16, 1988.

On that date, a fourth-year resident, Dr. Bridges, saw Corley in the orthopedic clinic. Bridges conducted a physical exam, which was normal, and started Corley on a conservative course of treatment for low back pain.

Dr. Mehta next saw Corley on April 20, 1988. Mehta's notes reflect that his physical exam of Corley was normal, but that he felt that Corley had a posture problem and referred him to physical therapy for correction of his posture. The notes do not reflect whether Mehta reviewed any of Corley's previous medical records, X-rays, or reports.

On September 14, 1988, Corley was seen by a fourth-year surgical resident, Dr. White, who, during the course of the examination, ordered a CT scan of Corley's low back. Dr. Ellis, a radiologist at the medical center, interpreted the CT scan as showing arthritis consistent with fibrosis or spinal stenosis and possible edema of the right L-5 nerve root, which, according to White, may or may not have been the cause of Corley's back pain. White did not review any of the previous medical records, X-rays, or reports. Corley's last visit to the medical center was September 21, 1988. On that date, White reviewed the results of the CT scan with Corley, continued him on an anti-inflammatory drug, and encouraged him to continue his back exercises.

On October 26, 1988, Corley, plagued by constant back pain and beginning to experience difficulty breathing, consulted Dr. Maxwell, a chiropractor, who did a full spinal X-ray that revealed a markedly diminished right lung area. Maxwell sent Corley to his father, also a chiropractor, who confirmed that there was a potential problem with Corley's right lung and recommended that he see a pulmonary specialist.

On October 31, 1988, Corley presented to Gremillion complaining of chest congestion and shortness of breath. Gremillion diagnosed him with bronchitis and implemented treatment. Corley returned to Gremillion on November 14, 1988, with complaints of shortness of breath and marked weight loss. Subsequent diagnostic testing confirmed the presence of a very large mass (cancer) in Corley's right chest. Prior to his death on January 23, 1990, Corley received radiation and chemotherapy treatment.

Corley's surviving spouse and son instituted a malpractice action seeking wrongful death and survival damages. The trial court rendered judgment in favor of the plaintiffs and against the medical center in the amount of $400,000. The defendants, the state, and medical center appealed.

Issue

The primary issue on appeal is whether the trial court committed error in finding that the physicians at the medical center deviated from the applicable standard of care by failing to properly diagnose Corley's condition, a large cancerous mass in his mediastinum, during the course of their treatment of his low back pain.

Finding

The physicians at the medical center fell below the standard of care when they failed to properly diagnose Corley's condition.

Reason

The evidence was in Gremillion's X-rays and medical report when Corley first arrived at the medical center. Simply put, these physicians failed to see what they should have seen. When Corley did not respond to conservative treatment, there had to be another explanation for his low back pain. The physicians ignored this and did not expand their inquiry, which they should have done under a differential diagnosis assessment. For this, Corley was deprived of a significant chance of survival. A physician is required to take a "thorough" history based upon a patient's presenting signs and symptoms. If the findings from the medical history and physical exam support a diagnosis, one should be made and treatment instituted. When, in treating a patient, a diagnosis cannot be made, at that time a differential diagnosis should be made, which includes all reasonable, plausible, and foreseeable causes for the signs and symptoms noted in the patient. After forming a differential diagnosis, it is the physician's duty to rule out all imminent, serious, and life-threatening causes for the signs and symptoms. Failure to eliminate these causes can subject a patient to a foreseeable risk of harm and would further constitute a breach of the applicable standards of care.

Discussion

1. Why is it important to be able to make differential diagnoses?
2. Why did the appellate court find that the trial court had not erred in finding that the physicians deviated from the applicable standard of care in their diagnosis and treatment of Corley?

Appendicitis

Misdiagnosis does not always end in a verdict for the plaintiff. Summary judgment was properly entered in dismissing an action alleging that a physician had been negligent in failing to diagnose a pregnant patient's appendicitis in *Fiedler v. Steger.*[37] The testimony of expert witnesses for both parties established that diagnosis of appendicitis during pregnancy is difficult, that it probably would not have been diagnosed on the dates in question, and that the appendix had probably ruptured postpartum.

Diabetic Acidosis

A case before the Mississippi Supreme Court, *Hill v. Stewart,*[38] involved a patient who became ill and was admitted to the hospital. The physician was advised of the patient's recent weight loss, frequent urination, thirst, loss of vision, nausea, and vomiting. Routine laboratory tests were ordered including a urinalysis, but not a blood glucose test. On the following day, a consultant diagnosed the patient's condition as severe diabetic acidosis. Treatment was given, but the patient failed to respond to the therapy and died. The attending physician was sued for failing to test for diabetes and for failing to diagnose and treat the patient on the first day in the hospital. The attending physician said in court that he suspected diabetes and admitted that when diabetes is suspected, a urinalysis and a blood sugar test should be performed. An expert medical witness testified that failure to do so would be a departure from the skill and care required of a general practitioner. The expert also stated that the patient in this case probably would have had a good chance of survival if treated properly. The state supreme court reversed the directed verdict for the physician by a lower court and remanded the case for retrial. There was sufficient evidence presented to permit the case to go to the jury for decision.

Once a physician concludes that a particular test is indicated, it should be performed and evaluated as soon as practicable. Delay may constitute negligence. The law imposes on a physician the same degree of responsibility in making a diagnosis as it does in prescribing and administering treatment.

FAILURE TO READ NURSING NOTES

A physician can breach his or her duty of care by failing to read nursing notes. In *Todd v. Sauls,*[39] Mr. Todd was admitted to Rapides General Hospital on October 3, 1988, and the next day, Dr. Sauls performed bypass surgery. Postoperatively, Todd sustained a heart attack. During the following days, Todd did not ambulate well and suffered a weight loss of 19½ pounds.

On October 17, the medical record indicated that Todd's sternotomy wound and the mid-lower left leg incision were reddened, and his temperature was 99.6. Sauls did not commonly read the nurses' notes but instead preferred to rely on his own observations of the patient. In his October 18 notes, he indicated that there was no drainage. The nurses' notes, however, show that there was drainage at the chest tube site. Contrary to the medical records showing that Todd had a temperature of 101.2 degrees, Sauls noted that the patient was afebrile.

On October 19, Sauls noted that Todd's wounds were improving and he did not have a fever. Nurses' notes indicated redness at the surgical wounds and a temperature of 100 degrees. No white blood count had been ordered. Again on October 20, the nurses' notes indicated a wound redness and a temperature of 100.8 degrees. No wound culture had yet been ordered. Dr. Kamil, one of Todd's treating physicians, noted that Todd's nutritional status needed to be seriously confronted and suggested that Sauls consider supplemental feeding. Despite this, no follow-up to his recommendation appears and the record is void of any action by Dr. Sauls to obtain a nutritional consult.

Todd was transferred to the intensive care unit on October 21 because he was gravely ill with profoundly depressed ventricular function. The nurses' notes for the following day describe the chest tube site as draining foul-smelling bloody purulence. The patient's temperature was recorded to have reached 100.6 degrees. This is the first time that Sauls had the test tube site cultured. On October 23, the culture report from the laboratory indicated a staph infection, and Todd was started on antibiotics for treatment of the infection.

On October 25, at the request of family, Todd was transferred to St. Luke's Hospital. At St. Luke's, Dr. Leatherman, an internist and invasive cardiologist, treated Todd. Dr. Zeluff, an infectious disease specialist, examined Todd's surgical wounds and prescribed antibiotic treatment. Upon admission to St. Luke's, every one of Todd's surgical wounds was infected. Despite the care given at St. Luke's, Todd died on November 2, 1988. The family brought a malpractice suit against the surgeon. The district court entered judgment on a jury verdict for the defendant, and the plaintiff appealed claiming the surgeon breached his duty of care owed to the patient by failing to: (1) aggressively treat the surgical wound infections; (2) read the nurses' observations of infections; and (3) provide adequate nourishment, allowing the patient's body weight to rapidly waste away.

The Louisiana Court of Appeal held that Sauls committed medical malpractice when he breached the standard of care he owed to Todd. He was effectively ineligible for a heart transplant, which was his only chance of survival due to the infections and malnourishment caused by Sauls' malpractice. Sauls' testimony convinced the court that he failed to aggressively treat the surgical wound infections, that he chose not to take advantage of the nurses' observations of infection, and that he allowed Todd's body weight to waste away, knowing that extreme vigilance was required because of Todd's already severely impaired heart. The awards of $4,975 for funeral expenses, $19,533.42 for medical expenses, $150,000 for Mrs. Todd, and $50,000 to each of his seven children for loss of love and affection were determined by the court to be appropriate.

In cases where a patient has died, the plaintiff need not demonstrate that the patient would have survived if properly treated. Rather, he or she need only prove that the patient had a chance of survival and that the chance of survival was lost as a result of the defendant/physician's negligence. The defendant/physician's conduct must increase the risk of a patient's harm to the extent of being a substantial factor in causing the result but need not be the only cause. Sauls's medical malpractice exacerbated an already critical condition and deprived Mr. Todd of a chance of survival.

Leatherman stated that it was the responsibility of the surgeon and cardiologist to pay closer attention to Todd's nutritional status and to have better managed his weight. He emphasized that wounds cannot heal when a patient is malnourished. Leatherman opined that Sauls deviated from the required standard of care he owed to Todd.

Zeluff stated that impaired nutritional status depresses the body's immune system and adversely affects the body's ability to heal wounds. In response to a hypothetical fact situation based on Todd's medical records at Rapides General, Zeluff opined that Sauls further deviated from the standard of care in failing to initiate parenteral or enteral nutrition by at least October 20.

Dr. Pipkin, an expert cardiac surgeon, corroborated the testimony of Leatherman and Zeluff on the negative effect that malnourishment has on the healing process and the body's ability to fight infection. Pipkin stated that it was Sauls' responsibility to make certain that Todd received adequate calories and proteins. After reviewing the records of Todd, Pipkin found that there was a general wasting of Todd in the postoperative period as evidenced by his steady loss of weight. Pipkin opined that Sauls deviated from the standard of care owed to Todd both with regard to wound infections and malnourishment.

MEDICATION ERRORS

Thousands of brand and generic drugs in use have led to an increase in medication errors. Such errors are a leading cause of patient injuries. Physicians should encourage the limited and judicious use of all medications and periodically document the reason for their continuation. They should be alert to any contraindications and incompatibilities between prescription, over-the-counter drugs, and herbal supplements.

The negligent administration of medications is often due to errors, such as the wrong medication, the wrong patient, the wrong dosage, and the wrong route.

Wrong Dosage

Expert testimony in *Leal v. Simon,*[40] a medical malpractice action, supported the jury's determination that the physician had been negligent when he reduced the dosage of a resident's psychotropic medication, Haldol. The resident, a 36-year-old individual who had been institutionalized his entire life, was a resident in an intermediate care facility. The drug was used for controlling the resident's self-abusive behavior. Expert medical testimony showed that the physician failed to familiarize himself with the resident's history, failed to secure the resident's complete medical records, and failed to wean the resident slowly off the medication.

Abuse in Prescribing Medications

The board of regents in *Moyo v. Ambach*[41] determined that a physician prescribed methaqualone fraudulently and with gross negligence to 20 patients. The board of regents found that the physician did not prescribe methaqualone in good faith or for sound medical reasons. His abuse in prescribing controlled substances constituted the fraudulent practice of medicine. Expert testimony established that it was common knowledge in the medical community that methaqualone was a widely abused and addictive drug. Methaqualone should not have been used for insomnia without first trying other means of treatment. On appeal, the court found that there was sufficient evidence to support the board's finding.

Medications Aggravate Preexisting Condition

Damages were awarded in *Argus v. Scheppegrell*[42] for the wrongful death of a teenage patient with a preexisting drug addiction. It was determined that the physician wrongfully supplied the patient with prescriptions for controlled substances in excessive amounts, with the result that the patient's preexisting drug addiction worsened, causing her death from a drug overdose. The Louisiana Court of Appeal held that the suffering of the patient caused by drug addiction and deterioration of her mental and physical condition warranted an award of $175,000. Damages of $120,000 were to be awarded for the wrongful death claims of the parents, who not only suffered during their daughter's drug addiction caused by the physician in wrongfully supplying the prescription, but who also were forced to endure the torment of their daughter's slow death in the hospital.

FAILURE TO FOLLOW DIFFERENT COURSE OF TREATMENT

Failure of an attending physician to recognize recommendations by consulting physicians—who determine a different diagnosis and recommend a different course of treatment in a particular case—can result in liability for damages suffered by the patient. This was the case in *Martin v. East Jefferson General Hospital*[43] in which the attending physician continued to treat the patient for a viral infection despite three other physicians' diagnoses of lupus and their recommendations that the attending physician treat the patient for collagen vascular disease. The trial court found that lupus had been more probable than not the cause of the patient's death and that her chances of recovery had been destroyed by the physician's failure to rule out that diagnosis. Damages totaling $150,000 were awarded to the plaintiff.

If a consulting physician has suggested a diagnosis with which the treating physician does not agree, it would be prudent to consider obtaining the opinion of a second consultant who could either confirm or disprove the first consultant's theory. Failure to diagnose and properly treat a suspected illness is an open door to liability.

FAILURE TO PROVIDE INFORMED CONSENT

The doctrine of informed consent is a theory of professional liability independent from malpractice. A physician's duty to disclose known dangers associated with a proposed course of treatment is imposed by law. The patient in *Leggett v. Kumar*[44] was awarded $675,000 for pain and disfigurement resulting from a mastectomy procedure. The physician in this case failed to advise the patient of treatment alternatives. He also failed to perform the surgery properly.

It is the physician's role to provide the necessary medical facts and the patient's role to make the subjective decision concerning treatment based on his or her understanding of those facts. Before subjecting a patient to a course of treatment, the physician has a duty to disclose information that will enable the patient to evaluate options available and the risks attendant to a specific procedure. A failure to disclose any known and existing risks of proposed treatment when such risks might affect a patient's decision to forgo treatment constitutes a prima facie violation of a physician's duty to disclose. If a patient can establish that a physician withheld information concerning the inherent and potential hazards of a proposed treatment, consent is abrogated. Consent for a medical procedure may be withdrawn at any time before the act consented to is accomplished.

In *Gates v. Jensen,*[45] a lawsuit was brought against Dr. Hargiss, an ophthalmologist, and others for failure to disclose to Mrs. Gates that her test results for glaucoma were borderline and that her risk of glaucoma was increased considerably by her high blood pressure and myopia. Hargiss failed to perform a field vision test and to dilate and examine the eye. He wrote off the patient's problem of difficulty in focusing and gaps in vision as being related to difficulties with her contact lenses. Gates visited the clinic 12 times during the following two years with complaints of blurriness, gaps in her vision, and loss of visual acuity. Gates eventually was diagnosed with glaucoma. By the time Gates was properly treated, her vision had deteriorated from almost 20/20 to 20/200. The court held that a duty of disclosure to a patient arises whenever a physician becomes aware of an abnormality that may indicate risk or danger. The facts that must be disclosed are those facts the physician knows, or should know that a patient needs to be aware of, to make an informed decision on the course of future medical care.

Once a physician concludes that a particular test is indicated, it should be performed and evaluated as soon as practicable. Delay may constitute negligence. The law imposes on a physician the same degree of responsibility in making a diagnosis as it does in prescribing and administering treatment.

SURGERY

The potential for negligence in the surgical setting seems to be the never-ending story, as illustrated in the cases described in this section. Wrong surgery, wrong site, wrong patient, foreign objects left in patients, and hidden mistakes all continue to be common occurrences.

The Phantom Surgeon

Here the list begins with the phantom surgeon. Watkins was referred to Dr. Eliachar, an attending surgeon, who diagnosed a deviated septum and advised that a surgical procedure be performed. When asked by the patient whether he would be performing the procedure, Eliachar testified that he would operate with the assistance of residents. On the morning of Watkins's surgery, Eliachar was scheduled to perform four elective surgeries in two adjoining operating rooms. The anesthesiologist was Dr. Popovich, who was also involved in more than one surgery at the time and, like Eliachar, moved between operating rooms during the patients' procedures. The nurse anesthetist, who assisted Popovich in Popovich's absence, was Woods. The chief resident of the ear, nose, and throat department, Dr. Guay, performed the surgery on Watkins. Eliachar, who was listed in the operative records and discharge summary as the performing surgeon, allegedly supervised Guay's work as he moved between the adjoining operating rooms.

Guay testified that he first met the patient on the day of the surgery in the preoperative holding area minutes before the patient was transported to the operating room. He also testified that Eliachar assigned the surgery to him and that Eliachar did not scrub up that morning. Guay, upon meeting the patient, told the patient that he would be operating on her with Eliachar. During the operation, which began at 7:30 A.M. and ended at 11:10 A.M., the patient was under a general anesthesia and was intubated by the nurse anesthetist. According to Eliachar, it was the surgeon's ultimate responsibility to ensure that the patient maintained an adequate airway during and after the operation—yet Eliachar could not recall whether he was present when the patient was extubated. He believed that the nurse anesthetist extubated the patient. Popovich was not present for the extubation and did not evaluate the patient between the operating room and the postanesthesia care unit (PACU). The nurse anesthetist stated that the patient was extubated at approximately 10:30 A.M. in the operating room and that he and Guay then transported the patient to PACU. On the way to the PACU at 10:35 A.M., the patient's heart rate was 85 beats per minute according to the records of nurse Woods—yet the nurse's notes from PACU indicate that at 10:35 A.M., when the patient was admitted to the PACU, her heart rate was 50 beats per minute. The nurse anesthetist's records also indicate that the patient was awake and responsive when he transported her to the PACU—yet the PACU records indicate that the patient was unresponsive, emitting a large amount of clear urine, and not moving. At 10:40 A.M., the nurse anesthetist's records indicate that the patient's heart rate was 78 to 80 beats per minute, while the PACU nurse's record states 30 beats per minute, a rate that is admittedly life threatening according to the nurse anesthetist. When the heart rate hit 30 beats per minute, the nurse anesthetist recalls, resuscitative measures were begun on the patient. The patient was given CPR and was reintubated at 10:50 A.M. The patient was left in a persistent vegetative state.[46]

The jury found for the plaintiffs on the fraud and battery. The evidence presented demonstrated Eliachar represented to Watkins that he would be operating on her. Watkins specifically asked Eliachar whether he would be performing the surgery. When making the representation to the patient, Eliachar knew that he was scheduled to perform simultaneous surgeries on that date; as the performing surgeon of record, he had the responsibility to monitor the patient throughout the entire operation, including the postoperative procedures on his patient. He admittedly knew the extubation parameters and would have prevented Watkins's premature extubation had he been the surgeon in the operating room at the time. Based on this evidence, the elements of fraud were demonstrated. The appeals court held that the trial court did not err in denying the motion for directed verdict on that issue.[47]

Wrong Surgical Procedure

In *Southwestern Kentucky Baptist Hospital v. Bruce,*[48] a patient admitted for conization of the cervix was taken mis-takenly to the operating room for a thyroidectomy. The physician was notified early during surgery that he had the wrong patient on the operating room table. The operation was terminated immediately. The thyroidectomy was not completed, and the incision was sutured. The patient filed an action for malpractice and recovered $10,000 from the physician and $90,000 from the hospital. That the patient mistakenly answered to the name of another patient who had been scheduled for a thyroidectomy did not excuse the failure of the surgeon, the anesthesiologist, and the surgical technician to determine the identity of the patient by examining her identification bracelet. The Kentucky Supreme Court held that the verdict was not excessive in view of the injuries, which consisted of a four-inch incision along the patient's neck, which became infected and required cosmetic surgery.

Correct Surgery–Wrong Site

The patient, in *Holdsworth v. Galler,*[49] had a two-centimeter cancerous tumor on the left side of his colon. Unfortunately, the surgeon erroneously performed right-sided colon surgery to remove the tumor. After the surgeon recognized the error, he performed the required left-sided abdominal surgery three days later. At the first surgery on the patient's right side, the surgeon removed the end of the patient's small intestine, his entire right colon, and the majority of his transverse colon; consequently, 40 to 45 percent of the colon was removed. Three days following the wrong-site surgery, the patient had to undergo left-sided surgery, after which he was left with approximately 20 percent of his colon. The patient developed complications and died six weeks thereafter.

Wrong Site: Surgery and Fraud

The physician-petitioner in *In re Muncan*[50] did not review either the patient's CT scan or MRI films prior to surgery. In addition, he did not have the films with him in the operating room on the day of surgery. Had he done so, he would have discovered that the CT scan report erroneously indicated that there was a mass in the patient's left kidney when in fact such mass was located in the patient's right kidney. During surgery, the physician did not observe any gross abnormalities or deformities in the left kidney and was unable to palpate any masses. Nonetheless, he removed the left kidney. The physician was later advised that he had removed a healthy kidney and that he may have removed the wrong kidney. The physician discharged the patient with a postoperative diagnosis of left renal mass, failing to note that he had in fact removed a tumor-free kidney. In September 1999, another CT scan revealed the presence of a six-centimeter by seven-centimeter mass in the patient's right kidney; the physician deemed this to be a new tumor that was not present on the CT scan conducted four months earlier. The diagnosis, however, appears highly suspect given the medical testimony that this new tumor was in the same location and had the same consistency and appearance as the tumor appearing in the prior CT study. The record also makes clear that it was highly unlikely that a tumor of this dimension could have achieved such size during the relatively brief period of time between the two CT studies.

A hearing committee of the state board for professional medical conduct sustained allegations that the physician practiced with gross negligence and negligence on more than one occasion. The committee suspended the physician's license to practice medicine for 48 months, stayed said suspension for 42 months, and placed the physician on probation. Upon appeal to the administrative review board for professional medical conduct (ARB), the ARB affirmed the committee's findings as to guilt and penalty and, further, sustained the specification alleging fraudulent practice. The physician commenced an action to annul that portion of the ARB's determination pertaining to the charge of fraudulent practice. The Supreme Court of New York, Appellate Division, Third Department held that the evidence was sufficient to support an inference of fraud. The physician knew he removed the wrong kidney and instead of taking steps to rectify the situation, intentionally concealed his mistake.

Foreign Objects Left in Patients

Physicians who change an organization's procedures governing surgical operations can be liable for those acts should they result in patient injury, even if they are performed by an organization's employees. In *Martin v. Perth Amboy General Hospital,*[51] a patient sued the hospital, cardiovascular surgeon, and nurses for leaving a laparotomy pad in his stomach. The surgeon, Dr. Lev, who performed the operation, was assisted by two other physicians as well as by a scrub nurse and a circulating nurse. Before the laparotomy pads were brought into the operating room, a strip of radiopaque material was embedded between the folds of the laparotomy pads that would show on an X-ray if a pad was left in the abdomen. Rings were attached to the laparotomy pads to prevent errors in counts made by the nurses; however, before the pads were used, the nurses, at the direction of the operating surgeon, removed the rings. The sponge count at the end of the operation indicated that no sponges were missing. Lev contended that the charge against him adopted the captain of the ship doctrine, which is not recognized by the state of New Jersey. If Lev had not ordered the rings to be removed by the nurses, the court would have agreed that the charge was contrary to state judicial decisions. By exercising control over the nurses to the extent of directing them to remove the rings and thus eliminating the safeguards provided by the hospital to ensure a proper count by its employees, the surgeon became the nurses' temporary or special employer with regard to their duties involving the laparotomy pads used during the operation. Thus, the surgeon was equally liable with the hospital for the nurses' subsequent negligence in counting the pads.

The most common methods of preventing operating room objects from being left in a surgical wound are

1. sponge and instrument counts

2. use of surgical sponges with radiopaque threads

3. use of X-rays for detecting foreign objects left in an operative wound

---

NEEDLE FRAGMENT LEFT IN PATIENT

Citation: *Williams v. Kilgore,* 618 So. 2d 51 (Miss. 1992)

Facts

On March 31, 1964, the patient-plaintiff was admitted to the medical center for treatment of metastatic malignant melanoma on her left groin. On April 6, 1964, an unknown resident performed a bone marrow biopsy. The needle broke during the procedure and a fragment lodged in the patient. The patient was told that the needle would be removed the following day, when surgery was to be performed to remove a melanoma from her groin. The operating surgeons, Dr. Peede and Dr. Kilgore, were informed of the presence of the needle fragment prior to surgery. A notation by Peede stated that the needle fragment had been removed.

The needle fragment, however, had not been removed. The patient remained asymptomatic until she was hospitalized for back pain in September 1985. During her hospitalization, the patient learned that the needle fragment was still in her lower back. The needle fragment was finally removed in October 1985. The physician's discharge report suggested that there was a probable linkage between the needle fragment and recurrent strep infections that the patient had been experiencing. Although the patient's treating physicians had known as early as 1972 that the needle fragment had not been removed, there was no evidence that the patient was aware of this fact.

The defendant physicians argued that the statute of limitations had tolled under Mississippi Code, thus barring the case from proceeding to trial. The circuit court entered a judgment for the physicians, and the plaintiff appealed.

Issue

Was the plaintiff's malpractice action time barred?

Holding

The Mississippi Supreme Court held that the plaintiff's action was not time barred and was, therefore, remanded for trial.

Reason

A patient's cause for action begins to accrue and the statute of limitations begins to run when the patient can reasonably be held to have knowledge of the disease or injury. In this instance, the patient began to experience infections and back pain in 1985. Moreover, this is the date she discovered that the needle was causing her problems, never having been informed previously that the needle from the 1964 biopsy procedure remained lodged within her.

Discussion

1. Describe under what circumstances the plaintiff's action would have been time barred by the statute of limitations.
2. Discuss the legal and ethical issues involved in this case (e.g., documentation in the medical record indicating that the needle fragment had been removed).

IMPROPER PERFORMANCE OF A PROCEDURE

In *Ozment v. Wilkerson,*[52] Mrs. Wilkerson was suffering from Crohn's disease, a chronic ailment that affects the colon and small intestine. Part of the treatment for the disease is to allow the patient's GI system to rest, and this means that the patient cannot eat. The patient is given a concentrated caloric solution intravenously. To deliver the needed nutritional solution, Dr. Ozment needed to place a central venous catheter into Wilkerson's body. Wilkerson's pericardial sac was punctured during the procedure. As a result, in a condition known as cardiac tamponade (accumulation of fluids in the pericardial sac) occurred. Wilkerson required emergency surgery to correct this condition and to repair the puncture. The defendants, following a jury verdict favorable to the plaintiffs, filed an appeal.

The Alabama Supreme Court held expert testimony supported the jury's finding that the catheter was inserted incorrectly. The plaintiff's expert, Dr. Moore, testified that the tip of the catheter should have been placed in the superior vena cava and should not have extended into the heart. Moore also stated that placing the tip of the catheter in the atrium, or against the wall of the atrium, was a deviation from the standard of care ordinarily exercised by a physician in the same line of practice under similar circumstances. Moore stated that the intravenous central line perforated the right atrium and caused the cardiac tamponade. Moore's testimony provided sufficient evidence from which the jury could determine that Ozment inserted the catheter incorrectly and had thereby breached his duty of care to Wilkerson.

FAILURE TO MAINTAIN AN ADEQUATE AIRWAY

In *Ward v. Epting,*[53] the anesthesiologist failed to establish and maintain an adequate airway and resuscitate properly a 22-year-old postsurgical patient, which resulted in the patient's death from lack of oxygen. Expert testimony based on autopsy and blood gas tests showed that the endotracheal tube had been removed too soon after surgery and that the anesthesiologist, in an attempt to revive the patient, reinserted the tube into the esophagus. The record on appeal was found to have contained ample evidence that the anesthesiologist failed to conform to the standard of care and that such deviation was the proximate cause of the patient's death.

PATHOLOGIST MISDIAGNOSES BREAST CANCER

On July 1, 1988, the patient, in *Anne Arundel Med. Ctr., Inc. v. Condon,*[54] underwent a routine mammogram ordered by her gynecologist, which revealed suspicious findings in her right breast. Advised by her physician that her breast needed further examination, the patient selected a surgeon to perform a biopsy. The biopsy was ultimately performed on July 19, 1988. Based on the pathology report, the surgeon advised the patient that she did not have cancer, but that she should undergo frequent mammograms. On February 7, 1990, the patient returned to her surgeon complaining of an inflammation of her right breast in the same area of her previous biopsy. The surgeon again recommended and performed a biopsy on February 15. Based on the second biopsy, the patient was advised that she was suffering from invasive carcinoma of the breast. On February 23, 1990, she underwent a bilateral modified radical mastectomy. The patient alleged that the first biopsy specimen was incorrectly interpreted by the pathologist and that the pathologist's failure to interpret invasive carcinoma was a departure from the standard of care required, and was the proximate cause of her injuries. On the eve of trial, December 9, 1992, counsel for the pathologist settled the claim against his client for $1 million.

AGGRAVATION OF A PREEXISTING CONDITION

Aggravation of a preexisting condition through negligence may cause a physician to be liable for malpractice. If the original injury is aggravated, liability will be imposed only for the aggravation, rather than for both the original injury and its aggravation. In *Nguyen v. County of Los Angeles,*[55] an eight month-old girl went to the hospital for tests on her hip. She had been injected with air for a hip study and suffered respiratory arrest. She later went into cardiac arrest and was resuscitated, but she suffered brain damage that was aggravated by further poor treatment. The Los Angeles Superior Court jury found evidence of medical malpractice, ordering payments for past and future pain and suffering as well as medical and total care costs that projected to the child's normal life expectancy.

The plaintiff in *Favalora v. Aetna Casualty & Surety Co.*[56] sued the hospital and the radiologist for injuries she sustained when she fell while undergoing an X-ray examination. The patient's personal physician admitted her to the hospital for a general checkup and a gastrointestinal (GI) series, when she complained about stomach pains, general fatigue, and fainting. The morning after her admission to the hospital, she was taken from her room in a wheelchair to the radiology department. When preparations for the GI series were complete, two technicians brought the patient to the X-ray room. She then waited for the arrival of the radiologist. When he arrived, she was instructed to walk to the X-ray table and stand on the footboard. The technician instructed her to drink a glass of barium. A second cup of barium was handed to her by the technician who then took the exposed film to a nearby pass box leading to the adjacent darkroom, obtained a new film, and repeated the X-ray process. While the technician was depositing the second set of exposed film in the pass box, the patient suddenly fainted and fell to the floor. The radiologist did not see the plaintiff fall, nor did he detect

any evidence of distress. The technician heard a noise, immediately turned on the lights, and found the patient lying on the floor. The patient was placed on the X-ray table, and X-rays were taken of those portions of her anatomy that indicated the possibility of injury. X-rays revealed a fracture of the neck and of the right femur that subsequently required open reduction and the insertion of a metal pin by an orthopedic surgeon. As a result, a preexisting vascular condition was aggravated, causing a pulmonary embolism, which, in turn, necessitated additional surgery. The failure of the radiologist to secure the patient's medical history before the X-ray examination was considered negligence, constituting the proximate cause of the patient's injuries.

A defendant generally is required to compensate a patient for only the amount of aggravation caused. However, it is often difficult to determine what monetary damages should be awarded to a plaintiff. In many instances, aggravation is a matter of conjecture.

LOSS OF CHANCE TO SURVIVE

In *Boudoin v. Nicholson, Baehr, Calhoun & Lanasa,*[57] expert testimony supported a finding of loss of chance to survive. A diagnostic radiologist's improper reading of a patient's X-ray resulted in a loss of chance to survive a chest-wall cancer. Boudoin had suffered a minor shoulder injury while lifting something at his job as a pipefitter. Because the pain did not subside after a few days, on May 19, he went to see Dr. Nicholson, the family practitioner who had treated him since he was 18. Based upon Boudoin's complaint of pain in the outer chest and a physical examination, Dr. Nicholson took a chest X-ray that, in his opinion, showed nothing remarkable and diagnosed Boudoin's injury as a muscle strain and prescribed accordingly. Nevertheless, he sent the X-ray to be evaluated by a diagnostic radiologist, Hendler. The radiology report returned to Nicholson read in part:

> CHEST: Cardiac, hilar, and mediastinal shadows do not appear unusual. Both lung fields and angles appear clear. A 3.5-cm. broad-based benign osteomatous projection is noted at the level of the vertebral border of the inferior aspect of the left scapula.
>
> IMPRESSION: 1—No evidence of active pulmonary or cardiac pathology.

Boudoin did not contact Nicholson again until January 1989, when he complained of discomfort in his neck as well as pain in his right shoulder blade and arm. Nicholson again ruled out serious injury through a cervical X-ray, resulting in a diagnosis of cervical spasm, degenerative discs, and bilateral spondylosis. On April 18, 1989, Boudoin returned to Nicholson complaining of night sweats, weight loss, and pain in his left chest. A chest X-ray showed a large abnormal mass. Boudoin was given both the 1988 X-ray and the one just taken, and was immediately sent to see a pulmonologist, Dr. Rosenberg. While Boudoin was undergoing a breathing test, Rosenberg called Mrs. Boudoin into his office and showed her the tumor as it appeared on the X-rays taken 11 months apart, and also had her read Hendler's May 1988 report. Rosenberg told Mrs. Boudoin that the tumor could have been removed easily when it was as small as it first appeared. Although the tumor initially appeared to be on Boudoin's left lung, innumerable tests and examinations established that the cancer was malignant and was in the pleura, the tissue lining the chest wall. No sign of metastasis was found in the lymph nodes of the chest or other tissues. Dr. Rigby surgically removed the tumor, now measuring $20 \times 17.5 \times 7$ centimeters, on May 10, 1989, along with a large portion of the chest wall and four ribs. Because a four- or five-millimeter metastatic deposit was found in Boudoin's right diaphragm, a section of that tissue also was removed. There was no sign of cancer on the lungs. A metal plate was implanted to replace the structural support lost with the removal of the ribs. After recovering from his surgery, Boudoin underwent concurrent radiation and chemotherapy. X-rays and examinations done every other month through March 1990 showed no signs of recurrence. Four months later, however, abnormalities were detected, and a second surgery performed on July 20, 1990, revealed that the tumor had spread. Due to the significant spread of cancer, the only tissue removed during surgery was a biopsy sample, which confirmed a malignant recurrence. Boudoin and his family were informed that even with chemotherapy, the prognosis was very poor. Further treatment was restricted to alleviating pain until Boudoin's death on December 18, 1990. Hendler appealed an award of $560,000 based upon a jury's finding that the physician's improper reading of Boudoin's X-ray resulted in a loss of chance to survive a chest-wall cancer. The appeals court affirmed the finding of liability and causation, but reduced the amount of the award.

The patient in *Downey v. University Internists of St. Louis, Inc.*[58] entered the hospital in December of 1996 for heart-bypass surgery. Two chest X-rays were taken during this hospitalization. The X-rays were interpreted as showing a lesion in the patient's left lung and that a neoplasm could not be completely ruled out. If clinically warranted, CT scanning could be performed. No further tests or evaluations were ordered in response to these reports. A jury found that the now-deceased patient had a material chance of surviving his cancer and that his chance of survival was lost due to the physician's negligence. The jury, however, did not award damages to compensate for the harm suffered. The Missouri Court of Appeals found that the verdict of no-damage award was inconsistent with the evidence, and remanded the case for a new trial.

POSSIBILITY OF SURVIVAL DESTROYED

On February 5, 1988, Mr. Griffett had been taken to the emergency department with a complaint of abdominal pain.[59] Two emergency department physicians evaluated him and ordered X-rays, including a chest X-ray. Dr. Bridges, a radiologist, reviewed the chest X-ray and noted in his written report that there was an abnormal density present in the upper lobe of Griffett's right lung. Griffett was referred to Dr. Ryan, a gastroenterologist, for follow-up care. Ryan admitted Griffett to the hospital for a 24-hour period and then discharged him without having reviewed the radiology report of the February 5 chest X-ray. On March 1, 1988, Griffett continued to experience intermittent pain. A nurse in Ryan's office suggested that Griffett go to the hospital emergency department if his pain became persistent.

In November 1989, Dr. Baker examined Griffett, who was complaining of pain in his right shoulder. Baker diagnosed Griffett's condition as being cancer of the upper lobe of his right lung. The abnormal density on the February 5, 1988 chest X-ray was a cancerous tumor that had doubled in size from the time it had been first observed. The tumor was surgically removed in February 1990, however, Griffett died in September 1990.

Dr. Muller, an internist and expert witness for the plaintiff, testified that Griffett would have had a greater likelihood of survival if Ryan had made an earlier diagnosis. The defendants objected to Muller's testimony, arguing that the plaintiff failed to establish that Muller was an expert witness capable of testifying as to the proximate cause of Griffett's alleged shorter life span. The trial court initially overruled the defendants' objection to Muller's testimony.

The jury returned a verdict for the plaintiff in the amount of $500,000. On a motion from the defendants, the trial court set aside the verdict, ruling that it erred by allowing Muller to testify as to causation. The plaintiff appealed, and the Virginia Supreme Court held that the plaintiff had sufficiently identified Muller as an expert witness capable of testifying as to the question of causation.

Evidence was sufficient to establish that the failure to diagnose lung cancer, in connection with the emergency department visit, was the proximate cause of the patient's death. The duty to review an X-ray contained in a patient's medical record should not vary between an internist and a gastroenterologist. Evidence showed that Ryan's negligence destroyed any substantial possibility of Griffett's survival.

LACK OF DOCUMENTATION

The importance of maintaining records of treatment rendered to a patient must not be underestimated. It may be many years after a patient has been treated before litigation is initiated; therefore, it is imperative that patient records of treatment in the physician's office, as well as in the health care facility, be maintained. A jury could consider lack of documentation as sufficient evidence for finding a physician guilty of negligence.

PREMATURE DISCHARGE

The premature discharge of a patient is risky business. The intent of discharging patients more expeditiously is often due a need to reduce costs. As pointed out by Dr. Nelson, an obstetrician and board member of the American Medical Association, such decisions "should be based on medical factors and ought not be relegated to bean counters."[60]

FAILURE TO FOLLOW UP

Failure to provide follow-up care can result in a lawsuit if such failure results in injury to a patient. In *Truan v. Smith*,[61] the Tennessee Supreme Court entered judgment in favor of the plaintiffs, who had brought action against a treating physician for damages alleged to have been the result of malpractice by the physician in the examination, diagnosis, and treatment of breast cancer. In January or February 1974, the patient noticed a change in the size and firmness of her left breast, which she attributed to an implant. She later noticed discoloration and pain on pressure. While being examined by the defendant on March 25, 1974, for another ailment, the patient brought her symptoms to the physician's attention but received no significant response, and the physician made no examination of the breast at that time. The patient brought her symptoms to the attention of her physician for the second time on May 6, 1974. She had been advised by the defendant to observe her left breast for 30 days for a change in symptoms, which at the time of the examination included discomfort, discoloration, numbness, and sharp pain. She was given an appointment for one month later. The patient, on the morning of her appointment, June 3, 1974, called the physician's office and informed the nurse that her symptoms had not changed and that she would like to know if she should keep her appointment. The nurse indicated that she would pass on her message to the physician. The patient assumed she would be called back if it was necessary to see the physician. By late June the symptoms became more acute, and the patient made an appointment to see the defendant physician on July 8, 1974. The patient also was scheduled to see a specialist on July 10, 1974, at which time she was admitted to the hospital and was diagnosed as having a malignant mass. A radical mastectomy was performed. Expert witnesses expressed the opinion that the mass had been palpable seven months before the removal. When the defendant undertook to give the plaintiff a complete physi-

cal examination and embarked on a wait-and-see program as an aid in diagnosis, the physician should have followed up with his patient, who died before the conclusion of the trial. The state supreme court held that the evidence was sufficient to support a finding that the defendant was guilty of malpractice in failing to inform his patient that cancer was a possible cause of her complaints and in failing to make any effort to see his patient at the expiration of the observation period instituted by him.

INFECTIONS

Nosocomial (hospital-acquired) infections are a leading cause of injury and unnecessary deaths. Such infections have been linked to unsanitary conditions in the environment and poor practices (e.g., hand-washing technique). The Centers for Disease Control and Prevention estimates that nearly 2 million patients annually get a hospital-acquired infection. There are estimates that as many as 90,000 of these patients die annually as a result of these infections.[62]

A Case for Best Practices

Making a case for using clinical guidelines is demonstrated in *McKowan v. Bentley*,[63] in which the patient, Mrs. Bentley, sought advice about gastric bypass surgery from Dr. McKowan in January 1993. On March 8, 1993, McKowan, assisted by Dr. Day, performed gastric bypass surgery on Bentley to alleviate her morbid obesity. Bentley was discharged from the hospital two days later with no indication of complications. On March 14, Bentley returned to see McKowan with redness and swelling around her incision. McKowan removed the sutures and found that Bentley had a wound infection. There was no indication that she had an intraabdominal infection at that time.

On March 15, the drainage from her wound changed in character and she was admitted to the hospital. McKowan operated on Bentley and drained the abscesses. Bentley had exploratory surgery on March 17 so that the doctors could see the extent to which the surgery had successfully reduced her infection. McKowan operated again and found no disruption of the wound site.

On March 18, another follow-up surgery was performed. Following that surgery, Bentley was placed on a ventilator and began receiving total parenteral nutrition intravenously. On March 22, surgery was again performed on Bentley. This time McKowan cut the front part of the stomach and placed a gastrostomy tube in the lower stomach. On March 26, purulent drainage was discovered around the gastrostomy tube. The gastrostomy site was repaired. Bentley showed some improvement on March 27.

At that point McKowan went on vacation and Dr. Day took over Bentley's care. On March 28, Day performed surgery to remove purulent material in the abdomen. On May 30, Bentley's sister transferred her to UAB Hospital in Birmingham, where she died.

Mr. Bentley filed a malpractice case. At trial, the plaintiff presented expert testimony from Dr. Kirchner, who testified that Bentley died because McKowan and Day did not properly manage her postoperative infection. Kirchner testified that the conduct of both physicians in managing the massive intraabdominal infection fell below the legally imposed standard of care in Alabama.

Testimony of the plaintiff's expert was emphatic, stating that the defendants disregarded obvious signs of grave complications; omitted obvious, simple, effective measures for stopping the infection that eventually killed the patient; and repeatedly applied inappropriate measures virtually certain to exacerbate the infection.

The jury awarded Mr. Bentley $2 million in punitive damages. The defendants contended that the award was excessive. The defendants' motion for a new trial was denied.

Infections a Recognized Risk

The mere fact that a patient contracted an infection after an operation will not, in and of itself, cause a surgeon to be liable for negligence. The reason for this, according to the Nebraska Supreme Court in *McCall v. St. Joseph Hospital*,[64] is as follows:

> Neither authority nor reason will sustain any proposition that negligence can reasonably be inferred from the fact that an infection originated at the site of a surgical wound. To permit a jury to infer negligence would be to expose every doctor and dentist to the charge of negligence every time an infection originated at the site of a wound. We note the complete absence of any expert testimony or any offer of proof in this record to the effect that a staphylococcus infection would automatically lead to an inference of negligence by the people in control of the operation or the treatment of the patient.[65]

Preventing Spread of Infection

A district court of appeals held in *Gill v. Hartford Accident & Indemnity Co.*[66] that the physician who performed surgery on a patient in the same room as the plaintiff should have known that the patient's infection was highly contagious. The failure of the physician to undertake steps to prevent the spread of the infection to the plaintiff and his failure to warn the plaintiff led the court to find that hospital

authorities and the plaintiff's physician caused an unreasonable increase in the risk of injury. As a result, the plaintiff suffered injuries causally related to the negligence of the defendant.

Poor Infection-Control Technique

A jury verdict in the amount of $300,000 was awarded in *Langley v. Michael*[67] for damages arising from the amputation of the plaintiff's thumb. Evidence that the orthopedic surgeon failed to deeply cleanse, irrigate, and debride the injured area of the patient's thumb constituted proof of a departure from that degree of skill and learning ordinarily used by members of the medical profession, and that failure directly contributed to the patient's loss of the distal portion of his thumb.

OBSTETRICS

One of the most vulnerable medical specialties with significant risk exposure to malpractice suits is obstetrics. Negligence claims in this specialty often stem from errors in physician judgment. The following cases illustrate why the risks are high.

C-Section Delay Causes Injury

The plaintiffs' experts in *Northern Trust Co. v. University of Chicago Hospitals and Clinics*[68] supported their contention that an obstetrical nurse's delay in placing a fetal monitor and an additional delay caused by the unavailability of a second operating room for a cesarean section caused an infant's mental retardation. Although there was contrary expert opinion, there was no error in the trial court's denial of the hospital's motion for judgment notwithstanding the verdict.

Failure to Perform Cesarean Section

A medical malpractice action was brought against two obstetricians, a pediatrician, and the hospital in *Ledogar v. Giordano*[69] because of a newborn infant's prenatal and postnatal hypoxia, which allegedly caused brain damage resulting in autism. The record contained sufficient proof of causation to support a verdict in favor of the plaintiff when an expert obstetrician testified that both obstetricians were negligent in failing to perform a cesarean section at an earlier time, that the hospital staff departed from proper medical standards of care by not monitoring the fetal heartbeat at least every 15 minutes, and that, with a reasonable degree of medical certainty, it was probable that the fetus suffered hypoxia during labor.

Failure to Attend Delivery: Fetus Decapitated

The plaintiff in *Lucchesi v. Stimmell*[70] brought an action against a physician for intentional infliction of emotional distress, claiming that the physician failed to be present during unsuccessful attempts to deliver her premature fetus, and that he thereafter failed to disclose to her that the fetus was decapitated during attempts to achieve delivery by pulling on the hip area to free the head. The judge instructed the jury that it could conclude that the physician had been guilty of extreme and outrageous conduct for staying at home and leaving the delivery in the hands of a first-year intern and a third-year resident, neither of whom was experienced in breech deliveries.

The intentional infliction of emotional distress requires that the following four elements be proven:

1. the defendant's conduct was intentional or reckless;

2. the conduct was extreme and outrageous;

3. the conduct caused emotional distress to the plaintiff; and

4. the emotional distress was severe.

All of these elements were present in *Lucchesi v. Stimmell*.

Failure to Perform Timely Cesarean Section

The attending physician in *Jackson v. Huang*[71] was negligent in failing to perform a timely cesarean section. The attending physician applied too much traction when he was faced with shoulder dyscotia, a situation in which a baby's shoulder hangs under the pubic bone, arresting the progress of the infant through the birth canal. As a result, the infant suffered permanent injury to the brachial plexus nerves of his right shoulder and arm. On appeal of this case, no error was found in the trial court's finding of fact when such finding was supported by testimony of the plaintiff's expert witness. The trial judge accepted the testimony of Dr. Forte, the expert witness, who testified that the defendant possessed the necessary skill and knowledge relevant to the practice of obstetrics and gynecology. The defendant, because of prolonged labor and weight of the baby, should have anticipated the possibility of shoulder dyscotia and performed a timely cesarean section.

Wrongful Death of Unborn Fetus

A medical malpractice action was filed against the physician in *Modaber v. Kelley*[72] for personal injuries and mental anguish caused by the stillbirth of a child. The circuit court entered judgment on a jury verdict against the obstetrician, and an appeal was taken. The Virginia Supreme Court held that the evidence was sufficient to support a finding that the obstetrician's conduct during the patient's pregnancy caused direct injury to the patient. Evidence at trial showed that the physician failed to treat the mother's known condition of toxemia, including the development of high blood pressure and the premature separation of the placenta from the uterine wall, and that the physician thereafter failed to respond in a timely fashion when the mother went into premature labor. The court also held that injury to the unborn child constituted injury to the mother and that she could recover for the physical injury and mental anguish associated with the stillbirth. The court found that the award of $750,000 in compensatory damages was not excessive.

PSYCHIATRY

The major risk areas of psychiatry include commitment, electroshock, duty to warn, and suicide. Matters relating to admission, consent, and discharge are governed by statute in most states.

Commitment

The recent emphasis on patient rights has had a major impact on the necessity to perform an appropriate assessment prior to commitment. The various state statutes often provide requirements granting an individual's rights to legal counsel and other procedural safeguards (e.g., patient hotline) governing the admission, retention, and discharge of psychiatric patients.

Most states have enacted administrative procedures that must be followed. The various statutes often require that two physicians certify the need for commitment. Physicians who participate in the commitment of a patient should do so only after first examining the patient and reaching their own conclusions. Reliance on another's examination and recommendation for commitment could give rise to a claim of malpractice. Commitment is generally necessary in those situations in which a person may be in substantial danger of injuring himself or herself or third persons.

Involuntary Commitment

In *In re Detention of Meistrell*,[73] proof of dangerousness was found adequate to support an order for involuntary commitment. There was testimony that on two occasions the patient jumped off a teeter-totter, causing his two small children to fall to the ground. A substantial risk of physical harm to others also was demonstrated by testimony that the patient threatened his wife's ex-husband.

Involuntary Commitment Ordered

There was clear and convincing evidence, in *Luis A. v. Pilgrim Psychiatric Center,*[74] that the patient remained extremely psychotic and delusional. This was manifested by his own testimony denying that the victim of the crime in which he participated in 1990 was dead. Further, he denied his attempted suicide on two prior occasions, his substance abuse problems, and his mental illness. The evidence showed that the patient believed that the reason he was reincarcerated upon violating his probation in 2000 was a conspiracy by certain individuals against him rather than the fact that he tested positive for marijuana and violated his curfew. The evidence demonstrated that the patient would likely relapse to his substance abuse. He posed a substantial threat of physical harm to himself and others if release from the care and control of the facility was permitted. Proof was demonstrated that if released, he intended to reside with his elderly mother, who had a significant history of mental illness herself and was incapable of properly caring for him out of an institutional setting, or of preventing deterioration in his mental health status. Expert medical opinion indicated that such would inevitably occur. The application to retain the respondent on an involuntary basis was granted.

Continuation of Commitment

In *In re Todd,*[75] a psychiatrist filed a petition for additional detention of a patient previously ordered admitted to a state hospital for pretrial psychiatric examination. The circuit court, after hearing testimony from the appellant's son, a social worker at the hospital, and the psychiatrist, ordered detention, and the detainee appealed. The episode that gave rise to the involuntary commitment occurred when the appellant threw eggs at a house and various businesses and also broke some windows at a house with a tire iron. She lightly bumped a police car and was charged with second-degree property damage. During her involuntary detention, she refused to take her medications, which were necessary because of her illness. The psychiatrist indicated his concern that, on release, she might harm her invalid husband. Additional detention was considered necessary until such time as the detainee's illness could be controlled by drugs. The court of appeals held that the testimony of the psychiatrist established clear and convincing evidence to meet a required standard that the detainee's actions presented risk of serious harm to herself or others.

Involuntary Commitment Invalid

In *In re Carl,*[76] a New York Supreme Court found a patient to be mentally ill and authorized his involuntary retention. On appeal, however, the New York Supreme Court, Appellate Division, held that the state had not shown by clear and convincing evidence that the patient's instability caused him to pose a substantial threat of physical injury to himself or others. The examining physician's testimony indicated that the patient did not pose a direct threat of physical harm to himself or others but that it was questionable whether he would be able to provide for the essentials of life. The patient testified that he was aware of food needs, of where to get food, and how he would pay for it. He indicated that he would not sleep outside and that he had a bed in a rooming house where he had been paying rent for two years.

Commitment by Spouse

The plaintiff's husband in *Bencomo v. Morgan*[77] filed a petition to have his wife declared incompetent. In a letter supporting the petition, the defendant physician, who had treated the wife 10 years previously, stated that she was badly in need of a psychiatric examination. The plaintiff/wife attempted to sue the physician for libel and slander. The court held that the plaintiff had no cause for action because it was her husband who initiated the commitment procedures.

Commitment by a Parent

The U.S. Supreme Court in *Parham v. J.R.*[78] held that the risk of error inherent in a parental decision to have a child institutionalized for mental health care is sufficiently great that an inquiry should be made by a neutral fact finder to determine whether statutory requirements for admission are satisfied. Although a formal or quasiformal hearing is not required and an inquiry need not be conducted by a legally trained judicial or administrative officer, such inquiry must probe a child's background using all available sources. It is necessary that a decision maker have the authority to refuse to admit a child who does not satisfy medical standards for admission. A child's continuing need for commitment also must be reviewed periodically by a similarly independent procedure.

Patient Due-Process Rights

The principles of due process were violated in *Birl v. Wallis*[79] when an involuntarily committed patient was conditionally released and once again confined without notice and opportunity for a hearing. Remand was required to permit the drafting of reconfinement procedures that would protect the patient's due-process rights.

Release Denied

In *State v. Wenk,*[80] Wenk was charged with one count of attempt to entice a child for immoral purposes in October

1977. He entered a plea of not guilty. While awaiting trial and out on bail, Wenk was charged with three additional felonies involving an 11-year-old boy: one count of abduction and two counts of first-degree sexual assault. Ultimately, Wenk withdrew his pleas of not guilty but maintained a plea of not guilty by reason of a mental disorder. The trial court agreed with Wenk and found him not guilty due to his mental disorder. The trial court also found him dangerous and needed to be committed. Wenk successfully petitioned for conditional release in 1979. He eventually succeeded in obtaining a conditional release. Five years later, Wenk waived his right to contest the motion seeking revocation of his conditional release after his probation agent instituted proceedings against him when it was discovered that Wenk failed to remain drug free and to abstain from contacting his ex-wife.

Wenk, at the age of 76, again petitioned the trial court seeking conditional release. As a result of his request, the trial court appointed two experts to examine Wenk: Palermo, a psychiatrist, and Smail, a psychologist. At the hearing, the state called Smail, who testified that Wenk could be released if certain conditions were placed on him. Also admitted into evidence were Palermo's report and the report of Chapman, a clinical psychologist employed by the state institution. Both of these reports recommended that Wenk be released, but only if certain conditions were placed upon him. Following the close of testimony, the assistant district attorney stated he was unsure whether he had met his burden of proof, but he urged the court to place conditions on Wenk if the trial court decided to release him.

The trial court, disagreeing with the doctors' ultimate recommendations, found that Wenk was still dangerous. He had a long-standing substance abuse problem, and although Wenk had not abused drugs while he was confined, the trial court believed his drug relapse that occurred during his earlier conditional release indicated he still posed a danger to the community if released. As a result, the trial court, in denying the petition, found that the state had met its burden of proof to a reasonable certainty by evidence that is clear and convincing that Wenk still remained dangerous.

Wenk argued that all the expert witnesses who examined him opined that he could be released under certain conditions. The court remained unpersuaded by his arguments. None of the doctors believed Wenk should be unconditionally released. Each recommended his release only under certain conditions. In Chapman's report, the doctor noted that Wenk had been previously diagnosed as suffering from bipolar disorder, as well as inhalant dependence. Chapman reasoned that Wenk could be conditionally released because Wenk's mental illness appeared to be in remission. With regard to Wenk's addiction to toluene, a paint thinner, Chapman acknowledged that Wenk used this drug when he engaged in his sexual criminal conduct, but Chapman's report contained the mistaken entry that during the four years Wenk was on conditional release, Wenk reported that he had no temptation to inhale. Wenk's records clearly show that Wenk

was recommitted, in part, as a result of his probation agent's discovery of his drug addiction. Consequently, the doctor's opinion that Wenk could be conditionally released was premised on his mistaken belief that Wenk had no difficulty with drugs during his previous release. Either Wenk minimized his toluene abuse when discussing his history with Chapman or Chapman failed to investigate the record.

Smail testified that Wenk's inhalant dependence was in remission. He did, however, admit that all of Wenk's criminal acts took place while he was under the influence of toluene. Smail's recommendation in favor of conditional release was also based on Wenk's statement to him that he had no personal concerns about resuming his abuse of inhalants. This self-serving opinion was not only overly optimistic but also, given Wenk's past conduct, not borne out by his history.

Palermo's report acknowledged that Wenk was abusing drugs when recommitted, but notwithstanding this history, Palermo recommended that Wenk be conditionally released, although he failed to set forth in his report any conditions that needed to be imposed on Wenk when he was released. This gaping hole in Palermo's report could easily have caused the trial court to lack confidence in the doctor's opinion.

The Wisconsin Court of Appeals determined that the trial court's decision was supported by the record. The differences of opinion between the doctors and the trial court lay with their prediction of Wenk's likely behavior when released. While the trial court acknowledged that predicting a person's future behavior is a difficult task, it pointed out that the past predictions of the psychiatric experts were wrong. Further, the trial court stated that its prediction for Wenk's future behavior was based on his past conduct, conduct that strongly suggested it was quite likely Wenk would again abuse drugs. The trial court was concerned that Wenk's pattern of abusing drugs posed too great a danger to the community to release him.

Recommended Discharge Denied

A trial court's decision that an insanity acquittee suffering from schizophrenia, paranoid type, in remission, failed to meet his burden of proving that he should be discharged, even though a psychiatric review board had recommended discharge. Two psychiatrists testified that as long as the patient was taking his medication, he was in no danger to himself or to others. The appeals court decision, based on the entire record found that the acquittee had not proven by a preponderance of the evidence that there was a mechanism in place to provide for continuation of the required medication if he was released from supervision. The court considered the violent nature of the underlying crimes (e.g., attempt to commit sexual assault in the first degree and kidnapping in the first degree), which was precipitated by the acquittee's mental illness. It was unclear whether the patient would continue to show the same progress after being discharged from the board's supervision.[81]

Electroshock

Most states have laws and regulations governing the use of electroshock and other treatments for psychiatric patients. Failure to abide by these statutory and regulatory guidelines may result in liability to the organization and treating physician.

Duty to Warn

In *Tarasoff v. Regents of the University of California,*[82] a former patient allegedly killed a third party after revealing his homicidal plans to his therapist. His therapist made no effort to inform the victim of the patient's intentions. The California Supreme Court held that when a therapist determines or reasonably should determine that a patient poses a serious danger of violence to others, there is a duty to exercise reasonable care to protect the foreseeable victims and to warn them of any impending danger. Discharge of this duty also may include notifying the police or taking whatever steps are reasonably necessary under the circumstances.

Under Nebraska law, the relationship between a psychotherapist and a patient gives rise to an affirmative duty to initiate whatever precautions are reasonably necessary to protect the potential victims of a patient. This duty develops when a therapist knows or should know that a patient's dangerous propensities present an unreasonable risk of harm to others.[83]

Exceptions to Duty to Warn

The Maryland Court of Special Appeals in *Shaw v. Glickman*[84] held that a plaintiff could not recover against a psychiatric team on the theory that they were negligent in failing to warn the plaintiff of the patient's unstable and violent condition. The court held that making such a disclosure would violate statutes pertaining to privilege against disclosure of communications relating to treatment of mental or emotional disorders. The court found that a psychiatrist may have a duty to warn the potential victim of a dangerous mental patient's intent to harm. However, the duty could be imposed only if the psychiatrist knew the identity of the prospective victim.

The psychiatrist in *Currie v. United States*[85] was found not to have had a duty to seek the involuntary commitment of a patient who evidenced homicidal tendencies. Absent control over the patient, the federal government could not be held liable for a murder that the patient committed at his former place of employment. The psychiatrist had warned the patient's former employer and law enforcement officials that he could be dangerous.

There was no duty on the part of the hospital or treating psychiatrists in *Sharpe v. South Carolina Department of Mental Health*[86] to warn the general public of the potential danger that might result from a psychiatric patient's release from a state hospital. There was no identifiable threat to a decedent who was shot by the patient approximately two months after the patient's release from voluntary commitment under a plan of outpatient care. In addition, there was nothing in the record indicating that the former patient and the decedent had known each other prior to the patient's release.

Suicidal Patients

Organizations have a duty to exercise reasonable care to protect suicidal patients from foreseeable harm. This duty exists whether the patient is voluntarily admitted or involuntarily committed. The District Court in *Abille v. United States*[87] held that evidence supported a finding that the attending physician had not authorized a change in status of a suicidal patient to permit him to leave the ward without an escort. The nursing staff allowed him to leave the ward, and he found a window from which he jumped. This constituted a breach of the standard of due care under the law in Alaska, where the act or omission occurred.

The attendant in *Fernandez v. State*[88] left a patient alone in her room for five minutes when the patient appeared to be asleep. During the attendant's absence, the patient injured herself in a repeated suicide attempt. The court found that even if the hospital assumed a duty to observe the patient continually, such a five-minute absence would not constitute negligence. Therefore, the hospital could not be held liable for the patient's injuries.

However, in a case in which a patient with a 14-year history of mental problems escaped from a hospital and committed suicide by jumping off a roof,[89] the record showed the patient was to be checked every 15 minutes. There was no evidence that such checks had been made. The appellate court ruled that the facts showed a prima facie case of negligence.

The New York Supreme Court, Appellate Division, in *Eady v. Alter*[90] held that an intern's notation on the hospital record that the patient tried to jump out the window was sufficient to establish a prima facie case against the hospital. The patient succeeded in committing suicide by jumping out the window approximately 10 minutes after having been seen by the intern. Testimony had been given that the patient was restrained inadequately after the reported attempted suicide.

Failure to Provide Appropriate Evaluation

John Doe was at his father's home seeking help in overcoming a heroin addiction. Doe was acting noticeably withdrawn and began vomiting. The plaintiff-father took his son to a local hospital to be evaluated for drug withdrawal. Doe tested negative for the presence of drugs in his blood and was discharged with instructions to attend a drug rehab program. The following day the father became aware that his son had attempted suicide. He called the office of a drug rehab program for help and was advised to take Doe to the hospital's crisis center.

The crisis center referred the father and his son to the hospital's emergency department. The father explained to the emergency department nurse that his son had attempted suicide by cutting his wrist. Doe's wrist was bandaged. The father and his son proceeded to the crisis center. Following an interview by a nurse and physician, the physician and nurse advised the father that his son was not suicidal but was "acting out" and looking for attention. Hospitalization was not offered, and the plaintiff was advised to follow up with a drug rehab program. Doe's medical records contain no information regarding voluntary hospitalization being recommended or offered, nor do the records reflect that the son refused any offer of voluntary hospitalization.

They returned home, and Doe went to bed. When the father checked Doe at about 6:00 A.M., he was gone. He telephoned the home of his ex-wife and was relieved to learn that his son was there. The father agreed to pick him up before the mother left for work. A few minutes later, the mother called and told the father that their son had left the house. The father immediately went to look for his son. While searching for his son, he noticed flashing lights on a nearby highway. When he went to see what was happening, he saw paramedics administering cardiopulmonary resuscitation (CPR) to his son. The father was told that his son jumped in front of a dump truck and was killed.

A lawsuit was filed against the defendants alleging negligence, malpractice, and infliction of emotional distress. At trial, the physician testified that the deceased declined voluntary admission to the hospital. However, in a deposition prior to trial, he testified that he could not recall whether Doe had declined voluntary admission or not. On cross-examination, the physician conceded that he had never specifically recommended hospitalization to Doe.

The nurse testified that voluntary hospitalization was offered as an option to the plaintiff and his son, but was not recommended. That option, if in fact offered, was not recorded in the hospital record.

The plaintiff's medical experts testified that: (1) because of Doe's two suicide attempts, he needed hospitalization; (2) additional steps should have been taken prior to ruling out major depression; (3) in all probability, Doe would not have killed himself had he been hospitalized earlier and put on medications; and (4) Doe's prior suicide attempts should have been taken more seriously. They opined that the failure to hospitalize Doe and keep him under close supervision was a deviation from accepted standards of medical practice. The defendants' expert testified to the contrary, but conceded on cross-examination that Doe had at least three high-risk factors for suicide.

The trial largely turned to a contest between the experts. The jury, by its verdict, accepted the opinions of the plain-tiff's experts. The court found, after a review of the record, no reason to disturb the jury's verdict. The plaintiff, as administrator of the estate of his late son, recovered a verdict of $425,000 against the defendants for their failure to provide appropriate evaluation and hospitalization of Doe.[91]

ABANDONMENT

The relationship between a physician and a patient, once established, continues until it is ended by the mutual consent of the parties, the patient's dismissal of the physician, the physician's withdrawal from the case, or agreement that the physician's services are no longer required. A physician who decides to withdraw his or her services must provide the patient with reasonable notice so that the services of another physician can be obtained. Premature termination of treatment is often the subject of a legal action for *abandonment;* the unilateral termination of a physician-patient relationship by the physician without notice to the patient. The following elements should be established in order for a patient to recover damages for abandonment:

- Medical care was unreasonably discontinued.

- The discontinuance of medical care was against the patient's will. Termination of the physician-patient relationship must have been brought about by a unilateral act of the physician. There can be no issue of abandonment if the relationship is terminated by mutual consent or by dismissal of the physician by the patient.

- The physician failed to arrange for care by another physician.

- Foresight indicated that discontinuance might result in physical harm to the patient.

- Actual harm was suffered by the patient.

PHYSICIAN-PATIENT RELATIONSHIP

The following suggestions can help to decrease the probability of malpractice suits:

- Personalize your treatment. A patient is more inclined to sue an impersonal physician than one with whom he or she has developed a good relationship.

- Conduct a thorough assessment/history and physical examination that includes, at a minimum, the following elements:

History

- chief complaint

- history of present illness

- past medical history

- family history

- allergies

- current medications

- social history

- review of systems

Physical

- general appearance

- vital signs

- mental status

- skin

- lymph nodes

- head, ears, eyes, nose, throat (HEENT)

- neck

- thorax, lungs

- breasts

- cardiovascular system

- abdomen

- genitalia

- rectum

- musculoskeletal

- neurologic

• Develop a problems list and comprehensive treatment plan that addresses the patient's problems.

• Provide sufficient time and care to each patient. Take the time to explain treatment plans and follow-up care to the patient, his or her family, and other professionals caring for your patient.

• Request consultations when indicated and refer if necessary.

• Closely monitor the patient's progress and, as necessary, make adjustments to the treatment plan as the patient's condition warrants.

• Maintain timely, legible, complete, and accurate records. Do not make erasures.

• Do not guarantee treatment outcome.

• Provide for cross-coverage during days off.

• Do not overextend your practice.

• Avoid prescribing over the telephone.

• Do not become careless because you know the patient.

• Seek the advice of counsel should you suspect the possibility of a malpractice claim.

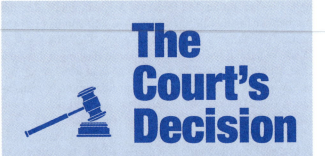

The Court's Decision

The Illinois Appellate Court held that the evidence was sufficient to support a determination that the defendant's negligence caused the plaintiff's pain and suffering.

CHAPTER REVIEW

1. A health care organization's bylaws set forth, among other things, the responsibilities of the medical staff. The committees of the staff review and analyze their responsibilities, clinical experiences, and opportunities for improvement.

2. In cases where a medical staff member's credentials are not screened properly, the health care organization can be held liable for injuries to patients as a result of the lack of investigation. The screening and appointment process involves many stages. These include the application, an evaluation of the applicant's physical and mental status, the applicant's release of information from third parties, the applicant's provision of a certificate of insurance, provision of evidence of an applicant's state licensure, a query of the National Practitioner Data Bank for information on the applicant, evaluation of the applicant's references, a thorough interview of the applicant, and approval by the governing body.

3. The medical staff must determine what procedures a physician is authorized to perform. This determination, known as *delineation of privileges,* is based on set criteria for credentials required to perform with competence the privileges requested.

4. To commence a court action for issues such as initial denial of medical staff privileges, grievances, and disciplinary actions, a physician must first exhaust all remedies set forth in the hospital's bylaws, rules, and regulations.

5. Physician monitoring is most effectively practiced through peer review. The governing body of a hospital has a duty to create a means through which the medical staff can evaluate, counsel, and, when appropriate, take action against a physician whose actions pose an unreasonable risk of harm to a patient.

6. A physician will not be held liable for exercising best judgment in following a course of treatment that is supported by a reputable, respected body of medical experts. However, a physician is at risk for liability if he or she uses an unprecedented procedure that results in harm.

7. A variety of malpractice issues discussed in this chapter include a failure to respond to emergency call; delaying treatment; performing inadequate history and physical examinations; failure to order diagnostic tests; failure to promptly review test results; failure to obtain a second opinion; failure to refer; practicing outside one's field of competence; misdiagnosis; failure to read nursing notes; medication errors; failure to follow a different course of treatment; failure to obtain informed consent; improper performance of a procedure; failure to maintain an adequate airway; aggravation of a preexisting condition; lack of documentation; premature discharge; failure to follow-up; and abandonment.

8. Among the duties held by mental health professionals is the duty to warn. If a therapist determines or should reasonably determine that a patient poses a serious threat of violence or danger to a third party, the therapist must exercise reasonable care to protect the third party and warn him or her of the impending danger.

9. In a malpractice case, the standard of care applied will be that pertaining to the specialty in which the physician is treating, regardless of whether or not that physician is credentialed in that specialty.

REVIEW QUESTIONS

1. Discuss the importance of delineating clinical privileges.
2. Why is it important that the governing body approve the appointment and reappointment of physicians to the medical staff?
3. What, if any, sanctions should be imposed upon an on-call physician who fails to respond to such call when requested? Discuss your answer.
4. Under what circumstances should a hospital be liable for a physician's negligence?
5. Describe what options a hospital has in disciplining a disruptive physician. What effect can a physician's disruptive behavior have on patient care?
6. When two physicians have opposing views as to a patient's medical needs, what course of action should the patient's attending physician follow?
7. Describe malpractice risks for radiologists and attending physicians.
8. Is a poor outcome always an indication of a negligent act? Explain.
9. When is a physician considered to have abandoned his or her patient?

NOTES

1. *Bombagetti v. Amine,* 627 N.E.2d 230 (Ill. App. Ct. 1993).
2. 42 C.F.R. § 482.12(a)(7).
3. *Szold v. Medical Board of California,* 127 Cal.App.4th 591, 25 Cal.Rptr.3d 665 (Cal. App. 2005).
4. 835 F.2d 1250 (8th Cir. 1987).
5. 645 P.2d 171 (Alaska 1982).
6. 301 N.W.2d 156 (Wis. 1981).
7. 211 N.E.2d 253 (Ill. 1965).
8. 394 N.E.2d 770 (Ill. App. Ct. 1979).
9. 540 P.2d 1398, 1400 (Or. 1975).
10. 130 Cal. App. 3d 970 (1982).
11. No. 04AP-72 (Ohio Ct. App. 2004).
12. *Warnick v. Natchez Community Hospital, Inc.,* No. 2003-CA-01513-SCT (Miss. 2004).

13. 218 N.W.2d 492 (Iowa 1928).

14. 520 N.Y.S.2d 751 (N.Y. App. Div. 1987).

15. *John v. Jarrard,* 927 F.2d 551 (11th Cir. 1991).

16. 737 S.W.2d 455 (Ark. 1987).

17. 291 A.D.2d 744, 738 N.Y.S.2d 137 (N.Y. App. Div. 2002).

18. 173 N.W.2d 881 (Neb. 1970).

19. No. WD63543 (Mo. Ct. App. 2004).

20. 85 Conn. App. 854 (Conn. App. 2004).

21. 294 F. Supp. 466 (D.S.C. 1968).

22. 865 F. Supp. 433 (N.D. Ohio 1994).

23. 632 A.2d 1333 (Pa. Super. Ct. 1993).

24. 235 A.2d 889 (N.J. 1967).

25. 568 N.W.2d 93 (Mich. App. 1997).

26. 594 A.2d 1309 (N.J. 1991).

27. 530 A.2d 1217 (D.C. 1987).

28. *Gomez v. Tri City Community Hosp.,* 4 S.W.3d 281 (Tex. App. 1999).

29. 531 A.2d 226 (D.C. 1987).

30. 653 A.2d 541 (Md. App.1995).

31. *Valentine v. Kaiser Found. Hosps.,* 15 Cal. Rptr. 26 (Cal. Ct. App.1961) (dictum).

32. 402 S.W.2d 855 (Ky. Ct. App. 1966).

33. 343 N.E.2d 589 (Ill. 1976).

34. No. CA 04-02238 (N.Y. App. Div. 2005).

35. 33 Cal. Rptr. 673 (Cal. Ct. App. 1963).

36. 666 F. Supp. 1511 (Ala. 1987).

37. 713 P.2d 773 (Wyo. 1986).

38. 209 So. 2d 809 (Miss. 1968).

39. 647 So. 2d 1366 (La. App. 3d Cir. 1994).

40. 542 N.Y.S.2d 328 (N.Y. App. Div. 1989).

41. 523 N.Y.S.2d 645 (N.Y. App. Div. 1988).

42. 489 So. 2d 392 (La. Ct. App. 1986).

43. 582 So. 2d 1272 (La. 1991).

44. 570 N.E.2d 1249 (Ill. App. Ct. 1991).

45. 595 P.2d 919 (Wash. 1979).

46. *Watkins v. Cleveland Clinic Foundation,* 719 N.E.2d 1052 (Ohio App. 1998) (April 1995).

47. *Watkins v. Cleveland Clinic Foundation,* 719 N.E.2d 1052 (Ohio App. 1998) (April 1995).

48. 539 S.W.2d 286 (Ky. 1976).

49. 785 A.2d 25 (2001).

50. 745 N.Y.S.2d 304 (N.Y. App. Div. 2002).

51. 250 A.2d 40 (N.J. Super. Ct. App. Div. 1969).

52. 646 So. 2d 4 (Ala. 1994).

53. 351 S.E.2d 867 (S.C. Ct. App. 1987).

54. 649 A.2d 1189 (1994).

55. No. C538628 (L.A. Co. Cal. Super. Ct.).

56. 144 So. 2d 544 (La. Ct. App. 1962).

57. 698 So. 2d 469 (La. App. 4 Cir. 1997).

58. No. ED83231 (Mo. App. 2004).

59. *Griffett v. Ryan,* 443 S.E.2d 149 (Va. 1994).

60. ANITA MANNING, *AMA Calls Drive-Thru Birth Risky,* USA TODAY, June 21, 1995, at 1.

61. 578 S.W.2d 73 (Tenn. 1979).

62. JP BURKE. *Infection Control-A Problem for Patient Safety.* NEW ENG. J. MED. 2003; 348; 651–656.

63. 773 So. 2d 990 (1999).

64. 165 N.W.2d 85 (Neb. 1969).

65. *Id.* at 89.

66. 337 So. 2d 420 (Fla. Dist. Ct. App. 1976).

67. 710 S.W.2d 373 (Mo. Ct. App. 1986).

68. No. 1-02-3838 (Ill. App. Ct. Rpt. 2004).

69. 505 N.Y.S.2d 899 (N.Y. App. Div. 1986).

70. 716 P.2d 1013 (Ariz. 1986).

71. 514 So. 2d 727 (La. Ct. App. 1987).

72. 348 S.E.2d 233 (Va. 1986).

73. 733 P.2d 1004 (Wash. Ct. App. 1987).

74. Nos. 2004-04404 & 2004-03036 (N.Y. App. Div. 2004).

75. 767 S.W.2d 589 (Mo. Ct. App. 1988).

76. 511 N.Y.S.2d 144 (N.Y. App. Div. 1987).

77. 210 So. 2d 236 (Fla. Dist. Ct. App. 1968).

78. 442 U.S. 584 (1979).

79. 619 F. Supp. 481 (D. Ala. 1985).

80. 637 N.W.2d 417 (2001).

81. *State v. Corr,* 867 A.2d 124, 87 (Conn. App. Ct. 2005).

82. 551 P.2d 334 (Cal. 1976).

83. See *Lipari v. Sears, Roebuck & Co.,* 497 F. Supp. 185 (D. Neb. 1980).

84. 415 A.2d 625 (Md. Ct. Spec. App. 1980).

85. 836 F.2d 209 (4th Cir. 1987).

86. 354 S.E.2d 778 (S.C. Ct. App. 1987).

87. 482 F. Supp. 703 (N.D. Cal. 1980).

88. 356 N.Y.S.2d 708 (N.Y. App. Div. 1974).

89. *Fatuck v. Hillside Hosp.,* 356 N.Y.S.2d 105 (N.Y. App. Div. 1974).

90. 380 N.Y.S.2d 737 (N.Y. App. Div. 1976).

91. *Vasilik v. Federbush,* 742 A.2d 591 (N.J. Super. Ct. App. Div. 1999).

CHAPTER 9

Nursing and the Law

It's Your Gavel ...

CHANCE OF SURVIVAL DIMINISHED

On the afternoon of May 20, the patient, Mr. Ard, began feeling nauseous. He was in pain and had shortness of breath. Although his wife rang the call bell several times, it was not until sometime later that evening that someone responded and gave Ard medication for the nausea. The nausea continued to worsen. Mrs. Ard then noticed that her husband was having difficulty breathing. He was reeling from side to side in bed. Believing that her husband was dying, she continued to call for help. She estimated that she rang the call bell for 1¼ hours before anyone responded. A code was eventually called. Unfortunately, Mr. Ard did not survive the code. There was no documentation in the medical records, on May 20 between 5:30 P.M. and 6:45 P.M., that would indicate any nurse or physician checked on Ard's condition. This finding collaborated Mrs. Ard's testimony regarding this time period.

A wrongful death action was brought against the hospital, and the district court granted judgment for Mrs. Ard. The hospital appealed.

Ms. Krebs, an expert in general nursing, stated that it should have been obvious to the nurses from the physicians' progress notes that the patient was a high risk for aspiration. This problem was never addressed in the nurses' care plan or in the nurses' notes.

On May 20, Ard's assigned nurse was Ms. Florscheim. Krebs stated that Florscheim did not perform a full assessment of the patient's respiratory and lung status. There was nothing in the record indicating that she completed such an evaluation after he vomited. Krebs also testified that a nurse did not conduct a swallowing assessment at any time. Although Florscheim testified that she checked on the patient around 6:00 P.M. on May 20, there was no documentation in the medical record.

Ms. Farris, an expert in intensive care nursing, testified for the defense. She disagreed with Krebs that there was a breach of the standard of care. However, on cross-examination, she admitted that if a patient was in the type of distress described by Mrs. Ard and no nurse checked on him for 1¼ hours, that would fall below the expected standard of care.[1]

WHAT IS YOUR VERDICT?

Each state has its own nurse practice act that defines the practice of nursing. Although most states have similar definitions of nursing, differences generally revolve around the scope of practice permitted. The scope of practice of a licensed practical nurse (LPN) is generally limited to routine patient care under the direction of a registered nurse (RN) or a physician.

An RN is one who has passed a state registration examination and has been licensed to practice nursing. The scope of practice of a registered professional nurse includes, for example, patient assessment, patient teaching, health counseling, executing medical regimens, and operating medical equipment as prescribed by a physician, dentist, or other licensed health care provider.

A *nurse practitioner* (NP) is an RN who has completed additional training beyond basic nursing education. The NP provides primary health care services in accordance with state nurse practice laws or statutes.

Nursing continues to change in response to advances in technology, changes in patterns of demand for health services, and the evolution of professional relationships among nurses, physicians, and other health professions. Although the actual authority of nurses to act varies considerably from state to state, the expanding scopes of nursing functions and licensure are illustrated clearly in the following examples:

- 1901—New York began to organize for passage of nurse practice legislation.

- 1903—North Carolina enacted the first nurse registration act.

- 1905—The development of the hospital economics course at Teachers College, Columbia University, ushered in a new era in preparation of nurse leaders in America. This one-year certificate course was extended to a two-year post-basic training program in 1905. The commitment of key nursing leaders to advancing educational preparation for nurse faculty fostered the subsequent development of baccalaureate education in nursing during the first quarter of the 20th century.

- 1937—The American Nurses Association (ANA) began recommending that nurses use their professional organization to improve every phase of their working lives.

- 1938—New York enacted the first exclusive practice act. This act required mandatory licensure of everyone who performed nursing functions as a matter of employment.

- 1946—The ANA convention adopted an economic security program and called for collective action on such items as a 40-hour workweek and higher minimum wages.

- 1952—All states, including the District of Columbia and U.S. territories, had enacted nurse practice acts.

- 1955—The ANA approved a model definition for nursing practice.

- 1957—The California Nurses' Association met with representatives of medical and hospital associations to draw up a statement supporting nurses in performing venipunctures.

- 1966—The Michigan Heart Association favored the use of defibrillators by coronary care nurses.

- 1968—The Hawaii nursing, medical, and hospital associations approved nurses performing cardiopulmonary resuscitation.

- 1970—The ANA amended its model definition for nursing practice to include nursing diagnosis.

- 1971—Idaho revised its nurse practice act by allowing diagnosis and treatment as part of the scope of practice for NPs.

- 1972—New York expanded its nurse practice act and adopted a broad definition of nursing.

- 1973—The first ANA guidelines for NPs were written for geriatric NPs. These were later modified and adapted to apply to other practitioners.

- 1975—Missouri revised statutes (1975) authorized a nurse to make an assessment of persons who are ill and to render a nursing diagnosis. The 1975 act not only described a much broader spectrum of nursing functions, but it also qualified this description with the phrase, "including, but not limited to."

- 1980—The ANA published a model nurse practice act for state legislators to provide for consistency in individual state nurse practice acts.

- 1985—New York revised its definition of nursing by providing that a registered professional nurse who has the appropriate training and experience may provide primary health care services as defined under the statutory authority of the public health law and as approved by the hospital's governing authority. The term *primary health care services* means taking histories and performing physical examinations, selecting clinical laboratory tests and diagnostic radiology procedures, and choosing regimens of treatment. These provisions do not alter a physician's responsibility for patient care.

- 1989—New York allowed NPs to diagnose, treat, and write prescriptions within their area of specialty with minimum physician supervision.

- 1990—The ANA again amended its model definition for nursing practice to include the advanced NP as well as the RN.

BROADENING SCOPE OF PRACTICE

The *scope of practice* refers to the permissible boundaries of practice for health care professionals, as is often defined in state statutes, which define the actions, duties, and limits of nurses in their particular roles. The role of the nurse continues to expand because of a shortage of primary care physicians in certain rural and inner-city areas, ever-increasing specialization, improved technology, public demand, and expectations within the profession itself.

Nurses are at risk for inappropriate professional relationships due to the broadening scope of nursing practice amidst rapid societal changes and pressures. The complexities of professional nursing relationships have outpaced awareness of ethical considerations of boundary issues. In addition, because professional nursing is founded on a caring ethic and nurses become intimately involved in life experiences of clients and families, nurses may be at risk for confusion over boundaries and inappropriate relationships. Boundaries which historically were unclear are increasingly recognized as an issue for the profession.[2]

A nurse who exceeds his or her scope of practice as defined by state nurse practice acts can be found to have violated licensure provisions or to have performed tasks that are reserved by statute for another health care professional. Because of increasingly complex nursing and medical procedures, it is sometimes difficult to distinguish the tasks that are clearly reserved for the physician from those that may be performed by the professional nurse. Nurses, however, generally have not encountered lawsuits for exceeding their scope of practice unless negligent conduct is an issue.

NURSING DIAGNOSIS

The defendant physicians in *Cignetti v. Camel*[3] ignored a nurse's assessment of a patient's diagnosis, which contributed to a delay in treatment and injury to the patient. The nurse testified that she told the physician that the patient's signs and symptoms were not those associated with indigestion. The defendant physician objected to this testimony, indicating that such a statement constituted a medical diagnosis by a nurse. The trial court permitted the testimony to be entered into evidence. Section 335.01(8) of the Missouri Revised Statutes (1975) authorizes an RN to make an assessment of persons who are ill and to render a nursing diagnosis. On appeal, the Missouri Court of Appeals affirmed the lower court's ruling, holding that evidence of negligence presented by a hospital employee, for which an obstetrician

was not responsible, was admissible to show the events that occurred during the patient's hospital stay.

NURSE LICENSURE

The common organizational pattern of nurse licensing authority in each state is to establish a separate board, organized and operated within the guidelines of specific legislation, to license all professional and practical nurses. Each board is in turn responsible for the determination of eligibility for initial licensing and relicensing; for the enforcement of licensing statutes, including suspension, revocation, and restoration of licenses; and for the approval and supervision of training institutions. A licensing board has the authority to suspend a license; however, it must do so within existing rules and regulations.

Requirements for Licensure

Formal professional training is necessary for nurse licensure in all states. The course requirements vary, but all courses must be completed at board-approved schools or institutions. Each state requires that an applicant pass a written examination, which is generally administered twice annually. A licensing board may draft examinations or a professional examination service or national examining board may prepare them. Some states waive their written examination for applicants who present a certificate from a national nursing examination board. Graduate nurses are generally able to practice nursing under supervision while waiting for the results of their examination. The four basic methods by which boards license out-of state nurses are (1) reciprocity, (2) endorsement, (3) waiver, and (4) examination.

Reciprocity

This is a formal or informal agreement between states whereby a nurse licensing board in one state recognizes licensees of another state if the board of that state extends reciprocal recognition to licensees from the first state. To have reciprocity, the initial licensing requirements of the two states must be essentially equivalent.

Endorsement

Although some nurse licensing boards use the term endorsement interchangeably with reciprocity, the two words have different meanings. In licensing by endorsement, boards determine whether out-of-state nurses' qualifications are equivalent to their own state requirements at the time of initial licensure. Many states make it a condition for endorsement that the qualifying examination taken in another state be comparable to their own. As with reciprocity, endorsement becomes much easier when uniform qualification standards are applied by the different states.

Waiver

Licensing out-of-state nurses can be accomplished by waiver and examination. When applicants do not meet all the requirements for licensure but have equivalent qualifications, the specific prerequisites of education, experience, or examination may be waived.

Examination

Some states will not recognize out-of state licensed nurses and make it mandatory that all applicants pass a licensing examination. Most states grant temporary licenses for nurses. These licenses may be issued pending a decision by a licensing board on permanent licensure or may be issued to out-of-state nurses who intend to be in a jurisdiction for a limited, specified time.

Graduates of schools in other countries are required to meet the same qualifications as are nurses trained in the United States. Many state boards have established special training, citizenship, and experience requirements for students educated abroad; others insist on additional training in the United States. Nurses who complete their studies in a foreign country are required to pass an English proficiency examination and/or a licensing examination administered in English. A few states have reciprocity or endorsement agreements with some foreign countries.

Suspension and Revocation of License

Nurse licensing boards have the authority to suspend or revoke the license of a nurse who is found to have violated specified norms of conduct. Such violations may include procurement of a license by fraud; unprofessional, dishonorable, immoral, or illegal conduct; performance of specific actions prohibited by statute; and malpractice.

Suspension and revocation procedures are most commonly contained in the licensing act; in some jurisdictions, however, the procedure is left to the discretion of the board or is contained in the general administrative procedure acts. For the most part, suspension and revocation proceedings are administrative, rather than judicial, and do not carry criminal sanctions.

Practicing Without a License

Health care organizations are required to verify that each nurse's license is current. The mere fact that an unlicensed practitioner is hired would not generally in and of itself impose additional liability unless a patient suffered harm as a result of the unlicensed nurse's negligence.

AMERICAN NURSES ASSOCIATION

The American Nurses Association (ANA) is a national professional organization of graduate RNs in the United States and its territories. ANA membership is available to all graduate nurses who are licensed in any jurisdiction of the United States. The purpose of the ANA is to

foster high standards of nursing practice and to promote the professional and educational advancement of nurses and the welfare of nurses to the end that all people may have better nursing care. The association helps provide health protection for the American people, aids nurses to become more effective members of their profession, and promotes quality health care.[4]

NATIONAL LEAGUE FOR NURSING

The National League for Nursing (NLN) is a membership organization of individuals and agencies organized for the purpose of fostering development and improvement of hospital, public health, and other organized nursing services and nursing education through the coordinated action of nurses, allied professional groups, citizens, agencies, and schools. The philosophy of the NLN is to bring together professional and paraprofessional health care workers and consumers to work toward improving nursing services and nursing education. The NLN is involved in nursing research, recruitment of students, testing services, workshops, conferences, seminars, consultation services, accreditation of nursing schools, fellowship aid, publications, and films. The NLN is funded through membership dues and grantors such as the American Hospital Association, the W. K. Kellogg Foundation, and the Rockefeller Fund.

NURSING NEGLIGENCE

Tables 9-1 and 9-2, as reported by the National Practitioner Data Bank, describe the number of malpractice occurrences and payments by malpractice reason for registered nurses, nurse anesthetists, nurse midwives, nurse practitioners,

TABLE 9-1 National Practitioner Data Bank, 2005 Annual Report

Number of Medical Malpractice Payment Reports by Malpractice Reason—Nurses (Registered Nurses, Nurse Anesthetists, Nurse Midwives, Nurse Practitioners, and Advanced Practice Nurses/Clinical Nurse Specialists)
National Practitioner Data Bank (September 1, 1990–December 31, 2005)

Malpractice Reason	RN (Professional) Nurse	Nurse Anesthetist	Nurse Midwife	Nurse Practitioner	Advanced Practice Nurse/ Clinical Nurse Specialist*	Total
Anesthesia related	128	915	1	8	1	1,053
Behavioral health related**	3	1	0	1	0	5
Diagnosis related	229	17	39	219	1	505
Equipment or product related	55	6	0	4	0	65
IV or blood products related	161	14	0	2	0	177
Medication related	555	29	3	62	1	650
Monitoring related	695	17	15	24	0	751
Obstetrics related	376	7	413	28	0	824
Surgery related	361	63	9	12	1	446
Treatment related	677	33	35	119	5	869
Miscellaneous	204	5	1	12	0	222
All reasons	**3,444**	**1,107**	**516**	**491**	**9**	**5,567**

This table includes only disclosable reports in the NPDB as of the end of the current year. Voided reports have been excluded. Medical malpractice payment reports that are missing data necessary to determine the malpractice reason (8 reports for RNs) are excluded.
*Reporting using the "Advanced Nurse Practitioner" category began on March 5, 2002. The "Advanced Nurse Practitioner" category was changed to "Clinical Nurse Specialist" on September 9, 2002. Prior to March 5, 2002, these nurses were included in the "RN (Professional Nurse)" category.
**The "Behavioral Health" category was added on January 31, 2004. Reports involving behavioral health issues filed before January 31, 2004 used other reporting categories. Cumulative data in this category includes only reports filed after January 31, 2004.

TABLE 9-2   National Practitioner Data Bank, 2005 Annual Report

Mean and Median Medical Malpractice Payment Amounts by Malpractice Reason, 2005 and Cumulative through 2005—Nurses (Registered Nurses, Nurse Anesthetists, Nurse Midwives, Nurse Practitioners, and Advanced Practice Nurses/Clinical Nurse Specialists) National Practitioner Data Bank (September 1, 1990–December 31, 2005)

| Malpractice reason | 2005 Only | | | Cumulative through 2005 | | | | |
| | Number of Payments | Mean Payment | Median Payment | Number of Payments | Actual | | Inflation-Adjusted | |
					Mean Payment	Median Payment	Mean Payment	Median Payment
Anesthesia related	68	$368,594	$110,938	1,053	$261,779	$100,000	$309,042	$123,867
Behavioral heath related**	3	$236,667	$60,000	6	$126,851	$37,500	$127,062	$37,810
Diagnosis related	80	$263,207	$100,000	504	$290,458	$125,000	$335,067	$140,494
Equipment or product related	6	$64,002	$61,695	65	$155,682	$40,000	$193,125	$43,667
IV or blood products related	6	$102,500	$67,500	177	$222,399	$75,000	$264,523	$79,332
Medication related	62	$406,830	$87,500	650	$267,366	$62,500	$306,440	$70,087
Monitoring related	97	$267,559	$100,000	751	$297,705	$95,000	$345,137	$107,040
Obstetrics related	90	$675,032	$288,750	824	$533,086	$249,832	$598,187	$264,483
Surgery related	52	$124,505	$60,000	446	$148,716	$50,000	$173,544	$55,471
Treatment related	99	$192,159	$75,000	869	$168,650	$50,000	$191,070	$61,934
Miscellaneous	23	$95,952	$47,500	222	$237,216	$40,000	$268,997	$49,547
All reasons	**586**	**$319,905**	**$100,000**	**5,567**	**$282,821**	**$90,000**	**$324,929**	**$102,482**

This table includes only disclosable reports in the NPDB as of the end of the current year. Voided reports have been excluded. Medical malpractice payment reports that are missing data necessary to determine the malpractice reason (8 reports cumulatively) are excluded.
**The "Behavioral Health" category was added on January 31, 2004. Reports involving behavioral health issues filed before January 31, 2004 used other reporting categories. Cumulative data in this category includes only reports filed after January 31, 2004.

and advanced practice nurses/clinical nurse specialists. The following narratives describe a variety of cases that illustrate some of the more common acts or failures to act that have led to lawsuits.

NURSE ANESTHETIST

Administration of anesthesia by a nurse anesthetist requires special training and certification. Nurse-administered anesthesia was the first expanded role for nurses requiring certification. Oversight and availability of an anesthesiologist are required by most organizations. The major risks for nurse anesthetists include improper placement of an airway, failure to recognize significant changes in a patient's condition, and the improper use of anesthetics (e.g., wrong anesthetic, wrong dose, wrong route).

NURSE ANESTHETIST: MEDICAL SUPERVISION REQUIRED

Citation: *Denton Reg'l Med. Ctr. v. LaCroix,* 947 S.W.2d 941 (Tex. Ct. App. 1997)

Facts

Mrs. LaCroix was admitted to the hospital's women's pavilion for the birth of her first child, Lawryn. She was admitted to the hospital under the care of Dr. Dulemba, her obstetrician. Prior to undergoing a cesarean section, LaCroix complained several times of breathing difficulty. When Dr. McGehee, the pediatrician, arrived, he noticed LaCroix appeared to be in respiratory distress and heard her say, "I can't breathe." McGehee asked Nurse Blankenship, a certified registered nurse anesthetist (CRNA), if LaCroix was OK. She responded that LaCroix was just nervous. Mr. LaCroix claimed his wife whispered to him that she could not breathe. Mr. LaCroix then shouted, "She can't breathe. Somebody please help my wife." Blankenship asked that Mr. LaCroix be removed from the operating room because his wife was having what appeared to her to be a seizure.

Blankenship could not establish an airway. She told one of the nurses: "Get one of the anesthesiol-

ogists here now!" Dr. Green, who was in his car, was paged. Upon receiving the page, he immediately drove to the women's pavilion, where Dulemba had already started the C-section. When Lawryn was delivered, she was not breathing, and McGehee had to resuscitate her. Meanwhile, Blankenship worked to establish an airway for LaCroix. The intubation was, however, an esophageal intubation. Dulemba stated that he thought that the intubation was esophageal. LaCroix's blood pressure and pulse dropped, and she went into cardiac arrest. A physician and nurse from the hospital's emergency department responded to a code for assistance. McGehee testified that the emergency department physician said that he did not know how to resuscitate pregnant women and left without providing any medical care. Dulemba and a nurse began cardiopulmonary resuscitation on LaCroix. McGehee, having finished treating Lawryn, took control of the code. LaCroix suffered irreversible brain damage.

Blankenship and Dr. Hafiz, the Denton Anesthesiology Associates (DAA), PA, anesthesiologist on call for the women's pavilion on the day of LaCroix's incident, settled with the LaCroixes by paying $500,000 and $750,000, respectively. The trial court entered a judgment against the hospital, awarding the LaCroixes approximately $8.8 million in damages.

Issue

Was the evidence sufficient to hold the hospital liable for medical negligence under a theory of corporate liability?

Holding

The evidence was sufficient to hold the hospital liable for medical negligence under a theory of corporate liability.

Reason

The evidence established that the hospital owed a duty to the plaintiff to have an anesthesiologist provide or supervise all anesthesia care, including having an anesthesiologist personally present or immediately available in the operating suite. The hospital's breach of this duty proximately caused the patient's brain damage.

The hospital's anesthesia department policies and procedures required that an anesthesiologist perform the preanesthesia evaluation, that an anesthesiologist discuss with the patient the anesthesia plan, and that an anesthesiologist supervise a CRNA by being "physically present or immediately available in the operating suite."

According to Dr. Via, chairman of the hospital's anesthesiology department in 1991, he complained to Mr. Ciulla, who was in charge of the DAA contract, about the lack of proper CRNA supervision in the women's pavilion. According to Ciulla, he renewed the contract in conjunction with the hospital's medical staff. According to Via, the hospital's medical executive committee recommended to Ciulla that he not renew DAA's contract and that he seek another anesthesia group for the women's pavilion. The hospital's board of directors renewed the contract anyway.

Discussion

1. Describe why this outcome occurred and how similar events can be prevented in the future.
2. Describe the role of the nurse anesthetist and anesthesiologist in this case.

NURSE PRACTITIONER

Nurse practitioners (NPs) are RNs who have completed the necessary education to engage in primary health care decision making. The NP is trained in the delivery of primary health care and the assessment of psychosocial and physical health problems such as the performance of routine examinations and the ordering of routine diagnostic tests. A physician may not delegate a task to an NP when regulations specify that the physician must perform it personally or when the delegation is prohibited under state law or by an organization's own policies.

The potential risks of liability for the NP are as real as the risks for any other nurse. The standard of care required most likely will be set by statute. If not, the courts will determine the standard based on the reasonable person doctrine (i.e., what would a reasonably prudent NP do under the similar circumstances?). The standard would be established through the use of expert testimony of other NPs in the field. Because of potential liability problems and pressure from physicians, hospitals have been historically reluctant to use NPs to the full extent of their training. Such reluctance has been diminishing as the competency of NPs has been well demonstrated in practice.

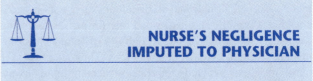

NURSE'S NEGLIGENCE IMPUTED TO PHYSICIAN

Citation: *Adams v. Krueger,* 856 P.2d 864 (Idaho 1993)

Facts

The plaintiff went to her physician's office for diagnosis and treatment. An NP who was employed by the physician performed her assessment and diagnosed the plaintiff as having genital herpes. The physician prescribed an ointment to help relieve the patient's symptoms. The plaintiff eventually consulted with another physician who advised her that she had a yeast infection, not genital herpes.

The plaintiff and her husband filed an action against the initial treating physician and his NP for their failure to correctly diagnose and treat her condition. The action against the physician was based on his failure to review the NP's diagnosis and treatment plan. The trial court found in favor of the plaintiff and the defendants appealed. The court of appeals affirmed and further appeal was made.

Issue

Did the trial court err by imputing the nurse's negligence to the physician?

Holding

The Idaho Supreme Court held that the negligence of the nurse was properly imputed to the physician.

Reason

The Idaho Supreme Court held that the physician and NP stood in a master-servant relationship and that the nurse acted within the scope of her employment. Consequently, her negligence was properly attributed to her employer/physician.

Discussion

1. Do you agree with the court's decision? Explain.
2. What might the physician/employer do to limit his liability in the future for the negligent acts of his professional employees?
3. If the NP has malpractice insurance, can the physician recover any of his losses from her insurance carrier?

CLINICAL NURSE SPECIALIST

A *clinical nurse specialist* (CNS) is a professional RN with an advanced academic degree, experience, and expertise in a clinical specialty (e.g., obstetrics, pediatrics, psychiatry). Further, the CNS acts as a resource for the management of patients with complex needs and conditions. The CNS participates in staff development activities related to his or her clinical specialty and makes recommendations to establish standards of care for those patients. The CNS functions as a change agent by influencing attitudes, modifying behavior, and introducing new approaches to nursing practice. The CNS collaborates with other members of the health care team in developing and implementing the therapeutic plan of care for patients.

NURSE MIDWIFE

Nurse midwives provide comprehensive prenatal care including delivery for patients who are at low risk for complications. For the most part, they manage normal prenatal, intrapartum, and postpartum care. Provided that there are no complications, normal newborns are also cared for by a nurse midwife. Nurse midwives often provide primary care for women's issues from puberty to postmenopause.

Practicing Without a License

The plaintiff in *Morris v. Dep't of Prof'l Regulation*[5] held herself out as a lay midwife in Illinois from 1983 through August 2001. The plaintiff performed prenatal exams on her patients, helped them deliver their babies at home, and provided postpartum and newborn care. The plaintiff was never

licensed to perform midwifery care and, therefore, failed to comply with the state nursing act's licensing requirements. The purpose of the nursing act is to promote the public health, safety, and welfare by ensuring that those individuals who engage in the conduct described in the Act are properly trained and licensed. The department of professional regulation ordered the plaintiff to cease and desist the practice of midwifery. The plaintiff's license was suspended, followed by probation and a fine. On appeal, the appellate court affirmed the orders requiring the nurse to cease and desist the practice of midwifery and suspending her nursing license and fining her.

Standard of Care Required of a Nurse Midwife

The plaintiff-appellant in *Ali v. Community Health Care Plan, Inc.,*[6] claimed that the trial court improperly charged the jury on the standard of care to be applied in the case. Specifically, the plaintiff contended that the effect of the trial court's charge was to establish a lower standard of care by which the jury would determine whether negligence existed in the case. The plaintiff asserted that the standard of care to be applied should have been that of a reasonably prudent professional engaged in the practice of obstetrics and gynecology, and not that of a reasonably prudent nurse-midwife engaged in the practice of obstetrics and gynecology. The defendant responded that the trial court's charge did not establish a lower standard of care and that the jury instruction was correct because it was in accordance with the actual evidence presented in the case. The Supreme Court of Connecticut, agreeing with the defendant, concluded that the trial court charged the jury with the correct standard of care. The question properly presented to the jury was whether defendant's conduct met the standard of care applicable to her as a nurse midwife.

NURSE MANAGERS

The *chief nursing officer* (CNO) is a qualified RN who has administrative authority, responsibility, and accountability for the function, activities, and training of the nursing staff. CNOs are generally responsible for maintaining standards of practice, maintaining current policy and procedure manuals, making recommendations for staffing levels based on need, coordinating and integrating nursing services with other patient care services, selecting nursing staff, and developing orientation and training programs.

A manager who knowingly fails to supervise an employee's performance or assigns a task to an individual whom he or she knows, or should know, is not competent to perform can be held personally liable if injury occurs. The employer will be liable under the doctrine of respondeat superior as the employer of both the manager and the individual who performed the task in a negligent manner. The manager is not relieved of personal liability even though the employer is liable under respondeat superior.

In determining whether a nurse with supervisory responsibilities has been negligent, the nurse is measured against the standard of care of a competent and prudent nurse in the performance of supervisory duties. Those duties include the setting of policies and procedures for the prevention of accidents in the care of patients.

Failure to Supervise

Nursing managers must properly supervise the care rendered to patients by their subordinates. Failure to do so can lead to disciplinary action by a state regulatory agency. This was the case in *Hicks v. New York State Department of Health*[7] in which the court held that evidence was sufficient to support a finding that a practical nurse was guilty of resident neglect for failing to ensure that the resident was properly cared for during her assigned shift. The record demonstrated that the petitioner was responsible for ensuring that the nursing aides' tasks were properly accomplished by conducting a visual check of each resident while making rounds at the end of her shift. The nurse's record indicated that a security guard found a resident lying in the dark, half in his bed and half still restrained in an overturned wheelchair. The nurse's record indicated that the resident was covered in urine and stool. The commissioner of health denied the petitioner's request to expunge the patient neglect report and assessed a penalty of $200, of which the petitioner was required to pay $50.

SPECIAL-DUTY NURSE

A *special-duty nurse* is a health care professional employed by a patient or patient's family to perform nursing care for the patient. An organization is generally not liable for the negligence of a special-duty nurse unless a master-servant relationship can be determined to exist between the organization and the special-duty nurse. If a master-servant relationship exists between the organization and the special-duty nurse, the doctrine of respondeat superior may be applied to impose liability on the organization for the nurse's negligent acts.

A special-duty nurse may be required to observe certain rules and regulations as a precondition to working in the organization. The observance of organization rules is insufficient, however, to establish a master-servant relationship between the organization and the nurse. Under ordinary circumstances, the patient employs the special-duty nurse and the organization has no authority to hire or fire the nurse. The organization does, however, have the responsibility to

protect the patient from incompetent or unqualified special-duty nurses.

FLOAT NURSE

A *float nurse* is health care professional who rotates from unit to unit based on staffing needs. "Floaters" can benefit an understaffed unit, but they also may present a liability as well if they are assigned to work in an area outside their expertise. If a patient is injured because of a floater's negligence, the standard of care required of the floater will be that required of a nurse on the assigned patient care unit.

NURSING ASSISTANT

A *nursing assistant* is an aide who has been certified and trained to assist patients with activities of daily living. The nursing assistant provides basic nursing care to patients in a safe and clean environment under the direction and supervision of an RN or LPN. The nursing assistant helps with positioning, turning, and lifting and performs a variety of tests and treatments. The nursing assistant establishes and maintains interpersonal relationships with patients and other hospital personnel while ensuring confidentiality of patient information.

Failure to Follow Policy: Patient Scalded

Ovitz, a 73-year-old resident of a convalescent center, died after immersion in a tub of hot water that had been prepared by a nursing assistant.[8] Ovitz had paralysis of his left side and could articulate only the words "yes" and "no." The nursing assistant checked the water with his hand and bathed the resident. Later in the day, a nurse noticed that the resident's leg was bleeding and his skin was sloughing off. The paramedics were contacted, and they transferred the resident to a hospital after determining that the patient had suffered third-degree burns. Dr. Drueck, the surgeon at the hospital, observed that Ovitz had suffered third-degree burns over 40 percent of his body, primarily on his back, buttocks, both sides, genitals, and lower legs.

Ovitz developed pneumonia during his hospitalization and died. There was testimony from Drueck that the cause of death was due to complications following the burns. The center's bathing policy to prevent accidents was to avoid making the water too hot. The center's daily temperature logs indicated that it knew that the water temperature in the system at times fluctuated above its bathing policy, sometimes exceeding 110°F, yet the center failed to take adequate measures to protect residents from exposure to excessive water temperatures. The center's own written policy was violated when the nursing assistant left the resident unattended in his bath. The appellate court held that revocation of the center's license was warranted in this case.

Failure to Follow Policy: Patient Fall

In *Bowe v. Charleston Area Medical Center*,[9] a nurse's aide brought an action against a medical center for retaliatory discharge and breach of contract. The nurse's aide assisted a patient to the bathroom and placed him on the commode. She left him unattended for about 10 minutes. When she returned, the patient was found lying on the floor in a pool of blood. The patient apparently hit his head on the sink when he fell. Following an investigation of the incident, the hospital found that the aide had been grossly negligent and thus terminated her employment. The human resources director had authorized the employee's termination because of a provision in the employee handbook that makes gross negligence a dischargeable offense. The aide claimed that she had been terminated because of her complaints about the lack of patient care on the oncology unit to which she had been assigned. There was no specific evidence that could substantiate that she filed a grievance regarding patient care.

The West Virginia Supreme Court of Appeals held that: (1) the evidence established that patient neglect by the plaintiff prompted an investigation that led to her subsequent discharge, and (2) the disclaimer in the employee handbook adequately shielded the employer from any contractual liability based on the employee handbook. The evidence showed that the aide, contrary to the medical center's policy, had assisted a patient in getting on a commode and then left him unattended, resulting in a fall and his subsequent death. Leaving the patient unattended for 10 minutes on the commode was clearly against hospital policy. The nurse's aide failed to establish that her discharge was a retaliatory act or that it contravened some public policy.

The hospital's disclaimer specifically stated that the employee handbook was not intended to create any contractual rights. Employment was subject to termination at any time by either the employee or employer. The disclaimer in the employee handbook read:

> Because of court decisions in some states, it has become necessary for us to make it clear that this handbook is not part of a contract, and no employee of the Medical Center has any contractual right to the matters set forth in this handbook. In addition, your employment is subject to termination at any time by either you or by the Medical Center.[10]

Failure to Safely Transfer Patient

The nursing assistant in *Kern v. Gulf Coast Nursing Home of Moss Point, Inc.*[11] was attempting to give a resident a whirlpool bath. The resident had been placed in a special rolling seat and was being lifted by a hydraulic lifting device that was used to place residents in the whirlpool. In the process of lifting the resident, the seat, which had been connected to the lift, disconnected. The resident fell to the floor, hitting her head and breaking her hip. The trial court entered a verdict in the amount of $20,000 for the plaintiff and the plaintiff appealed, stating that the award was inadequate. The Mississippi Supreme Court held that the verdict was not so low as to shock the conscience of the court.

Failure to Follow Safe Practice

The record in *Jones v. Axelrod*[12] indicated that a nurse's aide, while transferring nursing home patient to her bed from a wheelchair, left the patient sitting on the edge of the bed. The patient subsequently fell to the floor. The aide acknowledged that the patient required restraints. The supervisor testified that the act of leaving the patient unrestrained and unattended on the edge of the bed was improper and inconsistent with safe procedure. Sufficient evidence supported a determination by the commissioner of health that the conduct of the nurse's aide constituted patient neglect.

AGENCY STAFF

Health care organizations are at risk for the negligent conduct of agency staff. Because of this risk, it is important to be sure that agency workers have the necessary skills and competencies to carry out the duties and responsibilities assigned by the organization.

STUDENT NURSES

Student nurses are entrusted with the responsibility of providing nursing care to patients. They are personally liable for their own negligent acts, and the facility is liable for their acts on the basis of respondeat superior. A student nurse is held to the standard of a competent professional nurse when performing nursing duties. The courts, in several decisions, have taken the position that anyone who performs duties customarily performed by professional nurses is held to the standards of professional nurses. Every patient has the right to expect competent nursing services even if students provide the care as part of their clinical training. It would be unfair to deprive a patient of compensation for an injury simply because the nurse was a student.

MEDICATION ERRORS

Nurses are required to handle and administer a vast variety of drugs that are prescribed by physicians and dispensed by an organization's pharmacy. Medications may range from aspirin to highly dangerous drugs (e.g., potassium chloride) administered through IV solutions. Medications must be administered in the prescribed manner and dose to prevent serious harm to patients.

The practice of pharmacy includes the ordering, preparation, dispensing, and administration of medications. These activities may be carried out only by a licensed pharmacist by a person exempted from the provisions of a state's pharmacy statutes. Nurses are exempted from the various pharmacy statutes when administering a medication on the oral or written order of a physician.

Failure to Administer Drugs

The trial court in *Lloyd Noland Hospital v. Durham*[13] did not err in denying a hospital's motion for a new trial based on the hospital's argument that it did not breach an applicable standard of care in failing to administer a preoperative antibiotic to a patient. The record contained ample evidence of the existence of a standing order that required the nursing staff to administer preoperative antibiotics to patients prior to being treated.

In *Kallenberg v. Beth Israel Hospital*,[14] a patient died after her third cerebral hemorrhage because of the failure of the physicians and staff to administer necessary medications. When the patient was admitted to the hospital, her physician determined that she should be given a specific drug to reduce her blood pressure and make her condition operable. For an unexplained reason, the drug was not administered. The patient's blood pressure rose, and after the final hemorrhage, she died. The jury found the hospital and physicians negligent by failing to administer the drug and ruled that the negligence caused the patient's death. On appeal, the appellate court found that the jury had sufficient evidence to decide that the negligent treatment had been the cause of the patient's death.

Failure to Document Drug Wastage

The nurse in *Matthias v. Iowa Board of Nursing*[15] failed to conform to minimum standards of practice by neglecting to document the loss or wastage of controlled substances. The

minimum standard of acceptable practice requires nurses to count controlled substances each shift, to document all loss or wastage of controlled substances, and to obtain the signature of a witness to the disposal of controlled substances. Iowa Code section 147.\-55\-(2) allows a professional license to be suspended or revoked when the licensee engages in professional incompetency. Iowa Administrative Code section 655-4.\-19\-(2)\-(c), which regulates the actions of the board, defines professional incompetency as including "[w]illful or repeated departure from or failure to conform to the minimum standards of acceptable and prevailing practice of nursing in the state of Iowa."

Matthias argued that the board erred as a matter of law because it failed to find that she knowingly or willfully failed to conform to the minimum standards of practice regarding documentation of loss or wastage of controlled substances. The Iowa Court of Appeals found that there was substantial evidence supporting the board's finding that Matthias engaged in repeated departures from the minimum standards of nursing. The board, therefore, did not need to find that the departure was also willful.

Administering Unprescribed Drugs

In *People v. Nygren*,[16] evidence was considered sufficient to establish probable cause for charging the director of nursing and a charge nurse with second-degree assault in the administration of unprescribed doses of Thorazine to a resident at a time when the patient was incapable of providing consent. There was probable cause to believe that the defendants committed the offense charged and that it would have been established if the prosecution had been permitted to present its witnesses, two of which would have testified that the nurses administered the unprescribed doses of the drug. The treating physician told the special investigator from the attorney general's office that Thorazine never had been prescribed for the resident while he was in the nursing facility. The resident was mentally retarded and incapable of consenting to administration of the drug. Medical evidence of the amount of Thorazine in the resident's blood was consistent with stupor and impairment of physical and mental functions.

Administering the Wrong Drug

In *Abercrombie v. Roof*,[17] a solution was prepared by an employee and injected into the patient by a physician. The physician made no examination of the fluid, and the patient suffered permanent injuries as a result of the injection. An action was brought against the physician for malpractice. The patient claimed that the fluid injected was alcohol and that the physician should have recognized its distinctive odor. In finding for the physician, the court stated that he was not responsible for the misuse of drugs prepared by an employee unless the ordinarily prudent use of his faculties would have prevented injury to the patient.

Failure to Clarify Orders

A nurse is responsible for making an inquiry if there is uncertainty about the accuracy of a physician's medication order in a patient's record. In the Louisiana case of *Norton v. Argonaut Insurance Co.,*[18] the court focused attention on the responsibility of a nurse to obtain clarification of an apparently erroneous order from the patient's physician. The medication order, as entered in the medical record, was incomplete and subject to misinterpretation. Believing the order to be incorrect because of the dosage, the nurse asked two physicians present on the patient care unit whether the medication should be given as ordered. The two physicians did not interpret the order as the nurse did and therefore did not share the same concern. They advised the nurse that the attending physician's instructions did not appear out of line. The nurse did not contact the attending physician but instead administered the misinterpreted dosage of medication. As a result, the patient died from a fatal overdose of the medication.

The court upheld the jury's finding that the nurse had been negligent in failing to verify the order with the attending physician prior to administering the drug. The nurse was held liable, as was the physician who wrote the ambiguous order that led to the fatal dose. The court noted that it is the duty of a nurse to make absolutely certain what the physician intended, regarding both dosage and route. This clarification was not sought from the physician who wrote the order. This departure from the standard of competent nursing practice provided the basis for holding the nurse liable for negligence.

Administering the Wrong Dosage

The nurse in *Harrison v. Axelrod*[19] was charged with patient neglect because she administered the wrong dosage of the drug Haldol to a patient on seven occasions while she was employed at a nursing facility. The patient's physician had prescribed a 0.5 milligram dosage of Haldol. The patient's medication record indicated that the nurse had been administering dosages of 5.0 milligrams, the dosage sent to the patient care unit by the pharmacy. A department of health investigator testified that the nurse admitted that she administered the wrong dosage, and that she was aware of the facility's medication administration policy, which she breached by failing to check the dosage supplied by the pharmacy against the dosage ordered by the patient's doctor. The nurse denied that she made these admissions to the investigator. The commissioner of the department of health made a determination that the administration of the wrong dosage of Haldol on seven occasions constituted patient neglect.

On appeal, the New York Supreme Court, Appellate Division, held that the evidence established that the nurse administered the wrong dosage of the prescribed drug Haldol to the patient. This was a breach of the facility's medication administration policy and was sufficient to support the determination of patient neglect.

NEGLIGENT DRUG OVERDOSE

Citation: *Harder v. Clinton, Inc.,* 948 P.2d 298 (Okla. 1997)

Facts

Kayser was admitted to a nursing home on July 14, 1992. On the evening of September 30, she was transferred to a hospital after ingesting an overdose of tolbutamide, a diabetic medication. She was diagnosed as having a hypoglycemic coma caused by the lowering of her blood sugar from ingestion of the medication. An IV device was inserted in the dorsum area of her right foot to treat the coma. Gangrene later developed in the same foot, which eventually required an above-the-knee amputation.

As Kayser's guardian, Harder, Kayser's sister, brought a suit against the nursing home for harm caused to Kayser by an overdose of the wrong prescription administered to her while she was in the nursing home's care and custody. At the close of Harder's case, which followed a res ipsa loquitur pattern of proof, the trial court directed a verdict for the nursing home. The trial court ruled that Harder's evidence fell short of establishing a negligence claim because her proof failed to show all the requisite foundational elements for res ipsa loquitur.

Issue

Did the trial court err when it directed a verdict for the nursing home based on its ruling that Harder had not satisfied the requirements for a res ipsa loquitur submission?

Holding

By the evidence adduced at trial, Harder met the standards for submission of her claim based on the doctrine of res ipsa loquitur pattern of proof.

Reason

In light of the circumstances that surround the injurious event, it seems reasonably clear that Kayser's ingestion of a tolbutamide overdose would not have taken place in the absence of negligence by the nursing home's staff. The record shows that Kayser had not been prescribed any diabetes medication while a resident at the nursing home and that she had never been prescribed that type of hypoglycemic drug. It is uncontradicted that Kayser was at the nursing home when she ingested the prescribed medication. There is no direct evidence that anyone else supplied to her the harm-dealing dosage or that the substance in question was kept in her room (or elsewhere within her control). Neither is there indication that any other cause contributed to the coma. According to Dixon, the nursing home is responsible for the administration of medication to its residents. The administration of the wrong medication in an amount so excessive as to harm a resident is below the applicable standard of care.

Harder's evidence laid the requisite res ipsa loquitur foundation facts from which it could be inferred that the injury—from an overdose of the wrong prescription—was one that would not ordinarily occur in the course of controlled supervision and administration of prescribed medicine in the absence of negligence. Nothing in the record negates any of the critical elements for application of res ipsa loquitur. The responsibility for producing proof that would rebut the inferences favorable to Harder's legal position was thus shifted to the defendant.

Discussion

1. Describe the elements the plaintiff's attorney had to establish under the doctrine of res ipsa loquitur.
2. Describe what procedures you would implement to reduce the likelihood of similar occurrences.

Administering Drugs by the Wrong Route

The nurse in *Fleming v. Baptist General Convention*[20] negligently injected the patient with a solution of Talwin and Atarax subcutaneously, rather than intramuscularly. The patient suffered tissue necrosis as a result of the improper injection. The suit against the hospital was successful. On appeal, the court held that the jury's verdict for the plaintiff found adequate support in the testimony of the plaintiff's expert witness on the issues of negligence and causation.

Failure to Discontinue a Drug

A health care organization will be held liable if a nurse continues to inject a solution into a patient after noticing its ill effects. In the Florida case of *Parrish v. Clark*,[21] the court held that a nurse's continued injection of saline solution into an unconscious patient's breast after the nurse noticed ill effects constituted negligence. After something was observed to be wrong with the administration of the solution, the nurse had a duty to discontinue its use.

Failure to Identify the Correct Patient

A patient's identification bracelet must be checked prior to administering medications. To ensure that the patient's identity corresponds to the name on the patient's bracelet, the nurse should address the patient by name when approaching the patient's bedside to administer any medication. Should a patient unwittingly be administered another patient's medication, the attending physician should be notified and appropriate documentation placed on the patient's chart.

Failure to Note an Order Change

In *Larrimore v. Homeopathic Hospital Association*,[22] the physician wrote an instruction on the patient's order sheet changing the method of administration from intramuscular to oral. When a nurse on the patient unit who had been off duty for several days was preparing to medicate the patient by injection, the patient objected and referred the nurse to the physician's new order. The nurse, however, told the patient she was mistaken and administered the medication intramuscularly. The court went on to say that the jury could find the nurse negligent by applying ordinary common sense to establish the applicable standard of care.

NEGLIGENT INJECTION

In *Bernardi v. Community Hospital Association*,[23] a seven-year-old patient was in the hospital after surgery for the drainage of an abscessed appendix. The attending physician left a written postoperative order requiring an injection of tetracycline every 12 hours. During the evening of the first day after surgery, the nurse, employed by the hospital and acting under this order, injected the prescribed dosage of tetracycline in the patient's right gluteal region. It was claimed that the nurse negligently injected the tetracycline into or adjacent to the sciatic nerve, causing the patient to permanently lose the normal use of the right foot. The court did not hold the physician responsible. It concluded that if the plaintiff could prove the nurse's negligence, the hospital would be responsible for the nurse's act under the doctrine of respondeat superior. The physician did not know which nurse administered the injection because he was not present when the injection was given, and he had no opportunity to control its administration. The hospital was found liable under respondeat superior. The hospital was the employer of the nurse. Only it had the right to hire and fire her. Only it could assign the nurse to certain hours, designated areas, and specific patients.

FAILURE TO FOLLOW PHYSICIAN'S ORDERS

In July 1998, Kitchen became a resident of Wickliffe nursing home.[24] She had been a patient of the appellant, Dr. Muenster, since 1963. While Kitchen resided in the nursing home, Muenster continued to act as her treating physician. When Kitchen entered Wickliffe, she had been receiving Coumadin, a blood thinner that requires monitoring by specific blood tests on a periodic basis. These blood tests were needed in order to adjust the dosage of Coumadin if necessary. Muenster had written the orders for the nurses to conduct blood tests every Wednesday. On July 29, 1998, the nurses administered these tests and faxed the results to Muenster. Kitchen continued to receive Coumadin at the dosage prescribed by Muenster even though the nurses apparently failed to conduct subsequent weekly blood tests. Likewise, Muenster did not receive any reports concerning the blood test results. During this time, Muenster made no further effort to check up on the resident. On August 19, 1998, Kitchen was found in distress and was transported to a hospital, where she went into renal failure and later lapsed into a coma and died as a result of toxic levels of Coumadin.

The appellees filed suit against Muenster and Wickliffe, alleging negligence and wrongful death. After appellees settled with Wickliffe, the case proceeded against Muenster. Following trial, the jury returned a verdict in favor of the physician and the plaintiffs/appellees moved for a new trial. The appellees maintained that Muenster had a responsibility to follow up and make sure that his orders were fulfilled by the nurses. The appellees argued that if the jury found the nurses negligent in failing to follow the physician's orders, then the jury also should have found the physician negligent on the basis that he controlled the performance of the nurses.

Muenster claimed that there was absolutely no evidence to establish that he had a right to control or direct the performance of the nurses beyond the issuance of the orders in question. Thus, the negligence of the nurses could not be imputed to him. The trial court granted the appellees' motion for a new trial. The Ohio Court of Appeals found that there was substantial evidence, that beyond the issuance of treatment orders, there was no evidence presented that Muenster had the right to control and direct the performance of the nurses at the nursing home.

Evidence in *Redel v. Capital Reg. Med. Ctr.*[25] noted that nurses failed to follow the treating doctor's orders and established a submissible case of medical negligence against the hospital. It was established that, following bilateral knee replacement surgery, the action of nurses caused permanent drop foot to the patient. They failed to follow the doctor's *verbal orders* to watch the patient closely and to place him in one continuous passive motion machine at a time during physical therapy.

FAILURE TO RECORD PATIENT'S CARE

Contrary to the contention of a medical center, there was sufficient evidence at trial from which a jury could rationally conclude that the center departed from accepted medical and nursing practice in the administration of an intramuscular injection. The conflicting testimony of the parties and their medical experts presented issues of credibility to be resolved by the jury, which had the opportunity to observe and assess the witnesses and the evidence.[26]

The plaintiff in *Pellerin v. Humedicenters, Inc.,*[27] went to the emergency department at Lakeland Medical Center complaining of chest pain. An emergency department physician, Dr. Gruner, examined her and ordered a nurse to give her an injection consisting of 50 mg of Demerol and 25 mg of Vistaril. Although the nurse testified she did not recall giving the injection, she did not deny giving it, and her initials are present in the emergency department record. The nurse admitted that she failed to record the site and mode of injection in the emergency department records. She said she may have written this information in the nurse's notes, but no such notes were admitted into evidence.

The plaintiff testified that she felt pain and a burning sensation in her hip during the injection. The burning persisted afterward and progressively worsened over the next several weeks. The pain spread to an area approximately 10 inches in diameter around the injection site. She could not sleep on her right side, work, perform household chores, or participate in sports without experiencing pain. She also testified that she had a lump around the injection site and that her skin was numb in that area.

The appeals court found that there was sufficient evidence to support a jury finding that the nurse had breached the applicable standard of care in administering an injection of Vistaril into Pellerin's hip. The jury awarded the plaintiff $90,304.68 in total damages. The nurse admitted that she failed to record the site and mode of injection in the emergency department records. According to the testimony of two experts in nursing practice, failing to record this information is below the standard of care for nursing. Although these omissions could not have affected the administration of the injection, they tend to indicate that in this instance the nurse did not follow accepted procedure while performing her job.

FAILURE TO IDENTIFY CORRECT PATIENT

The plaintiff in *Meena v. Wilburn,*[28] injured her leg and developed an ulcer because of poor blood circulation. Due to the plaintiff's diabetic condition, the ulcer did not heal. Dr. Maples, a vascular surgeon, performed surgery. Two days following surgery, Dr. Meena was at the hospital covering for one of his partners, Dr. Petro, who had asked him to remove the staples from one of his patients, 65-year-old Slaughter. Slaughter shared a semiprivate room with the plaintiff. Meena testified that he went and picked up Slaughter's chart at the nurse's desk and asked one of the nurses which bed Slaughter was in. Meena claimed that he was led to believe that she was in the bed next to the window. He picked up the chart and asked Greer, a nurse, to accompany him to the plaintiff's room. Shortly thereafter, Meena received an emergency call at the nursing station. He said that he asked Greer to take out the staples, because he had to respond to an emergency call at another hospital. Greer conceded during her testimony that, before removing staples from a patient, a nurse should read the chart, be familiar with the chart, look at the patient's wrist band, and compare the arm band to the chart—all of which she failed to do. Greer rationalized her failure: "When the doctor I work for is standing at the foot of a patient's bed, I would have no doubt—no reason to doubt what he tells me to do."

Greer began to remove the plaintiff's staples. She soon realized that there was a problem. The plaintiff's skin split open, revealing the layer of fat under the skin. Greer stopped the procedure and left the room to check the medical records maintained at the nursing station. She realized that she had removed staples from the wrong patient. At that point, she encountered Maples and explained to him what had happened. Maples immediately restapled the skin.

Following discharge, the plaintiff's health began to falter and she developed a fever of 101°F. The tissue where the staples had been removed became infected. The plaintiff was ultimately readmitted to the hospital; she remained there for approximately 22 days. Her condition gradually improved and, presumably, she had recovered completely with the exception of some scarring and skin indention.

A complaint was filed against Meena and Greer. After four days of trial, the jury returned a verdict against Meena and assessed damages in the amount of $125,000. The jury declined to hold the nurse liable for the plaintiff's injuries. Meena appealed claiming that the jury's exoneration of the nurse, who removed the surgical staples, was grounds for a new trial on the issue of the physician's liability. Further, Meena argued the jury was bound to return a verdict against both defendants, inasmuch as the defendants were sued as joint tort-feasors. The Mississippi Supreme Court held that the jury's exoneration of Greer was not grounds for a new trial on the issue of the physician's liability.

This case was settled in 1992. In light of the Joint Commission's present day national patient safety goal requiring two forms of patient identification prior to rendering care or treatment, explain how the patient's injury might have been avoided (see Chapter 23).

BURNS

The negligent use of a Bovie plate led to liability in *Monk v. Doctors Hospital,*[29] in which a nurse had been instructed by the physician to set up a Bovie machine. The nurse placed the contact plate of the Bovie machine under the patient's right calf in a negligent manner and the patient suffered burns. The patient introduced instruction manuals, issued by the manufacturer, supporting a claim that the plate was placed improperly. These manuals had been available to the hospital. The trial court directed a verdict in favor of the hospital and the physician. The appellate court found that there was sufficient evidence from which the jury could conclude that the Bovie plate was applied in a negligent manner. There was also sufficient evidence, including the manufacturer's manual and expert testimony, from which the jury could find that the physician was independently negligent.

INFECTIONS

Failure to follow proper infection-control procedures (e.g., proper hand-washing techniques) can result in cross-contamination between patients, staff, and visitors. Staff members who administer to patients, moving from one patient to another, must wash their hands after changing dressings and carrying out routine procedures.

Cross-Contamination

The patient in *Helmann v. Sacred Heart Hospital*[30] was returned to his room following hip surgery. The patient's roommate complained of a boil under his right arm. A culture was taken of drainage from the wound and was identified as *Staphylococcus aureus.* The infected roommate was transferred immediately to an isolation room. Until this time, hospital employees administered to both patients regularly, moving from one patient to another without washing their hands as they changed dressings and carried out routine procedures. On the day the roommate was placed in isolation, the plaintiff's wound erupted, discharging a large amount of purulent drainage. A culture of the drainage showed it to have been caused by the presence of *Staphylococcus aureus*. The infection penetrated into the patient's hip socket, destroying tissue and requiring a second operation. The court ruled that there was sufficient circumstantial evidence from which the jury could have found that the patients were infected with the same *Staphylococcus aureus* strain and that the infection was caused by the hospital's employees' failure to follow sterile techniques in ministering to its two patients.

Failure to Notify Physician

The failure of nurses to follow adequate nursing procedures in treating decubitus ulcers was found to be a factor leading to the death of a nursing facility resident in *Montgomery Health Care v. Ballard*.[31] Two nurses testified that they did not know that decubitus ulcers could be life threatening. One nurse testified that she did not know that the patient's physician should be called if there were symptoms of infection. Such allegations would indicate that there was a lack of training and supervision of the nurses treating the patient. The seriousness of such failure was driven home when the court allowed $2 million in punitive damages.

INAPPROPRIATE CARE

The plaintiffs in *Morris v. Children's Hospital Medical Center*[32] alleged in their complaint that, while hospitalized at Children's Hospital Medical Center, the patient suffered a laceration to her arm as a result of treatment administered by the defendants and their agents that fell below the accepted standard of care. Morris alleged from personal observation that the laceration to her daughter's arm was caused by the jagged edges of a plastic cup that had been split and placed on her arm to guard an IV site. A nurse, in her affidavit, who stated her qualifications as an expert, expressed her opinion that the practice of placing a split plastic cup over an IV site as a guard constituted a breach of the standard of nursing care.

DELAY IN TREATMENT

On the morning of March 27, Howerton, in *Howerton v. Mary Immaculate Hospital, Inc.*,[33] was the only patient in the labor and delivery room. Dr. O'Connell, Howerton's obstetrician, directed hospital nurses to administer Pitocin (a drug to induce labor) to Howerton. When O'Connell examined her at 2:25 P.M., she thought that Howerton was in the early stages of labor and directed that Pitocin be continued. She did not expect Howerton's cervix to be sufficiently dilated for delivery for some time and left the hospital. At 3:00 P.M., Howerton testified that she experienced intense abdominal pains. Mr. Howerton went to the nurses' station and told the nurses that his wife was in severe pain. He was told that it would take a few minutes because the nurses were in the middle of a shift change. Later, Howerton's mother went to the nurses' station and stated that her daughter needed help now. She received the same response from the nurses. Two of the nurses finally came to the room at 3:15 P.M. after Howerton's father demanded that they do so. There was a further delay in contacting the doctor because one nurse suggested they not call the doctor yet. Then, at 3:23 P.M., another nurse, who disagreed with the first nurse, paged O'Connell. When the doctor answered the emergency page at 3:25 P.M., she was advised that the undelivered baby's heart rate was in the 60s to 70s (a normal heart rate being from 120 to 160) and that the mother was having abdominal pain. O'Connell, driving to the hospital, called the labor room at 3:30 P.M. and learned that the baby's heart rate remained in the 60s to 70s. O'Connell was able to deliver Howerton's daughter Kacie by C-section at 3:55 P.M. After Kacie's delivery, it was discovered that the mother's uterus had ruptured in three places during labor, resulting in extensive neurological damage to Kacie.

At trial, Holder, a nurse expert witness, opined that the labor and delivery room nurses should have immediately gone to Howerton when they were notified of the worsening pain, evaluated her condition, and notified her physician.

Dr. Juskevitch, who testified as an expert witness, stated that the intensity of labor pains prior to delivery of the baby could indicate a ruptured uterus or a separation of the placenta. A reasonably prudent physician should be prepared to perform any necessary C-section within 30 minutes of being informed of such complaints. Juskevitch also testified that Howerton's complaints of pain indicated that there was a rupture or tearing of the uterus that occurred at 3:00 P.M. Juskevitch opined that these knife-like instances of pain were associated with episodes of increased tearing. Juskevitch explained that these instances of tearing presented challenges to the unborn baby, which began when the first tear occurred at 3:00 P.M., and were evident at 3:17 P.M. when the nurses went into the room, and realized that the baby's heart rate was erratic. If these progressive tears had not ruptured the blood vessels from which the unborn baby received its necessary oxygen through the blood flowing through the mother's uterus to the placenta and from it to the baby, Juskevitch did not think that the baby would have suffered neurological damage provided it was delivered promptly after the tearing occurred.

Juskevitch opined that if O'Connell had been informed at 3:09 P.M., the baby should and would have been delivered by 3:39 P.M. Because O'Connell was not advised by the nurses of the change in the mother's condition until 3:25 P.M., the baby was not delivered until 3:55 P.M., 30 minutes after O'Connell responded to the delayed page.

This delayed delivery took place 46 minutes after the doctor should have been called at 3:09 P.M. and 16 minutes after the baby would have been delivered at 3:39 P.M., had the doctor been called at 3:09 P.M. According to Dr. White, a child neurologist called as an expert witness by the plaintiff, if the baby had been delivered 15 minutes before 3:55 P.M., or by 3:40 P.M., she would have sustained no neurological damage.

When the jury was unable to agree upon a verdict following deliberation for over two days, the court discharged the jury, declared a mistrial, and, after additional argument, finally struck the plaintiffs' evidence and entered summary judgment for the defendant, and the plaintiffs appealed.

The plaintiffs contend that their evidence was sufficient to show that the nurses were negligent in their delayed response and that this negligence was the proximate cause of Kacie's neurological disabilities. The defendant argued that the plaintiffs' evidence was insufficient to establish that such negligence was the proximate cause of the injuries sustained.

To support that claim, the defendant argued that even if the nurses were negligent between 3:00 and 3:11, there was no evidence that, had the necessary information been communicated to a reasonably prudent obstetrician during that period, anything he or she would or should have done would have changed the result to Kacie. The court did not agree with the defendant.

The defendant sought to confine the crucial period of its negligence to an 11-minute period, overlooking evidence in the record from which a jury could have found that its negligence extended over the 25-minute period before the nurses informed O'Connell of the mother's change of condition. The jury could have found that this 25-minute period, when combined with the 30-minute period it took O'Connell to deliver Kacie after the 25-minute delayed notification, effectively destroyed Kacie's chances of being delivered without neurological damage.

This was because White opined that the neurological damage to Kacie occurred 15 minutes before her birth at 3:55 P.M. and that no such damage would have occurred if Kacie had been delivered 16 minutes earlier, or by 3:39 P.M. Thus, the jury could have found that had O'Connell been notified by 3:09 P.M., she would have delivered Kacie without neurological damage by 3:39 P.M. Evidence was sufficient to raise a jury issue regarding the nurses' negligence and whether such negligence proximately caused Kacie's injuries. Judgment in favor of the defendant was reversed, and the case was remanded for a new trial.

FAILURE TO FOLLOW INSTRUCTIONS

Failure of a nurse to follow the instructions of a supervising nurse to wait for her assistance before performing a procedure can result in the revocation of the nurse's license. The nurse in *Cafiero v. North Carolina Board of Nursing*[34] failed to heed instructions to wait for assistance before connecting a heart monitor to an infant. The heart monitor was connected incorrectly and resulted in an electrical shock to the infant. The board of nursing, under the nursing practice act, revoked the nurse's license. The board had the authority to revoke the nurse's license even though her work before and after the incident had been exemplary. The dangers of electric cords are within the realm of common knowledge. The record showed that the nurse failed to exercise ordinary care in connecting the infant to the monitor.

TWO STANDARDS: WHICH IS RIGHT?

Given two standards of care, should a hospital adopt the least restrictive standard? This generally would not be a good idea. For example, in *Edwards v. Brandywine Hosp.,*[35] the plaintiff/appellant, Mr. Edwards, went to the emergency department complaining of pain in his hip. He was admitted and a heparin lock (a device that allows multiple IV fluids to be introduced at a common point) was placed in his left hand. The heparin lock was left in place for three or four days. This was in violation of regulations promulgated by the Pennsylvania Department of Health requiring hospitals to develop written standards regarding such antiseptic practices as changing IV catheter sites. The regulations state that these standards should comply with standards described in the American Hospital Association's publication entitled *Infection Control in the Hospital* (1979), which recommends that IV catheter sites be changed every 48 hours in order to reduce the risk of infection. The hospital was subject to corporate liability for adopting a 72-hour rule.

Following discharge, Edwards noticed a red spot at the site of the heparin lock. He returned that day to the hospital for physical therapy. His therapist referred him to the emergency department for evaluation. The emergency department physician examined Edward's hand and took a specimen of pus from the site of the heparin lock and sent it to the laboratory for evaluation. Edwards was provided with oral antibiotics and sent home. The laboratory results showed that Edwards had a staphylococcus infection. The emergency department physician entered this information on the patient's record.

Edwards returned to the hospital a few days later and was admitted with leg pains. A second laboratory test was ordered, which again showed the presence of a staph infection. The patient was treated over a period of time with

IV antibiotics and eventually discharged with a good bill of health, only to return a week later with pain and a fever. Following treatment and various hospitalizations over the next several years, Edwards's physicians decided to remove his artificial hip and treat him with massive doses of antibiotics. In order to be ambulatory, Edwards now needs the aid of assistive devices (e.g., crutches).

A suit was brought against the physicians and hospital. The trial court took notice of the health department's regulation regarding catheter site changing and ruled that the hospital's admitted failure to move the heparin lock for at least three days constituted negligence per se. The physicians settled with the plaintiff, leaving the hospital as the only defendant. At the close of the plaintiff's case, the trial court granted the defendant's motion for a directed verdict. The trial court held that although the negligence per se ruling established the hospital's breach of a duty to care, the plaintiff could not prove causation.

> The court reasoned that to establish legal causation, Edwards had to prove that staphylococcus bacteria entered his body at the heparin lock site at least 48 hours after the lock was installed, because it was only after 48 hours that the hospital became negligent in not moving the catheter. The court held that there is simply no evidence as to when this organism entered Edwards even if I did assume that it did enter through the heparin lock site. The jury would have to speculate as to when the organism entered the body and this I would not permit.[36]

The superior court reversed the trial court's directed verdict for the defendant, finding that the evidence presented at trial by the plaintiff was sufficient to allow the claim of causation to go to the jury. Evidence included:

1. failure to change placement of the catheter within 48 hours
2. testimony from an infectious diseases expert who testified to the same causal relationship
3. a discharge report that noted Mr. Edwards's staph infection was thought to be secondary to an abscess at the heparin lock site

The kind of causation evidence the trial court expects cannot be produced. No witness could possibly testify that she saw a *Staphylococcus aureas* bacterium crawl into Mr. Edwards's hand through the heparin lock site on his third day in the hospital and then multiply into the infection that spread to his artificial hip—yet the trial court's ruling implied that such showing was necessary to get to the jury.

Once a plaintiff has introduced evidence that a defendant's negligent act or omission increased the risk of harm to a person in the plaintiff's position, and that harm in fact

was sustained, it becomes a question for the jury as to whether or not that increased risk was a substantial factor in producing the harm.

Is there an issue of corporate negligence? Yes. The plaintiff claimed that the hospital was subject to corporate liability for adopting a 72-hour rule for changing placement of IV catheters. The plaintiff introduced evidence showing that a 48-hour rule was appropriate, but that the hospital adopted a rule allowing IVs to remain in place at the same site for 72 hours. If Edwards could prove that the 72-hour rule was inadequate, that the hospital should have known that it was inadequate, and that following this rule caused him harm, then he has made a proper claim for corporate negligence.

Should the nurse have been faulted for following hospital policy? No. A nurse following hospital rules cannot be faulted. If hospital policy required changing the site of the catheter every 48 hours and the nurse failed to do so, then the nurse could be held negligent and the hospital liable under the theory of respondeat superior.

When faced with the dilemma of two standards for rendering patient care, an organization may find it more attractive to adopt the one that is least restrictive or labor intensive. This could prove to be a costly decision for both the patient and the organization by increasing (1) the risk of patient injury and (2) the organization's exposure to corporate liability for any injury suffered from following the less restrictive standard.

FAILURE TO MONITOR VITAL SIGNS

In *McCann v. ABC Insurance Co.,*[37] an attempt to deliver a baby by forceps was unsuccessful. The obstetrician, Dr. Merrill, testified that he listened to the baby's heart tone immediately after the failed forceps delivery and the baby's heart rate was normal. The baby was then delivered by cesarean section. At birth the baby was not breathing and had no detectable heartbeat. The baby was resuscitated and transferred to another hospital where he was in a clinically brain-dead state within 24 hours. Evidence at trial established that during delivery the baby suffered a severe hypoxic event that caused the death. The plaintiffs instituted a lawsuit against the obstetrician; the hospital and the trial court granted a motion for a directed verdict at the end of the trial, dismissed Merrill, and an appeal was taken.

The plaintiffs' cause of action was dependent upon whether the plaintiffs could show that Merrill or the hospital was negligent in failing to timely diagnose the existence of the hypoxic event. The sole claim against Merrill was the allegation that he failed to properly monitor the baby's heartbeat or make sure that the nurse properly monitored the baby's heartbeat after the fetal monitor had been removed. Evidence presented indicated that the standard of care would require that fetal heartbeats be monitored every 10 minutes following removal of the fetal monitor. The evidence presented indicated that this did not occur. Both the defendants' and plaintiffs' medical experts agreed that Merrill did not breach the standard of care required in treating McCann. The plaintiffs' expert testified by deposition that the duty to monitor was a nursing responsibility.

Testimony was needed to show that Merrill breached the standard of care required in treating McCann. Because the plaintiffs failed to provide such testimony, the trial court was found to have correctly granted the directed verdict.

> Plaintiffs' cause of action against . . . Hospital was predicated primarily upon its failure to have policies and procedures regarding the continuous monitoring of fetal heart tones and its failure to adequately and continuously monitor the unborn infant. The basic thrust of the case was that none of the parties auscultated the baby every 10 minutes after the fetal monitoring device was removed, as required by the standards of the American College of Obstetrics and Gynecology (ACOG). Thus the issue in this case is not whether the baby would have died from other causes even if the Caesarean section had been performed faster, but rather the issue is whether the baby had lost a chance of survival . . . [Because] the nurses' negligent inaction has terminated any chance of survival, conjecture as to other possible causes of death is inadmissible.[38]

⚖ FAILURE TO REPEAT VITAL SIGNS

Citation: *Porter v. Lima Mem'l Hosp.*, 995 F.2d 629 (6th Cir. 1993)

Facts

During an automobile accident, Liesl, an infant, was thrown to the floor of her mother's car. Rescue squad personnel examined the infant and found nothing seriously wrong. Liesl was transported with her mother, Mrs. Porter, to Hospital A's emergency department. Ogelsbee, an RN, took Liesl's vital signs and recorded them on the medical chart. She reported the vital signs to Dr. Singh, the emergency room physician on duty. The only observable sign of injury was a small bruise on the right side of Liesl's head. Ogelsbee reported this to Singh, who found all of Liesl's extremities functioning normally and ordered several laboratory tests and X-rays. He did not, however order any spinal X-rays and failed to diagnose spinal instability. Ogelsbee did not repeat the vital signs during or after Singh's examination, claiming that she received no physician's instruction in this regard. After reviewing the X-rays and laboratory tests, Singh discharged Liesl and provided her mother with written instructions concerning her head injuries.

While awaiting a ride home, Liesl's mother reported a short period of irregular breathing by Liesl to one of the nurses. The nurse examined Liesl and determined that nothing was wrong. Porter testified that the nurse told her that "babies just breathe funny." When she reached home, Porter noted that Liesl's condition was worsening. She then decided to take Liesl to Hospital B, where physicians determined that Liesl's legs were not moving. They ordered X-rays and laboratory tests, and eventually another hospital staff physician diagnosed a subluxation at her first and second lumbar vertebrae, which resulted in Liesl's paralysis from the waist down. Experts who testified in trial agreed that Liesl suffered paralysis sometime after Singh's examination and before her arrival at Hospital B.

Singh was the primary person who could have prevented the spinal injury by diagnosing Liesl's unstable spine before it became critically injured. Singh settled for $2.5 million. The district court denied the hospital's motion for judgment, notwithstanding the verdict in favor of the mother, but ordered a new trial at which the jury found the hospital not liable for the infant's injuries. Both the hospital and the mother appealed.

Issue

Did the Lima nurses' conduct proximately cause the infant's paralysis?

Holding

The U.S. Court of Appeals for the Sixth Circuit held that the nurses' failure to repeat vital signs was legally insufficient to establish a connection between the failure to repeat vital signs and the eventual paralysis.

Reason

The experts on both sides generally agreed that the nurses had no independent duty, apart from a physician's instructions, to immobilize the infant. The plaintiff's experts made it clear that the physician is ultimately responsible for determining the patient's medical diagnosis and then to order the necessary and appropriate medical treatment. Singh did not diagnose any spinal cord injury and discharged the baby after examining and X-raying the infant. It was Singh who was responsible for treating Liesl's spinal cord injury, or at least he was responsible for ordering Liesl to be immobilized and hospitalized for further care and workup. The vital signs had no causal relationship to the paralysis.

Discussion

1. Discuss the importance of patient assessment and documentation.
2. Discuss the importance of collaboration of the transporting ambulance crew with the receiving hospital's nurses and physicians.

FAILURE TO REPORT PHYSICIAN NEGLIGENCE

An organization can be liable for failure of nursing personnel to take appropriate action when a patient's personal physician is clearly unwilling or unable to cope with a situation that threatens the life or health of the patient. In a California case, *Goff v. Doctors General Hospital*,[39] a patient was bleeding seriously after childbirth because the physician failed to suture her properly. The nurses testified that they were aware of the patient's dangerous condition and that the physician was not present in the hospital. Both nurses knew the patient would die if nothing was done, but neither contacted anyone except the physician. The hospital was liable for the nurses' negligence in failing to notify their supervisors of the serious condition that caused the patient's death. Evidence was sufficient to sustain the finding that the nurses who attended the patient and who were aware of the excessive bleeding were negligent and that their negligence

was a contributing cause of the patient's death. The measure of duty of the hospital toward its patients is the exercise of that degree of care used by hospitals generally. The court held that nurses who knew that a woman they were attending was bleeding excessively were negligent in failing to report the circumstances so that prompt and adequate measures could be taken to safeguard her life.

FAILURE TO QUESTION DISCHARGE

A nurse has a duty to question the discharge of a patient if he or she has reason to believe that such discharge could be injurious to the health of the patient. Jury issues were raised in *Koeniguer v. Eckrich*[40] by expert testimony that the nurses had a duty to attempt to delay the patient's discharge if her condition warranted continued hospitalization. By permissible inferences from the evidence, the delay in treatment that resulted from the premature discharge contributed to the patient's death. Summary dismissal of this case against the hospital by a trial court was found to have been improper.

SWOLLEN BEYOND RECOGNITION

Citation: *NKC Hosps., Inc. v. Anthony*, 849 S.W.2d 564 (Ky. Ct. App. 1993)

Facts

Mrs. Anthony was in her first pregnancy under the primary care of Dr. Hawkins, her personal physician. Anthony was in good health, 26 years of age, employed, and about 30 weeks along in her pregnancy. On September 5, 1989, Anthony's husband took her to the emergency department of Norton Hospital. She was experiencing nausea, vomiting, and abdominal pain. Because of her pregnancy, she was referred to the hospital's obstetrical unit. In the obstetrical unit, Anthony came under the immediate care of Moore, a nurse, who performed an assessment.

Hawkins was called and she issued several orders, including an IV start, blood work, urinalysis, and an antinausea prescription. Later that night, a second call was made to Hawkins, giving her the test results and informing her that the patient was in extreme pain. Believing that Anthony had a urinary tract infection, antibiotics were ordered along with an order for her discharge from the hospital.

That same night a third call was made to Hawkins because of the pain Anthony was experiencing, as observed by Moore. Mr. Anthony also talked with Hawkins about his wife's pain. Moore became concerned about Hawkins's discharge order. Although aware of Moore's evaluation, Hawkins prescribed morphine sulfate but was unrelenting in her order of discharge.

Love, the resident physician on duty, did not see or examine the patient, although a prescription for morphine was ordered and administered pursuant to the telephoned directions of Hawkins. At approximately 2:00 A.M., the morphine was administered to Anthony. She rested comfortably for several hours, but awakened in pain again. At 6:00 A.M., the patient was discharged in pain.

During trial testimony, Hale, a nursing supervisor, admitted that it was a deviation from the standard of nursing care to discharge a patient in significant pain. Moore, who was always concerned with the patient's pain, had grave reservations about her discharge. She suggested that Love examine Anthony. She even consulted her supervisor, Nurse Hale.

At approximately 10:00 A.M., Anthony was readmitted to the hospital. Upon readmission, Hawkins began personal supervision of her patient. It was determined that Anthony had a serious respiratory problem. The next day the patient was transferred to the hospital's intensive care unit (ICU).

The following day, the baby was delivered by cesarean section. It was belatedly determined at that time that Anthony's condition was caused by a perforation of the appendix at the large bowel, a condition not detected by anyone at the hospital during her first admission. Almost three weeks later, while still in Norton Hospital, Anthony died of acute adult respiratory distress syndrome, a complication resulting from the delay in the diagnosis and treatment of her appendicitis.

Judgment was brought against the hospital. At trial, Dr. Fields, an expert witness for the estate of Anthony, testified that the hospital deviated from the standard of care. Every patient who presents herself to the labor and delivery area, the emergency department, or any area of the hospital should be seen by a physician before anything is undertaken, and certainly before she is allowed to leave the institution. Further, to provide the patient with medication in the form of a prescription without the physician ever seeing the patient was below any standard of care with which Fields was acquainted. An award of more than $2 million was returned, with the apportionment of causation attributable to Hawkins as 65 percent and to the hospital as 35 percent. The hospital argued that the trial court erred in failing to grant its motions for directed verdict and for judgment notwithstanding the verdict because of the lack of substantial causation in linking the negligence of the hospital to Anthony's death.

Issue

Was the negligence of the hospital superseded by the negligence of the patient's primary care physician, and was the award excessive?

Holding

The Kentucky Court of Appeals held that negligence of the hospital was not superseded by the negligence of the patient's primary care physician, and that the award for pain and suffering was not excessive.

Reason

The hospital's negligence is based on acts of omission, by failing to have Mrs. Anthony examined by a physician and by discharging her in pain. The hospital should have foreseen the injury to Anthony because its own staff was questioning the judgments of Hawkins while at the same time failing to follow through with the standard of care required of it. The defense that the hospital's nurses were only following a "chain of command" by doing what

Hawkins ordered is not persuasive. The nurses were not the agents of Hawkins. All involved had their independent duty to Anthony.

The evidence presented a woman conscious of her last days on earth, swollen beyond recognition, tubes exiting almost every orifice of her body, in severe pain, and who deteriorated to the point where she could not verbally communicate with loved ones. Among the last things she did was write out instructions about the care for her newborn child. The trial court, when confronted with a motion for a new trial on excessive damages, must evaluate the award mirrored against the facts. It is said, if the trial judge does not blush, the award is not excessive. No question, the award was monumental, but so was the injury.

Discussion

1. Was Dr. Hawkins's "telephone" assessment of the patient appropriate?

2. How would you apportion negligence among the attending physician, resident, obstetrical nurse, nursing supervisor, and hospital?

3. What are the lessons that should be learned from this case?

4. What educational issues are apparent?

FAILURE TO NOTE CHANGES IN PATIENT'S CONDITION

Nurses have the responsibility to observe the condition of patients under their care and report any pertinent findings to the attending physician. Failure to note changes in a patient's condition can lead to liability on the part of the nurse and the organization. The recovery room nurse in *Eyoma v. Falco,*[41] who had been assigned to monitor a postsurgical patient, left the patient and failed to recognize that the patient stopped breathing. Nurse Falco had been assigned to monitor the patient in the recovery room. She delegated that duty to another nurse and failed to verify that another nurse accepted that responsibility.

Nurse Falco admitted she never got a verbal response from the other nurse, and when she returned there was no one near the decedent. She acknowledged that Dr. Brotherton told her to watch the decedent's breathing, but claimed she was not told that decedent had been given narcotics. She maintained that upon her return she checked the decedent and observed his respirations to be eight per minute.

Thereafter, Brotherton returned and inquired about the decedent's condition. Falco informed the doctor that the patient was fine. However, upon his personal observation, Brotherton realized that the decedent had stopped breathing.

• • • •

Decedent, because of oxygen deprivation, entered a comatose state and remained unconscious for over a year until his death.[42]

The jury held the nurse to be 100 percent liable for the patient's injuries. The court held that there was sufficient evidence to support the verdict.

PROMPT NOTIFICATION REQUIRED

In *Cuervo v. Mercy Hospital, Inc.,*[43] Cuervo was admitted to Mercy Hospital by Dr. Iglesias to undergo routine diagnostic cardiac tests. Iglesias had surgical privileges at Mercy Hospital and was authorized to perform a cardiac catheterization. After performing the catheterization on Cuervo, Iglesias decided to perform a balloon angioplasty procedure; Iglesias was not authorized to perform this procedure. Unfortunately, in carrying out this procedure, Iglesias inserted the catheter into the wrong artery in Cuervo's right leg. This compromised the blood flow to the leg, causing loss of pulse and sensation. This error was compounded when Mercy Hospital's nurses on Cuervo's floor were unable to reach Iglesias for six hours and never attempted to reach Dr. Milian, the backup physician, to alert them of Cuervo's deteriorating condition.

The following day, Dr. Pena attempted an arteriogram to treat the right leg. Regrettably, Pena accessed the wrong artery in the left leg, compromising the blood flow to that leg as well. Shortly thereafter, Cuervo began to lose pulse and sensation in his left leg. The hospital's nurses never reported this condition to the physicians. Sometime later, Milian performed surgery to attempt to restore circulation to the right leg; the surgery was unsuccessful. Two hours later, surgery was performed on the left leg; the surgery failed to restore circulation to that leg. Thereafter, both legs required amputation.

Cuervo sued the physicians and hospital, asserting that the hospital was negligent based on the nurses' failure to promptly notify a physician of his condition, and asserting corporate negligence against the hospital based on the unauthorized procedure. Cuervo's experts testified at deposition that except for the nursing staff's failure to contact a physician when the symptoms were first detected, the amputations would not have been necessary. Relying on the same experts' testimony, the hospital filed a motion for summary judgment, asserting that any acts or omissions of its nurses were not the proximate cause of Cuervo's injuries, and that the allegations in support of the corporate negligence count were also not the legal cause of Cuervo's injuries. The hospital's motion for summary judgment did not raise any issue as to whether the hospital breached its duty to Cuervo by allowing a medical doctor to perform unauthorized procedures or by failing to provide adequate nursing care. The hospital's motion solely disputed causation. The court granted the motion and entered final summary judgment in the hospital's favor.

On appeal, the court determined that when both parties to a lawsuit rely on testimony from the same experts and then draw diametrically opposed conclusions, the jury should be given opportunity to weigh the evidence and determine whether the hospital's conduct was the proximate cause of the patient's injuries. The case was remanded for trial by jury.

FAILURE TO REPORT DETERIORATING CONDITION

An organization's policies and procedures should prescribe the guidelines for staff members to follow when confronted with a physician or other health care professional whose action or inaction jeopardizes the well-being of a patient. Guidelines in place, but not followed, are of no value, as the following cases illustrate. Such was the case in *Goff v. Doctors General Hospital,*[44] in which the court held that nurses who knew that a woman they were attending was bleeding excessively were negligent in failing to report the circumstances so that prompt and adequate measures could be taken to safeguard her life.

The plaintiff in *Utter v. United Hospital Center, Inc.*[45] suffered an amputation that the jury determined resulted from the failure of the nursing staff to properly report the patient's deteriorating condition. The nursing staff, according to written procedures in the nursing manual, was responsible for reporting such changes. It was determined that deviation from hospital policy constituted negligence.

FAILURE TO REPORT PATIENT SYMPTOMS

In *Citizens Hospital Association v. Schoulin,*[46] an accident victim sued the hospital and the attending physician for their negligence in failing to discover and properly treat his injuries. The court held that there was sufficient evidence to sustain a jury verdict that the hospital's nurse was negligent in failing to inform the physician of all the patient's symptoms, to conduct a proper examination of the plaintiff, and

to follow the directions of the physician. Thus, as the nurse was the employee of the hospital, the hospital was liable under the doctrine of respondeat superior.

TIMELY REPORTING OF PATIENT SYMPTOMS

In *Hiatt v. Grace,*[47] on appeal by the hospital and the nurse, the Kansas Supreme Court held that there was sufficient evidence to authorize the jury to find that the nurse was negligent in failing to timely notify the physician that delivery of the plaintiff's child was imminent. This delay resulted in an unattended childbirth with consequent injuries. The trial court had awarded the plaintiff $15,000.

FAILURE TO REPORT DEFECTIVE EQUIPMENT

Failure to report defective equipment can cause a nurse to be held liable for negligence if the failure to report is the proximate cause of a patient's injuries. The defect must be known and not hidden from sight.

FAILURE TO CORRECTLY TRANSCRIBE TELEPHONE ORDERS

Failure to take correct telephone orders can be just as serious as failure to follow, understand, and/or interpret a physician's order(s). Nurses must be alert in transcribing orders because there are periodic contradictions between what physicians claim they ordered and what nurses allege they ordered. Orders should be read back, once transcribed, for verification purposes. Verification of an order by another nurse on a second telephone is helpful, especially if an order is questionable. Any questionable orders must be verified with the physician initiating the order. Physicians must authenticate their verbal order(s) by signing the written order in the medical record. Nurses who disagree with a physician's order should not carry out an obviously erroneous order. In addition, they should confirm the order with the prescribing physician and report to the supervisor any concerns they may have with a particular order.

SWITCHING OF INFANTS

The inadvertent or negligent switching of infants can lead to liability for damages. Damages in the amount of $110,000 were awarded for the inadvertent switching of two babies born at the same time in *De Leon Lopez v. Corporacion Insular de Seguros.*[48]

PATIENT FALLS

Patients are highly susceptible to falling, and the consequences of falling are generally more serious with older age groups. Among senior citizens, falls represent the fifth leading cause of death, and the mortality rate from falls increases significantly with age. For those aged 75 years and older, the mortality rate from falls is five times higher than for those in the 65- to 74-year age group, and the rate increases such that persons older than 80 years have an even greater chance of experiencing a fatal fall.

RESTRAINTS

Standards for the application of both physical and chemical restraints have been evolving over the past decade, and they are becoming more stringent. Because of patient rights issues, injuries, and the improper and indiscreet use of restraints, organizations are attempting to develop restraint-free environments.

Failure to Follow Policy

The plaintiffs, in *Estate of Hendrickson v. Genesis Health Venture, Inc.,*[49] filed an action for negligence, breach of contract, and negligent infliction of emotional distress against Genesis ElderCare Network Services, Inc. (GENS), among others.

Hendrickson suffered a massive stroke while she was a patient at a hospital in the summer of 1996. The stroke left her totally dependent on others for her daily care. During one of her admissions to Salisbury Center, a nursing home, operated by the defendant GENS, Ferguson went into Hendrickson's room while making rounds and found Hendrickson dead, her head wedged between the mattress and the adjacent bed rail.

A jury found that Hendrickson's death was caused by negligence. On appeal, GENS argued that the plaintiff failed to show that it knew or should have known of the risk of injury to Hendrickson from the side rails. The North Carolina Court of Appeals disagreed, finding there was evidence tending to show that nursing assistants employed by GENS were aware that Hendrickson, on several occasions before her death on October 30, had slid to the edge of the bed and became caught between the edge of the mattress and the bed rail. Plaintiffs offered evidence showing that GENS had a restraint policy in effect that required a restraint assessment form for any resident for whom the use of restraints was required. The nursing staff was required to document the effectiveness of less restrictive measures. The assessment was required to be reviewed by a restraint alternative team/committee. Evidence was offered showing that no restraint assessment form had been completed for Hendrickson. In addition, her medical records contained no nursing notes documenting the use of less restrictive measures than the bed rails. The defendant argued that the bed rails were required for positioning and safety and were not restraints, so that no restraint assessment was required. While the evidence was conflicting as to whether the bed rails were used as a restraint or as a safety measure, evidence indicated that the rails should have been considered a restraint in connection with Hendrickson's care, as per organization policy.

The court of appeals concluded that the plaintiffs offered sufficient evidence to sustain a finding by the jury that defendant GENS was negligent in failing to conform to its own policies with respect to the use of physical restraints and that such negligence was the proximate cause of Hendrickson's death.

Failure to Raise Bed Rails

The plaintiff in *Polonsky v. Union Hospital*[50] suffered a fall and fractured her hip after the administration of a sleeping medication commonly known by the trade name Dalmane. The superior court awarded damages in the amount of the statutory limit of $20,000, and the hospital appealed. The appeals court held that from the Dalmane warning provided by the drug manufacturer and the hospital's own regulation regarding bedside rails, without additional medical testimony, the jury could draw an inference that the hospital's nurse failed to exercise due care when she failed to raise the bed rails after administering Dalmane.

Patient Fall: Safe Procedures Followed

The fall of a patient is not always attributable to negligence. The New York Court of Appeals held that the evidence in *Stoker v. Tarentino*[51] did not support discipline of a nurse on a charge that a wheelchair resident was improperly left alone in the bathroom. The negligence charge against the petitioner was predicated on a wheelchair resident having been left alone in the bathroom after the petitioner assisted another nurse in moving the resident from the bed to the wheelchair to the bathroom. All the nurses who testified agreed that there was no order, written or verbal, requiring the nurse to remain with the resident while she was in the bathroom. Policies and procedures of the nursing facility and the health department contained no instructions concerning toilet procedures with respect to wheelchair residents. The court held that disciplinary action against the nurse should be annulled and expunged from the petitioner's personnel file.

Fall from Examination Table

A judgment for the plaintiff was affirmed in *Petry v. Nassau Hospital,*[52] which was an action to recover damages for personal injuries suffered by the plaintiff's wife. The patient had been placed on a narrow examination table in the emergency department of the defendant hospital and fell from the table. The table had no side rails in place to protect the patient from falling and the patient had been left unattended by the nurse in charge.

NEGLIGENT CARE

Bradshaw, in *Brandon HMA, Inc. v. Bradshaw*,[53] had been admitted to Rankin Medical Center (RMC) under the care of Dr. Bobo for treatment of bacterial pneumonia. She was prescribed oxygen and various medications. A general surgeon inserted a chest tube in Bradshaw's left side to drain some fluid that accumulated. Due to the pain and discomfort associated with a chest tube, Extra Strength Tylenol and Lorcet Plus were prescribed for pain. Bobo also prescribed Ativan to relieve anxiety. During the afternoon and evening following insertion of the chest tube, two nurses periodically checked Bradshaw, took her vital signs, and noted that she exhibited "no distress." Around 11:00 P.M., Lewis, an LPN, was assigned by Nail, the floor's charge nurse, to provide care to Bradshaw. Before checking on Bradshaw, Lewis reviewed the notes and a tape left by the previous nurse that detailed Bradshaw's condition. Around midnight, Lewis made his first visit to Bradshaw's room, took her vital signs, and noted she was experiencing some pain on her left side. Sometime before 1:00 A.M., a respiratory therapist checked on Bradshaw and did not notice any problems, but did note that Bradshaw was restless. Shortly after, at 1:00 A.M., Lewis made his second visit to Bradshaw's room. She continued to complain of pain in her chest. Lewis, however, did not take her vital signs. He gave her an Extra Strength Tylenol and made a note indicating that the patient was complaining of pain on the left side and appeared to be in distress. At 2:00 A.M. during Lewis's next visit, Bradshaw again complained that she could not sleep and that the pain had increased. Despite her complaints, Lewis again failed to take her vital signs. Instead, he consulted Nail and administered an injection of Ativan to relieve Bradshaw's anxiety and restlessness. Forty minutes later, Bradshaw again complained of increased pain. Lewis noticed that she was sitting up in bed and her respiration had become short and rapid. Feeling that the earlier Lorcet Plus was wearing off, Lewis administered another dose. Lewis again failed to check Bradshaw's vital signs.

Nail, while in Bradshaw's room at 3:00 A.M., did not note any problems. When Lewis returned to Bradshaw's room at 3:30 A.M., her condition had significantly worsened. She was nauseous, disoriented, covered in sweat, and did not follow verbal commands. Lewis checked her vital signs and found her temperature had fallen to 95.8 degrees. Realizing the seriousness of Bradshaw's condition, Lewis left the room to find Nail. At this point, testimony among RMC's employees varies. Lewis and Washington, a nurses' aide, testified that Lewis found Nail and Washington conversing in the hallway. According to the two testimonies, Nail and Lewis discussed Bradshaw's condition and returned to the room at 3:40 A.M.

When Lewis and Nail returned to the room, they found Bradshaw was cyanotic, had stopped breathing, and had no pulse. Nail called a "code" and started cardiopulmonary resuscitation (CPR). The code team arrived and revived Bradshaw by administering epinephrine. Bradshaw was transferred to ICU where she remained comatose for two weeks. She was eventually transferred to a rehabilitation center for treatment. While in treatment, MRIs of Bradshaw's brain were ordered and showed evidence of brain damage due to lack of oxygen. Bradshaw's present condition as a result of the cardiopulmonary arrest and hypoxic brain damage is permanent and severe. She has significant difficulty in moving due to rigidity in her muscles and is prone to bouts of spasms. Bradshaw cannot walk without assistance and often falls due to a lack of stability. She is unable to perform many daily activities without the aid of her mother or someone else, including dressing, brushing her teeth, driving a car, and going to the bathroom.

Bradshaw filed suit against Brandon HMA, Inc., for negligent nursing care. Bradshaw alleged that nursing personnel failed to properly monitor her, report vital information to her physician, and allowed her condition to deteriorate to a critical stage before providing urgently needed care and implementing life support. The jury found in favor of Bradshaw and awarded $9 million in damages. The judge entered a final judgment on the jury verdict and Brandon filed an appeal.

On appeal, the Supreme Court of Mississippi upheld the judgment of the circuit court. The court found that $9 million did not seem excessive. Bradshaw will live out her years with both emotional and physical pain, and her present existence will not remotely resemble her former life.

SURGERY: FOREIGN OBJECTS LEFT IN PATIENTS

There are many cases involving foreign objects left in patients during surgery. The hospital in *Ross v. Chatham County Hospital Authority*[54] was properly denied summary dismissal of an action in which a patient sought to recover damages for injuries suffered when a surgical instrument was left in the patient's abdomen during surgery. This incident occurred as a result of the failure of the operating room personnel to conduct an instrument and sponge count after surgery. The borrowed servant doctrine did not insulate the hospital from the negligence of its nurses because the doctrine applies only to acts involving professional skill and judgment. Foreign objects negligently left in a patient's body constitute an administrative act. A standard nursing check-off procedure should be used to account for all sponges and/or instruments used in the operating room. Preventative measures of this nature will reduce a hospital's risk of liability.

The decedent's estate in *Holger v. Irish*[55] sued the surgeon and the hospital that employed the nurses who assisted the surgeon during the operation performed upon the deceased. During the course of performing colon surgery, the surgeon placed laparotomy sponges in the decedent's abdomen. After he had removed the sponges at the end of surgery, the two nurses assisting him counted them and verified that they had all been removed. Two years later, a sponge was discovered in the patient's abdomen. It was removed, and the 92-year-old patient died. The jury decided in favor of the defendants, and the decedent's estate appealed. The court of appeals reversed, and the Oregon Supreme Court reviewed the case.

The Oregon Supreme Court held that the surgeon was not vicariously liable, as a matter of law, for the negligence of the operating room nurses. There was no evidence presented that the nurses were the defendants' employees or that they were under the supervision or control of the defendant regarding their counting of the sponges. It was their sole responsibility to count the sponges. The nurses had been hired and trained by the hospital, which paid for their services.

Nurses and Surgeons Responsible for Sponge Counts

Romero v. Bellina[56] describes how both nurses and surgeons are responsible for sponge counts. Bellina performed laser surgery on Romero at the hospital. During surgery, Bellina was assisted by Markey and Toups, surgical nurses employed by the hospital. Before the final suturing of the incision, the nurses erroneously informed Bellina that all the lap pads had been accounted for.

The day after the procedure, Romero complained of severe abdominal pain. A few months later, she discovered a mass in her abdomen near the area where the surgery was performed. She visited her treating physician, Dr. Blue, who determined through an X-ray that the mass in her abdomen was a lap sponge from the surgery with Bellina. Romero underwent corrective surgery with a different physician to remove the sponge.

The plaintiffs settled their claims with the hospital, and the case proceeded to trial against Bellin. After a bench trial, the trial court rendered judgment in favor of the plaintiffs for $170,966.41, and Bellina filed an appeal.

In ruling against Bellina, the trial court held that a surgeon's duty to remove foreign objects placed in a patient's body is an independent, nondelegable duty. The trial court found that Bellina was 70 percent at fault and the nurses employed by the hospital were 30 percent at fault. On appeal, Bellina argued that the trial judge erred in concluding that, in Louisiana, a surgeon cannot rely on surgical nurses to count sponges to make

sure none are left inside a patient. Prevailing case law, in Louisiana, however, holds that a surgeon has a nondelegable duty to remove all sponges placed in a patient's body.

The Louisiana Court of Appeals held that although nurses have an independent duty, apart from the surgeon's duty, to account for the sponges, and that they can be concurrently at fault with the surgeon for leaving a sponge in the patient's body, the nurses' count is a remedial measure that cannot relieve the surgeon of his or her nondelegable duty to remove the sponge in the first instance. Bellina had an independent, nondelegable duty to remove from the patient's body the foreign substance that he had placed into her.

Current jurisprudence more accurately reflects the modern team approach to surgery, whereby the nurses' count is a remedial measure that does not discharge the surgeon's independent duty to ensure that all sponges are removed before an incision is closed.

The lesson in this case illustrates the importance of building redundancy in the delivery of health care to protect patients from harm. The responsibility of accounting for sponges, instruments, and other foreign objects lies with both the surgeon and nurse, and in some instances, the operating room technician. Even though some jurisdictions may free the surgeon of such responsibility, organizations should adopt a higher standard, assigning responsibility to both the nurse and surgeon and, where applicable, the operating room technician.

IMPROPER STERILIZATION

The patient in *Howard v. Alexandria Hosp.*[57] brought a medical malpractice action against the hospital, seeking damages arising out of an operation performed with unsterile instruments. During her stay in the recovery room, the operating surgeon reported to the patient that she had been operated on with unsterile instruments. Allegedly, the nurse in charge of the autoclave used to sterilize the instruments did not properly monitor the sterilization process. Because of the patient's fear of a variety of diseases, she was administered several human immunodeficiency virus tests. The patient was evaluated by an infectious disease specialist and was administered antibiotics intravenously. Following her discharge, the patient was placed on several medications and, as a result, developed symptoms of pseudomembranous enterocolitis. Testimony described the patient's symptoms as resulting from the administration of the antibiotics. One expert testified that the patient had reason to be concerned for at least six months following the surgical procedure because of her risk of being infected with a variety of diseases. The hospital argued that the patient suffered no physical injury from the surgical procedure and the instruments utilized during the procedure. The circuit court entered summary judgment for the hospital on the grounds that no physical injury had been shown.

The Virginia Supreme Court held that the patient suffered injury resulting from measures taken to avoid infection following discovery of the use of unsterile instrumentation, even though the patient did not sustain any infection from use of the instruments. The case was reversed and remanded for a new trial on all issues.

Injury can be either physical or mental. It is clear that because of the hospital's use of inadequately sterilized instruments, the plaintiff sustained positive physical and mental injury. As the direct result of the wrong, IV tubes and needles invaded the plaintiff's body. She experienced physical pain and the discomforts of headache, nausea, vomiting, fever, chills, and unusual sweating.

NEGLIGENT PROCEDURE/ CUTTING AN IV TUBE

A nurse employed by the defendant in *Ahmed v. Children's Hospital of Buffalo*[58] amputated nearly one third of a one-month-old infant's index finger while cutting an IV tube with a pair of scissors. Surgery to reattach the amputated portion of the finger was unsuccessful. The plaintiffs were awarded $87,000 for past pain and suffering and $50,000 for future damages. The defendant moved to set aside the verdict and sought a new trial, claiming that damages were excessive. The trial court rejected much of the testimony presented by the plaintiffs.

An appeals court determined that it was the jury's function to assess the credibility of witnesses and to evaluate the testimony regarding the child's pain, suffering, and disability. The trial court was found to have improperly invaded the jury's province to evaluate the nature and extent of the injury. The appellate court found that the jury's award of damages did not deviate materially from what would be reasonable compensation. The jury's verdict was reinstated.

MONITOR ALARM DISCONNECTED

In *Odom v. State Department of Health and Hospitals,*[59] the appeals court held that the decedent's cause of death was directly related to the absence of being placed under the watch of a heart monitor. Jojo was born 12 weeks prematurely at the HPL Medical Center. Jojo remained in a premature infant's nursery and was eventually placed into two different foster homes prior to his admission to Pinecrest foster home. While Jojo was a Pinecrest resident, Mr. and Mrs. Odom adopted Jojo. He was unable to feed himself and was nourished via a gastrostomy tube. Because he suffered from obstructive apnea, he became dependent on a trach tube.

At Pinecrest, Jojo was assigned to Home 501. While making patient rounds, Ms. Means found Jojo with his trach out of the stoma. She called for help and Ms. Wiley, amongst others, responded. Wiley immediately took the CPR efforts under her control. She noticed that Jojo was breathless and immediately reinserted the trach. She then noticed that Jojo was still hooked to a monitor.

No one had heard the heart monitor's alarm sound. Means asserts that the monitor was on, because she saw that the monitor's red lights were blinking, indicating the heart rate and breathing rate. She stated that she took the monitor's leads off of Jojo to put the monitor out of the way, but the alarm did not sound. CPR efforts continued while Jojo was placed on a stretcher and sent by ambulance to HPL. Jojo was pronounced dead at HPL's emergency department at 7:02 P.M.

The Odoms filed a petition against Pinecrest, alleging that Jojo's death was caused by the negligence and fault of Pinecrest, its servants, and employees. Judgment was for the plaintiffs. The trial court's reasons for judgment was enlightening because it stated that the monitor should have been on but was, however, disconnected by the staff and this was the cause, in fact, of Jojo's injury. The appeals court found that the record supported the trial court's findings. There was overwhelming evidence upon which the trial court relied to find that the monitor was turned off, in breach of the various physicians' orders with which the nurses should have complied. The monitor was supposed to be on Jojo to warn the nurses of any respiratory distress episodes that he might experience. A forensic pathologist's report showed the cause of Jojo's death to be hypoxia, secondary to respiratory insufficiency, secondary to apnea episodes. Thus, Jojo's cause of death was directly related to the absence of being placed under the watch of a heart monitor.

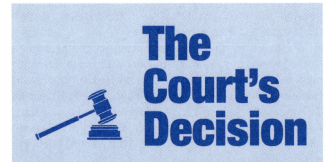

The Court's Decision

The court concluded there was ample evidence to support the trial judge's conclusion that the nursing staff breached the standard of care. Testimony indicated that Ard would have had a much better chance of survival if he had been transferred to the intensive care unit. The court raised the general damages award from $50,000 to $150,000.

CHAPTER REVIEW

1. Most states have similar definitions of nursing, but each state has its own individual *nurse practice act,* which defines the practice of nursing and outlines a nurse's authority to act in that state. The *scope of practice* defines the actions, duties, and limits of various health care professionals.

2. The nurse licensure process differs slightly from state to state, but each requires that an applicant receive formal professional training and pass a written examination.

3. The four basic methods by which boards license out-of state nurses are *reciprocity, endorsement, waiver,* and *examination.*

4. There are several positions for which nurses who have undergone the requisite training and certification can enjoy expanded roles. These include a:

   - *nurse anesthetist*—an RN who administers anesthesia

   - *clinical nurse specialist*—an RN with an advanced academic degree, experience, and expertise in a clinical specialty (e.g., obstetrics, pediatrics, psychiatry)

   - *nurse practitioner*—an RN who has completed the necessary education to engage in primary health care decision making

   - *nurse midwife*—an RN who provides comprehensive prenatal care including delivery for patients who are at low risk for complications

5. Among the common acts for which nurses can be found negligent include improper or inappropriate administration of medications, negligent injections, failure to follow a physician's orders, departure from acceptable practice, burns, infections, inappropriate care, delay in treatment, failure to follow instructions, failure to monitor vital signs, failure to report physician concerns, failure to question discharge, failure to note changes in a patient's condition, failure to report a patient's deteriorating condition, failure to report patient symptoms, failure to report defective equipment, failure to correctly transcribe telephone orders, infant mix-ups, patient falls, restraints, improper sterilization, and disconnecting monitor alarms.

REVIEW QUESTIONS

1. Describe how the scope of nursing is changing.
2. Describe how the roles of a nurse anesthetist, clinical nurse specialist, nurse practitioner, and nurse midwife differ.
3. Describe the various medication errors that can occur in the administration of medications.
4. If a nurse disagrees with a physician's written orders, discuss what action the nurse should take to protect the patient's safety.
5. Discuss why it is important to report significant changes in a patient's condition to the treating physician.
6. If a nurse knows that a piece of equipment is defective, should the nurse attempt to fix the problem? Discuss your answer.

NOTES

1. *Ard v. East Jefferson Gen. Hosp.,* 636 So. 2d 1042 (La. Ct. App. 1994).
2. *MNA Position Statement: Professional Relationships and Boundaries in Nursing Practice,* MNA Ethics Committee, June 3, 1996, Minnesota Nurses Association 9/98. www.mnnurses.org/index.asp?Type=B_BASIC &SEC=%7B33640DA6-C53B-454C-B408-2F195C79C3D2%7D.
3. 692 S.W.2d 329 (Mo. Ct. App. 1985).
4. E. SPALDING, PROFESSIONAL NURSING: TRENDS/RESPONSIBILITIES/ RELATIONSHIPS 351 (1959).
5. 824 N.E.2d 1151; 2005 (Ill. App. 2005).
6. 801 A.2d 775 (Ct. 2002).
7. 570 N.Y.S.2d 395 (N.Y. App. Div. 1991).
8. *Moon Lake Convalescent Center v. Margolis,* 535 N.E.2d 956 (Ill. App. Ct. 1989).
9. 428 S.E.2d 773 (W. Va. 1993).

10. *Id.* at 779.

11. 502 So. 2d 1198 (Miss. 1987).

12. 519 N.Y.S.2d 738 (N.Y. App. Div. 1987).

13. No. 1030422 (Supreme Court of Alabama 2005).

14. 357 N.Y.S.2d 508 (N.Y. App. Div. 1974).

15. No. 2-153/01-1019 (Iowa Ct. of App. 2002).

16. 696 P.2d 270 (Colo. 1985).

17. 28 N.E.2d 772 (Ohio 1940).

18. 144 So. 2d 249 (La. Ct. App. 1962).

19. 599 N.Y.S.2d 96 (N.Y. App. Div. 1993).

20. 742 P.2d 1087 (Okla. 1987).

21. 145 So. 2d 848 (Fla. 1933).

22. 181 A.2d 573 (Del. 1962).

23. 443 P.2d 708 (Colo. 1968).

24. *Kitchen v. Wickliffe Country Place,* No. 2000-L-051 (Ohio App. 11th 2001).

25. 165 S.W.3d 168 (Mo. App. 2005).

26. *Crockett v. Long Beach Medical Center,* No. 2003-04715 (N.Y. 2005).

27. 696 So. 2d 590 (La. App. 1997).

28. 603 So. 2d 866 (Miss. 1992).

29. 403 F.2d 580 (D.C. Cir. 1968).

30. 381 P.2d 605 (Wash. 1963).

31. 565 So. 2d 221 (Ala. 1990).

32. 597 N.E.2d 1110 (Ohio Ct. App. 1991).

33. 264 Va. 272, 563 S.E.2d 671 (2002).

34. 403 S.E.2d 582 (N.C. Ct. App. 1991).

35. 652 A.2d 1382 (Pa. Super. 1995).

36. *Id.* at 1385.

37. 640 So. 2d 865 (La. App. 4 Cir. 1994).

38. *Id.* at 872.

39. 333 P.2d 29 (Cal. Ct. App. 1958).

40. 422 N.W.2d 600 (S.D. 1988).

41. 589 A.2d 653 (N.J. Super. App. Div. 1991).

42. *Id.* at 655.

43. 694 So. 2d 98 (Fla. App. 1997).

44. 333 P.2d 29 (Cal. Ct. App. 1958).

45. 236 S.E.2d 213 (W. Va. 1977).

46. 262 So. 2d 303 (Ala. 1972).

47. 523 P.2d 320 (Kan. 1974).

48. 931 F.2d 116 (1st Cir. 1991).

49. 151 N.C. App. 139, 565 S.E.2d 254 (2002).

50. 418 N.E.2d 620 (Mass. App. Ct. 1981).

51. 478 N.E.2d 184 (N.Y. 1985).

52. 48 N.Y.S.2d 227 (N.Y. App. Div. 1944).

53. 809 So. 2d 611 (2001).

54. 367 S.E.2d 793 (Ga. 1988).

55. 851 P.2d 1122 (Or. 1993).

56. 798 So. 2d 279 (2001).

57. 429 S.E.2d 22 (Va. 1993).

58. 661 N.Y.S.2d 164 (N.Y. App. Div. 1997).

59. 733 So. 2d 91 (La. App. 3 Cir. 1999).

Liability by Departments and Health Care Professionals

It's Your Gavel ...

*DYING AT THE HOSPITAL'S DOOR: A CHILD LOST, TROUBLING QUESTIONS

While communications were breaking down among a child's parent, a 9-1-1 dispatcher, and hospital personnel, the child's condition was quickly deteriorating. Twelve hours later, the three year-old girl was brain dead, and she expired three days later. Although there are several central issues involved in this story, the frustrating dialogue that took place is particularly important.

The 9-1-1 dispatcher answers the phone.

Dispatcher: 9-1-1; is this an emergency?

Parent: Yes, it's an emergency. I need an ambulance. I have a 3-year-old daughter that's passed out on me.

Dispatcher: OK. Where do you need the ambulance?

Parent: I'm right in front of the emergency exit in . . . Hospital.

Dispatcher: You're right in front of the emergency exit?

Parent: Yes, that's exactly where I am. And they won't do a . . . thing in this place.

The dispatcher phones the hospital emergency department:

Dispatcher: There's a guy that says he's right outside your emergency exit. And he needs an ambulance. He says his 3-year-old daughter is passed out.

Hospital: This is a guy who wants to be seen quicker. We're busy—so he figured if he called 9-1-1 he'd be seen quicker.

Dispatcher: Well, he's saying he needs an ambulance right away. Is somebody going to go out there, or not?

Hospital: There's nothing we can do.[1]

WHAT IS YOUR VERDICT?

*MIAMI HERALD, April 16, 1995 by RONNIE GREEN. Copyright 1995 by MIAMI HERALD. Reproduced with permission of MIAMI HERALD in the format Textbook via Copyright Clearance Center.

This chapter presents an overview of selected departments and health care professions. Although it describes a variety of legal issues, there is no intensive review of any specific department or profession. Many of the cases presented in this chapter could have been discussed in more than one chapter. However, they were placed here to illustrate that no health care profession is exempt from the long arm of the legal system. Health care professionals are held to the prevailing standard of care required in their profession, which includes proper assessments, reassessments, diagnosis, treatment, and follow-up care.

Table 10-1 illustrates the number of malpractice reports by practitioner reported to the National Practitioner Data Bank for the years 1990–2005. The cases that follow illustrate a variety of acts or failures to act that have led to lawsuits.

CHIROPRACTOR

A chiropractor is required to exercise the same degree of care, judgment, and skill exercised by other reasonable chi-

TABLE 10-1 National Practitioner Data Bank, 2005 Annual Report

Practitioners with Reports
National Practitioner Data Bank (September 1, 1990–December 31, 2005)

Practitioner Type	Number of Practitioners with Reports	Number of Reports*	Reports per Practitioner
Acupuncturists	91	94	1.03
Chiropractors	6,359	7,896	1.24
Counselors	606	673	1.11
Dental assistants, technicians, hygienists	30	30	1.00
Dentists and dental residents	30,299	49,933	1.65
Denturists	10	10	1.00
Dieticians	9	9	1.00
Emergency medical practitioners	126	128	1.02
Homeopaths and naturopaths	11	11	1.00
Medical assistants	26	28	1.08
Nurses and nursing-related practitioners	19,918	21,125	1.06
Occupational therapists and related practitioners	70	72	1.03
Optical-related practitioners	618	741	1.20
Pharmacists and pharmacy assistants	2,457	2,810	1.14
Physical therapists and related practitioners	832	868	1.04
Physician assistants	1,132	1,267	1.12
Physicians (M.D., D.O., and interns and residents)	157,914	291,185	1.84
Podiatrists and podiatric-related practitioners	4,121	6,955	1.69
Prosthetists	5	5	1.00
Psychiatric technicians and aides	8	9	1.13
Psychology-related practitioners	1,243	1,540	1.24
Respiratory therapists and related practitioners	37	38	1.03
Social workers	185	202	1.09
Speech and language-related practitioners	45	49	1.09
Technologists	170	174	1.02
Other health care practitioners	8	8	1.00
Other individuals	12	14	1.17
Unspecified or unknown	325	336	1.03
All types	**226,667**	**386,210**	**1.70**

This table includes only disclosable reports in the NPDB as of the end of the current year. Voided reports have been excluded.
*"Number of Reports" include medical malpractice payment reports, adverse state licensure action reports, clinical privileges reports, professional society membership reports, drug enforcement administration reports, and Medicare/Medicaid exclusion reports. Only physicians and dentists are reported for adverse licensure, clinical privilege, and professional society actions.

ropractors under like or similar circumstances. He or she has a duty to determine whether a patient is treatable through chiropractic means and to refrain from chiropractic treatment when a reasonable chiropractor would or should be aware that a patient's condition will not respond to chiropractic treatment. Failure to conform to the standard of care can result in liability for any injuries suffered.

Immoral Conduct

The chief medical officer of the Nebraska Department of Health and Human Services Regulation and Licensure entered an order revoking Poor's license to practice as a chiropractor in the state of Nebraska.[2] Poor engaged in a conspiracy to manufacture and distribute a misbranded substance, and he introduced into interstate commerce misbranded and adulterated drugs with the intent to defraud and mislead. He was arrested for driving under the influence and was convicted of that offense. In addition, Poor knowingly possessed cocaine. He conceded that these factual determinations were understood as beyond dispute.

Both the district and appellate courts found that Poor's conduct was clearly immoral. The appellate court stated that Poor's denial now, after taking advantage of a plea bargain, that he committed any of the acts he admitted to in the U.S. district court is disturbing and is not consistent with the integrity expected by persons engaged in a professional occupation.

The Supreme Court of Nebraska determined that the seriousness of Poor's felony conviction and its underlying conduct, his subsequent lack of candor with respect to that conduct, as well as his lack of sound judgment demonstrated by his driving-under-the-influence conviction, concluded that revocation of Poor's license was an appropriate sanction.

DENTISTRY

Dental malpractice cases are generally related to patients who suffer from complications of a dental procedure. They can involve the improper treatment of dental infections or complications from the improper administration of anesthesia. Complications can also include damage to the nerves of the lower jaw, face, chin, lips, and tongue. Injuries can involve high-speed drills damaging the tongue and result in permanent loss of sensation or taste.

Drill Bit Left in Tooth

The patient, in *Mazor v. Isaacman*,[3] visited the defendant-dentist in August 1997 for routine root canal surgery. After the surgery, the patient began experiencing constant pain in the tooth in which the root canal was performed. The dentist told the patient that such pain was ordinarily felt after root canal surgery. In February 1999, the patient visited another dentist who discovered that a piece of a drill bit had been left inside the patient's tooth during the previous root canal. The patient filed a lawsuit against the defendant-dentist for dental malpractice. The defendant-dentist filed a motion to dismiss, arguing that the patient did not bring the claim within the one-year statute of limitations. This motion was granted and the patient appealed. The Tennessee Court of Appeals reversed the finding, holding that the patient had one year from the time she discovered or should have discovered the foreign object in which to file her lawsuit.

Tennessee Code Annotated § 29-26-116(a)(4) (2000) states that "where a foreign object has been negligently left in a patient's body . . . the action shall be commenced within one (1) year after the alleged injury or wrongful act is discovered or should have been discovered." This statute has been interpreted to require only that the plaintiff bring the action within one year after the foreign object was discovered or should have been discovered.

Failure to Refer

Dr. Smith told O'Neal that tooth number 14, an upper left molar, should be extracted. O'Neal advised Smith that another dentist warned her that tooth number 14 should not be pulled because it was embedded in the sinus. Smith responded that all of her top teeth were in the sinus and that extraction was no problem. O'Neal relented to Smith's judgment and tooth number 14 was extracted. Complications developed in the extraction process, resulting in an oral antral perforation of the sinus cavity wall. Four days after the extraction, Smith began root canal work, even though the antral opening wound was not healed. Three weeks after the extraction, a tissue mass developed in the tooth socket and the patient was referred to Dr. Herbert, an oral surgeon.

Herbert testified that the degree of infection inhibited proper healing and closure of the extraction site. After several more months, O'Neal was referred to Dr. Berman, an ear, nose, and throat specialist. Because of the continual deterioration, Berman performed a surgical procedure that sealed the extraction site. The surgery required hospitalization.

O'Neal brought a malpractice action against Smith.[4] The trial court entered judgment in favor of O'Neal. Smith appealed, arguing that the evidence was factually insufficient to support the judgment.

An expert witness testified that Smith was negligent for not referring the patient to an oral surgeon for the necessary extraction because of the known risks of roots embedded in the sinus floor. Smith was also negligent for not referring the patient to a specialist when the antral perforation first occurred and later by not referring her to a specialist when the fistula and the infection manifested itself. Expert testimony was found sufficient to support a jury finding that the defendant was negligent in the treatment of his patient.

Lack of Consent

The plaintiff in *Gaskin v. Goldwasser*[5] brought a suit against an oral surgeon, alleging dental malpractice. The oral surgeon had removed 19 of the teeth remaining in the plaintiff's mouth. The defendant admitted that 5 of the 19 teeth were removed without the consent of the patient. The circuit court entered a judgment for the plaintiff on a jury verdict for damages resulting from the extraction of the five lower teeth. On appeal, the appellate court held that the patient was entitled to have the allegation of willful and wanton misconduct and battery for unauthorized removal of the lower teeth submitted to the jury. The case was remanded for a new trial.

Failure to Prescribe Antibiotics

In *Pasquale v. Miller,*[6] the plaintiff brought a suit against the defendant, Dr. Miller, for dental malpractice. Miller treated the plaintiff for swollen gums. He removed tissue from the patient's gums and used sutures to control the bleeding. Although it was common practice to prescribe antibiotics prior to or following gum surgery, Miller failed to prescribe antibiotics in either case. The following May, after the plaintiff experienced a persistent fever, she was diagnosed as having contracted subacute bacterial endocarditis. The plaintiff was treated in the hospital for nearly a month. Miller claimed that the bacterial infection could have resulted from a number of causes. The trial court, upon a jury verdict, found for the plaintiff. An appeals court held that the evidence supported a finding of causation.

The plaintiff's expert witnesses testified that her endocarditis was related to the dental surgery and that one of the risks of not prescribing an antibiotic is that bacteria can flow through the bloodstream to the heart. The jury rejected testimony from Miller that endocarditis could have been caused by something other than failure to administer antibiotics prior to or following gum surgery.

Infection Control: Failure to Wear Protective Gloves

In *Kirschner v. Mills,*[7] there was sufficient evidence to support a charge that the dentist failed to wear protective gloves while performing a medical examination. That charge was supported by testimony of the patient, whom a hearing panel found to be credible, that the dentist did not wear gloves during the examination. The violation of accepted practice was also supported by the testimony of the dentist's own expert, a dentist, who opined that it was necessary to wear gloves any time you put your hands on a patient.

Practicing Outside Scope of Practice

Brown, in *Brown v. Belinfante,*[8] sued Dr. Belinfante and the Atlanta Orthofacial Surgicenter, LLC, after Belinfante performed several elective cosmetic procedures including a face lift, eyelid revision, and facial laser resurfacing. Belinfante is not a physician. He is licensed to practice dentistry in Georgia and was employed by the Surgicenter. Brown claims that after the cosmetic procedures, she could not close her eyes completely, developed chronic bilateral eye infections, and required remedial corrective surgery. Among other things, Brown alleged that Belinfante's performance of the cosmetic procedures constituted negligence per se because he exceeded the scope of the practice of dentistry.

The Georgia Court of Appeals held that cosmetic procedures of this nature do not fall within Georgia statutes. The primary purposes of the Georgia Dental Act are to define and regulate the practice of dentistry. The statute limits the scope of the practice of dentistry. Such limitation protects the health and welfare of patients who submit themselves to the care of dentists by guarding against injuries caused by inadequate care or by unauthorized individuals. Brown falls within that class of persons that the statute was intended to protect, and the harm complained of was of the type the statute was intended to guard against. In performing the elective cosmetic procedures, Belinfante violated the Dental Practice Act by exceeding the statutory limits of the scope of dentistry and therefore, committed negligence per se.

Dental Hygienist Administers Nitrous Oxide

A dental hygienist alleged that her employer-defendant allowed dental hygienists to administer nitrous oxide to patients. Under state law, dental hygienists may not administer nitrous oxide. The Department of Education's Office of Professional Discipline investigated the complaint by using an undercover investigator. The investigator made an appointment for teeth cleaning. At the time of her appointment, she requested that nitrous oxide be administered. Agreeing to the investigator's request, the dental hygienist administered the nitrous oxide. There were no notations in the patient's chart indicating that she had been administered nitrous oxide.

A hearing panel found the dental hygienist guilty of administering nitrous oxide without being properly licensed. In addition, the hearing panel found that the dental hygienist had failed to accurately record in the patient's chart that she administered nitrous oxide.

The New York Supreme Court, Appellate Division, held that the investigator's report provided sufficient evidence to support the hearing panel's determination. There is adequate evidence in the record to support a finding that the dentist's conduct was such that it could reasonably be said that he permitted the dental hygienist to perform acts that she was not licensed to perform.[9]

Failure to Supervise Dental Assistant

The plaintiff in *Hickman v. Sexton Dental Clinic*[10] brought a malpractice action against a dental clinic for a serious cut under her tongue. The dental assistant, without being supervised by a dentist, placed a sharp object into the patient's mouth, cutting her tongue while taking impressions for dentures. The court of common pleas entered a judgment on a jury verdict in favor of the plaintiff, and the clinic appealed. The court of appeals held that evidence presented was sufficient to infer without the aid of expert testimony that there was a breach of duty to the patient. The testimony of Dr. Tepper, the clinic dentist, was found pertinent to the issue of the common knowledge exception in which the evidence permits the jury to recognize breach of duty without the aid of expert testimony. Tepper presented the following testimony regarding denture impressions[11]:

Q. You also stated that you have taken, I believe, thousands?

A. Probably more than that.

Q. Of impressions?

A. Yes, sir.

Q. This never happened before?

A. No, sir, not a laceration.

Q. Would it be safe and accurate to say that if someone's mouth were to be cut during the impression process, someone did something wrong?

A. Yes, sir.

EMERGENCY DEPARTMENT

The courts recognize a general duty to care for all patients presenting themselves to hospital emergency departments. Not only must hospitals accept, treat, and transfer emergency department patients if such is necessary for the patients' well-being, but they must adhere to the standards of care they have set for themselves, as well as to national standards.

Hospitals under the Emergency Medical Treatment and Labor Act are required to provide either stabilizing treatment or appropriate transfer for patients with emergency medical conditions.

Emergency departments are high-risk areas that tend to be a main source of lawsuits for hospitals. Results of the Harvard Medical Practice Study revealed that the hospital emergency department is "a real hot spot" for negligence.[12] In this study, 70 percent of adverse events occurring in the emergency department were because of negligence. Hospital emergency departments heavily used by patients as primary care clinics are a major source of adverse events because of poor follow-up care. Suits that end up in a courtroom are few in comparison to the out-of-court settlements.

Both federal and state regulations, as well as the standards set by The Joint Commission, may be considered by the courts in finding a duty of hospital emergency departments to provide emergency care to those who present themselves with the need for such care.

Objectives of Emergency Care

The objectives of emergency care are the same regardless of severity. No matter how seemingly trivial the complaint, each patient must be examined. Treatment must begin as rapidly as possible, function is to be maintained or restored, scarring and deformity are to be minimized, and so forth. Every patient must be treated regardless of ability to pay.

As the Sixth Circuit points out, there are many reasons other than indigence that might lead a hospital to give less than standard attention to a person who arrives at the emergency room doors. These might include: prejudice against the race, sex, or ethnic group of the patient; distaste for the patient's condition (e.g., acquired immune deficiency syndrome [AIDS] patients); personal dislike or antagonism between medical personnel and the patient; disapproval of the patient's occupation; or political or cultural opposition. If a hospital refuses treatment to persons for any of these reasons, or gives cursory treatment, the evil inflicted would be quite akin to that discussed by Congress in the legislative history, and the patient would fall squarely in the statutory language.[13]

Emergency Department: No Duty to Patient Who Left

The chairman of the emergency department at University Hospitals of Cleveland, after reviewing the patient's medical records and consultation with Robinson Memorial Hospital (RMH), told the patient that he would only authorize the same tests already performed at RMH. He then told the patient that he would admit her to the hospital's mental health unit. The patient and her sister became upset and left the hospital and went home without proper discharge. The patient died two days later at home. The county coroner's office initiated a postmortem examination and determined that the patient died from meningoencephalitis. The patient made a conscious decision to leave the hospital on her own accord without the knowledge or permission of the hospital. She did not tell the doctors, nurses, or anyone else that she was leaving the emergency room; she just left the emergency room without informing anyone.

In a wrongful death medical malpractice action alleging negligence, the trial court properly granted summary judgment because under Ohio law, an emergency room nurse had no duty to interfere with an individual who left the emergency room without telling anyone and who refused treatment. A physician, nurse, or hospital commits a battery by treating a patient without the patient's consent. Under Ohio law, medical diagnoses, care, and treatment are beyond the scope of the nursing practice, and the evaluation of a patient's capacity to give consent is made by a doctor, not by a nurse.[14]

Failure to Admit

Roy went to the emergency department complaining of chest pains. The attending physician, Dr. Gupta, upon examination, determined that Roy exhibited normal vital signs. She showed no obvious physical abnormalities. Gupta performed an electrocardiogram that showed ischemic changes indicating a lack of oxygen to the heart tissue. He applied a transdermal nitroglycerin patch and gave her a prescription for nitroglycerin. After monitoring her progress, he sent her home. Several hours later, she returned to the emergency department, experiencing more chest pains. She was admitted to the hospital, and it was determined that she was having a heart attack. Three days later, Roy died of a massive myocardial infarction.

Gupta was found negligent in failing to hospitalize Roy or failing to inform her of the serious nature of her illness. The trial court found that had Roy been hospitalized on her first visit, her chances of survival would have been increased.

The Louisiana Court of Appeal held that Gupta was negligent by failing to advise Roy that she should be hospitalized for chest pains. All of the medical expert witnesses, except Dr. Kilpatrick, a defense witness, testified that Roy should have been admitted. Kilpatrick testified that such a decision varied greatly among physicians. The trial court disregarded his testimony because of his hostile responses to questioning.

The trial judge was not convinced by Gupta's explanation of why Roy was not hospitalized. He focused on Gupta's failure to have X-rays taken during the first visit, which might have allowed him to determine whether the ischemic changes were due to her hypertension medication or indicated the beginning of a heart attack. The relative simplicity of the technique and its obvious availability lent credence to the trial judge's belief that the requisite attention was not paid to Roy's complaints. The law does not require proof that proper

treatment would have been the difference between Roy's living or dying. It requires only proof that proper treatment would have increased her chances of survival.[15]

Documentation Sparse and Contradictory

An ambulance team found 26-year-old Feeney intoxicated, sitting on a street corner in South Boston. Feeney admitted to alcohol abuse but denied that he used drugs. He was physically and verbally combative, and he had trouble walking and speaking intelligibly. His condition interfered with conducting an examination, and he was transported by ambulance to the hospital.

Documentation at the hospital between 10:45 P.M. and 11:30 P.M. was sparse and contradictory. The minimum standard for nursing care required monitoring the patient's respiratory rate every 15 minutes. It was doubtful that this occurred. This monitoring would have more likely permitted the nursing staff to observe changes in the patient's breathing patterns and/or the onset of respiratory arrest. The emergency department physician failed to evaluate the patient and to initiate care within the first few minutes of Feeney's entry into the emergency facility. The emergency physician had an obligation to determine who was waiting for physician care and how critical the need was for that care. Had the standards been maintained, respiratory arrest might have been averted. According to the autopsy report, respiratory arrest was the sole cause of death.

The failure to provide adequate care rationally could be attributed to the staff nurse assigned to the area in which the patient lay, as well as to the physicians in charge. The hospital was implicated on the basis of the acts or omission of its staff.[16]

EMERGENCY MEDICAL TREATMENT UNDER EMTALA

In 1986, Congress passed the Emergency Medical Treatment and Active Labor Act (EMTALA) that forbids Medicare-participating hospitals from "dumping" patients out of emergency departments. The act provides that:

> [i]n the case of a hospital that has a hospital emergency department, if any individual (whether or not eligible for benefits under this subchapter) comes to the emergency department and a request is made on the individual's behalf for examination or treatment for a medical condition, the hospital must provide for an appropriate medical screening examination within the capability of the hospital emergency department, including ancillary services routinely available to the emergency depart-

ment, to determine whether or not an emergency medical condition . . . exists.[17]

Emergency Medical Condition Defined

The term *emergency medical condition* has been defined under EMTALA as:

> (A) a medical condition manifesting itself by acute symptoms of sufficient severity (including severe pain) such that the absence of immediate medical attention could reasonably be expected to result in (i) placing the health of the individual (or, with respect to a pregnant woman, the health of the woman or her unborn child) in serious jeopardy, (ii) serious impairment to bodily functions, or (iii) serious dysfunction of any bodily organ or part; or (B) with respect to a pregnant woman who is having contractions, (i) that there is inadequate time to effect a safe transfer to another facility before delivery, or (ii) that transfer may pose a threat to the health or safety of the woman or the unborn child.[18]

Limited to Actions Against Hospital

The decedent in *Ballachino v. Anders*[19] went to the hospital on May 15, 1990, with complaints of chest pain and repeated episodes of loss of consciousness. The physicians allegedly failed to provide an appropriate medical screening examination and failed to determine whether an emergency medical condition existed. The patient's survivor and representative brought an action against the hospital and physicians alleging violations of EMTALA and medical malpractice. EMTALA requires that a Medicare-provider hospital offer an appropriate medical screening examination to determine whether an emergency medical condition exists for any individual who presents to the emergency department seeking treatment. If the hospital determines that an emergency medical condition exists, then it must either stabilize the patient or provide for transfer of the patient to a facility capable of meeting the patient's medical needs.

A district court held that there is no private right of action against the individual physicians under EMTALA. However, the representative's complaint did state a claim against the hospital under EMTALA. The enforcement provision of EMTALA is explicitly limited to actions against a Medicare-participating hospital. Although the physicians were alleged to have acted in concert in rendering professional medical and surgical care and treatment to the decedent while at the hospital, the physicians importantly are nowhere alleged to have provided any emergency screening examination. The plaintiff clearly alleged that the defendants negligently failed to provide an appropriate medical screening examination and failed to determine whether an emergency medical condition existed for the decedent. The court was faced with the question of whether any emergency screening examination occurred at all. The plaintiff also alleged that the hospital failed in its stabilization and transfer procedures. The district court determined that all of the allegations taken together stated an EMTALA claim against the hospital.

Patient Screening Appropriate

On May 4, 2000, Nolen, pregnant with triplets, arrived at the hospital for a labor check at the direction of her physician, Dr. Zann. The hospital admitted Nolen as an outpatient about 20 minutes later. She complained of cramping and a mucous discharge that she feared signaled the onset of labor. After an initial assessment was performed, Zann arrived and performed an examination. Zann concluded that Nolen's lower uterine segment was consistent with what he expected from a normal pregnancy in this circumstance. Zann discharged Nolen from the hospital. He instructed Nolen to keep her scheduled appointment with her perinatologist, Dr. Scott, the next morning.

After leaving the hospital, Nolen's condition changed for the worse. She testified at deposition that she began cramping after leaving the hospital. She made no effort to contact Zann or the hospital after this change in condition. When she reached Scott's office the next morning, Nolen fully described the events of the previous day and her change in condition after leaving the hospital. Scott examined Nolen and sent her back to the hospital to suppress her preterm labor. Nolen was transferred on May 7 to Broward General Hospital where she went into preterm labor. Her first baby was stillborn, and her other two babies subsequently failed to survive.

Nolen contended that the hospital did not have a standard written screening procedure or, alternatively, that the hospital did not follow its screening procedure, either of which, she contends, violated the EMTALA.

Under EMTALA, hospital emergency rooms are subject to two principal obligations, commonly referred to as the *appropriate medical screening requirement* and the *stabilization requirement.* The appropriate medical screening requirement obligates hospital emergency rooms to provide an appropriate medical screening to any individual seeking treatment in order to determine whether the individual has an emergency medical condition. If an emergency medical condition exists, the hospital is required to provide stabilization treatment before transferring the individual.

The record shows that Nolen received superior care from the hospital. Nolen's treatment was provided primarily by her private physician, who provided care beyond the screening mandated by the EMTALA. Nolan's argument that the hospital was required to have a written screening procedure failed because a written procedure is not required by the terms of EMTALA.[20]

Stabilizing the Patient

Patients can be transferred only after they have been medically screened by a physician, stabilized, and cleared for transfer by the receiving institution. *Stabilized* means "with respect to an emergency medical condition . . . to provide such medical treatment of the condition as may be necessary to assure, within reasonable medical probability, that no material deterioration of the condition is likely to result from or to occur during the transfer of the individual from a facility."[21] A patient should not be transferred from the emergency department to another health care facility unless:

> (A)(i) the individual (or a legally responsible person acting on the individual's behalf) after being informed of the hospital's obligations . . . and of the risk of transfer, in writing requests a transfer to another medical facility, (ii) a physician . . . has signed a certification that based on the information available at the time of transfer, the medical benefits reasonably expected from the provision of appropriate medical treatment at another medical facility outweigh the increased risks to the individual and, in the case of labor, to the unborn child from effecting the transfer, or (iii) if a physician is not physically present in the emergency department at the time an individual is transferred, a qualified medical person . . . has signed a certification . . . after a physician . . . in consultation with the person, has made the determination . . . and subsequently countersigns the certification; and (B) the transfer is an appropriate transfer . . . to that facility.[22]

Alleged Delay in Patient Transfer

A hospital's motion for summary judgment would be denied where the hospital failed to establish prima facie evidence that an alleged delay in transferring the plaintiff's decedent from one hospital to another was not a departure from accepted medical standards. The expert's affirmation made no specific references to the care provided by the transferring hospital or, more significantly, to the nature and timeliness of the transfer from it to another hospital. Given its failure to make such a showing, the motion for summary judgment was denied regardless of the sufficiency of the plaintiff's papers in opposition.[23]

Discharge Found Appropriate

In *Holcomb v. Humana Med. Corp.,*[24] the administratrix of the estate of a deceased patient, Smith, sued the hospital alleging a violation of EMTALA. Smith entered the emer-gency department on May 4, 1990, a week after giving birth, with a complaint of a fever, aching, sore throat, and coughing. Both a physician's assistant (PA) and a physician examined Smith. The examination revealed that Smith had a temperature of 104.3°F, a pulse of 146, respirations of 32, and a blood pressure of 112/64. Diagnostic tests ordered included a white blood cell count, urine analysis, and chest X-ray. After reviewing the results of Smith's complaints and medical history, physical examination, and test results, the physician diagnosed the patient as having a viral infection. The physician ordered Tylenol and IV fluids as treatment. Smith was maintained in the emergency department overnight. The physician conducted a second physical examination during the night. By morning, Smith's vital signs had returned to normal. She was discharged with instructions for bed rest, fluids, and a request to return to the hospital if her condition worsened.

After returning home, Smith reported that she was feeling better, but then took a turn for the worse and was admitted to Jackson Hospital on May 6, 1990. She was diagnosed with endometritis and subsequently died on May 9, 1990.

Was the patient inappropriately discharged from the emergency department under provisions of EMTALA? The U.S. District Court for the Middle District of Alabama held that there was no EMTALA violation. The patient was appropriately examined and screened. The care rendered was standard for any patient based on the complaints given. In addition, the plaintiff failed to demonstrate that an emergency condition existed at the time the patient was discharged on May 4th.

Screening and Discharge Appropriate

Fifteen-year-old Nydia, in *Marshall v. East Carroll Parish Hospital Service District,*[25] was brought by ambulance to the hospital emergency department because she "wouldn't move" while at school after the bell rang. Upon her arrival, hospital personnel took her history and vital signs. She was unable to communicate verbally but cooperated with hospital staff. She was examined by Dr. Horowitz, who diagnosed Nydia as having a respiratory infection and discharged her. He informed Nydia's mother, Ms. Marshall, that her daughter's failure to communicate was of unknown etiology, and advised her to continue administering the medications that had been prescribed by the family physician on the previous day and to return to the emergency department if her condition deteriorated. The complaint alleged that, later that same day, Nydia's symptoms continued to worsen, and she was taken to the emergency department at a different hospital, where she was diagnosed as suffering from a cerebrovascular accident.

The action claimed that the hospital violated EMTALA by failing to provide Nydia with an appropriate medical screening examination and failing to stabilize her condition prior to discharge. The hospital moved for summary judgment and submitted supporting affidavits from Horowitz and a registered nurse who participated in Nydia's treatment in the hospital's emergency department. The district court granted summary judgment for the hospital on grounds that no material fact issues were in dispute.

Marshall, on appeal, claimed that hospital personnel knew that Nydia had an emergency medical condition and were concerned about the cursory examination provided by Horowitz and that Nydia should have been admitted to the hospital for observation of her unexplained altered mental status. Marshall argued that Horowitz committed malpractice by failing to accurately diagnose an emergency medical condition.

EMTALA was not intended to be used as a federal malpractice statute, but instead was enacted to prevent *patient dumping* (the practice of refusing to treat patients unable to pay for care). An EMTALA appropriate medical screening examination is not judged by its proficiency in accurately diagnosing a patient's illness, but rather by whether it was performed equitably in comparison to other patients with similar symptoms. If a hospital provides an appropriate medical screening examination, it is not liable under EMTALA even if the physician who performed the examination made a misdiagnosis that could subject him or her and the employer to liability in a medical malpractice action. The affidavits submitted by the hospital stated that Nydia was given an appropriate medical screening examination that would have been performed on any other patient, and that she was not diagnosed as having an emergency medical condition.

The court determined that the hospital was entitled to summary judgment as a matter of law because there was no material fact issue as to whether Horowitz conducted an appropriate medical screening examination. The stabilization and transfer provisions of EMTALA are triggered only after a hospital determines that an individual has an emergency medical condition. The hospital has no duty under EMTALA to stabilize a condition that was not diagnosed during an appropriate screening examination. The physician here did not diagnose an emergency situation. Therefore, this case is not an EMTALA issue. However, an issue in malpractice under the state's tort law can be raised.

Transfer Prior to Stabilizing Patient

The plaintiff in *Huckaby v. East Ala. Med. Ctr.*[26] brought an action against the hospital alleging that the patient was transferred from the hospital's emergency department before her condition was stabilized. The patient went to the hospital, suffering from a stroke. The complaint alleged that the patient's condition was critical and materially deteriorating. The attending emergency department physician, Dr. Wheat, informed the patient's family that she needed the services of a neurosurgeon, but that the hospital had problems in getting neurosurgeons to accept patients. Upon the recommendation of Wheat, the patient was transferred to another hospital where she expired soon after arrival. The plaintiff alleged

that Wheat did not inform the family regarding the risks of transfer and that the transfer of the patient in an unstable condition was the proximate cause of her death. Did the plaintiff have a cause of action under EMTALA?

The U.S. District Court held that the plaintiff stated a cause of action under EMTALA for which monetary relief could be granted. For the plaintiff to overcome the defendant's motion to dismiss the case, the plaintiff had to demonstrate that, under EMTALA, the patient: (1) went to the defendant's emergency department; (2) was diagnosed with an emergency medical condition; (3) was not provided with adequate screening; and, (4) was discharged and transferred to another hospital before her emergency condition was stabilized. The plaintiff met this standard.

Inappropriate Transfer

Failure to follow EMTALA can result in civil penalties. In addition, any individual who suffers personal harm as a direct result of a participating hospital's violation of a requirement may, in a civil action against the participating hospital, obtain those damages available for personal injury under the law of the state in which the hospital is located.

In *Burditt v. U.S. Department of Health and Human Services,*[27] EMTALA was violated by a physician when he ordered a woman with dangerously high blood pressure (210/130) and in active labor with ruptured membranes transferred from the emergency department of one hospital to another hospital 170 miles away. The physician was assessed a penalty of $20,000. Dr. Louis Sullivan, secretary of the Department of Health and Human Services at that time, issued this statement:

> This decision sends a message to physicians everywhere that they need to provide quality care to everyone in need of emergency treatment who comes to a hospital. This is a significant opinion and we are pleased with the result.[28]

The American Public Health Association, in filing an amicus curiae, advised the appeals court that if Burditt wants to ensure that he will never be asked to treat a patient not of his choosing, then he ought to vote with his feet by affiliating only with hospitals that do not accept Medicare funds or do not have an emergency department.

Wrong Record: Fatal Mistake

Terry Trahan, in *Trahan v. McManus,*[29] was taken to the hospital after being injured in an automobile accident. Lawrence and Marie, Terry's parents, were informed about the accident and asked to come to the hospital. Mrs. Trahan drove to the hospital and consulted with Dr. McManus, the emergency department physician who treated Terry. McManus assured Mrs. Trahan that it would be all right to take her son home because there was nothing more that could be done for him at the hospital. McManus advised Terry's mom to take him home and see that he got lots of rest.

Upon ordering discharge, however, McManus had not realized that he had made a grave and fatal mistake. McManus had looked at the wrong chart in determining Terry's status.

The chart McManus had looked at indicated that the patient's vital signs were normal. In fact, the correct chart showed that Terry had three broken ribs as a result of the accident. His blood pressure was 90/60 when he was admitted to the emergency department. Forty-five minutes after being admitted, Terry's blood pressure had dropped to 80/50, and his respiration rate had doubled. Terry's vital signs clearly indicated that he was suffering from internal hemorrhaging.

In the seven hours following his discharge, Terry's condition continued to worsen. Terry complained to his parents about severe pain. He could not turn from his back to his side without the aid of his father. Several hours after being brought home from the hospital, Lawrence Trahan noticed that Terry's abdomen was swelling. Mrs. Trahan immediately called the hospital. Mr. Trahan asked Terry if he wanted to sit up. Terry replied, "Well, we can try." Those were Terry's final words. Terry slumped in his father's arms and his head fell forward. When Mr. Trahan attempted to lift Terry's head, Terry's face was white. Mr. Trahan immediately laid his son down on the bed, realizing for the first time that his son was not breathing and had no pulse. He attempted CPR as Mrs. Trahan called for an ambulance. Mr. Trahan continued CPR until the ambulance arrived a few minutes later. Terry Trahan was pronounced dead on arrival at the hospital.

Subsequently, during a medical review panel proceeding in which the Trahans participated, McManus admitted liability by tendering his $100,000 limit of liability, pursuant to the Medical Malpractice Act.

A jury returned a verdict absolving McManus of any liability, finding that Terry's injuries would have occurred despite the physician's failure to use reasonable care in his treatment of Terry. The Trahans appealed.

On appeal, the jury's determination was found to be clearly erroneous when it concluded that the physician's actions were not the cause-in-fact of Terry's death. The record is replete with testimony, including McManus's own admissions, that he acted negligently when he discharged Terry, that his actions led to Terry's death, and that there was treatment available that could have made a difference.

Duty to Contact On-Call Physician

Hospitals are expected to notify specialty on-call physicians when their particular skills are required in the emergency department. A physician who is on call and fails to respond to a request to attend a patient can be liable for injuries suffered by the patient because of his or her failure to respond.

In *Thomas v. Corso*,[30] a patient had been brought to the hospital emergency department after he was struck by a car. A physician did not attend to him even though he had dangerously low blood pressure and was in shock. There was some telephone contact between the nurse in the emergency department and the physician who was providing on-call coverage. The physician did not act upon the hospital's call for assistance until the patient was close to death. Expert testimony was not necessary to establish what common sense made evident: the patient struck by a car may have suffered internal injuries and should have been evaluated and treated by a physician. Lack of attention in such cases is not reasonable care by any standard. The concurrent negligence of the nurse, who failed to contact the on-call physician after the patient's condition worsened, did not relieve the physician of liability for his failure to respond to his on-call duty. Because of the nurse's negligence, the hospital is liable under the doctrine of respondeat superior.

Failure to Respond to Call

Treatment rendered by hospitals is expected to be commensurate with that available in the same or similar communities or in hospitals generally. In *Fjerstad v. Knutson*,[31] the South Dakota Supreme Court found that a hospital could be held liable for the failure of an on-call physician to respond to a call from the emergency department. An intern who attempted to contact the on-call physician and was unable to do so for 3½ hours treated and discharged the patient. The hospital was responsible for assigning on-call physicians and ensuring that they would be available when called. The patient died during the night in a motel room as a result of asphyxia resulting from a swelling of the larynx, tonsils, and epiglottis that blocked the trachea. Testimony indicated that the emergency department's on-call physician was to be available for consultation and was assigned that duty by the hospital. Expert testimony also was offered that someone with the decedent's symptoms should have been hospitalized and that such care could have saved the decedent's life. The jury believed that an experienced physician would have taken the necessary steps to save the decedent's life.

Timely Response Required

Hospitals are not only required to care for emergency patients, but they also are required to do so in a timely fashion. In *Marks v. Mandel*,[32] a Florida trial court was found to have erred in directing a verdict against the plaintiff. It was decided that the relevant inquiry in this case was whether the hospital and the supervisor should bear ultimate responsibility for failure of the specialty on-call system to function properly. Jury issues had been raised by evidence that the standard for on-call systems was to have a specialist attending the patient within a reasonable time period of being called.

Notice of Inability to Respond to Call

In *Millard v. Corrado,*[33] the Missouri Appellate Court found that on-call physicians owe a duty to provide reasonable notice when they will be unavailable to respond to calls. Physicians who cannot fulfill their on-call responsibilities must provide notice as soon as practicable once they learn of the circumstances that will render them unavailable. Imposing a duty on on-call physicians to notify hospital staff of their unavailability does not place an unreasonable burden. In this case, a mere telephone call would have significantly reduced the 4-hour time period between an accident and life-saving surgery. Whatever slight inconvenience may be associated with notifying the hospital of the on-call physician's availability is trivial when compared to the substantial risk to patients.

Telephone Medicine Can Be Costly

The diagnosis and treatment of patients by telephone can be costly. *Futch v. Attwood*[34] points this out quite clearly. In this case, a suit was brought against Dr. Attwood and hospital seeking damages for a wrongful death action arising from negligent medical care rendered to Lauren Futch, the plaintiff's minor daughter.

The record shows that on the morning of February 28, 1990, Lauren, a four-year-old diabetic child, awoke her mother, Wanda. She had vomited two or three times and her glucose reading was high. Wanda administered Lauren's morning insulin and intended to feed her a light breakfast before bringing her to see Dr. Attwood, a pediatrician, at about 9:45 A.M. According to the plaintiff, Attwood did not check Lauren's blood sugar level or her urine to determine whether ketones were present. If Atwood had done so, Lauren's condition could have been quickly corrected by the simple administration of insulin. Instead of administering insulin, however, Attwood prescribed the use of Phenergan suppositories to address Lauren's symptoms. Lauren's symptoms of nausea continued, and she was taken the hospital emergency department. Hospital personnel contacted Attwood. Attwood returned the call and again prescribed a Phenergan injection. Attwood did not go to the hospital and had not been given Lauren's vital signs when he suggested such an injection, and further failed to order any blood or urine tests.

Wanda returned home with Lauren at approximately 8:00 P.M. and put her to bed, waking her around midnight to administer the prescribed medication. Lauren woke, but went back to sleep. Early the next morning, Wanda awoke and found Lauren with labored breathing. While attempting to wake up the four-year-old, the only responses, according

to plaintiff's brief, were "huh" followed by moaning. Wanda telephoned Attwood and informed him of her daughter's far-worsened condition. Attwood admitted Lauren to the hospital at 6:30 A.M. that morning.

Hospital records revealed that Lauren's glucose level was 507 at the time of admission with her blood acid revealing diabetic ketoacidosis. At approximately 9:13 A.M., Lauren went into respiratory arrest as a result of her brain swelling with rupturing into the opening at the base of her neck. Lauren was immediately transported by helicopter to Children's Hospital in New Orleans and diagnosed with ketoacidotic coma, cerebral edema, and bilateral pulmonary edema. She was pronounced dead at 5:07 P.M. on March 2, 1990.

Lauren and her mother were virtually inseparable, except when Wanda was at school. All of this changed in Lauren's last few days when she was rushed to New Orleans. During Lauren's 2½ days of illness, every moment seemed worse than the previous. The mother witnessed her daughter's decline in health and her protracted wait was punctuated only by various traumatic episodes: Lauren's respiratory intubation; her respiratory failure and consequent code blue; numerous medical staff scurrying in and out to see Lauren behind doors closed to Wanda; and, finally, Wanda's being asked to consider whether she would prefer to "pull the plug" on her daughter or to watch her linger indefinitely. Confronted with this dilemma, the young mother opted not to punish her daughter with more torment. She decided to let her go and did. For Wanda, the period following Lauren's death has been marked by the inevitable sense of loss of a daughter and by the guilt of a mother whose unrelenting loss compels her to ask what she might have done differently to save her child's life.

The trial court allocated $98,000 for the conscious pain and suffering of Lauren. The defendant complained that the award of $98,000 was excessive. On appeal, the appellate court could not find that the trial court had erred in concluding what sum was fair to both parties.

Prevention of Lawsuits in the Emergency Department

Emergency department lawsuits can be reduced by implementing and enforcing some fundamental commonsense policies, procedures, and programs:

- Develop and implement appropriate emergency department policies and procedures, including:

  - the necessity to treat each patient courteously and promptly

  - a requirement that all patients are to be treated, regardless of ability to pay

  - treatment priorities such as emergency cases to be treated first, followed by urgent and less serious cases

- on-call roster procedures

- consultation requirements for specialists

- consent procedures for both adults and minors

- disaster procedures

- transfer procedures

• Communicate with the patient and the patient's family to ensure that a complete and accurate picture of the patient's symptoms and complaints are obtained.

• Communicate among health care professionals. This is imperative. Each professional gains a certain amount of information from a patient's history. Such information must be communicated to the attending physician. Both the nurse and the physician must assume that each has certain pieces of information necessary for the proper care and treatment of the patient. A poor listener and a poor communicator have no place in the care of emergency department patients.

• Provide continuing education programs for all staff members.

• Institute a preventive maintenance program for emergency department equipment.

• Do not take lightly any patient's complaint. This may well be the single most fatal mistake of emergency departments.

• Those professionals who cannot accept the concept that all patients, regardless of ailment, must be treated need to search for placement outside the emergency department.

• Hospitals need to determine what types of patients and levels of care they can safely address. If there are several hospitals in a community, they must learn to communicate with one another and include emergency medical services personnel in addressing transport and care issues. For example, if Hospital A has a Level III emergency department, without a neurologist, neurosurgeon, or stroke team and Hospital B, one mile away has all of that plus a Level I trauma center, it would be fair to say that a suspected stroke victim should be transported to Hospital B. Failing to address such issues raises both ethical and legal concerns. As hospitals cooperate, plan, and prepare for major disasters involving many victims, they need to conduct the same planning process for addressing everyday emergency crises.

Emergency Rooms Vital to Public Safety

McBride, in *Simmons v. Tuomey Regional Medical Center,*[35] was involved in an accident while driving his moped. Upon learning of the accident, Simmons, McBride's daughter, rushed to the scene, where she found emergency service personnel attending to an injury to the back of her father's head. McBride was taken to Tuomey where Simmons signed an admission form for her father. The admission form contained the following provision:

> The Physicians Practicing in this Emergency Room are not Employees of the Tuomey Regional Medical Center They are Independent Physicians, as are All Physicians Practicing in this Hospital.

While in Tuomey's emergency department, Drs. Cooper and Anderson examined McBride. Despite McBride's confused state, the physicians decided to treat his contusions and release him from the hospital. The physicians, apparently attributing McBride's confusion to intoxication, did not treat his head injury.

The next day, McBride returned to Tuomey where his head injury was diagnosed as a subdural hematoma. Ultimately, McBride was transported to Richland Memorial Hospital. Approximately six weeks later, McBride died of complications from the hematoma.

When Simmons brought suit, Tuomey moved for summary judgment by alleging that it was not liable because the physicians were independent contractors. Tuomey relied on its June 1987 contract with Coastal Physicians Services, which set forth the procedures by which Coastal would provide emergency department physicians to Tuomey. The carefully worded contract referred numerous times to physicians as independent contractors and stated that Tuomey agreed not to exercise any control over the means, manner, or methods by which any Physician supplied by Coastal carries out his duties. The trial court accorded great weight to the Coastal-Tuomey contract when it granted Tuomey's motion for summary judgment. Simmons appealed, arguing that the trial court erred in granting summary judgment on the issues of actual agency, apparent agency, and nondelegable duty.

The operation of emergency departments is such an important activity to the community that hospitals should be liable for the negligence of emergency department caregivers. Few things are more comforting in today's society than knowing that immediate medical care is available around the clock at any hospital. As the Texas Court of Appeals astutely observed:

> Emergency rooms are aptly named and vital to public safety. There exists no other place to find immediate medical care. The dynamics that drive paying patients to a hospital's emergency rooms are known well. Either a sudden injury occurs, a child breaks his arm or an individual suffers a heart attack, or an existing medical condition worsens, a diabetic lapses into a coma, demanding immediate medical attention at the nearest emergency room. The catch phrase in legal nomenclature, "time is of the essence," takes on real meaning. Generally, one cannot choose to pass by the nearest emergency

room, and after arrival, it would be improvident to depart in hope of finding one that provides services through employees rather than independent contractors. The patient is there and must rely on the services available and agree to pay the premium charged for those services.[36]

The public not only relies on the medical care rendered by emergency departments, but also considers the hospital as a single entity providing all of its medical services. A set of commentators observed

> [T]he hospital itself has come to be perceived as the provider of medical services. According to this view, patients come to the hospital to be cured, and the doctors who practice there are the hospital's instrumentalities, regardless of the nature of the private arrangements between the hospital and the physician. Whether or not this perception is accurate seemingly matters little when weighed against the momentum of changing public perception and attendant public policy.[37]

Public reliance and public perceptions, as well as the regulations imposed on hospitals, has created an absolute duty for hospitals to provide competent medical care in their emergency departments. Hospitals contributed to the shift in public perception through commercial advertisements. By actively soliciting business, hospitals effectively removed themselves from the sterile world of altruistic agencies. The Alaska Supreme Court, the first American court to recognize a nondelegable duty in the hospital context, wrote:

> Not only is [finding a nondelegable duty] consonant with the public perception of the hospital as a multifaceted health care facility responsible for the quality of medical care and treatment rendered, it also treats tort liability in the medical arena in a manner that is consistent with the commercialization of American medicine.[38]

The real effect of finding a duty to be nondelegable is to render not the duty, but the liability, not delegable; the person subject to a nondelegable duty is certainly free to delegate the duty, but will be liable to third parties for any negligence of the delegatee, regardless of any fault on the part of the delegator.

Given the cumulative public policies surrounding the operation of emergency departments and the legal requirement that hospitals provide emergency services, hospitals must be accountable in tort for the actions of caregivers working in their emergency departments. The court in this case agreed with a New York court, which wrote:

> In this Court's opinion it is public policy, and not traditional rules of the law of agency or the

law of torts, which should underlie the decision to hold hospitals liable for malpractice which occurs in their emergency rooms. In this regard the observation of former U.S. Supreme Court Justice Oliver Wendell Holmes is apt: "The true grounds of decision are consideration of policy and of social advantage, and it is vain to suppose that solutions can be attained merely by logic and the general propositions of law which nobody disputes. Propositions as to public policy rarely are unanimously accepted, and still more rarely, if ever, are capable of unanswerable proof."[39]

The appeals court in Tuomey held that hospitals have nondelegable duty to render competent service to the patients of their emergency departments. The trial court's grant of summary judgment was reversed, and the case was remanded for further proceedings.

State Regulations

Legislation in many states imposes a duty on hospitals to provide emergency care. The statutes implicitly, and sometimes explicitly, require hospitals to provide some degree of emergency service.

If the public is aware that a hospital furnishes emergency services and relies on that knowledge, the hospital has a duty to provide those services to the public. Two Mexican children, burned in a fire at home, were refused admission or first aid by a local hospital. A lawsuit was filed claiming that additional injury occurred as a result of the failure to render care.[40] The trial court dismissed the suit. On appeal, the Arizona Court of Appeals found the defendants liable, claiming that it was the custom of the hospital to render aid in such a case. The Arizona Supreme Court, in finding the defendants liable, reasoned that state statutes and licensing regulations mandate that a hospital may not deny a patient emergency care.

State statutes, such as New York State Emergency Medical Services Act, provide that every hospital shall admit persons in need of immediate hospitalization. Any licensed medical practitioner who refuses to treat a person arriving at a general hospital for emergency medical treatment will be guilty of a misdemeanor and subject to up to one year in prison and a fine. Emergency medical technicians, paramedics, and ambulance drivers are expected to report any refusals by hospitals to treat emergency patients. Patients may be transferred only after they have been stabilized if it is deemed by the attending physician to be in the best interest of the patient.

LABORATORY

An organization must provide for clinical laboratory services to meet the needs of its patients. Each health care organization is responsible for the quality and timeliness of the services provided. Because it is often necessary to contract out certain tests, the organization should be sure that it is contracting for services with a reputable licensed laboratory.

An organization's laboratory provides data that are vital to a patient's treatment. Among its many functions, the laboratory monitors therapeutic ranges, measures blood levels for toxicity, places and monitors instrumentation on patient units, provides education for the nursing staff (e.g., glucose monitoring), provides valuable data utilized in research studies, provides data on the most effective and economical antibiotic for treating patients, serves in a consultation role, and provides valuable data as to the nutritional needs of patients.

Failure to Follow Recommended Transfusion Protocol

Fowler, in *Fowler v. Bossano,*[41] gave birth to twins on March 26, 1996. Due to premature birth, the twins were transferred to LCMH and were cared for by Bossano, a neonatologist. The infants experienced complications and problems associated with premature birth, including respiratory and feeding difficulties. The twins' treatment included blood transfusions. Bossano stated that the twins proceeded through these difficulties and began to make progress, but then Ryan (one of the twins) took a turn for the worse. According to Bossano, Ryan's condition generally continued to deteriorate until he died on May 25. Bossano stated that the most likely cause of death was a viral infection. At his urging, an autopsy was performed, and the pathologist found the presence of cytomegalovirus inclusion (CMV) disease. Bossano stated that he learned that the lab at the hospital did not, at that time, screen for the presence of the virus in the blood used for transfusions.

Ryan's parents instituted proceedings under the Medical Malpractice Act, convening a medical review panel against Bossano and LCMH. The panel determined that the evidence presented did not support a finding that Bossano breached the standard of care. As for the hospital, the panel found that the evidence showed that it failed to comply with the appropriate standard of care with regard to the testing of blood. The child most likely expired from an overwhelming CMV viral infection resulting from blood-product usage.

The hospital's blood bank formal policy for selecting components for neonatal transfusion provided: Special requests for blood products such as irradiated or CMV negative products are provided upon request, but are not routinely used. The American Association of Blood Banks' (AABB) 16th edition of *Standards for Blood Banks and Transfusion Services* provided in Section 18.500, that "Where transfusion-associated CMV disease is a problem, cellular components should be selected or processed to reduce that risk to infant recipients weighing less than 1200 grams at birth, when either the infant or the mother is CMV antibody-negative or that information is unknown."

The hospital's policy did not provide for compliance with the applicable AABB policy at that time so LCMH had the obligation to properly inform the medical staff and ensure that all such infants who might be affected could be readily identified. Bossano should have been able to make a correct medical assumption that all high-risk infants receiving blood products in the neonatal intensive care unit would receive CMV-negative blood products.

The Fowlers filed suit naming both Bossano and the hospital as defendants. They sought damages associated with a survival action and those for wrongful death. The plaintiffs and the hospital reached a settlement for $100,000, the limit of the hospital's statutory responsibility. The plaintiffs proceeded against the Louisiana Patient's Compensation Fund.

The jury found for the plaintiffs. LCMH breached the applicable standard of care by failing to test the blood used for this transfusion for CMV.

The evidence presented was sufficient to support the jury's determination that the hospital's breach of the standard of care was the cause of Ryan's death and the cause of damages in excess of $100,000. The Louisiana Court of Appeals found that the evidence of the experiences of both Ryan and his parents supported the awards made.

Mismatched Blood

A laboratory technician in *Barnes Hospital v. Missouri Commission on Human Rights*[42] had been discharged because of inferior work performance. On three occasions, the employee allegedly mismatched blood. The employee filed a complaint with the Commission on Human Rights, alleging racial discrimination as a reason for his discharge by the hospital. The hospital appealed, and the circuit court reversed the commission's order. The technician appealed to the Missouri Supreme Court, which held that the evidence did not support the ruling of racial discrimination by the Missouri Commission on Human Rights.

Refusal to Work with Certain Blood Specimens

A laboratory technician was found to have been properly dismissed from her job for refusing to perform chemical examinations on vials with AIDS warnings attached in *Stepp v. Review Board of the Indiana Employment Security Division.*[43] The court of appeals held that the employee was dismissed for just cause and that the laboratory did not waive its right to compel employees to perform assigned tasks.

LOST CHANCE OF SURVIVAL/ CHANGES IN PAP SMEAR

Citation: *Sander v. Geib, Elston, Frost Prof'l Ass'n,* 506 N.W.2d 107 (S.D. 1993)

Facts

The patient had several gynecological examinations, including Pap smears, in 1977, 1978, 1980, 1984, 1986, and 1987. The patient's physician performed the examinations. Specimens for the Pap test were submitted to a laboratory for evaluation. The laboratory procedure included a clerk assigning each specimen a number when it was received. A cytotechnologist would then screen the specimen. If the specimen was determined to be abnormal, it would be marked for review by a pathologist. Out of the Pap tests that were determined to be normal, only 1 in 10 was actually viewed by a pathologist. The pathologist made recommendations based on the classification of the Pap tests. A biopsy would be recommended if the Pap test was determined to be Class IV.

Except for the Pap test in 1987, which showed premalignant cellular changes, all of the patient's other Pap tests were determined to be negative. In 1986, the laboratory made a notation to the patient's physician that "moderate inflammation" was present. The patient's physician, who was treating her with antibiotics for a foot inflammation, thought that the medication would also treat the other inflammation. In September 1987, the patient returned to her physician complaining of pain, erratic periods, and tiredness. After completing a physical, her physician took a Pap test, which he sent to the laboratory. He also referred her to a gynecologist. The pathologist recommended a biopsy. Biopsies and further physical examinations revealed squamous cell carcinoma that had spread to her pelvic bones. Her Pap tests were reexamined by the laboratory, which reported that the 1986 smear showed that malignancy was highly likely. The patient was referred to the University of Minnesota to determine whether she was a viable candidate for radiation treatment. The cancer, however, had spread, and the patient was not considered a candidate for radiation treatment because she had no chance of survival. When the university reviewed all of the available slides, they found cellular changes back to 1984.

The patient sued in 1988, alleging that the laboratory failed to detect and report cellular changes in her Pap tests in time to prevent the spread of the cancer. Before trial, the patient died. Her husband and sister were substituted as plaintiffs, and the complaint was amended to include a wrongful death action. After trial, a jury awarded $3.7 million in damages, which were reduced to $1 million by the circuit court. The jury found against the laboratory and the laboratory appealed.

Issue

Was it erroneous for the trial court to submit to the jury the 1988 negligence claim based on the 1984 slide?

Holding

The South Dakota Supreme Court upheld the jury verdict and restored the $3.7 million damage award.

Reason

The court determined that evidence relating to negligence claims pertaining to Pap tests taken more than two years before filing the action were admissible because the patient had a continuing relationship with the clinical laboratory as a result of her physician submitting her Pap tests to the laboratory over a period of time.

Discussion

1. What changes in procedure should the laboratory take to help ensure that Pap tests are properly classified?
2. How might continuous quality-improvement activities improve the laboratory's operations?

MEDICAL ASSISTANT

The *medical assistant* is an unlicensed person who provides administrative, clerical, and/or technical support to a licensed practitioner. A licensed practitioner is generally required to be physically present in the treatment facility, medical office, or ambulatory facility when a medical assistant is performing procedures. Employment of medical assistants is expected to grow much faster than the average for all occupations as the health services industry expands. This growth is due in part to technological advances in medicine and a growing and aging population. Increasing use of medical assistants in the rapidly growing health care industry will most likely result in continuing employment growth for the occupation.

Medical assistants work in physicians' offices, clinics, nursing homes, and ambulatory care settings. The duties of medical assistants vary from office to office, depending on the location and size of the practice and the practitioner's specialty. In small practices, medical assistants usually are generalists, handling both administrative and clinical duties. Those in large practices tend to specialize in a particular area, under supervision. Administrative duties often include answering telephones, greeting patients, updating and filing patients' medical records, filling out insurance forms, handling correspondence, scheduling appointments, arranging for hospital admission and laboratory services, and handling billing and bookkeeping. Clinical duties vary according to state law and include assisting in taking medical histories, recording vital signs, explaining treatment procedures to patients, preparing patients for examination, and assisting the practitioner during examinations. Medical assistants collect and prepare laboratory specimens or perform basic laboratory tests on the premises, dispose of contaminated supplies, and sterilize medical instruments. They instruct patients about medications and special diets, prepare and administer medications as directed by a physician, authorize drug refills as directed, telephone prescriptions to a pharmacy, prepare patients for X-rays, perform electrocardiograms, remove sutures, and change dressings.

Medical assistants who specialize have additional duties. Podiatric medical assistants make castings of feet, expose and develop X-rays, and assist podiatrists in surgery. Ophthalmic medical assistants help ophthalmologists provide eye care. They conduct diagnostic tests, measure and record vision, and test eye-muscle function. They also show patients how to insert, remove, and care for contact lenses, and they apply eye dressings. Under the direction of the physician, ophthalmic medical assistants may administer eye medications. They also maintain optical and surgical instruments and may assist the ophthalmologist in surgery.[44]

Poor Communications

In 1987, the patient-plaintiff in *Follett v. Davis*[45] had her first office visit with Dr. Davis. In the spring of 1988, the plaintiff discovered a lump in her right breast and made an appointment to see Davis; however, the clinic had no record of her appointment. The clinic's employees directed her to radiology for a mammogram. The plaintiff was not offered an examination by Davis or any other physician at the clinic and she was not scheduled for an examination as a follow-up to the mammogram. A technician examined the plaintiff's breast and confirmed the presence of a lump in her right breast. After the mammogram, clinic employees told her that she would hear from Davis if there were any problems with her mammogram.

The radiologist explained in his deposition that the mammogram was not normal. Davis reviewed the mammogram report and considered it to be negative for malignancy. He was unaware about the lump in the patient's breast and there was no evidence that clinic employees informed him about it. The clinic, including Davis, never contacted the plaintiff about her lump or the mammogram. On April 6, 1990, the plaintiff called the clinic and was told that there was nothing to worry about unless she heard from Davis. On September 24, 1990, the plaintiff returned to the clinic after she had developed pain associated with the lump. A mammogram performed on that day gave results consistent with cancer. Three days later, Davis made an appointment for the plaintiff with a clinic surgeon for a biopsy and treatment. Davis subsequently transferred her care to other physicians. In October 1990, the biopsy confirmed the diagnosis of cancer. In August 1992, the plaintiff filed her complaint.

The Indiana Court of Appeals held that the statute of limitations did not begin to run until the patient's last visit to the clinic. When the plaintiff last visited Davis on September 24, 1990, and the clinic on September 27, 1990, the evidence demonstrated that, had clinic procedures been followed, Davis or another physician at the clinic would have had occasion to diagnose her problem before either of those dates. On August 20, 1992, the plaintiff timely filed her proposed complaint within two years of the last visits to Davis and the clinic.

MEDICAL IMAGING

Negligence in medical imaging tests and therapies often involve a failure to protect patients from falls and the negligent handling of equipment. The plaintiff, for example, in *Cockerton v. Mercy Hospital Medical Center*[46] was admitted to the hospital for the purpose of surgery to correct a problem with her open bite. Her physician ordered postsurgical X-rays for her head and face to be taken the next day. A hospital employee took the plaintiff from her room to the X-ray department by wheelchair. A nurse assessed her condition as slightly drowsy. An X-ray technician took charge of the plaintiff in the X-ray room. After the plaintiff was taken inside the X-ray room, she was transferred from a wheelchair to a portable chair for the procedure. Upon being moved, the plaintiff complained of nausea, and the technician observed that the plaintiff's pupils were dilated. The technician did not use the restraint straps to secure the plaintiff to the chair. At some point during the procedure, the plaintiff had a fainting seizure and the technician called for help. When another hospital employee entered the room, the technician was holding the plaintiff in an upright position; she appeared nonresponsive. The plaintiff only remembered being stood up and having a lead jacket placed across her back and shoulders. The technician maintains that the plaintiff did not fall. At the time the plaintiff left the X-ray room, her level of consciousness was poor. The plaintiff's physician noticed a deflection of the plaintiff's nose. Because the plaintiff had fainted in X-ray, an incident report was completed at the request of the plaintiff's physician. The following day, the deflection of the plaintiff's nose was much more evident. A specialist was contacted and an attempt was made to correct the deformity. The specialist made an observation that it would require a substantial injury to the nose to deflect it to that severity.

The plaintiff instituted proceedings against the hospital, alleging that the negligence of the nurses or technicians allowed her to fall during the procedure and subsequently caused injury. The trial court did not require expert testimony concerning the standard of care given by the technician. The jury concluded that the hospital was negligent in leaving the plaintiff unattended or failing to restrain her, which proximately caused her fall and injury. The jury rendered a verdict of $48,370, and the hospital appealed.

The Iowa Court of Appeals held that the patient was not required to present expert testimony on the issue of the hospital's negligence. The conduct in question was simply the way the technician handled the plaintiff during the X-ray examination. The X-ray technician testified that during the X-ray, the plaintiff appeared to have a seizure episode. She also testified that she left the plaintiff unattended for a brief period of time and that she did not use the restraint straps that were attached to the portable X-ray chair. Using the restraint straps would have secured the plaintiff to the portable chair during the X-ray examination. The court found that substantial evidence existed to establish a causal connection between the hospital's conduct and the plaintiff's injury.

X-RAY CASSETTE FALLS ON PATIENT'S HEAD

Citation: *Schopp v. Our Lady of the Lake Hospital, Inc.,* 739 So. 2d 338, 98 1382 (La. App. 1 Cir. 6/25/99)

Facts

On August 2, 1993, Sophie Schopp stumbled coming from her bathroom and fell, striking her head. She was unable to get up, so she lay on the floor until approximately 8:00 A.M., when a home health aide came to her home for her daily visit. Her doors were locked, but Schopp told Montgomery to go across the street and get a key, which she did. Emergency medical services arrived shortly thereafter and took Schopp to the hospital. Her friend and neighbor, Guwang, followed in her car. Schopp's friend, Haper, also came to the hospital that morning.

Schopp was taken for skull X-rays, and when she returned, the X-ray technologist, Coates, told Haper and Guwang that there had been "a little accident." Haper testified that Coates said that the X-ray plate fell on her head. He pointed to Schopp's head and showed Haper where it had fallen on her. Haper stated she saw no mark or bruise and thought nothing more of it. Guwang testified, however, that she pushed back Schopp's hair and saw a blue mark on the left side of her forehead.

A CT scan showed that Schopp had a large acute subdural hematoma. Dr. Perone, a board-certified neurosurgeon, performed surgery to evacuate the hematoma. Although Schopp seemed to improve initially following the surgery, her health declined thereafter, and she died on August 16, 1993.

Schopp's sons filed suit against the hospital (defendant) and two of the defendant's X-ray technologists, Coates and Smith. The plaintiffs later dismissed Coates and Smith but proceeded to jury trial against the hospital. The jury rendered a verdict in favor of the plaintiffs, and an appeal was taken for wrongful death.

Issue

Was Schopp's death caused by the negligence of hospital staff dropping an X-ray cassette on her head while undergoing a skull X-ray?

Holding

Schopp's death was caused by the negligence of hospital staff dropping an X-ray cassette on her head while undergoing a skull X-ray.

Reason

Although there was conflicting testimony as to the cause of death, Morris apparently gave the most convincing testimony regarding Schopp's injury. Morris stated that although he did not operate, he made the diagnoses that led to surgery. He pointed out he was the one who diagnosed the subdural hematoma. He stated that there was no doubt in his mind that the incident in the X-ray room caused the hematoma. He believed that the cartridge was dropped on Schopp's head based on her statements to him and the alarmed tone in the nurse's voice when she called him to report the X-ray incident. He saw the soft tissue swelling on Schopp's head and noted the hematoma was in the exact place she had shown him where the cartridge struck her.

In this case, there were two versions of the X-ray–room incident: either the cartridge tilted less than an inch and barely brushed Schopp's head, leaving no mark, or it was dropped from some distance and struck her with enough force to leave a soft-tissue injury. The jury chose to believe the second version.

Discussion

1. Do you agree with the court's findings? Discuss your answer.
2. What are the lessons to be learned from this case for employees?

NUTRITIONAL SERVICES

Health care organizations are expected to provide patients with diets that meet their individual needs. Failure to do so can lead to negligence suits. The daughter of the deceased in *Lambert v. Beverly Enterprises, Inc.*[47] filed an action claiming that her father had been mistreated. The deceased allegedly suffered malnutrition as a direct result of the acts or omissions of personnel, and that the plaintiff's father suffered actual damages that included substantial medical expenses and mental anguish due to the injuries he sustained. A motion to dismiss the case was denied.

PARAMEDIC

Many states have enacted legislation that provides civil immunity to paramedics who render emergency lifesaving services. The plaintiff in *Malone v. City of Seattle*[48] alleged that the defendant was negligent in providing care to the plaintiff after an automobile accident. The plaintiff, on appeal, contended that the trial court wrongfully instructed the jury regarding a 1971 civil immunity statute. The following is an excerpt from the relevant Washington statute:

> No act or omission of any physician's trained mobile intensive care paramedic . . . done or omitted in good faith while rendering emergency lifesaving service . . . to a person who is in immediate danger of loss of life shall impose any liability upon the trained mobile intensive care paramedic . . . or upon a . . . city or other local governmental unit. . . .[49]

One of the issues raised was whether the legislature intended the statute to apply only to the rendition of cardiopulmonary emergency treatment by a paramedic. The court of appeals indicated that although the definition contained in the statute places special emphasis on the paramedic's training in all aspects of CPR, the act does not limit the paramedic to CPR. The act implicitly recognizes that paramedics may encounter different emergencies.

In *Morena v. South Hills Health Systems*,[50] the Pennsylvania Supreme Court held that paramedics were not negligent in transporting a victim of a shooting to the nearest available hospital rather than to a hospital located five or six miles away where a thoracic surgeon was present. The paramedics were not capable of diagnosing the extent of the decedent's injury. Except for a children's center and a burn center, there were no emergency trauma centers specifically designated for the treatment of particular injuries.

Lidocaine Administered 44 Times Normal Dosage

In *Riffe v. Vereb Ambulance Service, Inc.*,[51] a wrongful death action was filed by appellants against Vereb Ambulance Service, St. Francis Hospital, and Custozzo. The complaint alleged that, while responding to an emergency call, defendant Custozzo, an emergency medical technician employed by Vereb began administering lidocaine to Anderson, as ordered over the telephone by the medical command physician at the defendant hospital. While en route to the hospital, Anderson was administered lidocaine 44 times the normal dosage. Consequently, normal heart function was not restored, and Anderson was pronounced dead shortly at the hospital shortly thereafter.

The superior court held that the liability of medical technicians could not be imputed to the hospital. The court noted the practical impossibility of the hospital carrying ultimate responsibility for the quality of care and treatment given patients by emergency medical services (EMS). The focus of training and monitoring of such services must lie with EMS regional and local councils pursuant to and subject to regulations promulgated by the department of health.

Although hospitals, as facilities, participate in the overall operation of EMS services, the hospital command facility derives its function from the law and regulations relating to the operation of EMS. The networking of EMS and command facilities is such that they have a common interrelated function that is apart from the administration of the hospitals to which they are attached. Because EMS may be involved with several hospitals depending on specialization, and even allowing for patients' directions, a hospital's legal responsibility for the operation of any given EMS becomes too tenuous.

Application for Licensure Denied

The South Dakota Board of Medical and Osteopathic Examiner was found not to have acted arbitrarily in denying the petitioner's application for a paramedic license. The record indicated that the board had considered petitioner's multiple felony convictions along with extensive evidence of her current conduct. Considering her six felony convictions, the board was not arbitrary and capricious in concluding that Benton did not meet her burden of proving good moral character and an absence of unprofessional or dishonorable conduct.

The appeals court was advised by counsel that the petitioner recently received a pardon for her convictions and that she has completed paramedic training in Nebraska. The board did not have the benefit of that information at the time it heard the matter, and those facts were not in the record. The appeals court could only deal with matters presented in the record and, therefore, remanded the matter to the circuit court with directions to remand to the board for further proceedings.[52]

PHARMACY

Because of the immense variety and complexity of medications now available, it is practically impossible for nurses or doctors to keep up with the information required for safe medication use. The pharmacist has become an essential resource in modern hospital practice.[53]

Among the nonoperative adverse events, medication errors are considered a leading cause of medical injury in the United States. Antibiotics, chemotherapeutic drugs, and anticoagulants are the three categories of drugs responsible for many drug-related adverse events. The prevention of medication errors requires recognition of common causes and the development of practices to help reduce the incidence of errors. With thousands of drugs, many of which look alike and sound alike, it is understandable why medication errors are so common. The following listing describes some of the more common type of medication errors:

- prescription errors
  - wrong patient
  - wrong drug
  - inappropriate drug ordered due to, for example, known drug allergies, drug-drug and food-drug interactions
  - wrong dose
  - wrong route
  - wrong frequency
  - transcription errors (often due to illegible handwriting and improper use of abbreviations)
  - inadequate review of medication for appropriateness
- dispensing errors
  - improper preparation of medication
  - failure to properly formulate medications
  - dispensing expired medications
  - mislabeling containers
  - wrong patient
  - wrong dose
  - wrong route
  - misinterpretation of physician order
- administration errors
  - wrong patient
  - wrong route
  - double-dosing (drug administered more than once)
  - failure to administer medications
  - wrong frequency
  - administering discontinued drugs
  - administering drugs without an authorized order
  - wrong dose (e.g., IV rate)
- documentation errors
  - transcription errors (often due to illegible handwriting and improper use of abbreviations)
  - inaccurate transcription to medication administration record (MAR)

- charted but not administered

- administered but not documented on the MAR

- discontinued order not noted on the MAR

- medication wasted and not recorded

The practice of pharmacy essentially includes preparing, compounding, dispensing, and retailing medications. These activities may be carried out only by a pharmacist with a state license or by a person exempted from the provisions of a state's pharmacy statutes. The entire stock of drugs in a pharmacy is subject to strict government regulation and control. The pharmacist is responsible for developing, coordinating, and supervising all pharmacy activities and reviewing the drug regimens of each patient.

Government Control of Drugs

The power and authority to regulate drugs, their products, packaging, and distribution rest primarily with federal and state governments. Consequently, there are often two sets of regulations and standards governing the same activity. In general, states have attempted to enact laws that comply with federal laws. For example, most states have adopted the Uniform Controlled Substances Act (UCSA). This uniform law is based on and is in conformity with the federal Controlled Substances Act. Several states have modified the UCSA in various ways, frequently setting more stringent standards than are required under the federal law.

Controlled Substances Act

The Comprehensive Drug Abuse Prevention and Control Act of 1970, commonly known as the Controlled Substances Act (CSA), was signed into law on October 27, 1970, as Public Law No. 91-513. This law replaced virtually all preexisting federal laws dealing with narcotics, depressants, and stimulants.

The CSA places all substances that are regulated under existing federal law into one of five schedules. This placement is based upon the substance's medicinal value, harmfulness, and potential for abuse or addiction. Schedule I is reserved for the most dangerous drugs that have no recognized medical use, while Schedule V is the classification used for the least dangerous drugs. The act also provides a mechanism for substances to be controlled, added to a schedule, decontrolled, removed from control, rescheduled, or transferred from one schedule to another.[54]

Federal Food, Drug and Cosmetic Act

The Federal Food, Drug and Cosmetic Act (FDCA) applies to drugs and devices carried in interstate commerce and to goods produced and distributed in federal territory. The act's requirements apply to almost every drug that would be dispensed from a pharmacy, because nearly all drugs and devices, or their components, are eventually carried in interstate commerce.

Section 502 of the act sets forth the information that must appear on the labels or the labeling of drugs and devices. The label must contain, among other special information: (1) the name and place of business of the manufacturer, packer, or distributor; (2) the quantity of contents; (3) the name and quantity of any ingredient found to be habit forming, along with the statement "Warning—may be habit-forming"; (4) the established name of the drug or its ingredients; (5) adequate directions for use; (6) adequate warnings and cautions concerning conditions of use; and (7) special precautions for packaging.

The regulation implementing the labeling requirements of Section 502 exempts prescription drugs from the requirement that the label bear "adequate directions for use for laymen" if the drug is in the possession of a pharmacy or under the custody of a practitioner licensed by law to administer or prescribe legend drugs.[55] This particular exemption applies only to prescription drugs meeting the other requirements. Ordinary household remedies in the custody or possession of a practitioner or pharmacist would not fall under the labeling exemption.

If the drug container is too small to bear a label with all the required information, the label may contain only the quantity or proportion of each active ingredient and the lot or control number. The prescription legend may appear on the outer container of such drug units. The lot or control number may appear on the crimp of a dispensing tube, and the remainder of the required label information may appear on other labeling within the package.

Besides the label itself, each legend drug must be accompanied by labeling, on or within the sealed package from which the drug is to be dispensed, bearing full prescribing information including indications; dosage; routes, methods, and frequency of administration; contraindications; side effects; precautions; and any other information concerning the intended use of the drug necessary for the prescriber to use the drug safely. This information usually is contained in what is known in the trade as the *package insert.*

State Regulations

Besides federal laws affecting the manufacture, use, and handling of drugs, the different states have controlling legislation. All states regulate the practice of pharmacy, as well as the operation of pharmacies. State regulations generally provide that:

1. each health care organization must ensure the availability of pharmaceutical services to meet the needs of patients

2. pharmaceutical services must be provided in accordance with all applicable federal and state laws and regulations

3. pharmaceutical services must be provided under the supervision of a pharmacist

4. space and equipment must be provided within the organization for the proper storage, safeguarding, preparation, dispensing, and administration of drugs

5. each organization must develop and implement written policies and procedures regarding accountability, distribution, and assurance of quality of all drugs

6. each organization must develop and follow current written procedures for the safe prescription and administration of drugs

State laws require that pharmacies be licensed and that they be under the supervision of a person licensed to practice pharmacy. The pharmacist usually can be either an employee of the organization or a consultant. The authority of an organization to operate a pharmacy is conditioned on compliance with licensing requirements affecting the pharmacy premises and its personnel. The statutes applying to pharmacies usually empower regulatory agencies, such as the state pharmacy board, to issue rules and regulations as necessary.

Each organization is subject to liability for the negligent acts of its professional and nonprofessional employees in the handling of drugs and medications within the organization. Both the pharmacist and the organization are subject to criminal liability, as well as civil liability, for the violation of statutory directives. Most states have regulations that dictate in detail the dispensing, distribution, administration, storage, control, and disposal of drugs within health care organizations.

Distribution, Dispensing, and Administration of Drugs

Distribution of medications is the movement of a legend drug from a community pharmacy or institutional pharmacy to a nursing service area while in the originally labeled manufacturer's container, labeled according to federal and state statutes and regulations.

The *dispensing of medications* is the processing of a drug for delivery or for administration to a patient pursuant to the order of an appropriately licensed health care practitioner. It consists of checking the directions on the label with the directions on the prescription or order to determine accuracy; selecting the drug from stock to fill the order; counting, measuring, compounding, or preparing the drug; placing the drug in the proper container; and adding to a written prescription any required notations.

The *administration of medications* is an act in which a single dose of a prescribed drug is given to a patient by an authorized person in accordance with federal and state laws and regulations governing such act. The complete act of administration includes removing an individual dose from a previously dispensed, properly labeled container (including a unit-dose container), verifying it with the physician's order, giving the individual dose to the proper patient, and recording the time and dose given.

Each dose of a drug administered must be recorded on the patient's clinical records. A separate record of narcotic drugs must be maintained. The record must contain a separate sheet for each narcotic of different strength or type administered to the patient. The narcotic record must contain the following information: date and time administered, physician's name, signature of person administering the dose, and the balance of the narcotic drug on hand.

In the event that an emergency arises requiring the immediate administration of a particular drug, the patient's record should be documented properly, showing the necessity for administration of the drug on an emergency basis. Procedures should be in place for handling emergency situations.

Storage of Drugs

Drugs must be stored in their original containers and must be labeled properly. The label should indicate the patient's full name, physician, prescription number, strength of the drug, expiration date of all time-dated drugs, and the address and telephone number of the pharmacy dispensing the drug. The medication containers must be stored in a locked cabinet at the nurses' station. Medications containing narcotics or other dangerous drugs must be stored under double lock (e.g., a locked box within the medicine cabinet). The keys to the medicine cabinet and narcotics box must be in the possession of authorized personnel. Medications for external use only must be marked clearly and kept separate from medications for internal use. Medications that are to be taken out of use must be disposed of according to federal and state laws and regulations.

Drug Substitution

Drug substitution may be defined as the dispensing of a different drug or brand in place of the drug or brand ordered. Several states prohibit this, and penal sanctions, including loss of license, are imposed for violation of the law.

Health care organizations use a *formulary system,* whereby physicians and pharmacists create a formulary listing drugs used in the institution. The formulary contains the brand names and generic names of drugs. Under the formulary system, a physician agrees that his or her prescription, which calls for a brand-name drug, may be filled with the generic equivalent of that drug (i.e., a drug that contains the same active ingredients in the same proportions).

Authorization for using a generic equivalent should be given by the physician at the time he or she prescribes a formulary drug and should be evidenced by a written consent on the face of the prescription. When a formulary system is in use, the prescribing physician can require the use of a particular brand-name drug, when he or she deems it necessary or desirable, by expressly prohibiting the use of the formulary system.

A pharmacist can be subject to liability for the mishandling or misuse of drugs. Failure to meet and maintain required standards in the handling of drugs can lead to criminal or civil liability and even to the revocation of a pharmacist's license.

Decreasing Medication Misadventures: Helpful Tips

- Be sure that your handwriting is legible; print if necessary.

- For clarity, do not use felt-tip pens.

- Abbreviations should be used according to hospital policy.

- Do not write ambiguous orders.

- Always add a zero prior to a decimal.

- Hold orders should be accompanied by a time frame.

- Know about the medication that you are prescribing.

- Be sure medications have been properly diluted before prescribing.

- Be sure that medications are being administered by the proper route.

Expanding Role of the Pharmacist

Historically, the role of the pharmacist was centered on the management of the pharmacy and the accurate dispensing of drugs. The duties and responsibilities of pharmacists have moved well beyond the concept of filling prescriptions and dispensing drugs. Schools of pharmacy have recognized the ever-expanding role of the pharmacist into the clinical aspects of patient care—so much so that educational requirements are getting more stringent, with emphasis on clinical education and application. Pharmacists now, among other duties, maintain patient medication profiles and monitor patient profiles, looking for incompatibilities between drug-drug and food-drug interactions.

Duty to Monitor Patient's Medications

In *Baker v. Arbor Drugs, Inc.,*[56] a Michigan court imposed a duty on a pharmacist to monitor a patient's medications. Three different prescriptions were prescribed by the same physician and filled at the same pharmacy. The pharmacy maintained a computer system that detected drug-drug interactions. The pharmacy advertised to consumers that it could, through the use of a computer-monitoring system, provide a medication profile for its customers that would alert its pharmacists to potential drug-drug interactions. Because the pharmacy advertised and used the computer system to monitor the medications of its customers, the pharmacist voluntarily assumed a duty of care to detect the harmful drug-drug interaction that occurred in this case.

Pharmacists have an ever-expanding clinical role in the delivery of patient care. For example, pharmacists often maintain a separate telephone line in hospitals for caregivers and practitioners to use to discuss medication usage. Pharmacists play an important role when they respond and participate in reviving patients in cardiac arrest. Their knowledge of drugs, potential drug interactions, and proper dosing can be the difference between life and death. Some hospitals have reported improved code outcomes when pharmacists attend and participate in patient codes.

Warning Patients About Potential for Overdose

A Pennsylvania court held that a pharmacist failed to warn the patient about the maximum dosage of a drug the patient could take.[57] This failure resulted in an overdose, causing permanent injuries. Expert testimony focused on the fact that a pharmacist who receives inadequate instructions as to the maximum recommended dosage has a duty to ascertain whether the patient is aware of the limitations concerning the use of the drug. The pharmacist should have contacted the prescribing physician to clarify the prescription.

Refusal to Honor a Questionable Prescription

In *Hooks v. McLaughlin,*[58] the Indiana Supreme Court held that a pharmacist had a duty to refuse to refill prescriptions at an unreasonably faster rate than prescribed pending directions from the prescribing physician. The Indiana code provides that a pharmacist is immune from civil prosecution or civil liability if he or she, in good faith, refuses to honor a prescription because, in his or her professional judgment, the honoring of the prescription would aid or abet an addiction or habit.[59]

Limited Duty to Warn

The rules and regulations promulgated by the Georgia State Board of Pharmacy require a generalized duty on the part of pharmacists to warn of every potentially adverse drug reaction. In this case, the pharmacy was properly granted summary judgment with respect to claims arising from a patient's extreme allergic reaction, namely, Stevens-Johnson syndrome, to a prescription drug, Daypro, which was a nonsteroidal anti-inflammatory drug, even though it was alleged that the pharmacist failed to warn the patient of the potential side effects of the drug.[60]

PHYSICAL THERAPY

Physical therapy is the art and science of preventing and treating neuromuscular or musculoskeletal disabilities through the evaluation of an individual's disability and rehabilitation potential; the use of physical agents (heat, cold, ultrasound, electricity, water, and light); and neuromuscular procedures that, through their physiologic effect, improve or maintain the patient's optimum functional level. Because of different physical disabilities brought on by various injuries and medical problems, physical therapy is an extremely important component of a patient's total health care.

Incorrectly Interpreting Physician's Orders

Pontiff, in *Pontiff v. Pecot & Assoc.*[61] filed a petition for damages against Pecot and Associates and Morris. Pontiff alleged Pecot and Associates had been negligent in failing to properly train, supervise, and monitor its employees, including Morris, and that Pecot and Associates was otherwise negligent. Pontiff alleged that employee Morris failed to exercise the degree of care and skill ordinarily exercised by physical therapists, failed to heed his protests that he could not perform the physical therapy treatments she was supervising, and failed to stop performing physical therapy treatments after he began to complain he was in pain. Pontiff claimed he felt a muscle tear while he was exercising on the butterfly machine, a resistive exercise machine.

Pontiff's expert, Boulet, a licensed practicing physical therapist, testified that Pecot deviated from the standard of care of physical therapists by introducing a type of exercise that, according to her, was not prescribed by Dr. deAraujo, the treating physician. She stated that Pecot added resistive or strengthening exercises to Pontiff's therapy and that these were not a part of the physician's prescription. Pecot argued that resistive exercises were implicitly part of the prescription, even if her interpretation of the prescription was not reasonable.

Legally, under Louisiana law, a physical therapist may not treat a patient without a written physical therapy prescription. Ethically, the Physical Therapists' Code of Ethics, Principle 3.4, states that any alteration of a program or extension of services beyond the program should be undertaken in consultation with the referring practitioner. Because resistive exercises were not set forth in the original prescription, Boulet stated that consultation with the physician was necessary before Pontiff could be advanced to that level. Only in the case where a physician has indicated on the prescription that the therapist is to evaluate and treat would the therapist have such discretion. There was no such indication on the prescription written by deAraujo.

Davis, a physical therapist in private practice and Pecot's expert witness, testified that the program that Pecot designed for Pontiff was consistent with how she interpreted the prescription for therapy that the physician wrote. Davis, however, did not at any time state that Pecot's interpretation was a reasonable one. In fact, Davis herself would not have interpreted the prescription in the manner that Pecot did. Davis testified only that Pecot's introduction of resistive exercises was reasonable based on her interpretation of the prescription.

It is clear that Pecot, as a licensed physical therapist, owed a duty to Pontiff, her client. Pecot's duty is defined by the standard of care of similar physical therapists and the Association of Physical Therapists of America. If Pecot found the prescription to be ambiguous, she had a duty to contact the prescribing physician for clarification. The appeals court found that the trial court was correct in its determination that Pontiff presented sufficient evidence to show that this duty was breached and that Pecot's care fell below the standard of other physical therapists.

Termination of Contracted Services

The physical therapist in *Armintor v. Community Hospital of Brazosport*[62] was properly enjoined from entering the hospital's premises after termination of an oral contract to furnish services to hospital patients in need of physical therapy. Substantial evidence supported the court's finding that the hospital's attempt to establish a hospital-based physical therapy program would have been disrupted if the independent therapist had been permitted to continue treating patients. The court considered the exclusion of a therapist an administrative matter within the board's discretion. The therapist's entering the hospital without the permission of a staff physician would constitute trespass and would be in violation of hospital policy.

Neglect

In *Zucker v. Axelrod*,[63] a physical therapist had been charged with resident neglect for refusing to allow an 82-year-old nursing facility resident to go to the bathroom before starting his therapy treatment session. Undisputed evidence at a hearing showed that the petitioner refused to allow the resident to be excused to go to the bathroom. The petitioner claimed that her refusal was because she assumed that the resident had gone to the bathroom before going to therapy and that the resident was undergoing a bladder training program. The petitioner had not mentioned when she was interviewed after the incident or during her hearing testimony that she considered bladder training a basis for refusing to allow the resident to go to the bathroom. It is uncontroverted that the nursing facility had a policy of allowing residents to go to the bathroom whenever they wished to do so. The court held that the finding of resident neglect was supported sufficiently by the evidence.

Physical Therapist License Revoked

The license of a physical therapist was found to have been properly revoked by the Bureau of Professional and Occupational Affairs, State Board of Physical Therapy after the therapist had been disciplined in other states. In New Jersey, the board of physical therapy denied Girgis a license to practice physical therapy. The Michigan Board of Physical Therapy imposed a $1000 fine on Girgis. The South Carolina Board of Physical Therapy suspended Girgis's license indefinitely. The New Hampshire Governing Board of Physical Therapy suspended Girgis's license for five months. The Montana Board of Physical Therapy Examiners revoked Girgis's license. The Medical Licensing Board of Indiana put Girgis's license on indefinite probation for no less than two years, and later indefinitely suspended it for no less than six months and imposed a $500 fine because Girgis failed to comply with the terms of his probation. The Hawaii Board of Physical Therapy suspended Girgis's license for five months. The Florida Department of Health accepted Girgis's voluntary relinquishment of his Florida license.

Whether Girgis was incompetent, negligent, or abusive, or a risk to patients in Pennsylvania, was found to be wholly irrelevant. The sole inquiry is whether his license to practice physical therapy was suspended, revoked, or otherwise disciplined in another jurisdiction. Because he does not dispute he was disciplined in eight states, the board did not err in disciplining him in Pennsylvania.[64]

PHYSICIAN'S ASSISTANT

One of the solutions to the shortage of physicians in certain rural and inner-city areas has been to train allied health professionals, such as a physician's assistant (PA), to perform the more routine and repetitive medical procedures. A physician may delegate to a PA such tasks as suturing minor wounds, administering injections, and performing routine history and physical examinations. A physician may not delegate a task to a PA in those instances where regulations specify that the physician must perform it or when the delegation is prohibited under state law or by the facility's own policies.

PAs are responsible for their own negligent acts. The employer of a PA can be held liable for the PA's negligent acts on the basis of respondeat superior. To limit the potential risk of liability for a PA's negligent acts, PAs should be monitored and supervised by a physician. Guidelines and procedures also should be established to provide a standard mechanism for reviewing a PA's performance.

PODIATRIST

The legal concerns of podiatrists, similar to those of surgeons, include misdiagnosis and negligent surgery. The podiatrist, for example, in *Strauss v. Biggs*[65] was found to have failed to meet the standard of care required of a podiatrist and that failure resulted in injury to the patient. The podiatrist, by his own admission, stated that his initial incision in the patient's foot had been misplaced. The trial court was found not to have erred in permitting the jury to consider additional claims that the podiatrist acted improperly by failing to refer the patient, stop the procedure after the first incision, inform the patient of possible nerve injury, and provide proper postoperative treatment. Testimony of the patient's experts was adequate to show that such alleged omissions violated the standard of care required of podiatrists.

RESPIRATORY THERAPIST

Respiratory therapy is the allied health profession responsible for the treatment, management, diagnostic testing, and control of patients with cardiopulmonary deficits. A respiratory therapist is a person employed in the practice of respiratory care who has the knowledge and skill necessary to administer respiratory care.

Respiratory therapists are responsible for their negligent acts. A respiratory therapist's employer is responsible for the negligent acts of the therapist under the legal doctrine of respondeat superior.

Failure to Remove Endotracheal Tube

The court in *Poor Sisters of St. Francis v. Catron*[66] held that the failure of nurses and an inhalation therapist to report to the supervisor that an endotracheal tube had been left in the plaintiff longer than the customary period of three or four days was sufficient to allow the jury to reach a finding of negligence. The patient experienced difficulty speaking and underwent several operations to remove scar tissue and open her voice box. At the time of trial, she could not speak above a whisper and breathed partially through a hole in her throat created by a tracheotomy. The hospital was found liable for the negligent acts of its employees and the resulting injuries to the plaintiff.

Multiple Use of Same Syringe

The respiratory therapist in *State University v. Young*[67] was suspended for using the same syringe for drawing blood from a number of critically ill patients. The therapist had been warned several times of the dangers of that practice and that it violated the state's policy of providing quality patient care.

Restocking the Code Cart

Dixon had been admitted to the hospital and was diagnosed with pneumonia in her right lung. Dixon's condition began to deteriorate and she was moved to the intensive care unit (ICU). A code blue was eventually called signifying that her cardiac and respiratory functions were believed to have ceased. During the code, a decision was made to intubate, which is to insert an endotracheal tube into Dixon so that she could be given respiratory support by a mechanical ventilator. As Dixon's condition stabilized, Dr. Taylor, Dixon's physician at that time, ordered that she gradually be weaned from the respirator. Blackham, a respiratory therapist employed by the hospital, extubated Dixon at 10:15 P.M. Taylor left Dixon's room to advise her family that she had been extubated. Blackham decided an oxygen mask would provide better oxygen to Dixon but could not locate a mask in the ICU, so he left ICU and went across the hall to the critical care unit (CCU). When Blackham returned to Dixon's room with the oxygen mask and placed it on Dixon, he realized that she was not breathing properly. Blackham realized that she would have to be reintubated as quickly as possible.

A second code was called. Shackleford, a nurse in the cardiac CCU, responded to the code. Shackleford recorded on the code sheet that she arrived in Dixon's room at 10:30 P.M. She testified that Blackham said he had too short of a blade and he needed a medium, a Number 4 MacIntosh laryngoscope blade, which was not on the code cart. The code cart is a cart equipped with all the medicines, supplies, and instruments needed for a code emergency. The code cart in the ICU had not been restocked after the first code that morning, so Shackleford was sent to obtain the needed blade from the CCU across the hall. When Shackleford returned to the ICU, the blade was passed to Taylor, who had responded to the code, and was attempting to reintubate Dixon. Upon receiving the blade, Taylor was able to quickly intubate Dixon. Dixon was placed on a ventilator, but she never regained consciousness. After the family was informed there was no hope that Dixon would recover the use of her brain, the family requested that no extraordinary measure be taken to prolong her life.

A medical negligence claim was filed against Taylor and the hospital. The jury found that Taylor was not negligent. Evidence presented at trial established that the hospital's breach of duty in not having the code cart properly restocked resulted in a three-minute delay in the intubation of Dixon. Reasonable minds could accept from the testimony at trial that the hospital's breach of duty was a cause of Dixon's brain death, without which the injury would not have occurred. Foreseeability on the part of the hospital could be established from the evidence introduced by the plaintiff that the written standards for the hospital require every code cart be stocked with a Number 4 MacIntosh blade. This evidence permits a reasonable inference that the hospital should have foreseen that the failure to have the code cart stocked with the blade could lead to critical delays in intubating a patient. Accordingly, there was substantial evidence that failure to have the code cart stocked with the proper blade was a proximate cause of Dixon's injuries.[68]

SECURITY

Hospitals have a duty to implement and maintain reasonable measures to protect patients from the criminal acts of third parties. However, if an attack and injury to a patient is not foreseeable, the hospital's actions cannot be the proximate cause of the patient's injuries.

The patient in *Lane v. St. Joseph's Regional Medical Center*[69] was sitting in the emergency department waiting room when a teenage boy, D.G., arrived with his mother. After they had all sat in the waiting room for a short period of time, D.G. walked up to Lane and began to hit her on her right arm and shoulder. Lane's son-in-law, who had accompanied her to the emergency room, jumped to her aid and struck D.G., knocking him to the floor. The attack stopped and nothing further happened. Lane suffered some injuries as a result of the attack.

The evidence in this case depicts a situation in which the attack upon Lane by D.G. was unexpected and that no other evidence was designated to the trial court from which it could have concluded that the specific actions of D.G. on the day in question were foreseeable. The court was bound to conclude that the attack and injury were not foreseeable, that the center's actions were not the proximate cause of Lane's injuries, and that the center is entitled to judgment as a matter of law.

FAILURE TO PROVIDE ADEQUATE SECURITY

Citation: *Hanewinckel v. St. Paul's Property & Liab.,* 611 So. 2d 174 (La. App. 1992)

Facts

The plaintiff, a nurse anesthetist, arrived at the hospital at approximately 5:25 A.M. After parking her car and before she shut off the engine, a man jumped into the driver's seat and began to drive off. The nurse jumped from the car but her attacker caught her and started to beat her. An employee pulling into the parking lot saw what was happening and alerted security. The plaintiff suffered a broken left wrist, 12 teeth either knocked out or broken, severe bruises on her face, and cuts on her legs and knees. She also suffered mental distress from which she had not recovered.

The nurse sued the owner of the parking lot and the security force for breach to protect her from a criminal attack committed on the premises. The trial court found that the defendant had a duty to provide reasonable and adequate security in the parking area, and that it had breached this duty. The plaintiff was awarded $733,000 and the defendant appealed.

Issue

Did the hospital breach a duty by failing to adequately patrol its parking lot?

Holding

The court of appeals affirmed the decision for the plaintiff, finding that the hospital breached its duty to the employee by failing to patrol the parking lot.

Reason

The hospital took on the responsibility of maintaining a security force to cover the parking lot. As such, the hospital assumed liability, giving a warranty that, through employment of a security service, their work would be carried out in a nonnegligent manner. The evidence indicated that other witnesses had seen the attacker in or near the parking lot five hours earlier in the day, yet no security personnel spotted him. Further, there were not enough security officers on duty that day to adequately patrol the parking lot. If they had been patrolling properly, the court concluded that the criminal would have been discovered and the attack prevented. The court found that the security force breached its duty by negligently failing to provide adequate security, which should have included random patrolling of all of the areas. After the attacker was reported to security earlier in the day, nothing other than a brief walk through the lot was done.

Discussion

1. Discuss the required duty to care and how it was breached in this case.
2. What are the implications of this case for health care organizations?

SEXUAL IMPROPRIETIES

A significant number of cases address health care professionals who have been involved in sexual relationships with their patients. Such cases are being litigated, in many instances, in both civil and criminal arenas. Health care professionals finding themselves in such unprofessional relationships must seek help for themselves as well as refer their patients to other appropriate professionals. Besides being subject to civil and criminal litigation, health care professionals also are subject to having their licenses revoked for sexual improprieties.

Dentist

Revocation of a dentist's license on charges of professional misconduct was properly ordered in *Melone v. State*

Education Department[70] on the basis of substantial evidence that while acting in his professional capacity, the dentist engaged in physical and sexual contact with five different male patients within a three-year period. Considering the dentist's responsible position, the extended time period during which the sexual contacts occurred, the age and impressionable nature of the victims (7 to 15 years of age), and the possibility of lasting effects on the victims, the penalty was not shocking to the court's sense of fairness.

Nurse

A nurse's sexual relations with a patient can give rise to disciplinary action resulting in the nurse's loss of license. In *Heineche v. Department of Commerce,*[71] a male nurse lost his license after having a sexual relationship with a patient, even though she was no longer a patient at the hospital where he had met her. The fact that the nurse resigned from the hospital and was living with the patient was not a defense sufficient to support such behavior.

Osteopath

The board of registration in medicine, after a full hearing before an administrative magistrate, properly revoked the license of an osteopath to practice medicine. The record supported findings that the osteopath had an extended personal and romantic relationship with one of his patients, conduct forbidden under then-current professional standards, and that he had attempted to obstruct the board's proceedings against him by threatening the complaint counsel and investigator with criminal prosecution. There was no merit to the osteopath's contentions that the board's authority to revoke a physician's license was limited to instances of gross misconduct or that specific intent to cause harm must be shown. Revocation was appropriate where the osteopath had a dual relationship with the patient that went on for over two years, including incidents of sexual intercourse, and where there was evidence that the patient suffered harm as a result of osteopath's misconduct.[72]

Physician

A hospital technologist in *Copithorne v. Framingham Union Hospital*[73] alleged that a staff physician raped her during the course of a house call. The technologist's claim against the hospital was summarily dismissed for lack of proximate causation. On appeal, the dismissal was found to be improper when the record indicated that the hospital had received notice of allegations that the physician assaulted patients on and off the hospital's premises. The hospital had instructed the physician to have another individual present when visiting female patients and had instructed nurses to keep an eye on him. The physician's sexual assault was foreseeable. There was evidentiary support for the proposition that failure to withdraw the physician's privileges caused the rape when the technologist asserted that it was the physician's good reputation in the hospital that led her to seek his services.

Psychiatrist

The sexual relationship a psychiatrist had with the spouse of a patient was found to be improper in *Richard v. Larry.*[74] California Civil Code Section 43.5, abolishing causes of action for alienation of affection, criminal conversation, and seduction of a patient over the age of consent, did not bar damages for emotional distress caused by the alleged professional negligence of the psychiatrist who had sexual relations with the plaintiff's wife. The psychiatrist owed a special duty to use due care for his patient's health. The statute was not intended to lower the standard of care that psychiatrists owed their patients. Besides an action against the psychiatrist, allegations that the psychiatrist was an agent of the hospital stated a cause of action against the hospital.

On April 10, 1998, the bureau of professional medical conduct charged the petitioner in *Goldberg v. De Buono,*[75] a licensed physician and psychiatrist, with moral unfitness, gross negligence and incompetence, negligence on more than one occasion, and incompetence by reason of his alleged sexual relationship with a patient. Following a hearing, a hearing committee of the state board for professional medical conduct sustained the specifications of moral unfitness and gross negligence and recommended revocation of the petitioner's license. The petitioner commenced a proceeding to annul the committee's determination and revocation of petitioner's license.

The New York Supreme Court, Appellate Division, rejected the petitioner's assertion that the committee erred in crediting the testimony of patient A and her daughter. Issues of credibility, even as to witnesses with psychiatric illnesses, are exclusively for the administrative fact finder to determine. Moreover, it is noteworthy that the petitioner conceded his sexual relationship with patient A but contended that the physician-patient relationship had been terminated at the time the sexual relationship occurred. Inasmuch as there was expert testimony that the relationship had not been terminated and the petitioner's relationship with patient A constituted a serious deviation from accepted standards of practice, the court was satisfied that the committee's determination was supported by substantial evidence.

SURGERY

Operating rooms, hidden behind closed doors, are often the scenes of negligent acts. A Wyoming man was awarded $1.175 million after doctors removed the wrong cervical disc during spinal surgery.[76] The following cases illustrate a variety of medical errors that have occurred during the course of surgery.

Improper Positioning of Arm

The plaintiff in *Wick v. Henderson*[77] experienced pain in her left arm upon awakening from surgery; an anesthesiologist told her that her arm was stressed during surgery. According to the plaintiff, she sustained an injury to the ulnar nerve in her left upper arm. A malpractice action was filed against the hospital and the anesthesiologist. The plaintiff sought recovery on theory of res ipsa loquitur. There was testimony that the main cause of the injury was the mechanical compression of the nerve by improper positioning of the arm during surgery. The trial court granted the defendants a directed verdict, resulting in dismissal of the case.

On appeal, the Iowa Supreme Court held that the res ipsa loquitur doctrine applied. The plaintiff must prove two foundational facts in order to invoke the doctrine of res ipsa loquitur. First, she must prove that the defendants had exclusive control and management of the instrument that caused her injury, and second, that it was the type of injury that ordinarily would not occur if reasonable care had been used. As to control, the plaintiff can show an injury resulting from an external force applied while she lay unconscious in the hospital. It is within common knowledge and experience of a layperson that an individual does not enter the hospital for gallbladder surgery and leave with ulnar nerve injury.

Sciatic Nerve Injury

The plaintiff in *Lacombe v. Dr. Walter Olin Moss Regional Hospital*[78] was admitted to the hospital for a bladder suspension operation. Upon regaining consciousness in the recovery room, the plaintiff began complaining of severe pain in her right buttock, shooting down the back of her right leg. The plaintiff was eventually diagnosed with sciatic nerve injury. It is undisputed that the injury is permanent. A medical malpractice claim was filed against the hospital and the physicians involved in the surgery. A medical review panel rendered a decision finding no breach of the standard of care. The plaintiff then filed a malpractice suit against the hospital and physicians. By the time of trial, all of the defendants except the hospital had been dismissed from the litigation. After trial, the trial judge rendered judgment in favor of the plaintiff. The trial judge found that, applying the doctrine of res ipsa loquitur to the evidence, the plaintiff had proven her case. Accordingly, he found the hospital responsible under the theory of respondeat superior for the negligent conduct of its agents (the personnel who prepared the plaintiff for surgery and the physicians who conducted the operation).

The hospital contended that the trial court incorrectly applied the doctrine of res ipsa loquitur. The facts established by the plaintiff must also reasonably permit the jury to discount other possible causes and to conclude it was more likely than not that the defendant's negligence caused the injury.

The Louisiana Court of Appeals held that the evidence warranted an inference of res ipsa loquitur. Expert testimony established that the plaintiff was suffering from a sciatic nerve injury and that the injury was permanent. Experts on both sides agreed that sciatic nerve injury was not a known risk of this surgery. The testimony indicated that the plaintiff went into the hospital without the injury and came out with it. After reviewing the record, the court agreed with the trial court that the evidence warranted an inference that negligence on the part of the defendant caused the injury.

CERTIFICATION OF HEALTH CARE PROFESSIONALS

The certification of health care professionals is the recognition by a governmental or professional association that an individual's expertise meets the standards of that group. Some professional groups establish their own minimum standards for certification in those professions that are not licensed by a particular state. Certification by an association or group is a self-regulation credentialing process.

LICENSING HEALTH CARE PROFESSIONALS

Licensure can be defined as the process by which some competent authority grants permission to a qualified individual or entity to perform certain specified activities that would be illegal without a license. As it applies to health care personnel, *licensure* refers to the process by which licensing boards, agencies, or departments of the several states grant to individuals who meet certain predetermined standards the legal right to practice in a health care profession and to use a specified health care practitioner's title. The commonly stated objectives of licensing laws are to limit and control admission to the different health care occupations and to protect the public from unqualified practitioners by promulgating and enforcing standards of practice within the professions.

The authority of states to license health care practitioners is found in their regulating power. Implicit in the power to license is the authority to collect license fees, establish standards of practice, require certain minimum qualifications and competency levels of applicants, and impose on applicants other requirements necessary to protect the general public welfare. This authority, which is vested in the legislature, may be delegated to political subdivisions or to state boards, agencies, and departments. In some instances, the scope of the delegated power is made specific in the legislation; in others, the licensing authority may have wide discretion in performing its functions. In either case, however, the authority granted by the legislature may not be exceeded.

SUSPENSION AND REVOCATION OF LICENSE

Licensing boards have the authority to suspend or revoke the license of a health care professional who is found to have violated specified norms of conduct. Such violations may include procurement of a license by fraud; unprofessional, dishonorable, immoral, or illegal conduct; performance of specific actions prohibited by statute; and malpractice.

Suspension and revocation procedures are most commonly contained in a state's licensing act; in some jurisdictions, however, the procedure is left to the discretion of the board or is contained in the general administrative procedure acts.

HELPFUL ADVICE FOR CAREGIVERS

- Abide by the ethical code of one's profession.
- Do not criticize the professional skills of others.
- Maintain complete and adequate medical records.
- Provide each patient with medical care comparable with national standards.
- Seek the aid of professional medical consultants when indicated.
- Obtain informed consent for diagnostic and therapeutic procedures.
- Inform the patient of the risks, benefits, and alternatives to proposed procedures.
- Do not indiscriminately prescribe medications or diagnostic tests.
- Practice the specialty in which you have been trained.
- Participate in continuing education programs.
- Keep patient information confidential.
- Check patient equipment regularly, and monitor it for safe use.

- When terminating a professional relationship with a patient, give adequate written notice to the patient.
- Authenticate all telephone orders.
- Obtain a qualified substitute when you will be absent from your practice.
- Investigate patient incidents promptly.
- Be a good listener, and allow each patient sufficient time to express fears and anxieties.
- Develop and implement an interdisciplinary plan of care for each patient.
- Safely administer patient medications.
- Closely monitor each patient's response to treatment.
- Provide education and teaching to patients.
- Foster a sense of trust and feeling of significance.
- Communicate with the patient and other caregivers.
- Provide cost-effective care without sacrificing quality

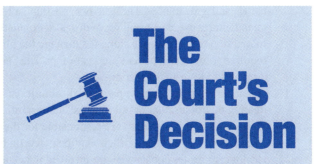

The Court's Decision

The parents were offered an out-of-court settlement totaling $200,000. This tragedy might have been prevented if the patient had been screened and triaged by a person competent to determine the patient's need for immediate care. Failure to assign triage responsibility to a competent individual can lead to lawsuits that involve not only the hospital, but also the supervisor who assigns responsibilities to unqualified staff members. First level managers who have knowledge of such practices and allow them to occur can also be held liable for negligence.

CHAPTER REVIEW

1. Health care professionals, regardless of field, are required to adhere to the prevalent standards of care required within their professions. This includes proper assessment, reassessment, diagnosis, treatment, and follow-up care.
2. Many lawsuits against hospitals arise from care administered in emergency departments. The vast majority of these lawsuits are the result of negligence. Many of these claims charge poor follow-up care and are brought by patients who use emergency departments as primary care clinics.
3. Some of the most common issues around which emergency department lawsuits are centered are improper and inappropriate administration of medication, failure to admit a patient, sparse or contradictory medical documentation, failure to render care, and inappropriate discharge or transfer.
4. In many states, hospitals are required by law to provide emergency care.
5. When the skills of a specialist are required in an emergency department, hospitals are required to notify an on-call specialty physician for assistance. A physician who is on call and does not respond to such a notification can be found liable for injuries to the patient resulting from his or her lack of response.
6. Health care organizations are responsible for the quality and timeliness of the services provided by their clinical laboratories. When services are contracted out, organizations must be sure that they are contracting with reputable licensed laboratories.
7. The nutritional needs of each patient must be met during his or her stay in an organization's facility. Organizations are responsible for the provision of nourishing, palatable, well-balanced diets. Each diet must meet the daily nutritional and special dietary needs of the respective patient.
8. Medication errors are common due to many factors, including the vast number of drugs available and their similar names and appearances. These errors constitute a leading cause of injury. In addition to federal laws regarding the manufacture, use, and handling of drugs, states also have legislation designed to regulate pharmacies.
9. In addition to their regular duties to manage the pharmacy and accurately dispense medications, pharmacists are required to maintain patient medication profiles and monitor these profiles for incompatibilities between drug-drug and food-drug interactions.
10. Physical therapists evaluate patients' disabilities and potential for rehabilitation for the purpose of preventing and treating neuromuscular or musculoskeletal disabilities.
11. Physician's assistants (PAs) are responsible for their own negligent actions and, in addition, their employers can also be held responsible for their negligent acts on the basis of respondeat superior.
12. Health care professionals who are involved in sexual improprieties are subject to civil and criminal litigation and, along with other criminal or civil penalties, may have their licenses revoked.
13. Licensure of health care professionals is the process through which licensing boards, agencies, or departments grant to individuals who meet certain criteria the legal right to practice in a health care profession and use the title of a health care practitioner.

REVIEW QUESTIONS

1. What was the reasoning for enacting the Emergency Medical Treatment and Active Labor Act?
2. Comment on the statement: A sexual impropriety committed by a health care practitioner should be handled in the institution, not in court.
3. Should medical advice be dispensed on the telephone? Explain your opinion.
4. Discuss why the prescribing, control, administration, and monitoring of medications has become a major area of legal concern for health care professionals.
5. Describe the difference between the certification and licensing of a health care professional.

NOTES

1. RONNIE GREEN, *Dying at the Hospital's Door: A Child Lost, Troubling Questions,* THE MIAMI HERALD, Apr. 16, 1995, at 14A.

2. *Poor v. State,* No. S-02-472, 266 Neb. 183 (Neb. 2003).

3. No. W2000-01485-COA-R3-CV (Tenn. App. 2002).

4. *Smith v. O'Neal,* 850 S.W.2d 797 (Tex. Ct. App. 1993).

5. 520 N.E.2d 1085 (Ill. App. Ct. 1988).

6. 599 N.Y.S.2d 58 (N.Y. App. Div. 1993).

7. 711 N.Y.S.2d 65 (N.Y. Sup. Ct., App. Div., 3d Dep't. 2000).

8. 557 S.E.2d 339 (2001).

9. *Lowenberg v. Sobol,* 594 N.Y.S.2d 874 (N.Y. App. Div. 1993).

10. 367 S.E.2d 453 (S.C. 1988).

11. *Id.* at 455–456.

12. THE ROBERT WOOD JOHNSON FOUNDATION, *Negligent Medical Care: What Is It, Where Is It, and How Widespread Is It?* ABRIDGE, Spring 1991, at 7.

13. *Cleland v. Bronson Health Care Group,* 917 F.2d 266, 272 (6th Cir. 1990).

14. *Griffith v. University Hospitals of Cleveland,* No. 84314 (Ohio Ct. of App. 2004).

15. *Roy v. Gupta,* 606 So.2d 940 (La. Ct. App. 1992).

16. *Feeney v. New England Medical Center, Inc.,* 615 N.E.2d 585 (Mass. App. Ct. 1993).

17. 42 U.S.C.A. § 1395dd(a) (1992).

18. 42 U.S.C.A. § 1395dd(e)(1) (1992).

19. 811 F. Supp. 121 (W.D. N.Y. 1993).

20. *Nolen v. Boca Raton Community Hospital, Inc.,* 373 F.3d 1151 (2004).

21. 42 U.S.C.A. § 1395dd(3)(A) (1992).

22. 42 U.S.C.A. § 1395dd(c)(1) (1992).

23. *Guerin v. North Shore University Hospital,* Nos. 2003-07769 & 2004-00199 (N.Y. App. Div. 2004).

24. 831 F. Supp. 829 (M.D. Ala. 1993).

25. 134 F.3d 319 (5th Cir. 1998).

26. 830 F. Supp. 1399 (M.D. Ala. 1993).

27. 934 F.2d 1362 (5th Cir. Tex. 1991).

28. *Courts Uphold Law, Regulations against Patient Dumping,* NATION'S HEALTH, Aug. 1991, at 1.

29. 689 So. 2d 696 (La. App. 1997).

30. 288 A.2d 379 (Md. 1972).

31. 271 N.W.2d 8 (S.D. 1978).

32. 477 So. 2d 1036 (Fla. Dist. Ct. App. 1985).

33. 14 S.W.3d 42 (Mo. App. 1999).

34. 698 So. 2d 958 (La. App. 1997).

35. 498 S.E.2d 408 (1998).

36. *Baptist Mem'l Hosp. Sys. v. Sampson,* 969 S.W.2d 945, 947 (Tex. 1998).

37. MARTIN C. McWILLIAMS, JR. & HAMILTON E. RUSSELL, III, *Hospital Liability for Torts of Independent Contractor Physicians,* 47 S.C. L. REV. 431, 473 (1996).

38. *Jackson v. Powei,* 743 P.2d 1376, 1385 (Alaska 1987).

39. *Martell v. St Charles Hosp.,* 523 N.Y.S.2d 342, 352 (N.Y. Sup. Ct. 1987).

40. *Guerrero v. Copper Queen Hosp.,* 537 P.2d 1329 (Ariz. 1975).

41. 797 So. 2d 160 (2001).

42. 661 S.W.2d 534 (Mo. 1983).

43. 521 N.E.2d 350 (Ind. Ct. App. 1988).

44. *Medical Assistants,* Bureau of Labor Statistics, U.S. Department of Labor, www.bls.gov/oco/ocos164.htm.

45. 636 N.E.2d 1282 (Ind. Ct. App. 1994).

46. 490 N.W.2d 856 (Iowa Ct. App. 1992).

47. 753 F. Supp. 267 (W.D. Ark. 1990).

48. 600 P.2d 647 (Wash. Ct. App. 1979).

49. 1971 Wash. Laws § 1783.

50. 462 A.2d 680 (Pa. 1983).

51. 650 A.2d 1076 (Pa. Super. 1994).

52. *In re Application of Benton,* No. 23232 (S.D. 2005).

53. INSTITUTE OF MEDICINE, *To Err Is Human: Building a Safer Health System,* supra note 1, at 194.

54. www.usdoj.gov/dea/agency/csa.htm.

55. 62. 21 C.F.R. § 1.106.

56. 544 N.W.2d 727 (Mich. Ct. App. 1996).

57. *Riff v. Morgan Pharmacy,* 508 A.2d 1247 (Pa. Super. Ct.1986).

58. 68. 642 N.E.2d 514 (Ind. 1994).

59. IND. CODE § 25-26-13-16(b)(3) (1993).

60. *Chamblin v. K-Mart Corp.,* No. A04A2203 (Ga. Ct. App. 2005).

61. 780 So. 2d 478 (2001).

62. 659 S.W.2d 86 (Tex. Ct. App. 1983).

63. 527 N.Y.S.2d 937 (N.Y. App. Div. 1988).

64. *Girgis v. Board of Physical Therapy,* No. 361 C.D 2004 (Pa. Cmwlth. 2004).

65. 525 A.2d 992 (Del. 1987).

66. 435 N.E.2d 305 (Ind. Ct. App. 1982).

67. 566 N.Y.S.2d 79 (N.Y. App. Div. 1991).

68. *Dixon v. Taylor,* No. 9224SC760 (Filed 20 July 1993).

69. No. 71A05-0310-CV-525 (Ind. App. 2004).

70. 495 N.Y.S.2d 808 (N.Y. App. Div. 1985).

71. 810 P.2d 459 (Utah 1991).

72. *Weinberg v. Board of Registration in Medicine,* 824 N.E.2d 38, 443 Mass. 679 (Mass. 2005).

73. 520 N.E.2d 139 (Mass. 1988).

74. 243 Cal. Rptr. 807 (Cal. Ct. App. 1988).

75. 711 N.Y.S.2d 81 (N.Y. App. Div. 2000).

76. Baldwin, *Medical News Summary: $1.175 million awarded in a medical malpractice case,* Casper Star Tribune, May 13, 2005. http://www.wrongdiagnosis.com/news/_1_175_million_awarded_in_a_medical_malpractice_case.htm.

77. 485 N.W.2d 645 (Iowa 1992).

78. 617 So. 2d 612 (La. Ct. App. 1993).

Information Management and Health Care Records

It's Your Gavel ...

FATAL HANDWRITING MIX-UP

Forty-two-year-old Vasquez died as a result of a handwriting mix-up on the medication prescribed for his heart. Vasquez had been given a prescrip-

tion for 20 mg of Isordil to be taken four times per day. The pharmacist misread the physician's handwriting and filled the prescription with Plendil, a drug for high blood pressure, which is usually taken at no more than 10 mg per day. As a result, Vasquez was given the wrong medication at eight times the recommended dosage. He died two weeks later from an apparent heart attack. The family filed a lawsuit.[1]

WHAT IS YOUR VERDICT?

To significantly reduce the tens of thousands of deaths and injuries caused by medical errors every year, health care organizations must adopt information technology systems that are capable of collecting and sharing essential health information on patients and their care, says a new report by the Institute of Medicine of the National Academies. These systems should operate seamlessly as part of a national network of health information that is accessible by all health care organizations and that includes electronic records of patients' care, secure platforms for the exchange of information among providers and patients, and data standards that will make health information uniform and understandable to all, said the committee that wrote the report.

News: Institute of Medicine, November 20, 2003

The effective and efficient delivery of patient care requires that an organization determine its information needs. Organizations that do not centralize their information needs will often suffer scattered databases, which may result in such problems as duplication of data gathering, inconsistent reports, and inefficiencies in the use of economic resources.

As the principal means of communication between health care professionals in matters relating to patient care, the medical record primarily provides documentation of a patient's illness, symptoms, diagnosis, and treatment, and is used as a planning tool for patient care. Practitioners also use medical records to document communication; assist in protecting the legal interests of the patient, the organization, and the practitioner; provide a database for use in statistical reporting, continuing education, and research; and provide information necessary for third-party billing and regulatory agencies. Health care organizations are required to maintain a medical record for each patient in accordance with accepted professional standards and practices.

State laws often contain provisions mandating that organizations maintain a complete medical record for each patient that contains all pertinent information regarding the daily care and treatment of that patient. Medical records must be complete, accurate, current, readily accessible, and systematically organized. This chapter reviews the legal aspects of patient and physician information, communications, and finances.

MANAGING INFORMATION

All organizations, regardless of mission or size, develop and maintain information management systems, which often include financial, medical, and human resource data. Information management is a process intended to facilitate the flow of information within and between departments and caregivers. An information management plan should:

- Determine customer needs, both internal and external (e.g., third-party payers).

- Set goals and establish priorities (e.g., the development of an integrated patient care record).

- Improve accuracy of data collection.

- Provide uniformity of data collection and definitions.

- Limit duplication of entries.

- Deliver timely and accurate information.

- Provide easy access to information.

- Maintain security and confidentiality of information.

- Enhance patient care activities.

- Improve collaboration across the organization through information sharing.

- Establish disaster plans for the recovery of information.

- Orient and train staff on the information management system.

- Provide an annual review of the information plan to include its scope, organization, objectives, and effectiveness.

CONTENTS OF THE MEDICAL RECORD

Because the medical record fulfills many crucial roles within a health care organization, practitioners must strive to fulfill all requirements to maintain the integrity and accuracy of the records. The inpatient medical record includes:

- The admission record, which describes pertinent data regarding the patient's age, address, reason for admission, Social Security number, marital status, religion, health insurance, and other information necessary to meet both federal and state requirements

- Consent and authorization-for-treatment forms allowing the health care facility to perform various procedures, such as routine diagnostic testing

- Advance directives

- Medical history and physical examination, including diagnosis, and findings that support the diagnosis

- Assessments (e.g., nursing, functional, nutritional, social, and discharge planning)

- Treatment plan

- Physicians' orders

- Progress notes

- Nursing notes (where an integrated record exists, nursing notes are often placed in the progress notes, along with the notes of other disciplines)

- Diagnostic reports (e.g., laboratory and imaging)

- Consultation reports

- Vital signs charts

- Fluid intake and output charts

- Pain management records

- Anesthesia assessment

- Operative reports

- Medication administration records

- Discharge planning/social service notes and reports

- Patient education

- Discharge summaries

OWNERSHIP AND RELEASE OF MEDICAL RECORDS

Health care providers who handle medical records must fully understand the related issues of ownership and privacy. Medical records are the property of the provider of care and are maintained for the benefit of the patient. Ownership resides with the organization or professional rendering treatment. Although medical records typically have been protected from public scrutiny by a general practice of nondisclosure, this practice has been waived under a limited number of specifically controlled situations. Some jurisdictions recognize that individuals have a right to privacy and to be protected from the mass dissemination of information pertaining to their personal or private affairs. The right of privacy generally includes the right to be kept out of the public spotlight. The Privacy Act of 1974 further defines an individual's right to privacy.

Privacy Act of 1974

The Privacy Act of 1974, codified at 5 U.S.C. 552, was enacted to safeguard individual privacy from the misuse of federal records, to give individuals access to records concerning themselves that are maintained by federal agencies, and to establish a Privacy Protection Safety Commission. Section 2 of the Privacy Act reads as follows:

[a] The Congress finds that (1) the privacy of an individual is directly affected by the collection, maintenance, use, and dissemination of personal information by Federal agencies; (2) the increasing use of computers and sophisticated information technology, while essential to the efficient operations of the Government, has greatly magnified the harm to individual privacy that can occur from any collection, maintenance, use, or dissemination of personal information; (3) the opportunities for an individual to secure employment, insurance, and credit, and his right to due process, and other legal protections are endangered by the misuse of certain information systems; (4) the right to privacy is a personal and fundamental right protected by the Constitution of the United States; and (5) in order to protect the privacy of individuals identified in information systems maintained by Federal agencies, it is necessary and proper for the Congress to regulate the collection, maintenance, use, and dissemination of information by such agencies. [b] The purpose of this Act is to provide certain safeguards for an individual against an invasion of personal privacy by requiring Federal agencies, except as otherwise provided by law, to (1) permit an individual to determine what records pertaining to him are collected, maintained, used, or disseminated by such agencies; (2) permit an individual to prevent records pertaining to him obtained by such agencies for a particular purpose from being used or made available for another purpose without his consent; (3) permit an individual to gain access to information pertaining to him in Federal agency records, to have a copy made of all or any portion thereof, and to correct or amend such records; (4) collect, maintain, use, or disseminate

any record of identifiable personal information in a manner that assures that such action is for a necessary and lawful purpose, that the information is current and accurate for its intended use, and that adequate safeguards are provided to prevent misuse of such information. . . .

RELEASE OF CONFIDENTIAL INFORMATION

Citation: *Proenza Sanfiel v. Department of Health,* 749 So. 2d 525 (Fla. App. 1999)

Facts

Sanfiel, a psychiatric nurse, had his professional license suspended for five years after he intentionally disclosed confidential patient information to the news media. Sanfiel testified that he knew the information he possessed was confidential and that he understood the danger in disclosing psychiatric records to unauthorized persons. He also knew that a nurse could be disciplined for disclosing such information, yet he intentionally released information to the news media. The state board of nursing suspended Sanfiel's nursing license and placed him on probation for five years for disclosing confidential patient information.

Issue

Was the state board of nursing authorized to suspend Sanfiel's license because of his disclosure of information to the news media?

Holding

Sanfiel's professional license was properly suspended for a five-year period after he intentionally disclosed confidential patient information to the news media.

Reason

Sanfiel obtained a computer, which was previously owned by Charter Behavioral Health System psychiatric hospital in Orlando. Charter's patient records were contained in the computer. Sanfiel testified that he reviewed this information and recalled that Charter was being investigated for defrauding the government. He contacted local law enforcement and the state attorney's office to initiate a criminal investigation. The agencies declined, telling him that the matter was outside their jurisdiction. Sanfiel then called the news media and allowed them to see the information concerning the patients. He asked that the patients' names be blurred to protect their identity. He told reporters that the hard drive contained the names of psychiatric patients, their admission dates, types of addiction, treatments, and psychiatric disorders. The story was broadcast along with the patients' names and diagnoses shown on the computer screen. One of the journalists located and interviewed a patient identified from Sanfiel's computer. The patient was distressed over the fact that his confidential medical information was being exposed to the public.

Sanfiel violated Florida Administrative Code by violating the confidentiality of information or knowledge concerning a patient. Florida Code Rule 59S-8.005 states in part that unprofessional conduct includes violating the confidentiality of information or knowledge concerning a patient. The board reasonably interpreted this provision to apply to the circumstances present in this case. Sanfiel knew that a nurse could be disciplined for disclosing such information, yet he intentionally released the information to the news media. It is reasonable to characterize Sanfiel's actions as unprofessional conduct.

Discussion

1. Describe why Charter patients had legal recourse for the unauthorized release of their medical information.
2. Describe what steps Charter could take to prevent similar occurrences in the future.

Requests by Patients

Patients have a legally enforceable interest in the information contained in their medical records and, therefore,

have a right to access their records. Patients may have access to review and obtain copies of their records, X-rays, and laboratory and diagnostic tests. Access to information includes that maintained or possessed by a health care organization or a health care practitioner who has treated or is treating a patient. Organizations and physicians can withhold records if the information could reasonably be expected to cause substantial and identifiable harm to the patient (e.g., patients in psychiatric hospitals, institutions for the mentally disabled, or alcohol- and drug-treatment programs).

Failure to Release Patient Records

Failure to release a patient's record can lead to legal action. The patient in *Pierce v. Penman*[2] brought a lawsuit seeking damages for severe emotional distress when physicians repeatedly refused to turn over her medical records. The defendants had rendered different professional services to the plaintiff for approximately 11 years. The patient moved and found a new physician, Dr. Hochman. She signed a release authorizing Hochman to obtain her records from the defendant physicians. Hochman wrote a letter for her records but never received a response. The defendants claimed that they never received the request. The patient changed physicians again and continued in her efforts to obtain a copy of the records. Eventually the defendants' offices were burglarized, and the plaintiff's records were allegedly taken. The detective in charge of investigating the burglary stated that he was never notified that any records were taken. The court of common pleas awarded the patient $2,500 in compensatory damages and $10,000 in punitive damages. On appeal, the superior court upheld the award.

Requests by Third Parties

The medical record is a peculiar type of property because there is a wide variety of third-party interests in the information contained in medical records. Health care organizations may not generally disclose information without patient consent. Policies regarding the release of information should be formulated to address the rights of third parties, such as insurance carriers processing claims, physicians, medical researchers, educators, and governmental agencies.

Privacy Exception: Psychiatric Records

The psychotherapist-patient privilege that exists under the federal rules of evidence can be overcome if the evidentiary need for a psychiatric history outweighs a privacy interest. This was the case in *United States v. Diamond*,[3] in which the privacy interests regarding the psychiatric history of the person, who initiated a criminal investigation against another individual, were outweighed by the interests of the accused. Because the credibility of the complainant/witness was the central issue at trial, his psychiatric history was relevant.

Privacy Exception: Criminal Investigations

Another exception to the restriction on disclosing information obtained in a confidential relationship may occur when a patient is the victim of a crime. The hospital in *In re Brink*[4] sought to quash a grand jury request for the medical records pertaining to blood tests administered to a person under investigation. The court of common pleas held that physician-patient privilege did not extend to medical records subpoenaed pursuant to a grand jury investigation. A proceeding before a grand jury is considered secret in nature, inherently preserving the confidentiality of a patient's records.

Privacy Exception: Medicaid Fraud

Patient records may also be obtained during investigations into such alleged criminal actions as Medicaid fraud. The grand jury in *People v. Ekong*[5] was permitted to obtain certain patient files and records that were in the possession of the physician who was under investigation for Medicaid fraud. The physician contended that he could not release the files because of physician-patient privilege.

Privacy Exception: Substance Abuse Records

The federal Drug Abuse and Treatment Act of 1972[6] and the federal regulations promulgated thereunder provide that patient records relating to drug and alcohol abuse treatment must be held confidential and not disclosed except in specific circumstances. Unlike other medical records, drug- and alcohol-abuse records cannot be released until the court has determined whether a claimed need for the records outweighs the potential injury to the patient, to the patient-physician relationship, and to the treatment services being rendered. Because of these strict requirements, the courts have been reluctant to order the release of such records unless absolutely necessary.

RETENTION OF RECORDS

Professionals handling medical records must not only maintain the privacy of documents for patients, but they must also ensure that medical records are retained for the proper time frame. The length of time medical records must be retained varies from state to state. A California court revoked the license of a nursing facility for failure to keep adequate records. In *Yankee v. State Department of Health*,[7] the facility claimed that the word adequate was unclear and therefore the requirement was invalid. The court stated that the word adequate is not so uncertain as to render a penal statute invalid. Health care organizations, with the advice of an attorney, should determine how long records should be maintained, taking into account patient needs, statutory requirements, future need for such records, and the legal considerations of having the records available in the event of a lawsuit.

Retention of X-Rays: Failure to Preserve

Rodgers, in *Rodgers v. St. Mary's Hosp. of Decatur*,[8] filed a medical malpractice action alleging the wrongful death of his wife, who died in the hospital two days after giving birth to their son. The defendants in the medical malpractice action were Mrs. Rodgers's obstetricians, her radiologists, and the hospital.

Rodgers filed a complaint for damages against the hospital, alleging that the hospital breached its statutory duty to preserve for five years all of the X-rays taken of his wife. He claimed that the X-rays were crucial to proving his case against the obstetricians and radiologists. On motion of the hospital, the circuit court dismissed the complaint. Rodgers amended his complaint and brought a medical malpractice action against the hospital, a day after he reached an $800,000 settlement with the obstetricians. In his complaint, Rodgers alleged that his wife's death was caused by a condition that appeared on an X-ray that the hospital had a duty to preserve. He alleged that the hospital's failure to preserve the X-ray was a breach of its duty arising from the state's X-ray retention act and from the hospital's internal regulations. Rodgers asserted that because the hospital failed to preserve the X-ray, he was unable to prove his case against the radiologists. The circuit court entered judgment in favor of the hospital, and Rodgers appealed.

The Illinois Supreme Court held that a private cause of action existed under the X-ray retention act, and that Rodgers stated a claim under the act. The act provides that hospitals must retain X-rays and other such photographs or films as part of their regularly maintained records for a period of five years.

The hospital argued that the statute is merely an administrative regulation to be enforced exclusively by the public health department. The court disagreed. Nothing in the statute suggested that the legislature intended to limit the available remedies to administrative ones.

The hospital also argued that the loss of one X-ray out of a series of six should not be considered a violation of the statute. The court disagreed, finding that the statute requires that all X-rays be preserved, not just some of them. Whether the missing X-ray proximately caused Rodgers to lose his case against the radiologists and to settle for less than the full amount of the judgment is a question for the trier of fact.

COMPUTERIZED RECORDS

Retaining all patient records for five years may seem unwieldy, but computers make the task feasible, while also increasing efficiency for many other information management processes. Computers are found in the admitting office, the business office, and even the operating room. They are in the laboratory, pharmacy, imaging, and medical records departments. They are fast and accurate and have an almost endless capacity to store data.

Health care organizations undergoing computerization must determine user needs, design an effective system, select appropriate hardware and software, develop user training programs, develop a disaster recovery plan (e.g., provide for emergency power systems and backup files), and provide for data security. Solid planning and design can lead to great achievements. Large medical centers are generating more than 100,000 orders a week. At the Brigham and Women's Hospital in Boston, laboratory and pharmacy results, pulmonary function, EEG, and many other results-generating areas are based around the system. A strong aspect of the order-entry capability is its use of medical logic and medical-expertise technology. The system flags cases where there have been duplicate physician orders and signals a patient-allergy alert, resulting in an order cancellation.[9] Clearly, computers offer many advantages to today's health care.

Advantages

Computers have become an economic necessity and play an important role in assisting health care providers to improve the quality of health care. In the health care community, computers:

- Retrieve demographic information and consultants' reports, as well as laboratory, radiology, and other test results

- Improve productivity and quality

- Reduce costs

- Support clinical research

- Play an ever-increasing role in the education process

- Allow for interactive computer-assisted diagnosis and treatment

- Allow for computer-generated prescriptions (integrated computer systems and clinical pharmacy services are

associated with reducing the incidence of medication errors)

- Generate reminders for follow-up testing

- Assist in the decision-making process

- Aid in standardizing treatment protocols

- Assist in the identification of drug-drug and food-drug interactions

- Are used in telecommunications around the world, transporting picture graphics (e.g., computed tomography scans) between nations

Disadvantages

Computers may be an economic necessity, but they are not perfect. Computerization increases the risk of lost confidentiality and unauthorized disclosure of information. The rapid growth of the Internet has led to an explosion of high-technology crime and related illegal activities. Increases in cyber crime have led to a need for high-end technology products and services to combat these problems. Billions of dollars are spent annually to protect networks and critical infrastructures from cyber-based threats.

Legal Issues

Protecting a patient's medical information is an ongoing challenge; many federal laws protect credit information, but few protect the computerized medical record.

In *Whalen v. Roe,*[10] the applicant, the New York commissioner of health, had been enjoined by a three-judge court from enforcing certain provisions of the New York State Public Health Law that required the name and address of each patient receiving a schedule II controlled substance to be reported to the applicant. Schedule II drugs are those considered to have a high potential for abuse but also have an accepted medical use. Under the law, a physician prescribes schedule II drugs on a special serially numbered prescription form, one copy of which goes to the office of the New York commissioner of health where the data, including the name and address of the user, is transferred from the prescription form to a centralized computer file. The respondent claimed that mandatory disclosure of the name of a patient receiving schedule II drugs violated the patient's right of privacy and interfered with the physician's right to prescribe treatment for his or her patient solely on the basis of medical considerations. The court held that the patient identification requirement was the product of an orderly and rational legislative decision about the state's broad police powers. The statute does not impair any private interest on its face and does not impair the right of physicians to practice medicine free from unwarranted state interference.

MEDICAL RECORD BATTLEGROUND

The contents of a medical record must not be tampered with once an entry has been made; therefore, it should be used wisely. Although the record should be complete and accurate, it should not be used as an instrument for registering complaints about another individual or the organization. Its purpose is to record the patient's course of care. Those individuals who choose to make derogatory remarks in a patient's record about others might find themselves in a court room trying to defend such notations in the record. Always consider that comments written during a time of anger may have been based on inaccurate information, which, in turn, could be damaging to one's credibility and future statements.

A nurse tends to access the medical record more often than other health care professionals, simply because of the greater amount of time spent with the patient. Because of the job description, the nurse monitors the patient's illness, response to medication, display of pain and discomfort, and general condition. The patient's care, as well as the nurse's observations, should be recorded on a regular basis. The nurse should comply promptly and accurately with the physician orders written in the record. A nurse who has doubt as to the appropriateness of a particular order should verify with the physician the intent of the prescribed order.

Licensure rules and regulations contained in state statutes generally describe the requirements and standards for the maintenance, handling, signing, filing, and retention of medical records. Failure to maintain a complete and accurate medical record reflecting the treatment rendered may affect the ability of an organization and/or physician to obtain third-party reimbursement (e.g., from Medicare, Medicaid, or private insurance carriers). Under federal and state laws, the medical record must reflect accurately the treatment for which the organization or physician seeks payment. Thus, the medical record is important to the organization for medical, legal, and financial reasons.

PATIENT OBJECTS TO RECORD NOTATIONS

As noted in *Dodds v. Johnstone,*[11] during a physical exam conducted on October 30, 2000, the appellee indicated in her progress notes that she believed the appellant had been using cocaine prior to her last office visit. Appellee's notes read: "I believe by physical exam the patient was using cocaine on Friday before her office visit." The appellant filed a complaint in which she alleged that the appellee was negligent in her diagnosis of the appellant and that as a result, she incurred a loss of compensation for her automobile accident claim and suffered severe emotional distress. The court reviewed the record of proceedings before the trial court and found that there was no genuine issue of material fact as to negligent infliction of severe emotional distress, loss of employment opportunities, or a decreased insurance settlement as a result of the notation in the patient's medical records.

FAILURE TO RECORD PATIENT'S CONDITION

The plaintiff, in *Gerner v. Long Island Jewish Hillside Med. Ctr.,*[12] gave birth to her infant son at the defendant medical center. Dr. Geller, the attending pediatrician, arrived at the hospital six hours later. Geller, having noted and confirmed a slightly jaundiced condition, ordered phototherapy for the baby. After three days of treatment, the child's bilirubin count fell to a normal level, and Geller ordered the patient discharged. The child today is brain damaged, with permanent neurological dysfunction.

The plaintiff alleged medical malpractice on the part of both the medical center and Geller for failing to diagnose and treat the jaundice in a timely manner. Following examination before trial, the medical center motioned and was granted summary judgment. The plaintiff and Geller appealed.

The New York Supreme Court, Appellate Division, held that questions of fact precluded summary judgment for the hospital. A number of allegations were raised as to negligence attributed solely to hospital staff. For example, notes of attending nurses at the nursery failed to record any jaundiced condition or any reference to color until the third day after birth, despite the parents' complaints to hospital personnel about the baby's yellowish complexion. Additionally, Geller ordered a complete blood count and bilirubin test as soon as he learned of the first recorded observation by a nurse of a jaundiced appearance. Test results, which showed a moderately elevated bilirubin count, were not reported by the laboratory until 10 hours after the blood sample was drawn, and another three hours passed before Geller's order for phototherapy was carried out. An issue was thus raised as to whether the 13-hour delay in commencement of the treatment was the proximate cause of the infant's injuries.

FALSIFICATION OF RECORDS

When handling medical records, professionals must recognize that intentional alteration, falsification, or destruction to avoid liability for medical negligence is generally sufficient to show actual malice. Punitive damages may be awarded whether or not the act of altering, falsifying, or destroying records directly causes compensable harm. The evidence in *Dimora v. Cleveland Clinic Foundation*[13] showed that the patient had fallen and broken five or six ribs; yet, upon examination, the physician noted in the progress notes that the patient was smiling and laughing pleasantly, exhibiting no pain upon deep palpation of the area. Other testimony indicated that she was in pain and crying. The discrepancy between the written progress notes and the testimony of the witnesses who observed the patient was sufficient to raise a question of fact. The court then considered the possible falsification of documents by the physician in an effort to hide the possible negligence of hospital personnel. The testimony of the witnesses, if believed, would have been sufficient to show that the physician falsified the record or intentionally reported the incident inaccurately in order to avoid liability for the negligent care of the patient.

Falsification of medical or business records is grounds for criminal indictment, as well as for civil liability. In *People v. Smithtown General Hospital,*[14] a motion to dismiss indictments against a physician and a nurse charged with falsifying business records in the first degree was denied. The surgeon was charged because he omitted to make a true entry in his operative report and the nurse was charged because she failed to make a true entry in the operating room log.

Another such incident occurred in a rest home, where employees attempted to cover up the death of an elderly woman who had wandered away from the home and was found frozen in a drainage ditch.[15] The deceased patient had been brought back into the home, was dressed in a nightgown, and placed in her bed. On the basis of the account given by employees, a physician signed the death certificate stating that the 77-year-old patient died in her sleep. An anonymous tip to the county examiner's office prompted an autopsy and the patient was found to have frozen to death.

FALSIFYING RECORDS

Citation: *Moskovitz v. Mount Sinai Med. Ctr.,* 635 N.E.2d 331 (Ohio 1994)

Facts

On November 10, 1987, Figgie removed a left Achilles tendon mass from Moskovitz. The tumor was found to be a rare form of cancer. A bone scan revealed that the cancer had metastasized.

Moskovitz's care was transferred to Figgie's partner, Makley, an orthopedic surgeon specializing in oncology at University Hospitals. Makley received Figgie's original office chart, which contained seven pages of notes documenting Moskovitz's course of treatment from 1985 through November 1987. Makley thereafter referred Moskovitz to radiation therapy at University Hospitals, and sent along a copy of page seven of Figgie's office notes to the radiation department at University Hospitals.

One month later, Makley's office forwarded the chart to Figgie's office; a copy was then sent to Moskovitz's psychologist. In January 1988, Makley's secretary requested that Figgie's office return the chart to Makley. At this time, it was discovered that the original chart had mysteriously vanished. The problem arose on October 21, 1988, when Moskovitz filed a complaint for discovery seeking to ascertain information relative to a potential claim for medical malpractice. Moskovitz claimed that she had never refused to have the tumor biopsied, but discrepancies in her medical record led to questions.

In his January 30, 1989, deposition, Makley produced a copy of page seven of Figgie's office chart. That copy was identical to the copy ultimately recovered by the plaintiff's counsel from the radiation department records at University Hospitals. The copy produced by Makley contained a typewritten entry dated September 21, 1987, which stated: "Mrs. Moskovitz comes in today for her evaluation on the radiographs reviewed with Dr. York. He was not impressed that [the mass on Moskovitz's left leg] was anything other than a benign problem, perhaps a fibroma. We [Figgie and York] will therefore elect to continue to observe."

However, Figgie's photostatic copy revealed that a line had been drawn through the sentence "We will therefore elect to continue to observe." The copy further revealed that beneath the entry Figgie had interlineated a handwritten notation: "As she does not want excisional Bx [biopsy] we will observe." The September 21, 1987, entry was followed by a typewritten entry dated September 24, 1987, which states: "I [Figgie] reviewed the X-rays with Dr. York. I discussed the clinical findings with him. We [Figgie and York] felt this to be benign, most likely a fibroma. He [York] said that we could observe and I concur." At some point, Figgie also had added to the September 24, 1987, entry a handwritten notation, "see above," referring to the September 21, 1987, handwritten notation that Moskovitz did not want an excisional biopsy.

Figgie, at his deposition on March 2, 1989, produced records, including a copy of page seven of his office chart. As his original chart had been lost between December 1987 and January 1988, Figgie had made this copy from the copy of the chart that had been sent Moskovitz's psychologist. The September 21, 1987, entry in the records produced by Figgie did not contain the statement "We will therefore elect to continue to observe." That sentence had been deleted (whited out) on the original office chart from which the psychiatrist's copy (and, in turn, Figgie's copy) had been made, in a way that left no indication on the copy that the sentence had been removed from the original records.

Figgie maintained that he did not discover the mass on the left Achilles tendon until February 23, 1987, and that Moskovitz continually refused a workup or biopsy.

During discovery, another copy of page seven of Figgie's office chart, identical to the copy produced by Makley during his deposition, showed that the final sentence in the September 21, 1987, entry had been deleted from Figgie's original office chart sometime between November and mid-December 1987, the alteration presumably occurring while Figgie possessed the original chart.

Eventually, Figgie's entire office chart was reconstructed from copies obtained through discovery. The reconstructed chart contains no indication that a workup or biopsy was recommended by Figgie and refused by Moskovitz at any time prior to August 10, 1987.

In a videotaped deposition before her death, Moskovitz claimed that she never refused to have the tumor biopsied. The panel found in favor of the defendants participating in that proceeding with the exception of Figgie, and the trial court agreed. A panel of arbitrators unanimously found that:

3. The evidence supported a finding that plaintiffs' . . . decedent had a very good chance of long-term survival if the tumor was found to be malignant at a time when it was less than one centimeter in size. The evidence supported the fact that the tumor had not grown in size as of May 7, 1987. If Dr. Figgie had performed a biopsy prior to this date, the cancer would not have metastasized and the decedent would have recovered.

4. Dr. Figgie's office chart, which is the primary reference material in analyzing a physician's conduct, is filled with contradictions and inconsistencies.

5. Even if Dr. Figgie was first informed of the growth on February 23, 1987, he still fell below acceptable standards of care because he did not conduct further investigation until . . . X-rays performed in September 1987. All handwritten entries which appear on or prior to September 24, 1987, indicating that a biopsy was recommended or that the decedent refused further workup were subsequent changes of the records done to justify Figgie's conduct. The sentence "We will therefore elect to continue to observe" on the September 21, 1987 entry was whited out and the handwritten entry "as she does not want excisional biopsy we will observe" was a subsequent alteration of the records. *Id.* at 338.

The court of appeals upheld the finding of liability against Figgie on the wrongful death and survival claims. The court of appeals found that the appellant was not entitled to punitive damages as a matter of law. The court of appeals reversed the judgment of the trial court as to the award of damages and remanded the case for a new trial only on the issue of compensatory damages.

Issue

Is an intentional alteration or destruction of medical records to avoid liability sufficient to show actual malice? Can punitive damages be awarded whether the act of altering or destroying records directly causes compensable harm?

Holding

The Ohio Supreme Court held that the evidence regarding the physician's alteration of the patient's records supported an award of punitive damages, regardless of whether the alteration caused actual harm.

Reason

The intentional alteration or destruction of medical records to avoid liability for medical negligence is sufficient to show actual malice, and punitive damages may be awarded whether the act of altering, falsifying, or destroying records directly causes compensable harm. The jury's award of punitive damages was based on Figgie's alteration or destruction of medical records. The purpose of punitive damages is not to compensate a plaintiff, but to punish and deter certain conduct. The court warned others to refrain from similar conduct through an award of punitive damages.

Figgie's alteration of records exhibited a total disregard for the law and the rights of Moskovitz and her family. Had the copy of page seven of Figgie's office chart not been recovered from the radiation department records at University Hospitals, the appellant would have been substantially less likely to succeed in this case. The copy of the chart and other records produced by Figgie would have tended to exculpate Figgie for his medical negligence while placing the blame for his failures on Moskovitz.

The intentional alteration or destruction of medical records to avoid liability for medical negligence is sufficient to show actual malice, and punitive damages may be awarded whether or not the act of altering, falsifying, or destroying records directly causes compensable harm.

Discussion

1. Discuss what procedure should be followed when clarifying an entry in a patient's medical record.
2. Is correction fluid helpful when clarifying medical record entries? Explain.

TAMPERING WITH RECORD ENTRIES

Closely related to falsification, tampering with records sends the wrong signal to jurors and can shatter one's credibility. Altered records can create a presumption of negligence. The court in *Matter of Jascalevich*[16] held:

> We are persuaded that a physician's duty to a patient cannot but encompass his affirmative obligation to maintain the integrity, accuracy, truth and reliability of the patient's medical record. His obligation in this regard is no less compelling than his duties respecting diagnosis and treatment of the patient since the medical community must, of necessity, be able to rely on those records in the continuing and future care of that patient. Obviously, the rendering of that care is prejudiced by anything in those records which is false, misleading or inaccurate. We hold, therefore, that a deliberate falsification by a physician of his patient's medical record, particularly when the reason therefore is to protect his own interests at the expense of his patient's, must be regarded as gross malpractice endangering the health or life of his patient.[17]

Dr. McCroskey faced a lawsuit for tampering with documents. The state board of medical examiners in a disciplinary hearing in *State Board of Medical Examiners v. McCroskey*[18] issued a letter of admonition to Dr. McCroskey based upon a series of incidents arising out of the care of a patient's stab wound. Although the patient's condition was initially thought to be stable, he bled to death several hours after his admission to the hospital. McCroskey was the attending surgeon on the date of the incident and, therefore, responsible for the accurate completion of the patient's medical record. McCroskey declined to accept the letter of admonition and a formal disciplinary hearing was held.

McCroskey erased and wrote over a preoperative note made by another physician concerning the patient's estimated blood loss. Specifically, the original record entry was completed by a surgical resident on the date of the patient's death and stated that the patient's blood loss just prior to surgery was "now greater than 3000 cc." Sometime after the autopsy, McCroskey changed the record to read that the patient's blood loss was "now greater than 2000 cc."[19] After listening to conflicting expert testimony, the administrative law judge (ALJ) concluded that the physician had not violated generally accepted standards of medical practice by adding the note to the patient's medical record days or weeks after the patient's death and then backdating the note to the date of the death.

On review of the ALJ's decision, the board accepted the ALJ's evidentiary finding that many physicians date a medical record entry to reflect the date of the medical event, rather than the date on which the entry was made. The board disagreed, however, with the ALJ's conclusion that this fact brought McCroskey's conduct within generally accepted standards of medical practice. Instead, the board determined that backdating a medical record entry falls below accepted standards of documentation. Having thus found two acts that fell below generally accepted standards of medical practice, the board concluded that McCroskey committed unprofessional conduct under and issued a letter of admonition. On appeal, the court of appeals held that the board erroneously rejected the ALJ's findings.

On further appeal by the board, the Colorado Supreme Court held that the findings of the board were supported by substantial evidence. Because of the expertise of the board, it was in a position to determine the seriousness of the physician's conduct by placing the events in their proper factual context.

> All three of the inquiry panel's witnesses testified that the generally accepted standard of practice requires that a medical record entry be dated with the date it is made. Even one of McCroskey's witnesses acknowledged that misdating the medical record was "certainly something that should not have been done." McCroskey did not simply backdate a trivial note in a patient's medical record. Instead McCroskey's actions took place in the context of a patient's death, which resulted in a coroner's autopsy, peer review activities, publicity, and several legal actions. McCroskey was the attending physician responsible for the accuracy of the patient's medical record, and yet he engaged in conduct that cast doubt upon the medical record's integrity. Under these circumstances, the Board was justified in considering McCroskey's conduct to violate the standard of care.[20]

INACCURATE RECORD ENTRIES

Dimora,[21] a 79-year-old woman, was preparing to be discharged from the Cleveland Clinic. After using the toilet with the assistance of a student nurse, she lost her balance and fell backward. Dimora's broken ribs were not diagnosed until the following day, when X-rays were taken at Marymount Hospital.

A claim for punitive damages alleges that the clinic intentionally falsified Dimora's medical records or inaccurately and improperly reported the fall incident to avoid liability for its medical malpractice or negligence. The jury awarded a verdict in favor of Dimora in the amount of $25,000 for compensatory damages and $25,000 in punitive damages.

On appeal, the judgment of the trial court was affirmed. At trial, three witnesses testified that Dimora was crying and in pain approximately 45 minutes after the incident while she was still in the hospital. Testimony was offered that broken ribs would be painful upon deep palpation. The progress note of the examining physician at issue states in part:

> Pt was in transport between walker and toilet seat according to student nurse. Pt was at walker and lost balance backward. The SN acted by holding the pt from the L side and gradually lowering her to the floor, and called for help. Pt was lifted back into wheelchair. On exam, pt has full use of all 4 extremities with good strength and no pain with movement. A small 5×8 cm area on the pts r posterior thorax was slightly scraped. It was not tender to deep palpations and no crepitus was noted. There were no other lacerations, bumps or abrasions noted. Head was traumatic. The abrasion on the thorax was treated with lotion and ice. The pt was smiling and laughing pleasantly during the exam.

The discrepancy between the written progress notes and the testimony of the witnesses who observed Dimora was sufficient to raise a question of fact as to the possible falsification of documents by the physician to minimize the nature of the incident and the injury of the patient due to the possible negligence of clinic personnel. The testimony of the witnesses, if believed, would be sufficient to show that the physician falsified the record or intentionally reported the incident inaccurately to avoid liability for negligent care. If such evidence is believed, the jury could award punitive damages.

REWRITING AND REPLACING NOTES

Another temptation health care professionals should not fall prey to is the desire to clarify and explain one's activities in the care of a patient. In a well-publicized case that involved the death of a child, the nurse replaced her original notes with a second set of notes that were much more detailed and indicated that she had seen the patient more frequently than was reported in her original notes.[22] Rewriting one's notes in a patient's medical record casts doubt as to the accuracy of other entries in the record. It is easier to explain why one did not chart all activities than it is to explain why a new entry was recorded and an original note replaced.

ILLEGIBLE ENTRIES

Perhaps the simplest but one of the most potentially dangerous problems with medical records is illegible entries. Illegible handwriting is as ancient as the first stylus. Unfortunately, poor penmanship can cause injury to patients. The American Medical Association encourages physicians to print, type, or computerize physicians' orders. Medical errors because of poor handwriting can lead to extended length of hospital stays and, in some cases, the death of patients. A Harvard study found that "penmanship was among the causes of 220 prescription errors out of 30,000 cases."[23]

FAILURE TO MAINTAIN RECORDS

As with illegible penmanship, failure to maintain patient records may occur when a healthcare professional is busy, overwhelmed, or preoccupied. A disciplinary hearing, in *Braick v. New York State Department of Health,*[24] involving a physician, was conducted by a hearing committee of the New York State Review Board for Professional Medical Conduct. The committee reviewed 122 specifications of misconduct, which included gross negligence, failure to adequately maintain patient records, and failure to obtain informed consent. The committee revoked the physician-petitioner's license. In reaching its decision, the committee found the bureau of professional medical conduct's expert credible, including his opinion that the physician was ultimately responsible for what happened to his patients during the relevant surgeries, and the committee rejected the efforts of the physician and his expert to shift responsibility to nurses.

The petitioner appealed to the administrative review board for professional medical conduct, which affirmed the committee's determination and penalty. On review by an appeals court, the physician's license was found to have been properly revoked.

IMPROPER RECORD KEEPING

Maintaining records, of course, does little good when the records are flawed with errors. In one such case, *Tulier-Pastewski v. State Board for Professional Medical Conduct,*[25] two hospital administrators testified and showed undisputed proof that the physician had recorded a patient was alert during the purported examination when the patient

was actually sedated and asleep. Evidence also indicated the physician failed to properly document medical histories and current physical status. Although the physician asserted that evidence of failure to document did not support findings of negligence because there was no expert testimony that her omissions actually caused or created a risk of harm to a patient, an expert witness testified that the missing information as to certain patients was needed for proper assessment of the patient's condition and choice of treatment. This testimony, together with the obvious importance of cardiac information when treating patients with chest pain, provided a rational basis for the conclusion by administrative review board for professional medical conduct that the physician's deficient medical recordkeeping could have affected patient care. The physician was found to be practicing medicine negligently on more than one occasion, and fraudulent practice was supported by the record.

CHARTING BY EXCEPTION

Some health care professionals institute a practice of charting by exception. On April 9, 1986, Borras, in *Lama v. Borras,*[26] while operating on Mr. Lama, discovered that the patient had an extruded disc and attempted to remove the extruded material. Either because Borras failed to remove the offending material or because he operated at the wrong level, the patient's original symptoms returned several days after the operation.

On May 15, Borras operated again, but did not order preoperative or postoperative antibiotics. On May 17, a nurse's note indicated that the bandage covering the patient's surgical wound was extremely bloody, which, according to expert testimony, indicates the possibility of infection. On May 18, the patient was experiencing local pain at the site of the incision, another symptom consistent with an infection. On May 19, the bandage was soiled again. A more complete account of the patient's evolving condition was not available because the hospital instructed nurses to engage in charting by exception, a system whereby nurses did not record qualitative observations for each of the day's three shifts, but instead made such notes only when necessary to chronicle important changes in a patient's condition.

On May 21, Dr. Piazza, an attending physician, diagnosed the patient's problem as discitis—an infection of the space between discs—and responded by prescribing antibiotic treatment. Lama was hospitalized for several additional months while undergoing treatment for the infection.

After moving from Puerto Rico to Florida, Lama filed a tort action in the U.S. District Court for the district of Puerto Rico. Although the plaintiff did not claim that the hospital was vicariously liable for any negligence on the part of Borras, he alleged that the hospital failed to prepare, use, and monitor proper medical records.

The jury returned a verdict awarding the plaintiff $600,000 in compensatory damages. The district court ruled that the evidence was legally sufficient to support the jury's findings, and an appeal was taken.

The U.S. Court of Appeals for the First Circuit upheld the decision of negligence based on the charting by exception policy, but the jury had to decide whether the violation of the regulation was a proximate cause of harm to Lama.

Before deciding the case, the jury considered several important factors. For example, the jury may have inferred from evidence that, as part of the practice of charting by exception, the nurses did not regularly record certain information important to the diagnosis of an infection, such as the changing characteristics of the surgical wound and the patient's complaints of postoperative pain. Further, because there was evidence that the patient's hospital records contained described possible signs of infection that deserved further investigation (e.g., an excessively bloody bandage and local pain at the site of the wound), the jury could have reasonably inferred that the intermittent charting failed to provide the sort of continuous danger signals that would most likely spur early intervention by the physician.

CHARTING AND REIMBURSEMENT

When charting, professionals should be familiar with diagnosis-related groups (DRGs). DRGs refer to a methodology developed by professors at Yale University for classifying patients in categories according to age, diagnosis, and treatment resource requirements. It is the basis for the prospective payment system, contained in the 1983 Social Security Amendments for reimbursing inpatient hospital costs for Medicare beneficiaries. The key source of information for determining the course of treatment of each patient and the proper DRG assignment is the medical record. Reimbursement is based on preestablished average prices for each DRG. As a result of this reimbursement methodology, poor record keeping can precipitate financial disaster for a hospital. The potential financial savings for Medicare are substantial. Under this system of payment, if hospitals can provide quality patient care at a cost less than the price established for a DRG, they keep the excess dollars paid. This is an incentive for hospitals to keep costs under control. There is, however, a continuing fear that patients may, to their detriment, be discharged too early, for financial reasons. This in turn leads to costly malpractice suits.

INCOMPLETE RECORDS: SUSPENSION OF PRIVILEGES

Not only must the chart be accurate, but health care professionals must promptly complete records after patients are

discharged. Persistent failure to conform to a medical staff rule requiring physicians to complete records promptly can be the basis for suspension of medical staff privileges, as was the case in *Board of Trustees Memorial Hospital v. Pratt*.[27]

LEGAL PROCEEDINGS AND THE MEDICAL RECORD

The ever-increasing frequency of personal injury suits mandates that health care organizations maintain complete, accurate, and timely medical records. The integrity and completeness of the medical record are important in reconstructing the events surrounding an alleged negligence in the care of a patient. Medical records aid police investigations, provide information for determining the cause of death, and indicate the extent of injury in workers' compensation or personal injury proceedings.

When health care professionals are called as witnesses in a proceeding, they are permitted to refresh their recollections of the facts and circumstances of a particular case by referring to the medical record. Courts recognize that it is impossible for a medical witness to remember the details of every patient's treatment. The record therefore may be used as an aid in relating the facts of a patient's course of treatment.

If the medical record is admitted into evidence in legal proceedings, then the court must be assured the information is accurate, was recorded at the time the event took place, and was not recorded in anticipation of a specific legal proceeding. When a medical record is introduced into evidence, its custodian, usually the medical records administrator, must testify as to the manner in which the record was produced and the way in which it is protected from unauthorized handling and change. The records purportedly relating to a patient's treatment in *Belber v. Lipson*[28] were not admissible as business records because the witness who had possession of them had no personal knowledge of the circumstances under which the records were prepared.

Whether such records and other documents are admitted or excluded is governed by the facts and circumstances of the particular case, as well as by the applicable rules of evidence. Admission of a business record requires "the testimony of the custodian or other qualified witness."[29] If a record can be shown to be inaccurate or incomplete or that it was made long after the event it purports to record, its credibility as evidence will be diminished.

CONFIDENTIAL AND PRIVILEGED COMMUNICATIONS

Beyond the medical record lies an even more complex issue within health care organizations: communication. The duty of an organization's employees and staff to maintain confidentiality encompasses both verbal and written communications and applies to consultants, contracted individuals, students, and volunteers. Information about a patient, regardless of the method in which it is acquired, is confidential and should not be disclosed without the patient's permission. All health care professionals who have access to medical records have a legal, ethical, and moral obligation to protect the confidentiality of the information in the records, as well as verbal communications between physicians and patients. Communication between individual physicians and communication that occurs in peer-review activities also fall under strict confidentiality procedures.

The Federal Health Care Quality Improvement Act of 1986[30] insulates certain medical peer-review activities affecting medical staff privileges from antitrust liability. Peer review is protected as long as there is reasonable belief that it is conducted in the furtherance of quality care. In enacting this legislation, Congress recognized that without such antitrust immunity, effective peer review may not be possible. Privileged communications statutes do not protect from discovery the records maintained in the ordinary course of doing business and rendering inpatient care. Such documents often can be subpoenaed after showing cause.

The burden to establish privilege is on the party seeking to shield information from discovery. The party asserting the privilege has the obligation to prove, by competent evidence, that the privilege applies to the information sought.

Breach of Physician-Patient Confidentiality

Patients enter the physician-patient relationship assuming that information acquired by physicians will not be disclosed, unless the patient consents or the law requires disclosure. Mutual trust and confidence are essential to the physician-patient relationship. An action alleging a breach of physician-patient confidentiality is analogous to invasion of privacy, and plaintiffs are entitled to recover damages, including emotional damages, for the harm caused by the physician's unauthorized disclosure.

In such a case, *Berger v. Sonneland,*[31] Berger revealed information during her initial appointment with Dr. Sonneland regarding her medical and personal history. When questioned about her personal history, Berger said that she had previously been married to Dr. Hoheim, a physician in Montana. She described her relationship with her ex-husband as extremely strained. After meeting with Berger, Sonneland contacted Hoheim and discussed Berger's use of pain medications. Based on information provided by Sonneland, Hoheim filed a motion in a Montana court seeking to modify the custody orders relating to the couple's two children.

Berger sought damages for Sonneland's breach of physician-patient confidentiality. The court granted Sonneland's motion for summary judgment based on the absence of damage evidence, concluding that Berger failed to establish any objective symptoms of emotional distress. Berger moved for reconsideration, urging the court to apply invasion of privacy principles rather than principles related to the tort of negligent infliction of emotional distress.

During the course of events in this case, an appellate court held that a tort action exists for damages resulting from the unauthorized disclosure of confidential information obtained within the physician-patient relationship. The court also held that there is sufficient evidence to raise a question of fact as to whether Berger was injured by Sonneland's unauthorized disclosure. The matter was remanded for further proceedings.

JOINT COMMISSION REPORTS PRIVILEGED FROM DISCOVERY

Citation: *Humana Hosp. Corp. v. Spears Petersen,* 867 S.W.2d 858 (Tex. Ct. App. 1993)

Issue

Are accreditation reports prepared by The Joint Commission privileged from discovery?

Facts

The plaintiff Garcia sued Dr. Garg for negligently performing an injection, battery, fraud, and lack of informed consent. Garcia also sued Humana Corporation for negligence in credentialing, supervising, and monitoring Garg's clinical privileges. The plaintiff's attorney requested documents from Humana, including reports prepared by The Joint Commission. The Joint Commission is a voluntary organization that surveys health care organizations for the purpose of accreditation.

Humana objected to releasing Joint Commission reports and filed for a protective order preventing disclosure. The Joint Commission reports contained recommendations describing the hospital's noncompliance with certain of its published standards. Humana argued that The Joint Commission reports are privileged information under Texas statute. Under Texas law, the records and proceedings of a medical committee are considered confidential and are not subject to a court subpoena. The plaintiff argued that the Joint Commission is not a medical committee as defined in the Texas statute. The hospital's chief operating officer testified that the accreditation process with the Joint Commission is voluntary, and the hospital chooses to have the accreditation survey. During the survey, the Joint Commission looks at certain quality care standards it has developed for hospitals. Humana argued that release of the Joint Commission's recommendations would do more than "chill" the effectiveness of such accreditation. The plaintiff argued that even if the information was privileged, it had already been disclosed to a third party, the hospital, thus waiving its rights to non-disclosure. The trial court denied Humana's motion for a protective order that, if granted, would have permitted it to withhold from discovery any information pertaining to credentialing, monitoring, or supervision practices of the hospital regarding its physicians. Humana appealed.

Holding

The Texas Court of Appeals held that the accreditation reports were privileged.

Reason

The purpose of privileged communications is to encourage open and thorough review of a hospital's medical staff and operations of a hospital with the objective of improving the delivery of patient care. The plaintiff argued that the Joint Commission is not a medical committee as defined in the Texas statute. The court of appeals found that: the determinative factor is not whether the entity is known as a "committee," or a "commission," or by any other particular term, but whether it is organized for the purposes contemplated by the statute and case law. The Joint Commission is a committee made up of representatives of various medical organizations and thus fits within the statutory definition. It is organized for the purposes of improving patient care. Both Texas statute and case law recognize that the open, thorough, and uninhibited review that is required for

such committees to achieve their purpose can only be realized if the deliberations of the committee remain confidential.

As to the Joint Commission's disclosing its report to the hospital, the only disclosure was to the hospital as the intended beneficiary of the committee's findings. The only disclosure made to the outside world was the accreditation certificate, which merely declares that the hospital has been awarded accreditation by the Joint Commission.

Discussion

1. Do you agree with the court's decision? Explain.
2. Discuss why privilege from discovery does not extend to all documents maintained in the normal course of business.

Privileged Information: Self-Evaluation

In *Estate of Hussain v. Gardner,*[32] discovery was sought regarding the statements given by a physician to the hospital's internal peer-review committee regarding the management and treatment of a patient. In this medical malpractice action, the plaintiff alleged that the defendant physician deviated from accepted medical standards in the care and treatment of the decedent during surgical procedures. The New Jersey Superior Court held that the statements given by the defendant were protected.

In a similar case, *Wylie v. Mills,*[33] the court adopted the privilege used in several federal jurisdictions that prevents disclosure of confidential, critical evaluative, and deliberative material whenever the public interest in confidentiality outweighs an individual's need for full discovery. In applying the privilege to information contained in a corporate report on an accident in which an employee was involved, the court held that self-evaluation privilege protected the report from discovery. Without such protection, candid expressions of opinion or suggestions as to future policy would not be forthcoming due to a fear that these statements may be used against the employer in a subsequent litigation. The standard used for disclosure of confidential investigative records sets forth the following factors, which should be taken into consideration: (1) the extent to which the information may be available from other sources; (2) the degree of harm that the litigant will suffer from its unavailability; and (3) the possible prejudice in the agency's investigation. The court adopted the holding that the plaintiffs had not made a strong showing of a particular need that outweighs the public interest in the confidentiality of the quality assessment committee. Because information is available from other sources, the court found that the information sought by the plaintiff was readily discoverable.

Credentialing Files Privileged

An action was filed against a health care provider in *Abels v. Ruf* [34] for the negligent credentialing of a physician who allegedly committed medical malpractice. The credentialing file relative to the physician in question was privileged. There was no dispute that the provider's credentialing documents fell within the scope of records of the provider's peer-review committee, and it was clear that the legislature had dictated that such documents were not obtainable from the provider. The Ohio Court of Appeals found that the trial court abused its discretion in ordering the appellant to provide certain credentialing documents to plaintiffs-appellees in discovery, which documents may have been generated by the appellant's peer review committee.

The trial court in *Hammonds v. Ruf* [35] erred when it ordered that certain portions of a physician's credentialing file be disclosed to medical malpractice plaintiffs because the documents were obtainable from original sources. The trial court abused its discretion in ordering the documents in question to be disclosed by the physician in violation of a clear statutory mandate prohibiting such disclosures.

Ordinary Business Documents

Privileged communications statutes do not protect from discovery the records maintained in the ordinary course of doing business and rendering inpatient care. Such documents often can be subpoenaed after showing cause.

Attorney-Client Privilege

Attorney-client privilege generally will preclude discovery of memorandums written to an organization's general counsel by the organization's risk management director. In *Mlynarski v. Rush Presbyterian–St. Luke's Medical Center*, [36] a memorandum written by the risk management coordinator to the hospital's general counsel was barred from discovery. There was undisputed evidence that the risk management coordinator had consulted with and assisted counsel in determining the legal action to pursue and the advisability of settling a claim that she had been assigned to investigate. Information contained in the memorandum was available from witnesses whose names and addresses were made available to the plaintiff. If the hospital later at trial decided to attempt to impeach those witnesses based on the coordinator's testimony, privi-

lege would be waived and the hospital would be required to produce the relevant reports.

Peer-Review Documents Discoverable

The identity of peer-review committee members and individuals who may have given information to such committees is not always considered privileged. A state, for example, may access peer-review reports relating to a physician suspected of criminal negligence. [37] In a civil action, a hospital may be required to identify all persons who have knowledge of an underlying event that is the basis of a malpractice action, whether or not they were members of a peer-review committee. [38]

The surgeon in *Robinson v. Magovern* [39] brought an action under the Sherman Antitrust Act, as well as under state law, seeking recovery because he had been denied hospital privileges. The plaintiff moved in the U.S. District Court for an order compelling the defendants and certain third-party witnesses to respond to discovery requests and deposition questions. The defendants objected, claiming that the information sought was privileged and that the Pennsylvania Peer Review Protection Act seeks to foster candor and discussion at medical review committee meetings through grants of immunity and confidentiality. The court held that although there was a powerful interest in confidentiality embodied in the Pennsylvania Peer Review Protection Act, the act would not be applied to shield from discovery events surrounding the denial of staff privileges, including what occurred at meetings of the hospital's credentials committee and executive committee. The need for evidence was greater than the need for confidentiality in this case. The defendants' objections were overruled, and the motion to compel was granted.

In a similar case, the physician in *Ott v. St. Luke Hospital of Campbell County, Inc.* [40] brought a civil rights suit because his application for medical staff privileges was denied. The physician contended that he was not invited to several peer-review committee meetings or given an opportunity to be heard. The hospital filed for a protective order that would bar discovery of the proceedings of the peer-review committee. The hospital argued that such committees would become ineffective if their deliberations were discoverable and that the privilege claimed by the hospital is recognized in Section 311.377 of the Kentucky Revised Statutes Annotated (1990). The U.S. district court held that where there was no real showing that the peer-review committee's functions would be impaired substantially, and where the benefit gained for correct disposal of the litigation by denying privilege was overwhelming, the hospital would not be permitted to assert privilege. The hospital's motion was therefore denied. The court indicated that it cannot permit the discharge of its responsibility to conduct a search for the truth to be thwarted by rules of privilege in the absence of strong countervailing public policies.

Some Committee Minutes Not Privileged

When a plaintiff seeks case information that does not regard a committee's action or its exchange of honest self-critical study, but merely factual accountings of otherwise discoverable facts, such information is not protected by any privilege because it does not come within the scope of information entitled to that privilege. This does not mean that the plaintiff is entitled to the entire study, because it may contain evidence of policy making, remedial action, proposed courses of conduct, and self-critical analysis that the privilege seeks to protect in order to foster the ability of hospitals to regulate themselves unhindered by outside scrutiny and unconcerned about the possible liability ramifications that their discussions might bring about. As such, the trial court must make an in-camera inspection of such records and determine to what extent they may be discoverable.

In one such case, the plaintiff, a patient, brought an action against a hospital seeking to recover for injuries he sustained as a result of a nosocomial infection he allegedly contracted at the hospital.[41] The plaintiff claimed that his infection was due to an act or omission on the part of the hospital in failing to protect him from such infections. During the discovery phase of the proceedings, the plaintiff filed a motion for production of documents seeking studies done by the hospital regarding the percentage of nosocomial infection rates per patients admitted. The hospital objected to this request, and the plaintiff obtained an order to compel the hospital to produce the documents. The court of appeal, on review, reversed the trial court's ruling, determining that statutes rendering hospital records confidential barred the information from disclosure.

The Louisiana Supreme Court, however, held that the records sought by the plaintiff were not entirely privileged from disclosure. The reliance of the court of appeal on La. R.S. 13:3715.3(A) and 44:7(D) was partially misplaced. These provisions were intended to provide confidentiality to the records and proceedings of hospital committees, not to insulate from discovery certain facts merely because they have come under the review of any particular committee. Such an interpretation could cause any fact that a hospital chooses to unilaterally characterize as privileged to be barred from discovery. The plaintiff sought facts relating to nosocomial infection rates in the defendant's hospital. A nosocomial infection is the same malady that gave rise to the plaintiff's injuries. Such facts would be highly relevant to the plaintiff's case or highly likely to lead to such evidence.

Staff Privileging Documents Discoverable: Illinois

In *May v. Wood River Township Hospital,*[42] the patient's guardian sued the hospital and physicians, alleging that the

hospital was negligent in providing care to the patient and in granting staff privileges to Dr. Marrese. The circuit court granted the guardian's motion, and ordered the hospital to answer certain interrogatories. The hospital appealed.

The hospital submitted a memorandum of law and an affidavit stating all documents concerning the granting of associate staff privileges to Marrese were kept for the purpose of improving the quality of patient care and were protected by the Illinois Code of Civil Procedure.

The trial court denied the hospital's motion for a protective order and granted the plaintiff's motion to compel, ordering the hospital to answer all of the plaintiff's interrogatories. The court determined that nothing related to work done, communications between executive committee members during their meetings, or discussions related to Marrese is protected, nor are the minutes of the committee protected as long as this information existed or was created before the actual decision to grant privileges to Marrese. The hospital urged on appeal, however, that no Illinois case has interpreted the code as being inapplicable to the credentialing process.

The Illinois Appellate Court held that the code of civil procedure did not protect information generated prior to the physician's application for staff privileges or his application for the privileges. The same is true of a host of materials that might be considered by the committee, for example:

- Whether staff privileges were granted, denied, or revoked at other hospitals

- Whether licenses to practice medicine were awarded, denied, suspended, or revoked in a given state

- Whether an applicant has ever been sued for malpractice.

These facts would exist independent of a peer-review process. That which is nonprivileged cannot be converted to being privileged simply by handing the facts to a committee. On the other hand, if the committee sought to generate new opinions or information for consideration by the committee, a privilege could attach. For example, if the committee interviewed a colleague of Marrese's to elicit an opinion on Marrese's ability as a physician, that opinion could be privileged. If, however, the same opinion had been stated earlier in a deposition in a malpractice case and the committee reviewed the deposition, no privilege could attach to conceal the deposition from the discovery process.

Staff Privileging Documents Not Discoverable: South Carolina

The underlying action in *McGee v. Bruce Hospital System*[43] involved a wrongful death claim. A circuit court order granted the plaintiffs a motion instructing the defendant, Bruce Hospital System, to produce the credentialing files and clinical privileges for each of the defendant physicians.

The defendant physicians contended that such documentation is protected by a South Carolina confidentiality statute, S.C. CODE ANN. § 40-71-20 (Supp. 1992). The trial judge found that the materials sought were discoverable.

On appeal, the South Carolina Supreme Court held that: (1) applications for staff privileges and supporting documents of appropriate training were protected by the confidentiality statute; (2) the confidentiality statute did not preclude discovery of general policies and procedures for staff monitoring; and (3) the patient could discover a listing of clinical privileges either granted or denied by the hospital. The overriding public policy of the confidentiality statute is to encourage health care professionals to monitor the competency and professional conduct of their peers in order to safeguard and improve the quality of patient care. The underlying purpose behind the confidentiality statute is not to facilitate the prosecution of civil actions, but to promote complete candor and open discussion among participants in the peer review process.

Section 40-71-20 of the South Carolina statute does not preclude the discovery of the general policies and procedures for staff monitoring. The information contained in the written rules, regulations, policies, and procedures for the medical staff would not compromise the statutory goal of candid evaluation of peers in the medical profession.

The outcome of the decision-making process is not protected. The confidentiality statute was intended to protect the review process, not to restrict the disclosure of the result of the process. Accordingly, the plaintiffs were entitled to a listing of clinical privileges either granted or denied by the hospital.

Search Warrant for Peer Review Documents: Michigan

In *In re Investigation of Liberman*,[44] long-term patient Liberman fell and injured her head while unattended. She later died, apparently as a result of complications from the fall. The attorney general (AG) commenced a criminal investigation into Liberman's death. More than 15 employees were questioned by the AG. The AG obtained and executed an investigatory search warrant for hospital documents. Before the documents left the hospital's premises, however, some of the documents were sealed because the hospital deemed them privileged peer-review documents.

A hearing was held in district court regarding the AG's motion for permission to unseal the documents. The district court was persuaded that the privilege statute asserted by the hospital did not apply because the documents were seized pursuant to a search warrant. The district court allowed the AG to unseal the documents, but the district judge stayed the decision to give the hospital an opportunity to appeal to the circuit court.

On appeal, the circuit court ruled that the peer-review documents were protected by peer-review privilege and that the privilege could be enforced even against documents seized pursuant to a search warrant. The court determined that the legislature intended the privilege to apply regardless of whether the documents were seized pursuant to a subpoena or a search warrant.

The Michigan statute MCL 333 § 21515 provides:

> (1) peer review information is confidential; (2) peer review information is to be used "only for the purposes provided in this article;" (3) peer review information is not to be a public record; and (4) peer review information is not subject to subpoena.

The legislation commands that a hospital maintain a peer-review process for the purpose of improving patient care. Allowing a prosecutor to obtain a hospital's peer-review materials pursuant to a search warrant would be to allow the prosecutor's general investigative powers to override the specific privilege of confidentiality that covers such materials. Accordingly, the Michigan Court of Appeals concluded that documents created by a peer-review body exclusively for peer-review purposes are not subject to disclosure pursuant to a search warrant in a criminal investigation.

HEALTH INSURANCE PORTABILITY AND ACCOUNTABILITY ACT

The Health Insurance Portability and Accountability Act (HIPAA) was enacted by Congress in 1996. According to the Centers for Medicare and Medicaid Services, Title I of HIPAA protects health insurance coverage for workers and their families when they change or lose their jobs. Title II of HIPAA, the administrative simplification (AS) provisions, requires the establishment of national standards for electronic health care transactions and national identifiers for providers, health insurance plans, and employers. The AS provisions also address the security and privacy of health information. The standards are meant to improve the efficiency and effectiveness of the nation's health care system by encouraging the widespread use of electronic data interchange in health care.

Privacy Provision

The HIPAA privacy provision took effect on April 14, 2003. Key privacy provisions include:

- Patients must be able to access their record and request correction of errors.

- Patients must be informed of how their personal information will be used.

- Patient information cannot be used for marketing purposes without the explicit consent of the involved patients.

- Patients can ask their health insurers and providers to take reasonable steps to ensure that their communications with the patient are confidential. For instance, a patient can ask to be called at his or her work number, instead of home or cell phone number.

- Patients can file formal privacy-related complaints to the U.S. Department of Health and Human Services (HHS) Office for Civil Rights.

- Health insurers or providers must document their privacy procedures, but they have discretion on what to include in their privacy procedure.

- Health insurers or providers must designate a privacy officer and train their employees.

- Providers may use patient information without patient consent for the purposes of providing treatment, obtaining payment for services, and performing the nontreatment operational tasks of the provider's business.

Security Provision

The HIPAA security provisions took effect April 20, 2005. The security provision complements the privacy provision. HIPAA defines three segments of security safeguards for compliance: administrative, physical, and technical. Key provisions are:

Administrative Safeguards

- Policies and procedures must be designed to clearly show how the entity will comply with the act.

- Entities that must comply with HIPAA requirements must adopt a written set of privacy procedures and designate a privacy officer to be responsible for developing and implementing all required policies and procedures.

- Policies and procedures must reference management oversight and organizational buy-in to comply with the documented security controls.

- Procedures should clearly identify employees or classes of employees who will have access to protected health information (PHI).

- Access to PHI in all forms must be restricted to only those employees who have a need for it to complete their job function.

- Procedures must address access authorization, establishment, modification, and termination.

- Entities must show that an appropriate ongoing training program regarding the handling of PHI is provided to employees performing health plan administrative functions.

- Covered entities that outsource some of their business processes to a third party must ensure that their vendors also have a framework in place to comply with HIPAA requirements.

- Care must be taken to determine if the vendor further outsources any data handling functions to other vendors, while monitoring whether appropriate contracts and controls are in place.

- A contingency plan should be in place for responding to emergencies.

- Covered entities are responsible for backing up their data and having disaster recovery procedures in place.

- The recovery plan should document data priority and failure analysis, testing activities, and change control procedures.

- Internal audits play a key role in HIPAA compliance by reviewing operations with the goal of identifying potential security violations.

- Policies and procedures should specifically document the scope, frequency, and procedures of audits.

- Audits should be both routine and event based.

- Procedures should document instructions for addressing and responding to security breaches that are identified either during the audit or the normal course of operations.

Physical Safeguards

- Responsibility for security must be assigned to a specific person or department.

- Controls must govern the introduction and removal of hardware and software from the network.

- When equipment is retired, it must be disposed of properly to ensure that PHI is not compromised.

- Access to equipment containing health information should be carefully controlled and monitored.

- Access to hardware and software must be limited to properly authorized individuals.

- Required access controls consist of facility security plans, maintenance records, and visitor sign-in and escorts.

- Policies are required to address proper workstation use.

- Workstations should be removed from high-traffic areas and monitor screens should not be in direct view of the public.

- If the covered entities utilize contractors or agents, they too must be fully trained on their physical access responsibilities.

Technical Safeguards

- Information systems housing PHI must be protected from intrusion.

- When information flows over open networks, some form of encryption must be utilized.

- If closed systems/networks are utilized, existing access controls are considered sufficient and encryption is optional.

- Each covered entity is responsible for ensuring that the data within its systems has not been changed or erased in an unauthorized manner.

- Data corroboration, including the use of check sum, double-keying, message authentication, and digital signature may be used to ensure data integrity.

- Covered entities must also authenticate entities with which it communicates.

- Authentication consists of corroborating that an entity is who it claims to be.

- Covered entities must make documentation of their HIPAA practices available to the government to determine compliance.

- Information technology documentation should also include a written record of all configuration settings on the components of the network because these components are complex, configurable, and always changing.

- Documented risk analysis and risk management programs are required.

CHARTING—SOME HELPFUL ADVICE

The medical record is the most important document in a negligence action. Both the plaintiff and defendant use it as a basis for their action and defense in a lawsuit. The following suggestions on documentation should prove helpful when charting in a patient's record.

- The medical record describes the care rendered to each patient. It should be sufficiently complete to allow those not treating a patient to review the record and assume continuing care when necessary.

- Medical record entries should be timely, legible, clear, and meaningful to a patient's course of treatment. Illegible medical records not only damage one's ability to

defend oneself, but also can have an adverse effect on the credibility of other health care professionals who read the record and act on what they read.

- The medical record should be complete. This is often a problem with progress notes when there is little new information to report. Progress notes should describe the symptoms or condition being addressed, the treatment rendered, the patient response, and the patient's status at the time treatment is discontinued.

- Long, defensive, or derogatory notes should not be written. Only the facts should be related. Criticism, complaints, emotional comments, and extraneous remarks have no place in the medical record. Such remarks can precipitate a malpractice suit.

- Erasures and correction fluid should not be used to cover up entries. Do not tamper with the chart in any form. A single line should be drawn through a mistaken entry, the correct information entered, and the correction signed and dated.

- Charts related to pending legal action should be placed in a separate file under lock and key. Legal counsel should be notified immediately of any potential lawsuit.

- A medical record has many authors. Entries made by others must not be ignored. Good patient care is a collaborative interdisciplinary team effort. Entries made by health care professionals provide valuable information in treating the patient.

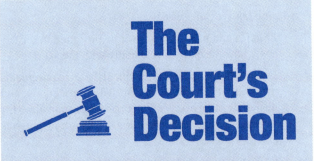

The Court's Decision

A West Texas jury ordered the physician, drugstore, and pharmacist to pay $225,000 to the family. The likelihood of similar occurrences is a growing danger as the number and variety of medications increase with similar names and look-alikes.

CHAPTER REVIEW

1. *Information management* is the process of facilitating the flow of information within and among departments and caregivers.
2. Health care organizations are required to maintain medical records for their patients in accordance with accepted professional standards and practices and the requirements for these records are often set forth within each state's public health laws. Records should be complete, accurate, current, readily accessible, and organized.
3. An admission record contains data including age, address, reason for admission, Social Security number, marital status, religious affiliation, and other information required under federal and state requirements. It includes general consent and authorization-for-treatment forms. Patient-specific medical information is recorded in the clinical record.
4. Third-party reimbursement may be denied to an organization or physician who has failed to maintain a complete and accurate medical record. To receive federal funding, health care organizations must meet minimum federal standards for record keeping.
5. *Diagnosis-related groups* (DRGs) are a method of classifying patients by categories according to age, diagnosis, and treatment resource requirements. DRGs are the basis for the prospective payment system and are assigned using information detailed in a patient's medical record. Failure to keep complete and accurate records could result in difficulty in obtaining reimbursement.
6. Medical records are maintained for the benefit of the patients and are considered the property of the health care provider. Generally, health care professionals and health care organizations do not release medical records to patients. Most courts, however, take the view that patients have a right to access their records, and some states have issued legislation granting this access.
7. Records can be used as important evidentiary tools. The integrity and completeness of a medical record can be crucial in reconstructing the events surrounding alleged negligence.
8. The employees and staff of health care organizations are required to maintain the confidentiality of verbal and written communications. This is in accordance with both laws protecting a patient's right to privacy and ethical standards for health care professionals.
9. Lack of trust and confidence in a physician can destroy the integrity of the physician-patient relationship and negatively affect the quality and appropriateness of the treatment administered. Patients can be awarded damages if it is proven that a physician disclosed confidential information without authorization and that this disclosure resulted in harm to the patient.
10. The requirements for the length of time medical records must be retained differ among states. In determining the length of time records should be retained, organizations, along with advice from legal counsel, should consider patient needs, statutory requirements, future need for the records, and legal considerations of record availability in the event of a lawsuit.
11. The intentional alteration, falsification, or destruction of medical records to avoid liability for negligence is usually sufficient to show malice. Punitive damages may be awarded whether or not the act resulted in compensable harm. Falsification of medical or business records is grounds for both criminal indictment and civil liability.
12. Information can be shielded from discovery if privilege can be established by the party that seeks to protect the information.
13. The restriction on disclosing patient information can be lifted under certain circumstances, including the information's relevance in a criminal investigation.
14. Although computers improve the ease and efficiency with which data are compiled and shared, they also pose confidentiality risks.
15. HIPAA requires the establishment of national standards for electronic health care transactions and national identifiers for providers, health insurance plans, and employers. HIPAA provisions also address the security and privacy of health information.

REVIEW QUESTIONS

1. What is information management as it relates to health care?
2. What are the basic purposes of the medical record?
3. Discuss the advantages and disadvantages of computer-generated medical records.
4. A medical record is the sole property of the patient and should never be released. Discuss your opinion on this statement.
5. What is the reasoning for the establishment of statutes that protect an organization's peer-review information?
6. Should statements given by a defendant to a hospital's internal peer-review committee be discoverable by a plaintiff? Explain your answer.
7. What records or parts thereof should be protected from discovery?
8. Should information gathered prior to a physician's application for staff privileges be privileged from discovery? Explain.
9. How long should patient records be maintained?

NOTES

1. *Doctor Held Liable for Fatal Handwriting Mix-up,* USA TODAY, Oct. 21, 1999.
2. 515 A.2d 948 (Pa. Super. Ct. 1986).
3. No. 91-1467 (2d Cir. June 1, 1992).
4. 536 N.E.2d 1202 (Ohio Com. Pl. 1988).
5. 582 N.E.2d 233 (Ill. App. Ct. 1991).
6. 21 U.S.C. § 1175 (1972).
7. 328 P.2d 556 (Cal. Ct. App. 1958).
8. 597 N.E.2d 616 (Ill. 1992).
9. John P. Glaser, *Brigham and Women's Wager on Huge PC Network Pays Solid Returns,* Health Management Technology, Oct. 1994, at 7.
10. 423 U.S. 1313 (1975).
11. No. L-03-1303 (Ohio App. 2004).
12. 609 N.Y.S.2d 898 (N.Y. App. Div. 1994).
13. 683 N.E.2d 1175 (Ohio App. 1996).
14. 402 N.Y.S.2d 318 (N.Y. Sup. Ct. 1978).
15. *Deceit Found in Fatality at Rest Home,* N.Y. Times, Feb. 5, 1995, at 35.
16. 442 A.2d 635 (N.J. Super. Ct. 1982).
17. *In re Jascalevich,* 182 N.J. Super. 445, 442 A.2d 635, 644–45 (1982).
18. 880 P.2d 1188 (Colo. 1994).
19. *Id.* at 1192.
20. *Id.* at 1196.
21. *Dimora v. Cleveland Clinic Found,* 683 N.E.2d 1175 (Ohio App. 8 ist. 1996).
22. Ronnie Greene, *Examiner: Treatment "Appropriate,"* The Miami Herald, April 16, 1995, at 14A.
23. Esme M. Infante, *Doctors' Rx: Write Right,* USA Today, June 14, 994, at 1.
24. No. 94189 (N.Y. App. Div 2004).
25. No. 94969 (Supreme Court of N.Y. App. Div. 2004).
26. 16 F.3d 473 (1st Cir. 1994).
27. 262 P.2d 682 (Wyo. 1953).
28. 905 F.2d 549 (1st Cir. 1990).
29. Federal Rules of Evidence, 28 § 803(6) (1988).
30. 42 U.S.C.A. § 11101–11152 (1989).
31. *Berger v. Sonneland,* 1 P.3d 1187 (2000).
32. 624 A.2d 99 (N.J. Super. Ct. App. Div. 1993).
33. 478 A.2d 1273 (N.J. Super. Ct. App. Div. 1984).
34. C. A. No. 22265 (Ohio App. 2005).
35. C. A. No. 22109 (Ohio Ct. App. 2004).
36. 572 N.E.2d 1025 (Ill. App. Ct. 1991).
37. *People v. Superior Court,* 286 Cal. Rptr. 478 (Cal. Ct. App. 1991).
38. *Moretti v. Lowe,* 592 A.2d 855 (R.I. 1991).
39. 521 F. Supp. 842 (W.D. Pa. 1981).
40. 522 F. Supp. 706 (E.D. Ky. 1981).
41. *Smith v. Lincoln Gen. Hosp.,* 605 So. 2d 1347 (La. 1992).
42. 629 N.E.2d 170 (Ill. App. Ct. 1994).
43. 439 S.E.2d 257 (S.C. 1993).
44. 646 N.W.2d 199 (Mich. App. 2002).

Patient Consent

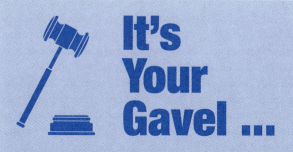

It's Your Gavel ...

THE LONG WAIT

On August 10, 1988, Matthews had gone unassisted to the emergency department (ED) of the hospital complaining of a burning pain in her upper chest that had radiated down her right side that evening, as well as the previous evening. Upon arriving at the hospital at about 11:25 P.M., Matthews was triaged by a nurse who took her vital signs, recorded her medical history, and made an assessment of her immediate medical needs. Although slightly elevated, Matthews's vital signs were within normal limits. The triage nurse classified Matthews as a "category two" patient, a nonthreatening condition. It was explained to her that she would have a long wait, as the ED was busy. A social services representative (SSR) testi-fied that he spoke to Matthews six or eight times during her wait in the ED. He indicated that she was in no apparent distress during those times that he spoke to her. Following a 4½-hour wait, Matthews decided to leave the ED without being treated. The SSR stated that he told Matthews that a treatment room was ready for her and that she would be attended to shortly. Matthews said that she had already waited long enough and she was leaving. The SSR stated that he pleaded with her to stay but she refused, claiming that she would see her own physician in the morning. Matthews went to work the following day without having seen her physician. She died on August 12, 1988. A malpractice action was brought against the hospital arising out of the death of Matthews. The DeKalb Superior Court granted the hospital's motion for summary judgment, and an appeal was taken.[1] Was the patient's subsequent death following her visit to the hospital's ED due to the hospital's negligence?

WHAT IS YOUR VERDICT?

INTRODUCTION

". . . no right is held more sacred, or is more care-
fully guarded, by the common law, than the right of
every individual to the possession and control of
his own person."

Union Pacific Ry. Co. v. Botsford[2]

Consent, in the health care setting, is the voluntary agreement by a person who possesses sufficient mental capacity
to make an intelligent choice to allow a medical procedure
and/or treatment proposed by another to be performed on
himself or herself. Consent changes a touching that otherwise would be nonconsensual to one that is consensual. Consent can be either express or implied.

Express consent can take the form of a verbal agreement,
or it can be accomplished through the execution of a written
document authorizing medical care.

Implied consent is determined by some act or silence,
which raises a presumption that consent has been authorized.

Consent must be obtained from the patient, or from a
person authorized to consent on the patient's behalf, before
any medical procedure can be performed. Every individual
has a right to refuse to authorize a touching. Touching of
another without authorization to do so could be considered
a battery. Not every touching results in a battery. When a
person voluntarily enters a situation in which a reasonably
prudent person would anticipate a touching (e.g., riding in
an elevator or rushing through a crowded subway), consent
is implied. Consent is not required for the normal, routine,
everyday touching and bumping that occurs in life. In the
process of caring for patients, it is inevitable that they will be
touched and handled. Most touching in the health care setting is considered routine. Typical routine touching includes
bathing, administering medications, dressing changes, and
so forth. This chapter reviews the many issues surrounding
consent in the health care setting.

INFORMED CONSENT

Whose Decision Is It?

The operation you get often depends on where
you live. One patient underwent a mastectomy
only to learn that a less-destructive alternative procedure was available in a region near her home.
The procedure, a lumpectomy, has the same survival rate as a mastectomy. The patient claims the
surgeon never informed her as to the alternative.

Informed consent is a legal doctrine that provides that a
patient has the right to know the potential risks, benefits, and
alternatives of a proposed procedure. Where there are two or
more medically acceptable treatment options, the competent
patient has the absolute right to know about and select from
the available treatment options after being informed of the
alternatives, risks, and benefits of each.

Informed consent is predicated on the duty of the physician to disclose to the patient sufficient information to enable
the patient to evaluate a proposed medical or surgical procedure before submitting to it. Informed consent requires that
a patient have a full understanding of that to which he or she
has consented. The informed consent doctrine provides that
a physician has a legal, ethical, and moral duty to respect
patient autonomy and to provide only such medical care as
authorized by the patient. An authorization from a patient
who does not understand to what he or she is consenting is
not effective consent.

The right to be free from unwanted medical treatment has
long been recognized by the courts. The right to control the
integrity of one's own body spawned the doctrine of informed
consent.[3] The U.S. Supreme Court, in *Cruzan v. Director,*
Missouri Dep't of Health,[4] held that a competent adult patient
has the right to decline any and all form of medical intervention, including lifesaving or life-prolonging treatment.

Florida statute § 766.103 (3) (a) (2) notes that reasonable
care on the part of a physician in obtaining the informed
consent for treatment consists of providing the patient information sufficient to give a reasonable person a general understanding of the proposed procedure, the medically acceptable alternative procedures, and the substantial risks and
hazards inherent in the proposed procedure that are recognized by other physicians in the same or similar community
who perform similar procedures. A physician is not under a
duty to elucidate upon all the possible risks, but only those
of a serious nature. Expert testimony is required to establish
whether a reasonable physician in the community would
make the pertinent disclosures under the same or similar
circumstances.

Hospitals generally do not have an independent duty to
obtain informed consent or to warn patients of the risks of a
procedure to be performed by a physician who is not an
agent of the hospital. It is the treating physician who has the
education, expertise, skill, and training necessary to treat a
patient and determine what information a patient should
have in order to give informed consent. Nurses and other
nonphysician hospital employees do not normally possess
the knowledge of a particular patient's medical history, diagnosis, or other circumstances that would enable the employee
to fully disclose all pertinent information to the patient.

ASSESSING DECISION-MAKING CAPACITY

A patient is considered competent to make medical decisions regarding his or her care unless a court determines
otherwise. Generally speaking, the determination of a patient's

decision-making capacity is made by medical personnel. The clinical assessment of decision-making capacity should include the patient's ability to

- understand the risks, benefits, and alternatives of a proposed test or procedure
- evaluate the information provided by the physician
- express his or her treatment preferences
- voluntarily make decisions regarding his or her treatment plan without undue influence by family, friends, or medical personnel

NURSES AND INFORMED CONSENT

In general, a nurse has no duty to advise a patient as to a surgical procedure to be employed; advise the patient as to the risks, benefits, and alternatives to the recommended procedure; or obtain a patient's informed consent to surgery merely because the physician directed a nurse to have the patient sign a consent form.

The plaintiff, Davis, in *Davis v. Hoffman*,[5] experienced pain in her lower abdomen and consulted Dr. Hoffman. He diagnosed her to be suffering from a fibroid uterus and prescribed a dilation and curettage procedure designed to remove the fibroids. Hoffman further suggested a laparoscopy and hysteroscopy to search for cancer. The physician's nurse, Puchini, conducted a presurgical interview with the plaintiff in which she described a video hysteroscopy, a dilation and curettage procedure, a resectoscopic removal of submucous fibroids, a laparoscopy, and a laser myomectomy. The plaintiff claimed that she specifically informed Hoffman and Puchini that she did not consent to a hysterectomy. They responded that they would awaken her during the operation to obtain her consent before proceeding to a hysterectomy. At no time did they inform the plaintiff that Hoffman intended to perform a hysterectomy. The plaintiff underwent a procedure that resulted in a hysterectomy, during which no one awakened Davis to discuss and explore possible alternatives. The plaintiff brought an action for lack of informed consent against Hoffman, Puchini, and the hospital.

In response to the plaintiff's allegation that the hospital committed battery by lack of informed consent to the hysterectomy, the hospital asserted that Pennsylvania law places no duty on a hospital to obtain a patient's consent to an operation. The hospital argued that Pennsylvania courts have applied the doctrine of informed consent only to physicians, not to hospitals.

The plaintiff responded that the hospital gratuitously undertook to obtain her consent prior to the operation. Although the consent form authored and printed by the hospital was used, there was no suggestion that the deficiency in consent was in any way causally inadequate in the form. Rather, any failure was attributed to the omissions in the

way the form was filled in, or in the way the patient was not informed as to the next phase of the operation. Thus, the form was causally irrelevant and could not be a basis for finding liability.

Because nurses do not have a duty to obtain informed consent in Pennsylvania, the plaintiff had not stated a claim for battery by lack of informed consent against Puchini. Pennsylvania law generally imposes no duty on persons other than surgeons to obtain informed consent before performing surgery.

PHYSICIANS AND INFORMED CONSENT

Physicians are expected disclose to their patients the risks, benefits, and alternatives of recommended procedures. Disclosure should include what a reasonable person would consider material to his or her decision of whether or not to undergo treatment. The patient-plaintiff in *Stover v. Surgeons*[6] suffered damage to her heart valves as a result of childhood rheumatic fever. Dr. Ford, one of a group of physicians that the patient consulted after her condition worsened, informed the patient she needed a heart-valve replacement. Testimony from Ford revealed that he briefly reviewed the details of the surgery with the patient. The plaintiff stated that she was never informed about the risks associated with installing mechanical valves, including the Beall valve that was implanted in her. Thromboemboli, strokes, and the lifelong use of anticoagulants, which are common side effects of valve replacements, were never discussed with her. Dr. Zikria performed the surgery and could not recall discussing any risks, other than clotting, associated with the implantation. After the surgery, the patient suffered severe, permanent brain damage from multiple episodes of thromboemboli directly caused by valve implantation. She then sued for lack of informed consent, and the jury returned a verdict for her. The physicians appealed.

The Pennsylvania Superior Court held that the physicians had to discuss alternative prostheses with the patient, where it represented medically recognized alternatives. Evidence that the heart valve actually implanted was no longer in general use at the time of operation was relevant and material to the issue of informed consent.

Although the physicians argued that the choice of prosthesis should belong to them, the court held that if there are other recognized, medically sound alternatives, the patient must be informed about the risks and benefits of them in order to make a sound judgment regarding treatment, including the desire to execute a waiver of consent. The agreement between the physician and the patient is contractual. Therefore, in order for valid consent to occur, there must be a finding that both parties understood the nature of the procedure, including what any possible as well as expected results would be. The consent is not valid if the patient did not understand the operation to be performed, its seriousness, the disease or incapacity, and possible results. In the instant case, the physicians failed to inform the patient about the recognized risks of the valve that was implanted.

Finally, the court reasoned that there were alternative valves available that were never discussed with the patient. To arrive at an informed decision concerning her treatment, it was material for her to have been told about the alternatives, risks, and benefits of the different valves available for use.

DUTY TO INFORM: DELICATE MEDICAL JUDGMENT

Citation: *Mathias v. St. Catherine's Hosp., Inc.,* 569 N.W.2d 330 (Wis. App. 1997)

Facts

Mathias, a patient of Dr. Witt's at St. Catherine's Hospital, delivered a full-term son by cesarean section on February 2, 1993, while she was under general anesthesia. In the operating room, Witt indicated that he needed a particular instrument that would be used in a tubal ligation. The nurses, Ms. Snyder and Ms. Perri, employees of St. Catherine's, looked at Mathias's chart. Snyder informed Witt that she did not see a signed consent form for that procedure. In deposition testimony, Snyder stated that Witt replied, "Oh, okay."

Witt performed a tubal ligation. Three days after the procedure had been done, a nurse brought Mathias a consent form for the procedure. This nurse told Mathias that the form was "just to close up our records." The nurse testified in her deposition that she signed Perri's name on that same consent form and backdated it to February 2, the day the surgery was performed. As the trial court noted in its oral decision granting summary judgment, these actions after the surgery are immaterial to the issue of the hospital's duty to Mathias. The trial court granted summary judgment dismissing St. Catherine's from the malpractice action. Mr. and Ms. Mathias appealed the summary judgment contending that the hospital owed a duty to Mathias to prevent her physician from performing a tubal ligation for which there was no signed consent.

Issue

Did the hospital owe a duty to Mathias to prevent her physician from performing a tubal ligation for which there was no consent? Did the trial court err in granting summary judgment to St. Catherine's?

Holding

St. Catherine's fulfilled its duty of ordinary care to Mathias and therefore is not liable. The trial court's grant of summary judgment was affirmed.

Reason

The duty to advise a patient of the risks of treatment lies with the physician and not the hospital. This duty is codified in Wis. Stat. § 448.30, which requires:

Any physician who treats a patient shall inform the patient about the availability of all alternate, viable medical modes of treatment and about the benefits and risks of these treatments. The physician's duty to inform the patient under this section does not require disclosure of:

1. information beyond what a reasonably well-qualified physician in a similar medical classification would know

2. detailed technical information that in all probability a patient would not understand

3. risks apparent or known to the patient

4. extremely remote possibilities that might falsely or detrimentally alarm the patient

5. information in emergencies where failure to provide treatment would be more harmful to the patient than treatment

6. information in cases where the patient is incapable of consenting

This statute is the cornerstone of the hospital's duty in this case. The court noted that the legislature limited the application of the duty to obtain informed consent to the treating physician. Although the record is littered with semantic arguments about whether this is a case of nonconsent or lack of informed consent, what the Mathiases sought was to extend the duty of ensuring informed consent to the hospital.

The duty to inform rests with the physician and requires the exercise of delicate medical judgment. It is the physician—not the hospital—who has the duty of obtaining informed consent. The surgeon, not the hospital, has the education, training, and experience necessary to advise each patient of risks associated with a proposed procedure. The physician is in the best position to know the patient's medical history and to evaluate and explain the risks of a particular operation in light of the particular medical history.

Discussion

1. Do you agree with the court's finding that the hospital had no legal duty to ensure that Witt obtain informed consent from Mathias? Explain.

2. What issues do you see in another nurse's decision to sign Perri's name on the consent form and then backdate it to February 2, 1993?

consented to bed rest if she had been informed of the probable effect on the quality of her life.

The New Jersey Supreme Court held that it is necessary to advise a patient when considering alternative courses of treatment. The physician should have explained medically reasonable invasive and noninvasive alternatives, including the risks and likely outcomes of those alternatives, even when the chosen course is noninvasive.

In an informed consent analysis, the decisive factor is not whether a treatment alternative is invasive or noninvasive, but whether the physician adequately presents the material facts so that the patient can make an informed decision. That conclusion does not imply that a physician must explain in detail all treatment options in every case. For example, a physician need not recite all the risks and benefits of each potential appropriate antibiotic when writing a prescription for treatment of an upper respiratory infection. Conversely, a physician could be obligated, depending on the circumstances, to discuss a variety of treatment alternatives, such as chemotherapy, radiation, or surgery, with a patient diagnosed with cancer. Distinguishing the two situations are the limitations of the reasonable patient standard, which need not unduly burden the physician-patient relationship. The standard obligates the physician to disclose only that information material to a reasonable patient's informed decision.[8]

If the patient's choice is not consistent with the physician's recommendation, the physician has the option of withdrawing from the case. The patient then has the option to seek another physician who is comfortable with the alternative treatment preferred by the patient.

COURSE OF TREATMENT: PATIENT'S DECISION

The plaintiff-patient in *Matthies v. Mastromonaco,*[7] an elderly woman living alone in a senior citizens' residence, fell and fractured her hip and was taken to the hospital. An orthopedic surgeon, the defendant, reviewed the patient's history, condition, and X-rays, and decided that, rather than utilizing a pinning procedure for her hip involving the insertion of four steel screws, it would be better to adopt a conservative course of treatment, bed rest.

Prior to her injury, the plaintiff maintained an independent style of living. She did her own grocery shopping and other household duties and had been able to climb steps unassisted.

Expert testimony at trial indicated that bed rest was an inappropriate treatment. The defendant was of the opinion that given the frail condition of the patient and her age, she would be best treated in a nursing home and, therefore, opting for a more conservative treatment. At the heart of the informed consent issue was the plaintiff's assertion that she would not have

LACK OF CONSENT

Four children, in *Riser v. American Medical Intern, Inc.,*[9] brought a medical malpractice action against Lang, a physician who performed a femoral arteriogram on their 69-year-old mother, Riser, who subsequently died of a stroke 11 days following the procedure. Riser had been admitted to De La Ronde Hospital experiencing impaired circulation in her lower arms and hands. The patient had multiple medical diagnoses, including diabetes mellitus, end-stage renal failure, and arteriosclerosis. Her physician, Dr. Sottiurai, ordered bilateral arteriograms to determine the cause of the patient's impaired circulation. Because De La Ronde Hospital could not accommodate Sottiurai's request, Riser was transferred to Dr. Lang, a radiologist at St. Jude Hospital. Lang performed a femoral arteriogram, not the bilateral brachial arteriogram ordered by Sottiurai. The procedure seemed to go well, and the patient was prepared for transfer back to De La Ronde Hospital. However, shortly after the ambulance departed the hospital, the patient suffered a seizure in the ambulance and was returned to St. Jude. Riser's condition deteriorated and she died 11 days later. The plaintiffs claimed in their lawsuit that Riser was a poor risk for the procedure. The district court ruled for the plaintiffs, awarding damages in the amount of $50,000 for Riser's pain and suffering and $100,000 to each child. Lang appealed.

The Louisiana Court of Appeal held that Lang breached the standard of care by subjecting the patient to a procedure that would have no practical benefit to the patient, that Lang failed to obtain informed consent from the patient, and that the damage award was not excessive.

Testimony revealed that Lang breached the standard of care by performing a procedure that he knew or should have known would have had no practical benefit to the patient or her referring physician. The defendant himself, as well as the expert witnesses in this case, testified that it is a breach of the standard of care for any physician to subject a patient to a particular test or procedure that has any risk of injury, however small, associated with it if that physician knows or reasonably should know that the procedure will be of no benefit to the patient.

As to informed consent, a reasonably prudent person in the position of Riser would have refused to undergo the procedure if he or she had known of the strong possibility of a stroke. Informed consent requires that the physician reveal to the patient all material risks. The patient's consent to an arteriogram was vitiated by Lang's failure to disclose such a possibility. The consent form itself did not contain express authorization for Lang to perform the femoral arteriogram. Sottiurai ordered a brachial arteriogram, not a femoral arteriogram. Riser was under the impression that she was about to undergo a brachial arteriogram, not a femoral arteriogram. Two consent forms were signed; neither form authorized the performance of a femoral arteriogram. O'Neil, one of Riser's daughters, claimed that her mother said following the arteriogram, "Why did you let them do that to me?"[10] Although Lang claims that he explained the procedure to Riser and O'Neil, the trial court, faced with this conflicting testimony, chose to believe the plaintiffs. The appeals court found no error in the trial court's decision. The defendants argued that the plaintiffs had not established a causal connection between the arteriogram and the stroke. There was conflicting testimony between the pathologists who testified at trial as to the cause of the patient's death. The judge chose to believe the pathologist's testimony that it was more probable than not that the stroke resulted from the arteriogram performed by Lang.

INFORMATION TO BE DISCLOSED

A physician should provide as much information about treatment options as is necessary based on a patient's personal understanding of the physician's explanation of the risks of treatment and the probable consequences of the treatment. The needs of each patient can vary depending on age, maturity, and mental status.

Some courts have recognized that the condition of the patient may be taken into account to determine whether the patient has received sufficient information to give consent. The individual responsible for obtaining consent must weigh the importance of giving full disclosure to the patient against the likelihood that such disclosure will seriously and adversely affect the condition of the patient.

The courts generally utilize an "objective" or "subjective" test to determine whether a patient would have refused treatment if the physician had provided adequate information as to the risks, benefits, and alternatives of the procedure. In the objective test, the plaintiff must prove that a "reasonable person" would not have undergone the procedure if he or she had been properly informed. Under the subjective test theory, the court examines whether the "individual patient" would have chosen the procedure if he or she had been fully informed. As described in the following cases, the courts favor the objective test.

Warren, in *Warren v. Schecter,*[11] was diagnosed as having a stomach ulcer. Schecter recommended surgery to remove the portions of the stomach containing the ulcer. One of the significant risks of gastric surgery is decreased calcium absorption, leading to early and severe metabolic bone disease (osteoporosis, osteomalacia, or bone pain). It was Schecter's role as the surgeon to advise Warren of the risks of surgery in order to obtain her informed consent. He did not discuss these risks with her. He did, however, advise Warren that she might experience bowel obstructions, dumping syndrome involving nausea, and the slight risk of death from anesthesia. Based on the risks disclosed to Warren, she consented to the surgery, which Schecter performed.

Following surgery, Warren developed dumping syndrome, a side effect that occurs in about 1 percent of the patients who undergo this procedure. Warren also developed alkaline reflux gastritis, a condition involving the movement of alkaline fluid back into the stomach.

After Warren was diagnosed with these complications, she returned to Schecter, who recommended a second surgery to relieve the pain and discomfort from the first surgery. The second surgery would enhance the risk of bone disease. However, Schecter again failed to advise Warren of the risk of metabolic bone disease.

Warren was taken to a hospital emergency department for care. There she was advised that she had suffered a fracture of one of her lumbar vertebrae and that previous surgeries had caused the osteoporosis that led to the fracture. A bone density scan confirmed that Warren's bones were brittle.

Warren filed an action for medical negligence, alleging that Schecter was liable under an informed consent theory for performing surgery without advising her of the risk of bone disease. Warren claimed that had Schecter warned her of the risk of metabolic bone disease, she would not have consented to surgery. The jury decided that: (1) Schecter did not disclose to Warren all relevant information that would enable her to make an informed decision regarding surgery; (2) a reasonably prudent person in Warren's position would not have consented to surgery if adequately informed of all the significant perils; and (3) Schecter's negligence was a cause of injury to Warren.

On appeal, the plaintiff was found entitled to compensation for all damages proximately resulting from the physician's failure to give full disclosure of the risks of surgery. The patient was entitled to recover because she would not have consented to any surgery had the true risk been disclosed.

A plaintiff meets the burden of establishing a causal relationship between the physician's failure to inform and the injury to the plaintiff by demonstrating that a prudent person in the plaintiff's position would have declined the procedure if adequately informed of the risks. The objective standard, which in effect equates the plaintiff with a reasonable person, is appropriate because it protects the defendant-physician from the self-serving testimony of a plaintiff who inevitably will assert at trial that he or she would have refused the procedure if duly advised of the risk. The objective test required of the plaintiff does not prevent the physician from showing, by way of defense, that even though a reasonably prudent person might not have undergone the procedure if properly informed of the perils, this particular plaintiff still would have consented to the procedure. Under the objective standard, Warren had only to prove that a prudent person in her position would not have consented if adequately informed of the risks. Schecter failed to provide Warren with the risks and benefits of the surgical procedures prior to obtaining her consent for the operations, and Warren testified that she would not have consented to either surgery if duly advised of the risk.

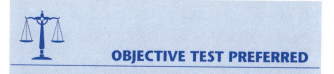

OBJECTIVE TEST PREFERRED

Citation: *Ashe v. Radiation Oncology Assocs.,* 9 S.W.3d 119 (Tenn. 1999)

Facts

The plaintiff, Ashe, was diagnosed with breast cancer in 1988. She underwent a double mastectomy and chemotherapy. In 1993, she began experiencing problems with a cough and a fever. She returned to her oncologist, Dr. Kuzu, where she presented a variety of symptoms, including fever, cough, weight loss, and decreased appetite. A chest X-ray and a computerized tomography (CT) scan revealed the presence of a mass in her left lung.

Ashe underwent surgery, and the upper portion of her left lung was removed. She underwent chemotherapy and was referred to the defendant, Dr. Stroup, for consideration of radiation therapy.

Stroup prescribed radiation treatment for Ashe. She received a daily dose of 200 centigray for 25 days. Ashe sustained radiation myelitis caused by a permanent radiation injury to her spinal cord. She is now a paraplegic.

Stroup did not inform Ashe that the radiation treatment might result in a permanent injury to her spinal cord. According to Stroup, the risk that she would sustain a spinal cord injury was less than one percent. Ashe's expert, Dr. Perez, stated that the risk of spinal cord injury was one to two percent. Perez testified that the applicable standard of care required physicians to warn patients about the risk of radiation injury to the spinal cord.

Ashe filed an action alleging claims for medical malpractice and lack of informed consent. At trial, she testified that she would not have consented to radiation therapy had she been informed of the risk of paralysis. On cross-examination, defense counsel pointed out that the plaintiff did equivocate in her deposition on the issue of consent. Her deposition testimony indicated that she did not know what she would have done had she been warned about the risk of spinal cord injury. She then testified on redirect examination that if Stroup had said to her, "Patty, if you do this, there is a risk that you will be in a wheelchair six months from now," I would have told him, "I will take my chances." I would not have it done.

The trial court found that the plaintiff's trial testimony conflicted with her deposition testimony regarding whether she would have consented to the procedure had she been warned of the risk of spinal cord injury. The trial court, therefore, struck the trial testimony and granted the defendant a directed verdict on the informed consent claim. The plaintiff's malpractice claim went to the jury. The jury was unable to reach a verdict, and a mistrial was declared.

The plaintiff appealed to the court of appeals. The court of appeals held that as part of the plaintiff's informed consent claim she was required to prove that a reasonable person knowing of the risk for spinal cord injury would have decided not to have the procedure performed. The court held that the discrepancy between the trial and deposition testimony went to the issue of credibility and that the trial testimony should not have been stricken. The court of appeals reversed the trial court's grant of a directed verdict on the informed consent claim and remanded the case for a new trial.

Issue

What is the appropriate standard to be employed when assessing the issue of causation in a medical malpractice informed consent case?

Finding

Causation in informed consent cases is better resolved on an objective basis. The standard to be applied in informed consent cases is whether a reasonable person in the patient's position would have consented to the procedure or treatment in question if adequately informed of all significant perils.

Reason

In Tennessee, the plaintiff in an informed consent medical malpractice case has the burden of proving: (1) what a reasonable medical practitioner in the same or similar community would have disclosed to the patient about the risk posed by the proposed procedure or treatment; and (2) that the defendant departed from the norm.

The issue with which the court was confronted was whether an objective, subjective, or a hybrid subjective/objective test should be employed when assessing causation in informed consent cases. The majority of jurisdictions in Tennessee having addressed this issue follow an objective standard.

Subjective Standard

The subjective standard relies solely on the patient's testimony. Patients must testify and prove that they would not have consented to the procedure(s) had they been advised of the particular risk in question. Proponents of the subjective standard argue that a patient should have the right to make medical decisions regarding his or her care regardless of whether the determination is rational or reasonable. The subjective standard, however, potentially places the physician in jeopardy of the patient's hindsight and bitterness. The subjective standard is premised on the credibility of a patient's testimony.

Objective Standard

When applying the objective standard, the finder of fact may also take into account the characteristics of the plaintiff, including the plaintiff's idiosyncrasies, fears, age, medical condition, and religious beliefs. Accordingly, the objective standard affords the ease of applying a uniform standard and yet maintains the flexibility of allowing the finder of fact to make appropriate adjustments to accommodate the individual characteristics and idiosyncrasies of an individual patient. The standard to be applied in informed consent cases is whether a reasonable person in the patient's position would have consented to the procedure or treatment in question if adequately informed of all significant perils.

Under the objective analysis, the plaintiff's testimony is only one factor when determining the issue of informed consent. The issue is not whether Ashe would herself have chosen a different course of treatment. The issue is whether a reasonable patient in Ashe's position would have chosen a different course of treatment. The jury, therefore, should have been allowed to decide whether a reasonable person in Ashe's position would have consented to the radiation therapy had the risk of paralysis been disclosed.

HOSPITAL'S ROLE IN INFORMED CONSENT

There are specific cases in which hospitals have a duty to provide patients with informed consent. The patient-plaintiff Keel, in *Keel v. St. Elizabeth Medical Center, Ky.,*[12] filed a medical malpractice action alleging that the hospital failed to provide him with informed consent when he went to there for a CT scan. The scan involved the injection of a contrast dye material. Prior to the test, Keel was given no information concerning any risks attendant to the procedure. The dye was injected and the scan was conducted. However, the plaintiff developed a thrombophlebitis at the site of the injection.

The plaintiff argued that expert medical testimony was not required in order to prove the absence of informed consent. The hospital argued that the question of informed consent, like the question of negligence, must be determined against the standard of practice among members of the medical profession.

The circuit court granted summary judgment to the hospital on the grounds that the plaintiff failed to present expert testimony on the issue. The plaintiff appealed.

The Kentucky Supreme Court held that expert testimony was not required to establish lack of informed consent, and that the hospital had a duty to inform the patient of the risks associated with the procedure. Responsibility did not lie solely with the patient's personal physician. The circuit court's summary judgment for the hospital was reversed, and the matter was remanded for further proceedings.

In most cases, expert medical evidence will likely be a necessary element of a plaintiff's proof in negating informed consent. In view of the special circumstances of this case, the court found it significant that the hospital offered Keel no information whatsoever concerning any possible hazards of this particular procedure, while at the same time the hospital admits that it routinely questions every patient about to undergo a dye injection as to whether he or she has had any previous reactions to contrast materials. Failure to adequately inform the patient need not be established by expert testimony if the failure is so apparent that laypersons may easily recognize it or infer it from evidence within the realm of common knowledge. A juror might reasonably infer from the nontechnical evidence that the hospital's utter silence as to the risks amounted to an assurance that there were none. The hospital's own questions to patients regarding reactions to the CT scan procedure demonstrated that the hospital recognized the substantial possibility of complications. These inconsistencies are apparent without recourse to expert testimony.

ADEQUACY OF CONSENT

When questions arise as to whether adequate consent has been given, some courts take into consideration the information that is ordinarily provided by other physicians. A physician must reveal to his or her patient such information as a skilled practitioner of good standing would provide under similar circumstance. A physician must disclose to the patient the potential of death, serious harm, and other complications associated with a proposed procedure. The scope of a physician's duty to disclose, as noted in *Wooley v. Henderson,*[13] is to be measured by those communications that a reasonable medical practitioner in that branch of medicine would make under the same or similar circumstances.

A patient suffering from hypertension could very well receive a modified disclosure if the attending physician has reason to believe that a full explanation of a contemplated treatment could aggravate the hypertension, which, in turn, could have a detrimental effect on the body systems already impaired by age or illness. Such disclosure consistent with the patient's condition may be adequate if it can be shown that other physicians in the community also would have made a modified disclosure.

The plaintiff in *Ramos v. Pyati*[14] brought a medical malpractice action, alleging that the physician performed surgery on his hand outside the scope of surgery to which he consented. The plaintiff had injured his thumb while at work. He was referred to the defendant after seeing three other physicians. The plaintiff was diagnosed as having a ruptured thumb tendon. The plaintiff consented to a surgical repair of the thumb. During surgery, the defendant discovered that scar tissue had formed, causing the ends of the tendons in the thumb to retract. As a result, the surgeon decided to use a donor tendon to make the necessary repairs to the thumb. He chose a tendon from the ring finger. On discovering additional disability from the surgery, the plaintiff filed a suit alleging that his hand was rendered unusable for his employment as a mechanic and that the defendant had breached his duty by not advising him of the serious nature of the operation, by not exercising the proper degree of care in performing the operation, and by failing to discontinue surgery when he knew or should have known that the required surgery would most likely cause a greater disability than the already injured condition of the thumb. The plaintiff testified that although he signed a written consent form authorizing surgery on his thumb, he did not consent to a graft of his ring finger tendon or any other tendon. The plaintiff's expert witness testified that the ring finger is the last choice of four other tendons that could have been selected for the surgery. The circuit court entered a judgment for the plaintiff, and the defendant appealed. The appellate court upheld the judgment for the plaintiff, finding that the plaintiff had not consented to use of the ring finger tendon for repair of the thumb tendon.

VERBAL CONSENT

Verbal consent, if proved, is as binding as written consent, for there is, in general, no legal requirement that a patient's consent be in writing. However, oral consent is more difficult to corroborate.

Verbal Consent to Surgery Sufficient

The plaintiff in *Siliezar v. East Jefferson General Hospital*[15] argued that the defendants breached the standard of care by failing to obtain written consent for a surgical procedure. The trial judge found that the plaintiff failed to sustain her burden of proof that the defendants were liable to her for damages. On appeal, the appellees admitted that they breached hospital policy by failing to obtain written consent prior to surgery. The physician testified that he explained the surgical procedure, as well as the risks of the procedure. He testified that after he explained the procedure and its risks, he left a written consent for the patient to sign. He explained that while it is the policy of the clinic to obtain a written consent prior to performing surgery, the patient did not sign the consent form. The surgeon testified that he did not know why the form was not signed, but that the patient did not refuse to sign the form.

At trial, a nurse testified that she placed the patient in an operating room and prepared her for surgery. Although she was not in the room when the surgeon discussed the surgical procedure with the plaintiff, she testified that she was in the next room and was able to hear the physician explain the procedure to the plaintiff. The nurse also had no explanation as to why the consent was not signed. She did state that the patient never said she did not want surgery nor did she ask the physician to stop the procedure. The nurse testified that as the physician performed the surgery, he explained to the patient what he was doing.

Louisiana statutes do not require that a patient's consent be written. Verbal consent was sufficient. The verbal consent included the information required by statute and the patient was given an opportunity to ask questions and those questions were answered. The plaintiff claimed that she was told that surgery would not be performed. The trial judge did not find her testimony to be credible. The appellate court found that the defendants did not commit malpractice by failing to obtain written consent prior to surgery.

WRITTEN CONSENT

A written consent form should be executed when a proposed treatment may involve some unusual risk(s) to the patient. A list of procedures and treatments requiring written consent should be maintained and appropriate consent forms used by the organization's staff. Written consent provides visible proof of a patient's wishes. Because the function of a written consent form is to preserve evidence of informed consent, the nature of the treatment, the risks, the benefits, and the consequences involved should be incorporated into the consent form. States have taken the view that consent, to be effective, must be informed consent. An informed consent form should include the following elements:

- the nature of the patient's illness or injury
- the procedure or treatment consented to
- the purpose of the proposed treatment
- the risks and probable consequences of the proposed treatment
- the probability that the proposed treatment will be successful
- any alternative methods of treatment and their associated risks and benefits
- the risks and prognosis if no treatment is rendered
- an indication that the patient understands the nature of any proposed treatment, the alternatives, the risks involved, and the probable consequences of the proposed treatment
- the signatures of the patient, physician, and witnesses
- the date the consent is signed

Health care professionals have an important role in the realm of informed consent. They can be instrumental in averting major lawsuits by being observant as to a patient's doubts, changes of mind, confusion, or misunderstandings expressed by a patient regarding any proposed procedures he or she is about to undergo.

CONSENT FOR ROUTINE PROCEDURES

Many physicians and health care organizations have relied on consent forms worded in such general terms that they permit the physician to perform almost any medical or surgical procedure believed to be in the patient's best interests. There is little difference between a surgical patient who signs no authorization and one who signs a form consenting to whatever procedure the physician deems advisable.

Consent forms signed at the time of admission should be executed at the time of a patient's admission. This form generally records the patient's consent to routine services, general diagnostic procedures, medical treatment, and the everyday routine touchings of the patient. The danger from its use arises from the potential of unwarranted reliance on it for specific, potentially high-risk procedures or treatments.

CONSENT FOR SPECIFIC PROCEDURES

There are a variety of consent forms found in the health care setting designed to more specifically describe the risks, benefits, and alternatives of particular invasive and non-invasive procedures. Such forms include consent for:

- anesthesia
- surgery
- blood and blood byproducts
- CT and MRI scans
- cardiac catheterization
- radiation therapy
- chemotherapy
- endoscopy and colonoscopy

TEMPORARY CONSENT

Temporary or interim consent forms authorize, for example, school officials, teachers, and camp counselors to act on the parent(s)' or legal guardian's behalf when seeking emergency care for injured students or campers. Such consent for treatment provides limited protection in the care of a particular child. Temporary consent indicates a parent's or guardian's intent to have a school official, teacher, or counselor seek emergency treatment when necessary. Such consent allows the health care facility to initiate emergency treatment while an attempt is being made to reach the parents or legal guardian for consent.

IMPLIED CONSENT

Although the law requires consent for the intentional touching that stem from medical or surgical procedures, exceptions do exist with respect to emergency situations. Implied consent will generally be presumed when immediate action is required to prevent death or permanent impairment of a patient's health. If it is impossible in an emergency to obtain the consent of the patient or someone legally authorized to give consent, the required procedure may be undertaken without liability for failure to procure consent.

Unconscious patients are presumed under law to approve treatment that appears to be necessary. It is assumed that such patients would have consented if they were conscious and competent. However, if a conscious patient expressly refuses to consent to certain treatment, such treatment may not be instituted after the patient becomes unconscious.

Similarly, conscious patients suffering from emergency conditions retain the right to refuse consent.

If a procedure is necessary to protect one's life or health, every effort must be made to document the medical necessity for proceeding with medical treatment without consent. It must be shown that the emergency situation constituted an immediate threat to life or health.

In *Luka v. Lowrie*,[16] a case involving a 15-year-old boy whose left foot had been run over and crushed by a train, consultation by the treating physician with other physicians was an important factor in determining the outcome of the case. On the boy's arrival at the hospital, the defending physician and four house surgeons decided it was necessary to amputate the foot. The court said it was inconceivable that, had the parents been present, they would have refused consent in the face of a determination by five physicians that amputation would save the boy's life. Thus, despite testimony at the trial that the amputation may not have been necessary, professional consultation before the operation supported the assertion that a genuine emergency existed and could be implied consent.

Consent also can be implied in nonemergency situations. For example, a patient may voluntarily submit to a procedure, implying consent, without any explicitly spoken or written expression of consent. In the Massachusetts case of *O'Brien v. Cunard Steam Ship Co.*,[17] a ship's passenger who joined a line of people receiving injections was held to have implied his consent to a vaccination. The rationale for this decision is that individuals who observe a line of people and who notice that injections are being administered to those at the head of the line should expect that if they join and remain in the line, they will receive an injection. The voluntary act of entering the line and the plaintiff's opportunity to see what was taking place at the head of the line were accepted by the jury as manifestations of consent to the injection. The O'Brien case contains all the elements necessary to imply consent from a voluntary act: The procedure was a simple vaccination, the proceedings were visible at all times, and the plaintiff was free to withdraw up to the instant of the injection.

Whether a patient's consent can be implied is frequently asked when the condition of a patient requires some deviation from an agreed-on procedure. If a patient expressly prohibits a specific medical or surgical procedure, consent to the procedure cannot be implied. The same consent rule applies if a patient expressly prohibits a particular extension of a procedure even though the patient voluntarily submitted to the original procedure.

STATUTORY CONSENT

Many states have adopted legislation concerning emergency care. An emergency in most states eliminates the need for consent. When a patient is clinically unable to give consent to a lifesaving emergency treatment, the law implies consent on the presumption that a reasonable person would consent to lifesaving medical intervention.

When an emergency situation does arise, there may be little opportunity to contact the attending physician, much less a consultant. The patient's records, therefore, must be complete with respect to the description of his or her illness and condition, the attempts made to contact the physician as well as relatives, and the emergency measures taken and procedures performed. If time does not permit a court order to be obtained, a second medical opinion, when practicable, is advisable.

JUDICIAL CONSENT

Judicial consent may be necessary in those instances where there is concern as to the absence or legality of consent. Judicial intervention is periodically necessary to grant consent on an emergency basis when a court is not in session. A judge should be contacted only after alternative methods have been exhausted and the matter cannot wait for a determination during the normal working hours of the court. Some courts (e.g., Massachusetts trial courts) require an attorney to initiate the call to the justice and to certify that there are no alternatives, other than a judicial response, available in the matter.

WHO MAY CONSENT

Consent of the patient ordinarily is required before treatment. However, when the patient is either physically unable or legally incompetent to consent and no emergency exists, consent must be obtained from a person who is empowered to consent on the patient's behalf. The person who authorizes treatment of another must have sufficient information to make an intelligent judgment on behalf of the patient.

Competent Patients

A competent adult patient's wishes concerning his or her person may not be disregarded. The court in *In re Melideo*[18] held that every human being of adult years has a right to determine what shall be done with his or her own body and cannot be subjected to medical treatment without his or her consent. When there is no compelling state interest that justifies overriding an adult patient's decision, that decision should be respected.

In *Fosmire v. Nicoleau*,[19] the New York Supreme Court, Suffolk County, issued an order authorizing blood transfusions for a patient who had refused them. The plaintiff applied for an order vacating the court's order.

The appeals court held that the patient's constitutional rights of due process were violated when the trial court issued an order authorizing blood transfusions in the absence of notice or opportunity for the patient or her representatives to be heard. The right of a competent patient to refuse medical treatment, even if premised on fervently held religious beliefs, is not unqualified and may be overridden by compelling state interests. However, a state's interest in preserving a patient's life is not inviolate, and in and of itself may not, under certain circumstances, be sufficient to overcome the patient's express desire to exercise her religious belief and forgo blood transfusion. The appellate division held in part that the state's interest would be satisfied if the other parent survived.

The New York Court of Appeals, New York's highest court, went further by stating that the citizens of the state have long had the right to make their own medical care choices without regard to their medical condition or status as parents. The court of appeals held that a competent adult has both a common-law and statutory right under public health law to refuse lifesaving treatment. Citing the state's authority to compel vaccination to protect the public from the spread of disease, to order treatment for persons who are incapable of making medical decisions, and to prohibit medical procedures that pose a substantial risk to the patient alone, the court of appeals did note that the right to choose is not absolute. However, if there is no compelling state interest to justify overriding a patient's refusal to consent to a medical procedure because of religious beliefs, states are reluctant to override such a decision.

Guardianship

A *guardian* is an individual who by law is vested with the power and charged with the duty of taking care of a patient by protecting the patient's rights and managing the patient's estate. Guardianship is often necessary in those instances in which a patient is incapable of managing or administering his or her private affairs because of physical and/or mental disabilities or because he or she is under the age of majority.

Temporary guardianship can be granted by the courts if it is determined that such is necessary for the well-being of the patient. Temporary guardianship was granted by the court in *In re Estate of Dorone*.[20] In this case, the physician and administrator petitioned the court on two occasions for authority to administer blood. A 22-year-old male patient brought to the hospital center by helicopter after an automobile accident was diagnosed as suffering from an acute subdural hematoma with a brain contusion. It was determined that the patient would die unless he underwent a cranial operation. The operation required the administration of blood to which the parents would not consent because of their religious beliefs. After a hearing by telephone, the court of common pleas appointed the hospital's administrator as temporary guardian, authorizing him to consent to the performance of blood transfusions during emergency surgery. A more formal hearing did not take place because of the emergency situation that existed. Surgery was required a second time to remove a blood clot, and the court once again granted the administrator authority to authorize administration of blood. The superior court affirmed the orders, and the parents appealed.

The Pennsylvania Supreme Court held that the judge's failure to obtain direct testimony from the patient's parents and others concerning the patient's religious beliefs was not in error when death was likely to result from withholding blood. The judge's decisions granting guardianship and the authority to consent to the administration of blood were considered absolutely necessary in the light of the facts of this case. Nothing less than a fully conscious contemporary decision by the patient himself would have been sufficient to override the evidence of medical necessity.

Consent for Minors

When a medical or surgical procedure is to be performed on a minor, the question arises as to whether the minor's consent alone is sufficient and, if not, from whom consent should be obtained. The courts have held, as a general proposition, that the consent of a minor to medical or surgical treatment is ineffective and that the physician must secure the consent of the minor's parent or someone standing in loco parentis, otherwise, he or she will risk liability. Although parental consent should be obtained before treating a minor, treatment should not be delayed to the detriment of the child.

Parental consent is not necessary when the minor is married or otherwise emancipated. Most states have enacted statutes making it valid for married and emancipated minors to provide effective consent. Several courts have held the consent of a minor to be sufficient authorization for treatment in certain situations. In any specific case, a court's determination that the consent of a minor is effective and that parental consent is unnecessary will depend on such factors as the minor's age, maturity, mental status, and emancipation and the procedure involved, as well as public policy considerations.

In *Carter v. Cangello,*[21] the California Court of Appeals held that a 17-year-old girl who was living away from home, in the home of a woman who gave her free room and board in exchange for household chores, and who made her own financial decisions, legally could consent to medical procedures performed on her. The court made this decision knowing that the girl's parents provided part of her income by paying for her private schooling and certain medical care. The physician was privileged under statute to act on the minor's consent to surgery, and such privilege insulated him from liability to the parents for treating their daughter without their consent.

Many states have recognized by legislation that treatment for such conditions as pregnancy, venereal disease, and drug dependency does not require parental consent. State legislatures have reasoned that a minor is not likely to seek medical assistance when parental consent is demanded. Insisting on parental consent for the treatment of these conditions would increase the likelihood that a minor would delay or do without treatment to avoid explanation to the parents.

Incompetent Patients

The ability to consent to treatment is a question of fact. The attending physician, who is in the best position to make the determination, should become familiar with his or her state's definition of legal incompetence. In any case in which a physician doubts a patient's capacity to consent, the consent of the legal guardian or next of kin should be obtained. If there are no relatives to consult, application should be made for a court order that would allow the procedure. It may be the duty of the court to assume responsibility of guardianship for a patient who is non compos mentis. The most frequently cited conditions indicative of incompetence are mental illness, mental retardation, senility, physical incapacity, and chronic alcohol or drug abuse.

A person who is mentally incompetent cannot legally consent to medical or surgical treatment. Therefore, consent of the patient's legal guardian must be obtained. When no legal guardian is available, a court that handles such matters must be petitioned to permit treatment.

Subject to applicable statutory provisions, when a physician doubts a patient's capacity to consent, even though the patient has not been judged legally incompetent, the consent of the nearest relative should be obtained. If a patient is conscious and mentally capable of giving consent for treatment, the consent of a relative without the consent of the competent patient would not protect the physician from liability.

SPOUSAL CONSENT

Citation: *Greynolds v. Kurman,* 632 N.E.2d 946 (Ohio Ct. App. 1993)

Facts

On July 29, 1987, Mr. Greynolds suffered from a transient ischemic attack (TIA), a sudden loss of neurological function caused by vascular impairment to the brain. As a result of the TIA, Greynolds had garbled speech and expressive and perceptive aphasia (a medical term used to describe the loss of the power of expression by speech, writing, or signs, or of comprehending spoken or written language). Greynolds was taken to an emergency department where he was met by Dr. Litman, a cardiologist. At Litman's request, he was examined by Dr. Rafecas, a cardiologist. Rafecas determined that because of Greynolds's past medical history, which included previous TIAs, he was at a high risk for a stroke, and sought to pinpoint the exact source of vascular insufficiency to the brain.

On August 3, 1987, after receiving the results of noninvasive tests, Rafecas ordered a cerebral angiogram. Dr. Kurman performed the angiogram. During the procedure, Greynolds suffered a stroke that left him severely disabled.

Greynolds and his wife filed a medical malpractice action against Rafecas and Kurman, asserting that Rafecas negligently recommended the procedure and that Kurman performed the procedure without obtaining the informed consent of the patient.

Kurman argued that the trial court erred by refusing to enter judgment for him consistent with the answer to jury question number three (*Id.* at 949):

Question No. 1: Do you find there was a failure to obtain informed consent?

Answer: Yes.

Question No. 2: If you answered Interrogatory No. 1 yes, then state specifically in what manner Dr. Kurman's care fell below the recognized standards of the medical community.

Answer: Mr. Greynolds was not in our estimation capable of comprehending the consent form. Therefore, Dr. Kurman should have obtained consent from the next-of-kin, specifically, Mrs. Greynolds.

Question No. 3: If you answered yes to interrogatory No. 1 and you found that Mr. Greynolds did not consent to the procedure, do you find

that a reasonable person would have consented to the procedure?

Answer: Yes.

Kurman moved the trial court to grant him a judgment notwithstanding the verdict because the jury's answer to interrogatory number three was inconsistent with the jury's general verdict. The trial court overruled Kurman's motion and entered judgment for the plaintiffs, and Kurman appealed.

Issue

Was there sufficient evidence to support a judgment for the plaintiffs?

Holding

The court of appeals held that the evidence was sufficient to support a judgment in favor of the patient and his wife.

Reason

The jury needed to determine that the risks involved in the cerebral angiogram were not disclosed to Greynolds, that the risks involved in the procedure materialized and caused his stroke, and that a reasonable person in the position of Greynolds would have decided against having the angiogram had the risks associated with the procedure been disclosed to him. The jury concluded that Greynolds did not consent to the angiogram because he "was not . . . capable of comprehending the consent form," and further noted that Kurman should have sought consent from the next of kin, specifically, the spouse. Given the evidence of Greynolds's condition when he signed the consent forms, his past medical history, and the fact that he was at an increased risk to suffer complications during an angiogram, the court found that there was sufficient evidence to support a finding of lack of informed consent.

Discussion

1. What would constitute informed consent?
2. Who should describe the risks associated with a procedure to the patient?

RIGHT TO REFUSE TREATMENT

"the individual's right to make decisions vitally affecting his private life according to his own conscience . . . is difficult to overstate . . . because it is, without exaggeration, the very bedrock on which this country was founded."

Wons v. Public Health Trust[22]

Adult patients who are conscious and mentally competent have the right to refuse medical care to the extent permitted by law, even when the best medical opinion deems it essential to life. If a patient rejects treatment, the hospital should take all reasonable steps to inform the patient of the risks of refusing treatment. Such a refusal must be honored whether it is grounded in religious belief or mere whim. Every person has the legal right to refuse to permit a touching of his or her body. Failure to respect this right can result in a legal action for assault and battery. Coercion through threat, duress, or intimidation must be avoided.

A patient's right to make decisions regarding his own health care is addressed in the Patient Self-Determination Act of 1990.[23] The act provides that each person has a right under state law (whether statutory or as recognized by the courts of the state) to make decisions concerning his or her medical care, including the right to accept or refuse medical or surgical treatment.

A competent patient's refusal to consent to a medical or surgical procedure must be adhered to, whether the refusal is grounded on lack of confidence in the physician, fear of the procedure, doubt as to the value of a particular procedure, or mere whim. The U.S. Supreme Court stated that the "notion of bodily integrity has been embodied in the requirement that informed consent is generally required for medical treatment" and the "logical corollary of the doctrine of informed consent is that the patient generally possesses the right not to consent, that is, to refuse treatment."[24] The common law doctrine of informed consent is viewed as generally encompassing the right of a competent individual to refuse medical treatment.

The question of liability for performing a medical or surgical procedure without consent is separate and distinct from any question of negligence or malpractice in performing a procedure. Liability may be imposed for a nonconsensual touching of a patient, even if the procedure improved the patient's health. The eminent Justice Cardozo, in *Schloendorff v. Society of New York Hospital,* stated:

> Every human being of adult years and sound mind has a right to determine what shall be done with his own body and a surgeon who performs an operation without his patient's consent commits an assault, for which he is liable in damages, except in cases of emergency where the patient is unconscious and where it is necessary to operate before consent can be obtained.[25]

The courts perform a balancing test to determine whether to override a competent adult's decision to refuse medical treatment. The courts balance state interests, such as preservation of life, protection of third parties, prevention of suicide, and the integrity of the medical profession against a patient's rights of bodily integrity and religious freedom. The most frequently used state right to intervene in a patient's decision-making process is for the protection of third parties. In *In re Fetus Brown,*[26] the state of Illinois asserted that its interest in the well-being of a viable fetus outweighed the patient's rights to refuse medical treatment. The state argued that a balancing test should be used to weigh state interests against patient rights. The appellate court held that it could not impose a legal obligation upon a pregnant woman to consent to an invasive medical procedure for the benefit of her viable fetus.

Religious Beliefs

As part of their religious beliefs, Jehovah's Witnesses generally have refused the administration of blood, even in emergency situations. Case law over the past several decades has developed to a point where any person, regardless of religious beliefs, has the right to refuse medical treatment.

The plaintiff, Bonita Perkins, in *Perkins v. Lavin,*[27] was a Jehovah's Witness. She gave birth at the defendant-hospital on September 26, 1991, and was discharged two or three days later. After going home, she began hemorrhaging and returned to the hospital. She specifically informed the defendant's employees that she was not to be provided any blood or blood derivatives and completed and signed a form to that effect:

> I request that no blood or blood derivatives be administered to (plaintiff) during this hospitalization, notwithstanding that such treatment may be deemed necessary in the opinion of the attending physician or his assistants to preserve life or promote recovery. I release the attending physician, his assistants, the hospital and its personnel from any responsibility whatever for any untoward results due to my refusal to permit the use of blood or its derivatives.[28]

Due to the plaintiff's condition, it became necessary to perform an emergency dilation and curettage on her. She continued to bleed, and her condition deteriorated dramatically.

Her blood count dropped, necessitating administration of blood products as a lifesaving measure. Her husband, who was not a Jehovah's Witness, consented to a blood transfusion, which was administered. The plaintiff recovered and filed an action against the defendant for assault and battery and intentional infliction of emotional distress. The plaintiff's claim as to assault and battery was sustained. The claim as to the intentional infliction of emotional distress was overruled.

The plaintiff specifically informed the defendant that she would consider a blood transfusion an offensive contact. The plaintiff submitted sufficient evidence to the trial court to establish that there was, at least, a genuine issue as to whether the defendant intentionally invaded her right to be free from offensive contact. Because of the plaintiff's recognition that the defendant acted to save her life, a jury may find that she is entitled to only nominal damages.

RELEASE FORM

A patient's refusal to consent to treatment, for any reason, religious or otherwise, should be noted in the medical record, and a release form should be executed. The completed release provides documented evidence of a patient's refusal to consent to a recommended treatment. A release will help protect the organization and physicians from liability should a suit arise as a result of a failure to treat. The best possible care must be rendered to the patient at all times within the limits imposed by the patient's refusal.

Should a patient refuse to sign the release, documentation of the refusal should be placed on the form and the form should be included as part of the patient's permanent medical record. Advice of legal counsel should be sought in those cases where refusal of treatment poses a serious threat to a patient's health. With the advice of legal counsel, the organization should formulate a policy regarding treatment when consent has been refused. An administrative procedure should be developed to facilitate application for a court order when one is necessary and there is sufficient time to obtain one.

EXCULPATORY AGREEMENTS

An exculpatory agreement is an agreement that relieves one from liability when he or she has acted in good faith. Exculpatory agreements in the medical setting are generally considered invalid.

In *Cudnik v. William Beaumont Hospital,*[29] Mr. Cudnik underwent radiation therapy in March and April 1985 after undergoing surgery for prostate cancer. Before receiving therapy, he signed a consent document that provided in part:

Further, my physician has fully explained to me the possibilities of reactions and the possible side effects of the treatment. I understand that there is no guarantee given to me as to the results of radiation therapy. Understanding all of the foregoing, I hereby release the physicians and staff of the Department of Radiation Oncology and William Beaumont Hospital from all suits, claims, liability, or demands of every kind and character which I or my heirs, executors, administrators [sic] or assigns hereafter can, shall, or may have arising out of my participation in the radiation therapy treatment regimen.[30]

In early 1989, Cudnik returned to the hospital complaining of back discomfort, whereupon he was diagnosed as suffering from a postradiation ulcer burn at the site where he previously received radiation treatment. An action was brought against the hospital claiming that the negligent administration of radiation therapy contributed to Cudnik's death. The defendant moved for summary judgment and the Oakland Circuit Court granted the hospital's motion after concluding that the exculpatory agreement between the parties precluded the plaintiff's claims. The plaintiff appealed, claiming that the hospital should be held vicariously liable for the medical malpractice of its employees or agents. As a general proposition, the parties to a contract may enter into an exculpatory agreement provided that it does not violate the law or contravene public policy. The question in this case is whether the plaintiff's claim of medical malpractice is precluded by the exculpatory agreement between the two parties.

The court of appeals held that the exculpatory agreement executed by the patient prior to receiving radiation therapy was invalid and unenforceable to absolve a medical care provider from liability for medical malpractice. The agreement in this case is clearly against public policy. Further, the majority of jurisdictions have held that exculpatory agreements involving patient care are unenforceable.

Some exculpatory agreements in the medical setting are considered valid. For example, experimental procedures may require a different standard, because, by their very nature, they require a deviation from generally accepted medical practices. In a case involving the patient's last hope of survival, the New York Supreme Court held that "the parties may covenant to exempt the physician from liability for those injuries which are found to be the consequences of the nonnegligent, proper performance of the procedure."[31] The Cudnik case does not appear to involve an experimental procedure.

CLAIMS: PROVING LACK OF CONSENT

The burden of establishing proof on a complaint of lack of informed consent is on the plaintiff. The plaintiff must establish that: (1) a reasonably prudent person in the patient's position would not have undergone the treatment if fully informed; and (2) the lack of informed consent is the proximate cause of the injury or condition for which recovery is sought.

In a lawsuit, testimony would be necessary to establish the extent of the patient's actual knowledge and understanding of the treatment rendered. It is possible for a patient, after treatment, to claim a lack of advance knowledge about the nature of a physician's treatment—and it is possible that a jury will believe the patient and impose liability on the physician and/or the organization.

CLAIMS: AVAILABLE DEFENSES

Several defenses are available to defendants who have been sued on the basis of failure to provide their patients with sufficient information to make an informed decision. Some of the defenses include:

- The risk not disclosed is too commonly known to warrant disclosure.

- The patient assured the medical practitioner that he or she would undergo the treatment, procedure, or diagnosis regardless of the risk involved, or the patient assured the medical practitioner that he or she did not want to be informed of the matters to which he or she would be entitled to be informed.

- Consent by or on behalf of a patient was not reasonably possible.

- The medical practitioner, after considering all of the attendant facts and circumstances, used reasonable discretion as to the manner and extent to which such alternatives or risks were disclosed to the patient because the practitioner reasonably believed that the manner and extent of such disclosure could reasonably be expected to adversely and substantially affect the patient's condition.

A patient's condition during surgery may be recognized as different from that which had been expected and explained, requiring a different procedure than the one to which the patient initially consented. The surgeon may proceed to treat the new condition; however, the patient must have been aware of the possibility of extending the procedure. The patient in *Winfrey v. Citizens & Southern National Bank*[32] brought a suit against the deceased surgeon's estate, alleging that during exploratory surgery, the surgeon performed a complete hysterectomy without the patient's consent. The superior court granted summary judgment for the surgeon's estate, and the patient appealed. The court of appeals held that even though the patient may not have read the consent document, when no legally sufficient excuse appeared, she was bound by the terms of the consent document that she voluntarily executed. The plain wording of the binding con-

sent authorized the surgeon to perform additional or different operations or procedures that he might consider necessary or advisable in the course of the operation. Relevant sections of the consent signed by the patient included the following[33]:

1. I authorize the performance on (patient's name) of the following operation/laparoscopy, possible laparotomy. . . .

2. I consent to the performance of operations and procedures in addition to or different from those now contemplated, which the above named doctor or his associates or assistants may consider necessary or advisable in the course of the operation. . . .

• • • •

7. I acknowledge that the nature and purpose of the operation, possible alternative methods of treatment, the risks involved, and the possibility of complications have been fully explained to me.

INFORMED CONSENT: DIALOGUE BETWEEN PHYSICIAN AND PATIENT

Informed consent requires physicians to disclose the risks, benefits, and alternatives of a procedure to their patients. It is not merely a tool to avoid lawsuits; rather it is designed to allow patients to make an *informed* decision. The emphasis of *informed* must not be to avoid a lawsuit by meeting some legal requirement, with little regard to the patient's level of understanding of informed consent. The use of consent forms in this manner has contributed to the view that what was intended as a process of dialogue and discussion has developed into an event in which papers are signed and minimal legal requirements are satisfied. The consent form is often as a legal protection for the physician for unforeseen mishaps that might occur during surgery.

The ethical rationale underlying the doctrine of informed consent is firmly rooted in the notions of liberty and individual autonomy. Informed consent protects the basic right of the patient is make the ultimate informed decision regarding the course of treatment to which he knowledgeably consents. The focus of informed consent must involve the patient receiving informed consent as a result of active personal interaction with the physician. Consent forms should be used as supplement to the oral disclosure of risks, benefits, and alternatives to the proposed procedure that a physician normally gives. Ideally, the consent should be the result of an active process of dialogue between the patient and physician.

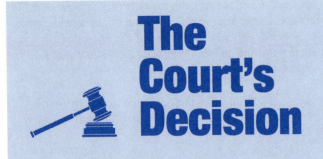

The Court's Decision

Matthews left the hospital on her own cognizance at a time when the hospital's emergency department physician was about to see her. She went to work the following morning without seeing her own physician, as she had indicated that she would. The elements that a plaintiff must establish in a malpractice case are duty to care, breach of duty, injury, and causation. The fact that Matthews voluntarily terminated her relationship with the emergency department personnel effectively severed any causal relationship that might have existed between the hospital's act of classifying Matthews as a category 2 patient and her death. Accordingly, the hospital could not be held liable for the death of the patient.

CHAPTER REVIEW

1. Patients have a right to make decisions regarding their own health care. These rights include the ability to refuse or accept medical or surgical treatment.

2. *Consent* is voluntary agreement by a person to allow something proposed by another to be performed on him- or herself. A person can consent to something only if he or she has sufficient mental capacity to make an intelligent choice. A verbal or written agreement provides express consent. In cases in which an act or silence indicates that performance of an act has been authorized, the consent is referred to as implied consent. Consent may be given either by an individual or by someone authorized to consent on the individual's behalf.

3. The legal concept that protects a patient's right to know the potential risks, benefits, and alternatives of a proposed procedure is referred to as *informed consent.*

4. Under the *subjective standard,* informed consent is determined by patient testimony. Conversely, the *objective standard* resolves the issue of informed consent in terms of what a reasonably prudent person in the patient's position would have decided if suitably informed of the risks, benefits, and alternatives of the procedure.

5. Liability for performing a medical or surgical procedure without consent is distinct from a question of negligence or malpractice in performing the procedure. A physician can be found liable for imposing nonconsensual treatment, even if that treatment improved the patient's health.

6. Oral consent, although binding, is often difficult to corroborate, whereas written consent provides visible proof of a patient's wishes.

7. *Temporary consent* is an agreement that allows the health care facility to initiate emergency treatment while an attempt is being made to reach the family or other appropriate party for consent. Temporary consent is often provided by people who work with children, such as school officials, teachers, and camp counselors.

8. *Special consent* forms are obtained when a proposed treatment exposes a patient to unusual risks. These forms should be signed, dated, and witnessed at the time that the physician explains the procedure and associated risks to the patient.

9. *Implied consent* is generally presumed when immediate action is required to prevent death or permanent impairment of a patient's health. In such cases, documentation justifying the need to treat before obtaining consent should be maintained.

10. *Statutory consent* provides that when a patient is clinically unable to give consent to a lifesaving emergency treatment, the law implies consent on the presumption that a reasonable person would consent to lifesaving medical intervention.

11. *Judicial consent* may be necessary in those instances where there is concern as to the absence or legality of consent.

12. Generally, the consent of a minor is not sufficient to proceed with medical or surgical treatment. However, parental consent, or the consent of another party standing in loco parentis, is not required if the minor is married or otherwise emancipated.

13. If an individual is found incompetent to give consent, and if there are no relatives or other parties from whom to obtain consent, an application should be made for a court order that would allow the procedure.

14. Any person, regardless of religious beliefs, has the right to refuse medical treatment. If a patient refuses treatment, that refusal should be noted in the patient's medical record and a release form should be executed.

15. An *exculpatory agreement* is an agreement that relieves one from liability when he or she has acted in good faith. However, these are generally considered invalid in the medical setting.

REVIEW QUESTIONS

1. Who should be responsible for reviewing with the patient the risks, benefits, and alternatives of a proposed diagnostic test or treatment?

2. Describe what information a patient should be provided prior to undergoing a risky procedure in order for consent to be informed.

3. Why is it important to obtain consent from a patient prior to proceeding with a risky procedure?

4. Can a patient consent to a procedure and then withdraw it?

5. Can a parent refuse to consent to a lifesaving procedure for his or her child? Discuss your answer.

6. Discuss how much information is sufficient in order for informed consent to be effective (e.g., consider your answer here from both the objective and subjective forms of consent).

7. Discuss the implications of the following statement: "Patients are generally persons unlearned in the medical sciences and, therefore, except in rare instances, the knowledge of patient and physician is not in parity."

NOTES

1. *Matthews v. DeKalb County Hosp. Auth.,* 440 S.E.2d 743 (Ga. Ct. App. 1994).
2. 141 U.S. 250, 251 (1891).
3. *In re Duran,* 769 A.2d 497 (Pa. 2001).
4. 497 U.S. 261 (1990).
5. 972 F. Supp. 308 (D.C. Pa. 1997).
6. 635 A.2d 1047 (Pa. Super. Ct. 1993).
7. 733 A.2d 456 (1999).
8. *Id.* at 461.
9. 620 So. 2d 372 (La. Ct. App. 1993).
10. *Id.* at 380.
11. 67 Cal. Rptr. 2d 573 (Cal. App. 1997).
12. 842 S.W.2d 860 (Ky. 1992).
13. 418 A.2d 1123 (Me. 1980).
14. 534 N.E.2d 472 (Ill. App. Ct. 1989).
15. No. 04-CA-939 (La. Ct. App. 5 Cir. 1/11/05).
16. 136 N.W. 1106 (Mich. 1912).

17. 28 N.E. 266 (Mass. 1891).
18. 390 N.Y.S.2d 523 (N.Y. Sup. Ct. 1976).
19. 536 N.Y.S.2d 492 (N.Y. App. Div. 1989).
20. 534 A.2d 452 (Pa. 1987).
21. 164 Cal. Rptr. 361 (Cal. Ct. App. 1980).
22. 500 So. 2d 679, 687 (Fla. Dist. Ct. App. 1987), aff'd 541 So. 2d 96 (Fla. 1989).
23. Public Law 101-508, November 5, 1990, sections 4206 and 4751 of the Omnibus Budget Reconciliation Act.
24. *Cruzan v. Director, Missouri Dep't of Health,* 497 U.S. 261, 269 (1990).
25. 105 N.E. 92, 93 (N.Y. 1914).
26. 689 N.E.2d 397 (Ill. App. Ct. 1997).
27. 648 N.E.2d 839 (Ohio App. 9 Dist. 1994).
28. *Id.* at 840.
29. 525 N.W.2d 891 (Mich. App. 1994).
30. *Id.* at 893.
31. *Colton v. New York Hosp.,* 414 N.Y.S.2d 866 (1979).
32. 254 S.E.2d 725 (Ga. Ct. App. 1979).
33. *Id.* at 727.

CHAPTER 13

Legal Reporting Requirements

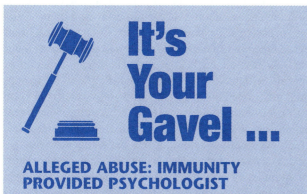

It's Your Gavel ...

ALLEGED ABUSE: IMMUNITY PROVIDED PSYCHOLOGIST

Two children were placed in the temporary custody of a foster family. One child was referred to a licensed psychologist for evaluation. After two interviews, the psychologist formed a professional opinion that the child had been sexually molested. Based in part on statements made by the child, the psychologist further believed that the perpetrator of the suspected molestation was the father. At a hearing before a juvenile court, the court determined that the evidence did not support a finding that the child had been abused by his father. Custody was returned to the parents. The child's parents subsequently initiated an action for medical malpractice against the psychologist. The psychologist claimed immunity from liability as provided by a state child abuse reporting statute. The parents argued that the immunity provisions of the statute do not apply to the psychologist because she was not a "mandatory reporter" under that statute.[1]

WHAT IS YOUR VERDICT?

This chapter provides an overview of a variety of reporting requirements mandated by both federal and state regulatory agencies. Through such reporting, appropriate measures can be taken to safeguard the health of the nation's population. Most states have legislative reporting requirements for diseases that pose a threat to public health and safety. Although most statutory reporting requirements do not contain an express immunity from liability for disclosure without the permission of the person affected, as a general rule, a person making a report in good faith and under statutory command is protected.

CHILD ABUSE

The physically abused or neglected child presents a medical, social, and legal problem. What constitutes an abused child is difficult to determine because it is often impossible to ascertain whether a child was injured intentionally or accidentally.

What Is Child Abuse and Neglect?

An *abused child* is one who has suffered intentional serious mental, emotional, sexual, and/or physical injury inflicted by a family or other person responsible for the child's care. Some states extend the definition to include a child suffering from starvation. Other states include moral neglect in the definition of abuse. Others mention immoral associations; endangering a child's morals; and the location of a child in a disreputable place or in association with vagrant, vicious, or immoral persons. Sexual abuse also is enumerated as an element of neglect in the statutes of some states.

The Child Abuse Prevention and Treatment Act defines the term "child abuse and neglect" as, any recent act or failure to act on the part of a parent or caretaker, which results in death, serious physical or emotional harm, sexual abuse or exploitation, or an act or failure to act which presents an imminent risk of serious harm.[2]

Who Should Report?

Presently, all states have enacted laws to protect abused children. Most states protect the persons required to report cases of child abuse. In a few states, certain identified individuals who are not required to report instances of child abuse, but who do so, are protected. Child abuse laws may provide penalties for failure to report. Persons in the health care setting who are required to report, or cause a report to be made, when they have reasonable cause to suspect that a child has been abused include administrators, physicians, interns, registered nurses, chiropractors, social service workers, psychologists, dentists, osteopaths, optometrists, podiatrists, mental health professionals, and volunteers in residential facilities.

Detecting Abuse

An individual who reports child abuse should be aware of the physical and behavioral indicators of abuse and maltreatment that appear to be part of a pattern (e.g., bruises, burns, and broken bones). In reviewing the indicators of abuse and maltreatment, the reporter does not have to be absolutely certain that abuse or maltreatment exists before reporting. Rather, abuse and maltreatment should be reported whenever they are suspected, based on the existence of the signs of abuse and maltreatment and in light of the reporter's training and experience. Behavioral indicators include, but are not limited to, substantially diminished psychological or intellectual functioning, failure to thrive, no control of aggression, self-destructive impulses, decreased ability to think and reason, acting out and misbehavior, or habitual truancy. Such impairment must be clearly attributable to the unwillingness or inability of the person responsible for the child's care to exercise a minimum degree of care toward the child.

Good-Faith Reporting

Any report of suspected child abuse must be made with a good-faith belief that the facts reported are true. The definition of good faith as used in a child abuse statute may vary from state to state. However, when a health care practitioner's medical evaluation indicates reasonable cause to believe a child's injuries were not accidental and when the health care practitioner is not acting from his or her desire to harass, injure, or embarrass the child's parents, making the report will not result in liability. Statutes generally require that when a person covered by a statute is attending a child and suspects child abuse, the staff member must report such concerns. Typical statutes provide that an oral report be made immediately,

followed by a written report. Most states require the report to contain the following information:

- the child's name and address

- the person(s) responsible for the child's care

- the child's age

- the nature and extent of the child's injuries (including any evidence of previous injuries)

- any other information that might be helpful in establishing the cause of the injuries, such as photographs of the injured child, and the identity of the alleged perpetrator

A minor child and his mother brought an action for damages against physicians for failing to diagnose disease and filing erroneous child abuse reports in *Awkerman v. Tri-County Orthopedic Group*.[3] The Wayne County Circuit Court granted the physicians' motions for partial summary judgment, and the plaintiffs appealed. The Michigan Court of Appeals held that the child abuse reporting statute provides immunity to persons who file child abuse reports in good faith even if the reports were filed because of negligent diagnosis of the cause of the child's frequent bone fractures, which eventually was diagnosed as osteogenesis imperfecta. The court of appeals also held that damages for shame and humiliation were not recoverable pursuant to Michigan statute. Immunity from liability did not extend to damages for malpractice that may have resulted from the failure to diagnose the child's disease as long as all the elements of negligence are present.

The psychologist in *E.S. by D.S. v. Seitz*[4] was immune from liability in a suit charging her with negligence in formulating and reporting her professional opinion to a social worker that a father had sexually abused his three-year-old daughter. The psychologist made the report in compliance with the Wisconsin statute, after having examined the child in the course of her professional duties as a mental health professional.

The patient in *Marks v. Tenbrunsel*[5] had been assured that anything he disclosed during his treatment sessions would remain confidential. During the treatment sessions, the patient disclosed that he had fondled two children under the age of 12. As a result of that disclosure, two psychologists made a good-faith report to Child Protective Services. The report caused the patient to be prosecuted for his admitted sexual misconduct. Because the patient admitted to the abuse of two children, the psychologists had reasonable cause to believe that the children currently were being abused. The psychologists were found immune from both civil and criminal liability as a result of their good-faith report.

Failure to Report Child Abuse

The criminal and civil risks for health care professionals do not lie in good-faith reporting of suspected incidents of child abuse, but in failing to report such incidents. Most states have legislated a variety of civil and criminal penalties for failure to report suspected child abuse incidents.

Psychologist

The Minnesota Board of Psychology was found to have acted properly when it placed the license of a psychologist on conditional status.[6] The psychologist argued that he was not required to report past abuse that was not ongoing, that a report made five weeks after the incident was not untimely, and that the reporting laws were unconstitutional because they violated the privacy rights of clients and the privilege against self-incrimination. The psychologist had failed to report incidents of sexual child abuse. The court held that there was no merit to the psychologist's contentions that the child abuse reporting laws were unclear and that they did not apply to one patient who was a grandfather responsible for the child's care at the time of the incident in question.

Nurse

In *State v. Brown*[7], rescue personnel were summoned to the scene of an emergency found a two-year-old foster child unconscious, not breathing, and "posturing," which is an abnormal rigidity of the body and a sign of brain damage. While performing emergency medical treatment, rescue personnel discovered a series of small, round, dime- to quarter-sized bruises running parallel along child's spine. They also noticed a red bruise under his eye. This information was relayed to the flight crew who airlifted the child to the hospital. The flight crew then reported the information to a nurse employed at the hospital. The child recovered after treatment and was released from the hospital on August 14, 2002. Four days later, on August 18, the child was returned to the hospital where he died of abusive head trauma.

The nurse did not document the bruises or call the state's child abuse hotline because the boy's foster mother said the bruises were the result of the boy leaning back in a booster seat. In February 2003, the prosecutor alleged that the nurse had reasonable cause to suspect that the child had been abused or neglected. She was charged with failure to report child abuse to the division of family services under section 210.115.1, Revised Statutes of Missouri, and to a physician under section 210.120, RSMo. The nurse sought to dismiss the charges, alleging the statutes were unconstitutionally vague. In September 2003, the court held that the sections were unconstitutionally vague and dismissed the case. The state appealed. The appellate court determined that the statutes were not vague. The test for determining whether a law is void for vagueness is whether its language conveys to a person of ordinary intelligence a sufficiently definite warning as to the proscribed conduct when measured by common understanding and practices. The statute criminalizing a health professional's failure to report child abuse upon "reasonable cause to

suspect" abuse was not unconstitutionally vague. The phrase "reasonable cause to suspect" has been in use for more than a century and is understandable by ordinary persons.

Physician

A physician who was not the initial reporter of suspected child abuse, but who performed a medical examination of a child at the request of the department of children and families to determine whether reasonable cause existed to suspect child abuse, was entitled to the immunity from liability provided by statutory law. It was clear that the physician, a mandated reporter under the law, examined the child in the ordinary course of his employment in the emergency department. He complied with applicable statutes when he relayed his findings that there was a reasonable suspicion of child abuse to the department. Inasmuch as the plaintiffs did not allege that the physician acted in bad faith during the examination and reporting process, his actions constituted a report of suspected child abuse protected by statutory law. The trial court, therefore, properly granted the medical defendants' motion for summary judgment.[8]

ELDER ABUSE AND NEGLECT

Elder abuse is any form of mistreatment that results in harm or loss to an older person. It can involve physical abuse (that results in bodily injury, pain, or impairment and includes assault, battery, and inappropriate restraint); sexual abuse (nonconsensual sexual contact of any kind with an older person); domestic violence (an escalating pattern of violence by an intimate partner where the violence is used to exercise power and control); psychological abuse (the willful infliction of mental or emotional anguish by threat, humiliation, or other verbal or nonverbal conduct); financial abuse (the illegal or improper use of an older person's funds, property, or resources).[9] *Neglect* is the failure to provide the care necessary to avoid physical harm (e.g., the failure of staff to turn a patient periodically to prevent pressure sores) or mental anguish.

Most states have enacted statutes mandating the reporting of elder abuse. In general, elder abuse is less likely to be reported than child abuse. Physical and emotional neglect, as well as verbal and financial abuse, are perceived as the most prevalent forms of elder abuse. Seniors often fail to report incidents of abuse because they fear retaliation and not being believed. Threats of placement in a nursing home or shame that a family member may be involved often prevents the elder from seeking help. In addition, proving such charges is often difficult. Signs of abuse or neglect include:

- Unexplained or unexpected death

- Development of pressure sores

- Heavy medication and sedation used in place of adequate nursing staff

- Occurrence of broken bones

- Sudden and unexpected emotional outbursts, agitation, or withdrawal

- Bruises, welts, discoloration, burns, and so on

- Absence of hair and/or hemorrhaging below scalp

- Dehydration and/or malnourishment without illness-related cause

- Hesitation to talk openly

- Implausible stories

- Unusual or inappropriate activity in bank accounts

- Signatures on checks and other written materials that do not resemble the patient's signature

- Power of attorney given, or recent changes or creation of a will, when the person is incapable of making such decisions

- Missing personal belongings such as silverware or jewelry

- An untreated medical condition

- Patient is unable to speak for himself or herself, or see others, without the presence of the caregiver (suspected abuser)

Policies and Procedures

Policies and procedures that include prohibition of mistreatment, description of reporting procedures regarding alleged abuse, maintenance of evidence of alleged abuse, investigation of alleged abuse, and prevention of further potential abuse while an investigation is in progress should be developed.

Documentation

Caregivers who suspect abuse are expected to report their findings. Symptoms and conditions of suspected abuse should be defined clearly and objectively.

- Witnesses: Reporters of abuse must describe statements made by others as accurately as possible; what actions were taken, by whom, when, where, and so forth. Information should be included about how witnesses may be contacted.

- Photographs: It may be necessary to photograph wounds or injuries. A hospital emergency room or the police department can be asked to photograph in emergency situations.

COMMUNICABLE DISEASES

Most states have enacted laws that require the reporting of actual or suspected cases of communicable diseases. The need for statutes requiring the reporting of communicable diseases is clear: If a state is to protect its citizens' health through its power to quarantine, it must ensure the prompt reporting of infection or disease.

BIRTHS AND DEATHS

All births and deaths are reportable by statute. Births occurring outside of a health care facility should be reported by the legally qualified physician in attendance at a delivery or, in the event of the absence of a physician, by the registered nurse or other attendant. The physician who pronounces death must sign the death certificate. Statutes requiring the reporting of births and deaths are necessary to maintain accurate census records.

SUSPICIOUS DEATHS

Greater than a state's interest in the recording of all births and deaths is the state's desire to review suspicious deaths that may be the result of some form of criminal activity. Unnatural deaths must be referred to the medical examiner for review. Such cases include violent deaths, deaths caused by unlawful acts or criminal neglect, and deaths that may be considered suspicious or unusual. The medical examiner may make an investigation of such cases and issue an autopsy report. The purpose of a medical examiner's investigation is to determine the actual cause of death and thereby provide assistance for any further criminal investigation that may be considered necessary.

HEALTH CARE QUALITY IMPROVEMENT ACT

The Health Care Quality Improvement Act of 1986 (HCQIA)[10] was signed by President Reagan on November 14, 1986. Congress enacted the HCQIA in order to improve the quality of medical care by encouraging physicians to participate in peer review and by restricting incompetent physicians' ability to move from state to state without disclosure or discovery of their previous substandard performance or unprofessional conduct. The HCQIA was enacted in part to provide those persons giving information to professional review bodies and those assisting in review activities limited immunity from damages that may arise as a result of adverse decisions that affect a physician's medical staff privileges. Prior to enacting the HCQIA, Congress found that "[t]he increasing occurrence of medical malpractice and the need to improve the quality of medical care . . . [had] become nationwide problems," especially in light of "the ability of incompetent physicians to move from State to State without disclosure or discovery of the physician's previous damaging or incompetent performance."[11] The problem, however, could be remedied through effective professional peer review combined with a national reporting system that made information about adverse professional actions against physicians more widely available. HCQIA was enacted by Congress to facilitate the frank exchange of information among professionals conducting peer review inquiries without the fear of reprisals in civil lawsuits. The statute attempts to balance the chilling effect of litigation on peer review with concerns for protecting physicians improperly subjected to disciplinary action.

NATIONAL PRACTITIONER DATA BANK

The HCQIA law established the National Practitioner Data Bank (NPDB), to be operated under the authority of the secretary of the Department of Health and Human Services (DHHS). The NPDB was created by Congress as a national repository of information with the primary purpose of facilitating a comprehensive review of physicians' and other health care practitioners' professional credentials. Hospitals are required to report to the NPDB professional review actions that are related to a physician's competence or conduct and that adversely affect clinical privileges for more than 30 days, and a physician's voluntary surrender or restriction of clinical privileges.

Responsibility for data bank implementation resides in the Bureau of Health Professions, Health Resources and Services Administration of the DHHS. The act authorizes the data bank to be used to collect and release information on the professional competence and conduct of physicians, dentists, and other health care practitioners. Reporting and disclosure requirements for the NPDB also are set out in the regulations.[12]

The regulations are intended to encourage good-faith professional review activities. The data bank was established because of the increasing occurrence of medical malpractice and the need to improve the quality of medical care, the need to restrict the ability of incompetent physicians who move from state to state without disclosure or discovery of their previous damaging or incompetent performance,

and the overriding need to provide incentive and protection for physicians engaging in professional peer review.[13]

The NPDB presents a number of challenges to health care institutions. A major one is to educate the medical staff so that the data bank will not erode medical staff participation in risk management. The purpose of the data bank is not punishment; rather, it is prevention and deterrence.

Reporting Requirements

The regulations establish reporting requirements applicable to hospitals; health care entities; boards of medical examiners; professional societies of physicians, dentists, or other health care practitioners that take adverse licensure or professional review actions (e.g., reduction, restriction, suspension, revocation, or denial of clinical privileges or membership in a health care entity of 30 days or longer); and individuals and entities (including insurance companies) making payments as a result of medical malpractice actions or claims. A *medical malpractice action* (or claim) has been defined as a written complaint or claim demanding payment based on a health care practitioner's provision of or failure to provide health care services, including the filing of a cause of action based on tort law, brought in any state or federal court or other adjudicative body.

Required Queries and Medical Staff Privileges

Health care organizations must query the data bank every two years on the renewal of staff privileges of physicians and dentists. The data bank serves as a flagging system whose principal purpose is to facilitate a more comprehensive review of professional credentials. As a nationwide flagging system, it provides another resource to assist state licensing boards, hospitals, and other health care entities in conducting extensive independent reviews of the qualifications of health care practitioners they seek to license or hire or to whom they wish to grant clinical privileges.

Who Should Report?

For those health care providers who question whether they are covered under this law, DHHS defines the term entity broadly, rather than attempting to focus on the myriad health care organizations, practice arrangements, and professional societies, to ensure that the regulations include all entities within the scope of the statute. A health care entity is an entity that provides health care services and engages in professional review activity through a formal peer-review process for the purpose of furthering quality health care or a committee of that entity. Health care practitioners include all health care practitioners authorized by a state to provide health care services by whatever formal mechanism the state uses (e.g., certification, registration, and licensure).

Data Bank Queries

Data bank queries can be made by state licensing boards, hospitals, other health care entities, and professional societies that have entered or may be entering employment or affiliation relationships with a physician, dentist, or other health care practitioner who has applied for clinical privileges or appointment to a medical staff. A plaintiff's attorney is permitted to obtain information from the data bank when a malpractice action has been filed and the practitioner on whom information has been sought is named in the suit.

Data Bank Query Fees

Under data bank rules, there is a nominal fee for data bank queries each time a physician and dentist apply for medical staff privileges at their facilities.[14]

Penalties for Failing to Report

Hospitals or other health care entities that fail to report adverse professional review actions limiting the clinical privileges of physicians or dentists lasting more than 30 days can lose immunity protection provided by Title IV of the HCQIA for a three-year period.

Confidentiality of Data Bank Information

Information reported to the data bank is considered strictly confidential and cannot be disclosed except as specified in the NPDB regulations. Individuals and entities that knowingly and willfully report to or query the data bank under false pretenses or fraudulently access the data bank computer directly are subject to civil penalties. The data bank follows the following guidelines on disclosure:

> Information reported to the Data Bank is considered confidential and shall not be disclosed outside the Department of Health and Human Services, except as specified in Sec. 60.10, Sec. 60.11 and Sec. 60.[15] Persons and entities which receive information from the Data Bank either directly or from another party must use it solely with respect to the purpose for which it was provided. Nothing in this paragraph shall prevent the disclosure of information by a party which is authorized under applicable State law to make such disclosure. . . .

> Any person who violates [the above] shall be subject to a civil money penalty of up to $10,000 for each violation. . . .[16]

The Privacy Act of 1974 protects the contents of federal systems of records such as those contained in the NPDB from disclosure, unless the disclosure is for a routine use of the system of records as published annually in the *Federal Register*. The published routine uses of NPDB information do not allow for disclosure of information to the general public.

INCIDENT REPORTING

Incident reports contain statements made by employees and physicians regarding a deviation from acceptable patient care. Some state health codes provide that hospitals and nursing facilities must investigate incidents regarding patient care and require that certain incidents must be reported in a manner prescribed by regulation. Reportable incidents often include such things as those incidents that have resulted in a patient's serious injury or death, an event such as fire or loss of emergency power, certain infection outbreaks, and strikes by employees.

Incident reports should not be placed in the medical record. They should be directed to counsel for legal advice. This will help prevent discovery on the basis of client-attorney privilege. There is conflicting case law in that some courts will not permit incident reports to be discovered whereas others will allow discovery. A Florida appeals court ruled that incident reports prepared in anticipation of litigation are not discoverable, even though the information contained in the report was not available by any other means.[17] In *Berg v. Des Moines General Hospital Co.*,[18] the Iowa Supreme Court ruled that, because of the time lapse between the actual incident and the inability of the nurses to recall the incident, discovery of the written incident report was allowed.

Hospital Incident/Occurrence Reports Discoverable

Occurrence reports in *Columbia/HCA Healthcare Corp. v. Eighth Judicial District Court*[19] were found to have been prepared in the ordinary course of the hospital's business, and were therefore not protected by the "work product doctrine." The hospital's petition implicitly admitted that it required its personnel to fill out preprinted forms in the event of an unexpected occurrence. Occurrence reports consisted of a four-page form, which was completed by a hospital employee who had information regarding an unusual event that occurred at the hospital. The hospital further admitted that the purpose, at least in part, for creating occurrence reports was to improve the quality of care given at the hospital. The hospital documents did not become privileged by injecting an attorney into the investigative process. The investigation occurred in the ordinary course of business. The Nevada legislature never intended to exempt occurrence reports from discovery under Nev. Rev. Stat. § 49.265.

Occurrence reports, which the hospital admitted are nothing more than factual narratives, contain the very type of information that will most likely be uncovered through traditional discovery procedures. In those instances where the information can be obtained only through the occurrence report, prospective plaintiffs should not be denied access. Allowing Nev. Rev. Stat. § 49.265 to become an impenetrable bulwark of damaging factual information defeats the very purposes of Nevada's evidence code for which Nev. Rev. Stat. § 49.265 is a part: "The purposes of this [evidence code is] to secure fairness in administration . . . to the end that truth may be ascertained and proceedings justly determined."[20] The court concluded that the occurrence reports are neither work product nor protected by the peer-review privilege embodied in Nev. Rev. Stat. § 49.265.

State Reportable Incidents

State reportable events include the reporting of communicable diseases, infections, and unusual or an unexpected cluster of patients with symptoms/diseases or exposures suggestive of a health emergency or terrorism event.

Many states have enacted legislation requiring hospitals to report incidents that result in patient injury. The new Pennsylvania Medical Care Availability and Reduction of Error Act (MCARE Act) reporting requirements, for example, are intended to help reduce and eliminate medical errors by identifying problems and implementing solutions to improve patient safety. The MCARE Act requires health care facilities to report serious events and incidents to a newly established patient safety authority. The act defines a *serious event* as an event, occurrence, or situation involving the clinical care of a patient in a medical facility that results in death or compromises patient safety and results in an unanticipated injury requiring the delivery of additional health care services to the patient.

Physicians are also required to report complaints, disciplinary actions, and criminal offenses to the professional licensure board. Physicians are required to report the following events:

- Medical professional liability actions filed against the physician.

- Disciplinary actions by a health care licensing authority of another state.

- Convictions for offenses above summary offenses.

- Arrests for a felony (criminal homicide, aggravated assault, sexual offenses) or an offense under the Con-

trolled Substance, Drug, Devise and Cosmetic Act (www.physiciansnews.com/law/902torrance.html).

A patient affected by a serious event must be notified of the event in writing by the medical facility through a designated individual at the facility.

Managers must be aware of specific state reporting requirements. Hospital procedures for reporting patient care incidents must comply with state regulations. As with Joint Commission requirements, the Pennsylvania law prohibits retaliatory action against the health care worker for reporting patient care incidents and provides for written notification to patients.

Individuals designated to report incidents must do so if required by a state's statute. The director of nursing at a nursing facility in *Choe v. Axelrod*[21] was fined $150 for failure to report an instance of patient neglect. An anonymous telephone call had been placed with the department of health regarding two incidents of alleged patient neglect. In one incident, a patient had been left unattended in a shower by an orderly, and the patient sprayed himself with hot water, which resulted in second-degree burns on his forehead. On a second occasion, a similar incident occurred, but no one was injured. On investigation by the department of health, a determination was made that both incidents constituted patient neglect and that failure to report these incidents was a violation of New York public health law. After a hearing by an administrative law judge, the charge in the first incident was sustained and in the second incident was dismissed. The director of nurses petitioned to annul the administrative determination. She contended that the department of health failed to establish a prima facie case of patient neglect, that the incident was an unavoidable accident, and that the department of health's proof was based on hearsay evidence. The court held that evidence supported a finding that the director of nurses failed to report an incident of patient neglect as required by statute. On the question of hearsay evidence:

> It is . . . well established that an agency can prove its case through hearsay evidence. . . . In the final analysis, the evidence showed that the patient was left unattended, albeit momentarily, O'Brien (the orderly) was disciplined for that act, and petitioner did not report the incident. The finding is thus supported by the kind of evidence on which reasonable persons are accustomed to rely in serious affairs.[22]

Although it may not always be clear as to when an incident report should be filed, appropriate procedures should be in place addressing how questionable events should be handled.

SENTINEL EVENTS AND THE JOINT COMMISSION

The Joint Commission encourages health care organizations to self-report sentinel events. The Joint Commission defines a *sentinel event* as "an unexpected occurrence involving death or serious physical or psychological injury, or the risk thereof. Serious injury specifically includes loss of limb or function. The phrase, 'or the risk thereof,' includes any process variation for which a recurrence would carry a significant chance of a serious adverse outcome."[23] Sentinel events subject to review by the Joint Commission include the following occurrences:

- The event has resulted in an unanticipated death or major permanent loss of function, not related to the natural course of the patient's illness or underlying condition or the event is one of the following (even if the outcome was not death or major permanent loss of function unrelated to the natural course of the patient's illness or underlying condition)[24]:

  - Suicide of any patient receiving care, treatment, and services in a staffed around-the-clock-care setting or within 72 hours of discharge

  - Unanticipated death of a full-term infant

  - Abduction of any patient receiving care, treatment, and services

  - Infant abduction or discharge to the wrong family

  - Rape

  - Hemolytic transfusion reaction involving administration of blood or blood products having major blood-group incompatibilities

  - Surgery on the wrong patient or wrong body part

  - Unintended retention of a foreign object in a patient after surgery or other procedure

- Severe neonatal hyperbilirubinemia . . .

- Prolonged fluoroscopy . . .

Frequently reported sentinel events include patient suicides, medication errors, deaths due to delays in treatment, operative/postoperative complications, and surgical procedures on the wrong site.

Although the Joint Commission encourages but does not require the reporting of sentinel events, it does expect organizations to conduct a root-cause analysis when sentinel events occur.

Root-Cause Analysis

A root cause analysis (RCA) is a chronological review of an event to identify what, how, why, when, and where an unwanted event occurred in order to prevent reoccurrence of the event. RCAs focus on systems and processes, not individual performance.

. . . a process for identifying the basic or causal factors that underlie variation in performance, including the occurrence or possible occurrence of a sentinel event. A root cause analysis focuses primarily on systems and processes, not on individual performance. It progresses from special causes in clinical processes to common causes in organizational processes and systems and identifies potential improvements in processes or systems that would tend to decrease the likelihood of such events in the future or determines, after analysis, that no such opportunities exist.[25]

The basic purpose of an RCA is to improve organizational performance outcomes. Organizations are often concerned with the possibility that RCAs could be subject to discovery by a plaintiff's attorney and could then be used against them in civil trials. To address this concern and minimize the risks of additional liability exposure, the Joint Commission continues to work on ways to prevent the disclosure of the substance of RCAs.

The RCA process involves:

- thoroughly investigating an unfortunate occurrence to determine the main cause of the event

- conducting a thorough and credible analysis

- investigating both general and special causes instigating the event

- researching and reviewing the literature

- searching for best practices on the Internet

- contacting and consulting with other organizations that have implemented best practices to limit the likelihood of such events from occurring in the future

- identifying changes that can be made to reduce or eliminate the likelihood of similar occurrences in the future

- identifying who will be responsible for implementing changes

- pilot testing the new design/best practice prior to full implementation

- determining a time line for implementing changes

- determining how changes will be communicated to those who will be working under the new design

- educating staff, who will be responsible for operating under the newly designed practice

- determining how implementation of new processes will be monitored and evaluated

Reporting sentinel events, conducting root-cause analyses, and sharing that information with the Joint Commission will be helpful to all organizations in improving patient care. For helpful Web site information on sentinel events and root-cause analyses in health care, see www.sentinel-event.com/credible.php.

CORPORATE COMPLIANCE PROGRAMS

The federal government's initiative to investigate and prosecute health care organizations for criminal wrong-doing, coupled with strong sanctions imposed after conviction, has resulted in health care organizations establishing corporate compliance programs. These programs establish internal mechanisms for preventing, detecting, and reporting criminal conduct. Sentencing incentives are in place for organizations that establish such programs. The following paragraphs describe the elements of an effective corporate compliance program:

An "effective program to prevent and detect violations of the law" means a program that has been reasonably designed, implemented, and enforced so that it generally will be effective in preventing and detecting criminal conduct. Failure to prevent or detect the instant offense, by itself, does not mean that the program was not effective. The hallmark of an effective program to prevent and detect violations of law is that the organization exercised due diligence in seeking to prevent and detect criminal conduct by its employees and other agents. Due diligence requires that an organization will at the very least have implemented the following[26]:

(1) The organization must have established compliance standards and procedures to be followed by its employees and other agents that are reasonably capable of reducing the prospect of criminal conduct.

(2) Specific individual(s) within high-level personnel of the organization must have been assigned overall responsibility to oversee compliance with such standards and procedures.

(3) The organization must have used due care not to delegate substantial discretionary authority to individuals whom the organization knew, or should have known through the exercise of due diligence, had a propensity to engage in illegal conduct.

(4) The organization must have taken steps to communicate effectively its standards and procedures to all employees and other agents, e.g., by requiring participation in training programs or by disseminating publications that explain in a practical manner what is required.

(5) The organization must have taken reasonable steps to achieve compliance with its standards, e.g., by utilizing monitoring and auditing systems reasonably designed to detect criminal conduct by its employees and other agents and by having in place and publicizing a reporting system whereby employees and other agents could report criminal conduct by others within the organization without fear of retribution.

(6) The standards must have been consistently enforced through appropriate disciplinary mechanisms, including, as appropriate, discipline of individuals responsible for the failure to detect an offense. Adequate discipline of individuals responsible for an offense is a necessary component of enforcement; however, the discipline that will be appropriate will be case specific.

(7) After an offense has been detected, the organization must have taken all reasonable steps to respond appropriately to the offense and to prevent similar offenses—including any necessary modifications to its program to prevent and detect violations of the law.

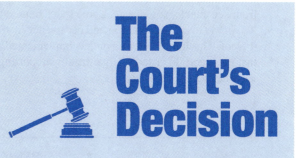

The Court's Decision

The Georgia Court of Appeals held that the statute's grant of immunity from liability extended to the psychologist. The evidence did not establish bad faith on the part of the psychologist so as to deprive her of such immunity. The statute provides that any person participating in the making of a report, or participating in any judicial proceeding or any other proceeding resulting in a report of suspected child abuse, is immune from any civil or criminal liability that might otherwise be incurred or imposed, provided such participation pursuant to the statute is made in good faith. The grant of qualified immunity covers every person who, in good faith, participates over time in the making of a report to a child welfare agency. There was no competent evidence that the psychologist acted in bad faith.

CHAPTER REVIEW

1. An *abused child* is defined as one who has suffered intentional and serious mental, emotional, sexual, and/or physical injury inflicted by a parent or other person charged with the child's care.
2. Child abuse laws differ from state to state, but, in most states, persons required to report cases of child abuse are protected. The person reporting abuse does not have to be absolutely certain that abuse has taken place before he or she reports, but reports must be made with a good-faith belief that the facts reported are true.
3. Generally, senior abuse is less likely to be reported than child abuse and proving senior abuse charges is often difficult.
4. The prompt reporting of infection or disease is necessary in order for states to protect citizens' health by invoking the power to quarantine.
5. All births and deaths are reportable by statute. Unnatural deaths are to be referred to the medical examiner to determine the actual cause of death and provide related assistance for further criminal investigation, when necessary.
6. The *National Practitioner Data Bank* is used to collect and release information on the professional competence and conduct of physicians, dentists, and other health care practitioners.
7. Information in the data bank is considered strictly confidential. Data bank queries can be made by state licensing boards, hospitals, other health care organizations, and professional societies that have entered or may be entering into employment or affiliation relationships with a physician, dentist, or other health care practitioner who has applied for clinical privileges or appointment to a medical staff.
8. Incident reports include statements from employees and physicians regarding significant or noteworthy deviation from acceptable patient care. Some states require the reporting of specific incidents.
9. A *sentinel event* is an unexpected occurrence involving death or serious physical or psychological injury, or the risk thereof. The Joint Commission has implemented a policy that requires organizations to self-report sentinel events that meet certain criteria. Organizations reporting sentinel events must conduct *root-cause analyses* to determine why the events occurred.

REVIEW QUESTIONS

1. What is child abuse?
2. Who should report child abuse?
3. Describe the signs of elder abuse.
4. Why was the Health Care Quality Improvement Act of 1986 enacted?
5. Describe the purpose of the National Practitioner Data Bank.
6. What is a sentinel event?
7. Discuss the process of conducting a root-cause analysis.
8. Describe the basic elements of an effective corporate compliance program.

NOTES

1. *Michaels v. Gordon,* 439 S.E.2d 722 (Ga. Ct. App. 1993).

2. U.S. Code, Title 42, Chapter 67, Subter 1, § 5106g.

3. 373 N.W.2d 204 (Mich. Ct. App. 1985).

4. 413 N.W.2d 670 (Wis. Ct. App. 1987).

5. No. 1031515 (Ala. 2005).

6. 415 N.W.2d 436 (Minn. Ct. App. 1987).

7. 140 S.W.3d 51 (Mo. banc).

8. *Manifold v. Ragaglia,* No. SC 17150 (Conn. 2004).

9. *What is Elder Abuse,* National Committee for the Prevention of Elder Abuse, www.preventelderabuse.org/elderabuse/elderabuse.html

10. PUB. L. No. 99-660, tit. IV (1986).

11. 42 U.S.C. § 11101[0].

12. 45 C.F.R. § 60.1 (1991).

13. 42 U.S.C. § 11101 (1991).

14. There is a guidebook that is meant to serve as a resource for the users of the National Practitioner Data Bank. It is one of a number of efforts to inform the U.S. health care community about the data bank and what is required to comply with the requirements established by the HCQIA. The data bank Help Line (1-800-767-6732) is a toll-free telephone service that provides health care entities and health care practitioners with information about the data bank.

15. 456 N.W.2d 173 (Iowa 1990).

16. 45 C.F.R. § 60.13 (1991).

17. 551 So. 2d 532 (Fla. Dist. Ct. App. 1990).

18. 456 N.W.2d 173 (Iowa 1990).

19. 936 P.2d 844 (Nev. 1997).

20. Nev. Rev. Stat. § 47.030.

21. 534 N.Y.S.2d 739 (N.Y. App. Div. 1988).

22. *Id.* at 741.

23. *2007 Comprehensive Manual for Hospitals: The Official Handbook,* Joint Commission on Accreditation of Healthcare Organizations, at SE-1.

24. *Id.* at SE-3.

25. *Id.* at SE-2.

26. 56 Fed. Reg. 22,762 (May 16, 1991).

CHAPTER 14

Issues of Procreation

It's Your Gavel ...

S.D. ABORTION BILL TAKES AIM AT *ROE*

South Dakota lawmakers approved a far-reaching ban on abortion. The measure, which passed the state senate, makes it a felony for doctors to perform any abortion, except to save the life of a pregnant woman. The bill was designed to challenge the Supreme Court's ruling in *Roe,* which in 1973 recognized a right of women to terminate pregnancies.[1] As of 2005, there have been more than 47 million abortions since the U.S. Supreme Court Supreme Court issued its *Roe v. Wade* decision legalizing abortion on January 22, 1973.[2]

WHAT IS YOUR VERDICT?

This chapter reviews a variety of issues of procreation. Primary emphasis is placed on abortion. Discussed to a lesser extent are issues relating to sterilization, artificial insemination, and wrongful birth, wrongful life, and wrongful conception.

ABORTION

Abortion is the premature termination of pregnancy. It can be classified as spontaneous or induced. It may occur as an incidental result of a medical procedure or it may be an elective decision on the part of the patient. In addition to having substantial ethical, moral, and religious implications, abortion has proven to be a major political issue and will continue as such in the future. More laws will be proposed, more laws will be passed, and more lawsuits will wind their way up to the U.S. Supreme Court.

The Right to Abortion

Roe v. Wade in 1973 gave strength to a woman's right to privacy in the context of matters relating to her own body, including how a pregnancy would end.[3] However, the Supreme Court also has recognized the interest of the states in protecting potential life and has attempted to spell out the extent to which the states may regulate and even prohibit abortions.

In *Roe v. Wade,* the U.S. Supreme Court held the Texas penal abortion law unconstitutional, stating: "[s]tate criminal abortion statutes . . . that except from criminality only a lifesaving procedure on behalf of the mother, without regard to the stage of her pregnancy and other interests involved, is violating the Due Process Clause of the Fourteenth Amendment."[4]

First Trimester

During the first trimester of pregnancy, the decision to undergo an abortion procedure is between the woman and her physician. A state may require that abortions be performed by a physician licensed pursuant to its laws. However, a woman's right to an abortion is not unqualified because the decision to perform the procedure must be left to the medical judgment of her attending physician. "For the stage prior to approximately the end of the first trimester, the abortion decision and its effectuation must be left to the medical judgment of the pregnant woman's attending physician."[5]

Second Trimester

In *Roe v. Wade,* the Supreme Court stated, "[f]or the stage subsequent to approximately the end of the first trimester, the State, in promoting its interest in the health of the mother, may, if it chooses, regulate the abortion procedure in ways that are reasonably related to maternal health."[6] Thus, during approximately the fourth to sixth months of pregnancy, the state may regulate the medical conditions under which the procedure is performed. The constitutional test of any legislation concerning abortion during this period would be its relevance to the objective of protecting maternal health.

Third Trimester

The Supreme Court reasoned that by the time the final stage of pregnancy has been reached, the state has acquired a compelling interest in the product of conception, which would override the woman's right to privacy and justify stringent regulation even to the extent of prohibiting abortions. In the *Roe* case, the Court formulated its ruling as to the last trimester in the following words: "[f]or the stage subsequent to viability, the State in promoting its interest in the potentiality of human life, may, if it chooses, regulate, and even proscribe, abortion except where it is necessary, in appropriate medical judgment for the preservation of the life or health of the mother."[7]

Thus, during the final stage of pregnancy, a state may prohibit all abortions except those deemed necessary to protect maternal life or health. The state's legislative powers over the performance of abortions increase as the pregnancy progresses toward term.

State Requirements: Not an Undue Burden

1992: In *Planned Parenthood v. Casey,*[8] the Supreme Court affirmed Pennsylvania law restricting a woman's right to abortion. The Court was one vote shy of overturning *Roe v. Wade.* The Supreme Court ruling, as enunciated in *Roe v. Wade,* reaffirmed:

- the constitutional right of women to have an abortion before viability of the fetus, as first enunciated in *Roe v. Wade*

- the state's power to restrict abortions after fetal viability, as long as the law contains exceptions for pregnancies that endanger a woman's life or health

- the principle that the state has legitimate interests from the outset of the pregnancy in protecting the health of the woman and the life of the fetus

The Supreme Court rejected the trimester approach in *Roe v. Wade,* which limited the regulations states could issue on abortion depending on the development stage of the fetus. In place of the trimester approach, the Court will evaluate the permissibility of state abortion rules based on whether they unduly burden a woman's ability to obtain an abortion. A rule is an undue burden if its purpose or effect is to place a substantial obstacle in the path of a woman seeking an abortion before the fetus attains viability. The Supreme Court ruled that it is not an undue burden to require that

- a woman be informed of the nature of the abortion procedure and the risks involved

- a woman be offered information on the fetus and on the alternatives to abortion

- a woman give her informed consent before the abortion procedure

- parental consent be given for a minor seeking an abortion, providing for a judicial bypass option if the minor does not wish or cannot obtain parental consent

- there be a 24-hour waiting period before any abortion can be performed

Abortion Counseling

1983: The Supreme Court in *City of Akron v. Akron Center for Reproductive Health*[9] voted six to three that the different states cannot (1) mandate what information physicians give abortion patients or (2) require that abortions for women more than three months pregnant be performed in a hospital. With respect to a requirement that the attending physician must inform the woman of specified information concerning her proposed abortion, it is unreasonable for a state to insist that only a physician is competent to provide the information and counseling relative to informed consent. A state may not adopt regulations to influence a woman's informed choice between abortion and childbirth. With regard to a second-trimester hospital requirement, this could significantly limit a woman's ability to obtain an abortion. This is especially so in view of the evidence that a second-trimester abortion may cost more than twice as much in a hospital as in a clinic.

Prohibition of Abortion Counseling Not Unconstitutional

1991: Federal regulations that prohibit abortion counseling and referral by family planning clinics that receive funds under Title X of the Public Health Service Act were found not to violate the constitutional rights of pregnant women or Title X grantees in a five-to-four decision by the Supreme Court in *Rust v. Sullivan.*[10] Proponents of abortion counseling argued that the regulations impermissibly burden a woman's privacy right to abortion. Prohibiting the delivery of abortion information, even as to where such information could be obtained, the regulations deny a woman her constitutionally protected right to choose under the First Amendment. The question arises: How can a woman make an informed choice between two options when she cannot obtain information as to one of them? In *Sullivan,* however, the Supreme Court found that there was no violation of a woman's or provider's First Amendment rights. The Court extended the doctrine that government need not subsidize the exercise of the fundamental rights to free speech. The plaintiff argued that the government may not condition receipt of a benefit on the relinquishment of constitutional rights.

24-Hour Waiting Period Not Burdensome

1993: The Utah Abortion Act Revision, Senate Bill 60, provides for informed consent by requiring that certain information be given to the pregnant woman at least 24 hours prior to the performance of an abortion. The law allows for exceptions to this requirement in the event of a medical emergency.

The Utah Women's Clinic, in *Utah Women's Clinic, Inc. v. Leavitt,*[11] filed a 106-page complaint. The plaintiffs' case was referred to the magistrate judge, who determined that the 24-hour waiting period does not impose an undue burden on the right to an abortion.

On appeal, the U.S. District Court for the district of Utah held that the Utah abortion statute's 24-hour waiting period and informed consent requirements do not render the statute unconstitutionally vague.

In 1992, the Supreme Court in *Planned Parenthood of Southeastern Pennsylvania v. Casey*[12] determined that in asserting an interest in protecting fetal life, a state may place some restrictions on previability abortions, as long as those restrictions do not impose an "undue burden" on the woman's right to an abortion. The Court determined that the 24-hour waiting period, the informed consent requirement, and the medical emergency definitions did not unduly burden the right to an abortion and were therefore constitutional. In the instant case, because Senate Bill 60 is less restrictive than the Pennsylvania abortion statute, the plaintiffs may not prevail unless they can show material differences between the circumstances of Utah and Pennsylvania.

It would be extremely difficult in light of the *Casey* decision to bring a good-faith facial challenge to the constitutionality of Utah's 24-hour waiting period and informed consent requirements. In an emergency situation, there is no a requirement of informed consent or a 24-hour waiting period. The plaintiffs' contention that Senate Bill 60 when read together with provisions from Utah's 1991 abortion law do not clearly provide that a woman can obtain an abortion in a medical emergency, is without merit.

> The abortion issue is obviously one that invokes strong feelings on both sides. Individuals are free to urge support for their cause through debate, advocacy, and participation in the political process. The subject also might be addressed in the courts so long as there are valid legal issues in dispute. Where, however, a case presents no legitimate legal arguments, the courthouse is not the proper forum. Litigation, or the threat of litigation, should not be used as economic blackmail to strengthen one's hand in the political battle. Unfortunately, the court sees little evidence that this case was filed for any other purpose.[13]

> Senate Bill 60, the duly enacted law of the people of Utah, has not been enforced for nearly nine months. That will change today. The court hereby adopts the report and recommendation of the magistrate judge, lifts the injunction, and dismisses plaintiffs' case in its entirety with prejudice.[14]

Abortion Committee Requirement Too Restrictive

1973: The Supreme Court delineated what regulatory measures a state lawfully may enact during the three stages of pregnancy. In the companion decision, *Doe v. Bolton,*[15] where the Court considered a constitutional attack on the Georgia abortion statute, further restrictions were placed on state regulation of the procedure. The provisions of the Georgia statute establishing residency requirements for women seeking abortions and requiring that the procedure be performed in a hospital accredited by The Joint Commission were declared constitutionally invalid. In considering legislative provisions establishing medical staff approval as a prerequisite to the abortion procedure, the Court decided that "interposition of the hospital abortion committee is unduly restrictive of the patient's rights and needs that . . . have already been medically delineated and substantiated by her personal physician. To ask more serves neither the hospital nor the State."[16]

The Court was unable to find any constitutionally justifiable rationale for a statutory requirement of advance approval by the abortion committee of the hospital's medical staff. Insofar as statutory consultation requirements are concerned, the Court reasoned that the acquiescence of two copractitioners has no rational connection with a patient's needs and, further, unduly infringes on the physician's right to practice.

Thus, by using a test related to patient needs, the Court in *Doe v. Bolton* struck down four preabortion procedural requirements commonly imposed by state statutes: (1) residency, (2) performance of the abortion in a hospital accredited by the Joint Commission, (3) approval by an appropriate committee of the medical staff, and (4) consultations.

Spousal Consent: Requirement Unconstitutional

1975: A Florida statute required written consent of the husband before a wife could be permitted to obtain an abortion. The husband's interest in the baby was held to be insufficient to force his wife to face the mental and physical risks of pregnancy and childbirth.[17]

In *Doe v. Zimmerman*,[18] the court declared unconstitutional the provisions of the Pennsylvania Abortion Control Act, which required that the written consent of the husband of a married woman be secured before the performance of an abortion. The court found that these provisions impermissibly permitted the husband to withhold his consent either because of his interest in the potential life of the fetus or for capricious reasons. The natural father of an unborn fetus in *Doe v. Smith*[19] was found not to be entitled to an injunction to prevent the mother from submitting to an abortion. Although the father's interest in the fetus was legitimate, it did not outweigh the mother's constitutionally protected right to an abortion, particularly in the light of the evidence that the mother and father had never married. The father had demonstrated substantial instability in his marital and romantic life. The father was able to beget other children and, in fact, did produce other children.

In the 1992 decision of *Planned Parenthood v. Casey,* the Supreme Court ruled that spousal consent would be an undue burden on the woman.

Parental Consent

1976: The Supreme Court ruled in *Danforth v. Planned Parenthood*[20] that a Missouri statute requiring all women under 18 to obtain written consent of a parent or person in loco parentis prior to an abortion is unconstitutional. The Court, however, failed to provide any definitive guidelines as to when and how parental consent may be required if the minor is too immature to fully comprehend the nature of the procedure.

1979: The Supreme Court in *Bellotti v. Baird*[21] ruled eight to one that a Massachusetts statute requiring parental consent before an abortion could be performed on an unmarried woman under 18 was unconstitutional. Justice Stevens, joined by Justices Brennan, Marshall, and Blackmun, concluded that the Massachusetts statute was unconstitutional, because under that statute as written and construed by the Massachusetts Supreme Judicial Court, no minor, no matter how mature and capable of informed decision making, could receive an abortion without the consent of either both parents or a superior court judge, thus making the minor's abortion subject in every instance to an absolute third-party veto.

Notice Requirement for Immature Minor Constitutional

1981: The Supreme Court, in *H. L. v. Matheson,*[22] by a six-to-three vote, upheld a Utah statute that required a physician to "notify, if possible" the parents or guardian of a minor on whom an abortion was to be performed. In this case, the physician advised the patient that an abortion would be in her best medical interest but, because of the statute, refused to perform the abortion without notifying her parents. The Supreme Court ruled that although a state may not constitutionally legislate a blanket, unreviewable power of parents to veto their daughter's abortion, a statute setting out a mere requirement of parental notice when possible does not violate the constitutional rights of an immature, dependent minor.

Consent Not Required for Emancipated Minor

1987: The trial court in *In re Anonymous*[23] was found to have abused its discretion when it refused a minor's request for waiver of parental consent to obtain an abortion. The record indicated that the minor lived alone, was within one month of her 18th birthday, lived by herself most of the time, and held down a full-time job.

Parental Notification Not Required

2000: The issue in *Planned Parenthood v. Owens*[24] is whether the Colorado Parental Notification Act, Colo. Rev. Stat. §§ 12-37.5-101, et seq. (1998), which requires a physician to notify the parents of a minor prior to performing an abortion upon her, violates the minor's rights protected by the U.S. Constitution. The act generally prohibits physicians from performing abortions on an unemancipated minor until at least 48 hours after written notice has been delivered to the minor's parent, guardian, or foster parent.

The plaintiffs claim the act is unconstitutional because it fails to provide an exception to the notice requirement when necessary to protect the health of minors short of imminent death. It was uncontested that there are situations when a physician must act promptly to protect the health or life of the minor. As a consequence, and as both parties agreed, delay in the abortion inherent in the act's notification process will result in adverse health consequences for some minors. The U.S. District Court decided that the act violated the rights of minor women protected by the Fourteenth Amendment.

Incompetent Persons

1987: An abortion was found to have been authorized properly by a family court in *In re Doe*[25] for a profoundly retarded woman. She became pregnant during her residence in a group home as a result of a sexual attack by an unknown person. The record supported a finding that if the woman had been able to do so, she would have requested the abortion. The court properly chose welfare agencies and the woman's guardian ad litem as the surrogate decision makers, rather than the woman's mother. The mother apparently had little contact with her daughter over the years.

Funding

Some states have placed an indirect restriction on abortion through the elimination of funding. Under the Hyde Amendment, the U.S. Congress, through appropriations legislation, has limited the types of medically necessary abortions for which federal funds may be spent under the Medicaid program. Although the Hyde Amendment does not prohibit states from funding nontherapeutic abortions, this action by the federal government opened the door to state statutory provisions limiting the funding of abortions.

Not Required for Elective Abortions

1977:[26,27] In *Beal v. Doe,*[28] the Pennsylvania Medicaid plan was challenged on the basis of denial of financial assistance for nontherapeutic abortions. The Supreme Court held that Title XIX of the Social Security Act (the Medicaid program) does not require the funding of nontherapeutic abortions as a condition of state participation in the program.[29] The state has a strong interest in encouraging normal childbirth, and nothing in Title XIX suggests that it is unreasonable for the state to further that interest. The Court ruled that it is not inconsistent with the Medicaid portion of the Social Security Act to refuse to fund unnecessary (although perhaps desirable) medical services.

1977: In *Maher v. Roe,*[30] the Supreme Court considered the Connecticut statute that denied Medicaid benefits for first trimester abortions that were not medically necessary. The Court rejected the argument that the state's subsidy of medical expenses incident to pregnancy and childbirth created an obligation on the part of the state to subsidize the expenses incident to nontherapeutic abortions. The Supreme Court voted six to three that the states may refuse to spend public funds to provide nontherapeutic abortions for women.

Not Required for Therapeutic Abortions

1980: In *Harris v. McRae,*[31] the Supreme Court upheld five to four the Hyde Amendment, which restricts the use of federal funds for Medicaid abortions. Under this case, the different states are not compelled to fund Medicaid recipients' medically necessary abortions for which federal reimbursement is unavailable, but may choose to do so.

Funding Bans Unconstitutional in California

The California Supreme Court held funding bans were unconstitutional; the court asked rhetorically:

> If the state cannot directly prohibit a woman's right to obtain an abortion, may the state by discriminatory financing indirectly nullify that constitutional right? Can the state tell an indigent person that the state will provide him with welfare benefits only upon the condition that he join a designated political party or subscribe to a particular newspaper that is favored by the government? Can the state tell a poor woman that it will pay for her needed medical care but only if she gives up her constitutional right to choose whether or not to have a child?[32]

Discrimination in Funding Prohibited in Arizona

The Arizona Supreme Court in *Simat Corp. v. Arizona Health Care Cost Containment Sys.,*[33] found that the state's constitution does not permit the state and the Arizona Health Care Cost Containment System (AHCCCS) to refuse to fund medically necessary abortion procedures for pregnant women suffering from serious illness while, at the same time, funding such procedures for victims of rape or incest or when the abortion was necessary to save the woman's life (A.R.S. § 35-196.02. AHCCCS). After the state has chosen to fund abortions for one group of indigent, pregnant women for whom abortions are medically necessary to save their lives, the state may not deny the same option to another group of women for whom the procedure is also medically necessary to save their health. An example is cancer, for which chemotherapy or radiation therapy ordinarily cannot be provided if the patient is pregnant, making an abortion necessary before proceeding with the recognized medical treatment. Other therapy regimens that must at times be suspended during pregnancy include heart disease, diabetes, kidney disease, liver disease, chronic renal failure, inflammatory bowel disease, and lupus. In many of the women suffering from these diseases, suspension of recognized therapy during pregnancy will have serious and permanent adverse effects on their health and lessen their life span. In such a situation, the state is not simply influencing a woman's choice but is actually conferring the privilege of treatment on one class and withholding it from another.

A woman's right to choose preservation and protection of her health, and therefore, in many cases, her life, is at least as compelling as the state's interest in promoting childbirth. The court's protection of the fetus and promotion of childbirth cannot be considered so compelling as to outweigh a woman's fundamental right to choose and the state's obligation to be even-handed in the design and application of its health care policies. The majority of states that have examined similar Medicaid funding restrictions have determined that their state statutes or constitutions offer broader protection of individual rights than does the U.S. Constitution, and they have found that medically necessary abortions should be funded if the state also funds medically necessary expenses related to childbirth. The case was remanded to the trial court for further proceedings consistent with this opinion.

States May Protect Viable Fetus

1979: The Supreme Court in *Colautti v. Franklin*[34] voted six to three that the states may seek to protect a fetus that a physician has determined could survive outside the womb. Determination of whether a particular fetus is viable is, and must be, a matter for judgment of the responsible attending physician. State abortion regulations that impinge on this determination, if they are to be constitutional, must allow the attending physician the room that he or she needs to make the best medical judgment.

Viability Tests Required

1989: *Webster v. Reproductive Health Services*[35] began the Court's narrowing of abortion rights by upholding a Missouri statute providing that no public facilities or employees should be used to perform abortions and that physicians should conduct viability tests before performing abortions.

Partial-Birth Abortion

Plan Constitutionally Vague

1998: The Supreme Court in *Women's Medical Professional Corp. v. Voinovich*[36] denied certiorari for the first

partial-birth case to reach the federal appellate courts. This case involved an Ohio statute that banned the use of the intact dilation and extraction (D&X) procedure in the performance of any pre- or postviability abortion. The Sixth Circuit Court of Appeals held that the statute banning any use of the D&X procedure was unconstitutionally vague. It is likely that a properly drafted statute will eventually be judged constitutionally sound.

Partial-Birth Abortion Ban Act Unconstitutional

1999: The defendants in *Little Rock Family Planning Services v. Jegley*[37] appealed a district court decision holding Arkansas's Partial-Birth Abortion Ban Act of 1997 unconstitutional. The act prohibited knowingly performing a partial-birth abortion. Arkansas code defines *partial-birth abortion* as an abortion in which the person performing the abortion partially vaginally delivers a living fetus before taking the life of the fetus and completing the delivery. Under this definition, any physician who knowingly partially vaginally delivered a living fetus, then takes the life of the fetus, and completes delivery, would have violated the act. Because both the D&E procedure and the suction-curettage procedure used in second trimester abortions often include what the act prohibits, physicians performing those procedures would have violated the act. The act provided that, in addition to committing a felony, a physician who knowingly performed a partial-birth abortion would be subject to disciplinary action by the state medical board. The federal district court held the act unconstitutional because it was unconstitutionally vague, imposed an undue burden on women seeking abortions, and it did not adequately protect the health and lives of pregnant women. The circuit court agreed, holding the act unconstitutional.

Partial-Birth Abortion Statute Vague

2000: New Jersey's partial-birth abortion statute was void for vagueness, in that it did not define the proscribed conduct with certainty and could be easily construed to ban the safest, most common, and readily available conventional abortion procedures. The statute also was unconstitutional as creating an undue burden on a woman's right to obtain an abortion, in that its broad language covered many conventional, constitutionally permissible methods of abortion, and it failed to contain a health exception.[38]

Partial-Birth Abortion: Ban Unconstitutional

2002: The U.S. Supreme Court in *Stenberg v. Carhart*[39] struck down a Nebraska ban on partial-birth abortion, finding it an unconstitutional violation of *Roe v. Wade.* The court found these types of bans to be extreme descriptive attempts to outlaw abortion—even early in pregnancy—that jeopardizes women's health. Following *Stenberg v. Carhart,* a Virginia statute that attempted to criminalize partial birth abortion was also held to be unconstitutional, under the 14th Amendment where it lacked an exception to protect a woman's health.[40]

Partial Birth Abortion Act: First Federal Restrictions

2003: President George W. Bush, on November 6, signed the first federal restrictions banning late-term partial-birth abortions. The ban is referred to as the Partial Birth Abortion Act of 2003. Both houses of Congress passed the ban. The ban permits no exceptions when a woman's health is at risk or the fetus has life-threatening disabilities.

Partial-Birth Abortion Act: Supreme Court Asked to Review

2005: On September 26, 2005, the Bush administration asked the Supreme Court to review an appellate court's decision holding the Partial Birth Abortion Act of 2003 unconstitutional.

Gag Rule Reimposed

2001: On January 22, 2001, on his first business day in office (and the 28th anniversary of *Roe v. Wade*), President George W. Bush reimposed the Global Gag Rule on the U.S. Agency for International Development (USAID) population program. This policy restricts foreign nongovernmental organizations (NGOs) that receive USAID family-planning funds from using their own, non-U.S. funds to provide legal abortion services, lobby their own governments for abortion law reform, or provide medical counseling or referrals regarding abortion.[41]

Revised Gag Rule

The White House directed the DHHS to make an exception to the gag rule, which bars abortion counseling at federally funded clinics, by revising the rule to allow physicians to discuss and provide medical information regarding abortions to their patients. The U.S. Circuit Court of Appeals held that the revised gag rule, making an exception for physicians in abortion counseling, was adopted illegally. The court held that the White House must provide opportunity for public comment prior to ordering an exception to the

rule. As anticipated, the gag rule was rescinded during the first week of the Clinton administration.

Employee Refusal to Participate in Abortions

1975: Individuals have a right to refuse to participate in abortions and can abstain from involvement in abortions as a matter of conscience or religious or moral conviction. In a Missouri case, *Doe v. Poelker,*[42] the city was ordered to obtain the services of physicians and personnel who had no moral objections to participating in abortions. The city also was required to pay the plaintiff's attorneys' fees because of the wanton disregard of the indigent woman's rights and the continuation of a policy to disregard and/or circumvent the U.S. Supreme Court's rulings on abortion.

Pharmacists' Refusal to Fill Prescriptions

Some pharmacists' religious beliefs prohibit abortion or the use of birth control. They believe that dispensing such medications to others is an infringement on their freedom of religion. Eleven states are considering conscience-clause laws that would permit pharmacists to refuse to fill certain prescriptions. Four states have laws specifically allowing pharmacists to refuse to fill prescriptions that violate their beliefs. Legislators in South Dakota, Arkansas, and Georgia hope to strengthen existing laws so pharmacists would be able to refuse to transfer or refer prescriptions for contraceptives to other pharmacies.

Those who object to these laws believe that pharmacists have an obligation to fill all prescriptions and that refusing to fill them violates the patients' freedom of conscience. Four states are considering laws that would explicitly require pharmacists to fill all prescriptions.

The First Amendment protects individual free exercise of religion. Does requiring pharmacists to fill prescriptions that conflict with their religious beliefs violate their rights under the First Amendment? Some say yes, because people whose religious beliefs prohibit birth control or abortion cannot freely exercise their religion if they are forced to dispense these medications. Others say no, because the patients' need to obtain their medication outweighs the pharmacists' rights.[43]

Physicians Feeling the Heat

Physicians are feeling the heat and are concerned about the ongoing abortion controversy. In *Beverly v. Choices Women's Medical Center,*[44] a physician, whose picture was published in an abortion calendar without her consent, brought a civil rights action against the for-profit medical center for publication of her picture. The calendar was disseminated to the public by the center. The center, among other things, performs abortions from which it derives approximately 50 percent of its income. The plaintiff was awarded $50,000 in compensatory damages and $25,000 in punitive damages. The physician testified that the publication of her picture caused her to suffer physical and mental injury. She also testified as to the effect of the publication on her lifestyle and career decisions.

Use of Force Against Demonstrators

In March 1989, the San Diego police became aware that Operation Rescue planned to stage several antiabortion demonstrations in the city.[45] The purpose of the demonstrations was to disrupt operations at the target clinics and ultimately to cause the clinic to cease operations. In each of the three demonstrations at issue, protesters converged on a medical building, blocking entrances, filling stairwells and corridors, and preventing employees and patients from entering.

For each arrest, the officers warned the demonstrators that they would be subjected to pain-compliance measures if they did not move, that such measures would hurt, and that they could reduce the pain by standing up, eliminating the tension on their wrists and arms. The officers then forcibly moved the arrestees by tightening Orcutt police nonchakus (two sticks of wood connected at one end by a cord used to grip a demonstrator's wrist) around their wrists until they stood up and walked. All arrestees complained of varying degrees of injury to their hands and arms. Several subsequently filed suit, claiming that the police violated the Fourth Amendment by using excessive force in executing the arrests. The judge allowed the case to proceed to the jury to determine whether any particular uses of force were unconstitutional. After viewing a videotape of the arrests, the jury concluded that none involved excessive force and returned a verdict for the city. An appeal was taken.

The U.S. Court of Appeals for the Ninth Circuit held that the police did not use excessive force. The videotape created an extensive evidentiary record: "Thanks to videotaped records of the actual events, plus the testimony of witnesses on both sides, the jury had more than a sufficient amount of evidence presented to them from which they could formulate their verdicts. The extensive use of video scenes of exactly what took place removed much argument and interpretation of the facts themselves."[46] The city clearly had a legitimate interest in quickly dispersing and removing the lawbreakers with the least risk of injury to police and others. The arrestees were part of a group of more than 100 protesters operating in an organized and concerted effort to invade private property, obstruct business, and hinder law enforcement.

PICKETING PHYSICIANS' RESIDENCES: A PRIVACY ISSUE

Citation: *Murray v. Lawson,* 642 A.2d 338 (N.J. 1994).

Facts

Two physicians brought separate actions to obtain injunctions against antiabortion protesters who had been picketing their residences. In the first case, the defendant discovered the personal address of Dr. Murray and visited the house, where the physician's 14-year-old son answered the door. The defendant told the son to tell his father to stop performing abortions. A month later, the defendant told the police that he and 50 other people were going to picket the physician's home. After being warned about the picketing, Murray sent his family away. However, he stayed in the house that day, managing, from his home, two of his patients who were in labor. The picketers walked on the sidewalk in front of Murray's home, carrying posters stating among other things, that he scars and kills women and their unborn children. They also told neighbors that he was a killer. Murray filed suit seeking damages and injunctive relief, testifying that the picketing deprived him and his family of their family time, harmed his ability to practice because he had to manage his patients from home, and caused his wife to suffer from nervousness and depression. After the hearing, the medical center where Murray performed abortions was burned to the ground. In spite of a telephone bomb threat, police never determined who called in the threat or burned the building. After the bomb threat, the defendant and another picketer protested in front of the Murray house. Murray called the police, who arrived and told him to stay in the house. He came out, however, and took a swing at the defendant. He was later convicted of assault.

The chancery division ordered a permanent injunction prohibiting the defendant and all others from picketing within 300 feet of the Murray home. The defendants appealed, claiming that the injunction impinged upon their freedom of speech. The appellate division affirmed, finding that the injunction did not violate freedom of speech.

In the second case, Dr. Boffard performed abortions at a clinic, which had been subjected to protests two years prior to the protests at Murray's home. In 1990, the protesters appeared at the front of Boffard's residence. The picketers carried signs, some of which read, "Thou Shalt Not Kill." Other signs contained pictures of bloody fetal parts. The demonstrators yelled at the physician's wife that her husband was a murderer.

Subsequently, a suit was brought in the chancery division to enjoin the defendants from picketing. The court issued a temporary restraining order prohibiting picketing within 200 feet of the physician's home, from referring to Boffard as a killer, and from depicting fetuses on posters. The court made the injunction permanent five months later, stopping the picketing within "the immediate vicinity" of Boffard's home. Again, as in the Murray case, the appellate division upheld the injunction. Both cases were appealed to the New Jersey Supreme Court.

Issue

Did the defendants' free speech rights outweigh the plaintiffs' residential privacy interests?

Holding

The New Jersey Supreme Court upheld the injunction in the Murray case, but remanded the Boffard injunction for a more precise definition of the spatial scope of the ban, finding that "within the immediate vicinity" was too vague.

Reason

Residential privacy represents a sufficient public policy interest to justify injunctive restrictions. Moreover, the chancery division had the power to enjoin the nonviolent, noncriminal activity of the defen-

dants to protect the plaintiffs' residential privacy. The court determined that the injunctions in both cases were content neutral because they could be justified without referring to the content of the defendants' speech. They prohibited any and all picketing, regardless of the type of speech, within a certain distance of the residences. The court further held that because a state has a significant interest in protecting the residential privacy of its citizens, it is justified in imposing injunctive relief.

Discussion

1. What do you see as the rationale behind a court balancing free speech rights against residential privacy rights in abortion protest cases?
2. Do you agree with the court's decision? Explain.

Trespass: Obstructing Access to Abortion Clinics

Abortion clinics and others sought enforcement of an injunction precluding antiabortion groups from blockading or obstructing access to abortion clinics. The order required the defendants to appear before the court to show cause why each of them should not be cited for contempt for violating and inducing others to violate an injunction order. The defendants Tucci, Terry, and Mahoney, spoke at a rally. Tucci was introduced as a leader of Operation Rescue National and spoke about how the group successfully had closed down clinics. He also solicited funds for his organization. Terry said that they needed contributions to keep their work going. The defendants appeared before the court at two hearings to show cause why they should not be cited in contempt for violating the court's injunction.[47] The questions posed are: (1) Can antiabortion leaders and groups be fined for violating an injunction barring them from blockading or obstructing access to abortion clinics? and (2) Can antiabortion groups be ordered to pay damages to compensate an abortion clinic for property damage resulting from an abortion clinic blockage that violated an injunction?

The U.S. District Court for the District of Columbia held that leaders and groups would be fined for violating the injunction. In addition, antiabortion groups are liable to abortion clinics for property damages resulting from blockades. The defendants violated provisions of the injunction "barring all defendants and those acting in concert with them 'from inducing, encouraging, directing, aiding, or abetting others' to trespass on, blockade, or obstruct access to or egress from facilities at which abortions are performed and other medical services are rendered."[48] In blockading the clinics, the defendants violated District of Columbia trespass law, which states, "Any person who, without lawful authority, shall enter, or attempt to enter, any public or private dwelling . . . against the will of the lawful occupant or of the person lawfully in charge thereof . . . shall be guilty of a misdemeanor" (D.C. Code § 22-3102).

The participants in the blockades were under court order not to trespass on the clinics and were ordered by clinic personnel and the police at the time of the blockades to leave the property. Their presence on the property clearly constituted trespass.

Continuing Controversy

While prochoice advocates are arguing the rights of women to choose, they are also pointing out the fact that legalized abortions are safer. In 1972, for example, the year before *Roe v. Wade* was upheld, the number of deaths from abortions in the United States is estimated to have reached the thousands; by 1985, the figure was six.[49] In addition, prochoice advocates argue that women who have a right to an abortion when pregnancy threatens the life of the mother also have the right to an abortion when pregnancy is the result of incest or rape.

Right-to-Life advocates argue that life comes from God and that no one has a right to deny the right to life.

There will most likely be a continuing stream of court decisions, as well as political and legislative battles, well into the 21st century. Given the emotional, religious, and ethical concerns, as well as those of women's rights groups, it is unlikely that this matter will be resolved anytime soon.

STERILIZATION

Sterilization is the termination of the ability to produce offspring. Sterilization often is accomplished by either a vasectomy for men or a tubal ligation for women. A *vasectomy* is a surgical procedure in which the vas deferens is severed and tied to prevent the flow of the seminal fluid into the urinary canal. A *tubal ligation* is a surgical procedure in which the fallopian tubes are cut and tied, preventing passage of the ovum from the ovary to the uterus. Sterilizations are often sought because of

- economic necessity to avoid the additional expense of raising a child

- therapeutic purposes to prevent harm to a woman's health (e.g., to remove a diseased reproductive organ)

- genetic reasons to prevent the birth of a defective child

Elective Sterilization

Voluntary or elective sterilizations on competent individuals present few legal problems, as long as proper consent has been obtained from the patient and the procedure is performed properly. Civil liability for performing a sterilization of convenience may be imposed if the procedure is performed in a negligent manner. The physician in *McLaughlin v. Cooke*[50] was found negligent for mistakenly cutting a blood vessel in the patient's scrotum while he was performing a vasectomy. Excessive bleeding at the site of the incision was found to have occurred because of the physician's negligent postsurgical care. On appeal, the jury's finding of negligence was supported by testimony that the physician's failure to intervene sooner and to remove a hematoma had been the proximate cause of tissue necrosis.

The parents in *Goforth v. Porter Medical Associates, Inc.*[51] brought a medical malpractice action for expenses resulting from the negligence of the physician in performing a sterilization. The physician assured the plaintiff that she was sterile. The patient subsequently became pregnant and delivered a child. The plaintiff argued that as a result of the physician's negligence, she incurred $2,000 in medical bills and will incur $200,000 for the future care of the child. The district court dismissed the case. On appeal, the Oklahoma Supreme Court held that the parents could not recover the expenses of raising a healthy child; however, they could maintain an action for expenses resulting from the negligent performance of sterilization and the unplanned pregnancy.

Regulation of Sterilization for Convenience

Like abortion, voluntary sterilization is the subject of many debates over its moral and ethical propriety. Some health care institutions have adopted policies restricting the performance of such operations at their facilities. The U.S. Court of Appeals for the First Circuit ruled in *Hathaway v. Worcester City Hospital*[52] that a governmental hospital may not impose greater restrictions on sterilization procedures than on other procedures that are medically indistinguishable from sterilization with regard to the risk to the patient or the demand on staff or facilities. The court relied on the Supreme Court decisions in *Roe v. Wade*[53] and *Doe v. Bolton*,[54] which accorded considerable recognition to the patient's right to privacy in the context of obtaining medical services. The extent to which hospitals may prohibit or substantially limit sterilization procedures is not clear, but it appears likely that hospitals will be allowed considerable discretion in this matter.

Kansas enacted legislation declaring that hospitals are not required to permit the performance of sterilization procedures, and physicians and hospital personnel may not be required to participate in such procedures or be discriminated against for refusal to participate. Such legislation, which more frequently is enacted in relation to abortion procedures, often is referred to by the term *conscience clause* and was not found objectionable in Supreme Court decisions striking down most state abortion laws.

Therapeutic Sterilization

If the life or health of a woman may be jeopardized by pregnancy, the danger may be avoided by terminating her ability to conceive or her husband's ability to impregnate. Such an operation is a *therapeutic sterilization*—one performed to preserve life or health. The medical necessity for sterilization renders the procedure therapeutic. Sometimes a diseased reproductive organ has to be removed to preserve the life or health of the individual. The operation results in sterility, although this was not the primary reason for the procedure. Such an operation technically should not be classified as a sterilization because the sterilization is incidental to the medical purpose.

Involuntary/Eugenic Sterilization

The term *eugenic sterilization* refers to the involuntary sterilization of certain categories of persons described in statutes, without the need for consent by, or on behalf of, those subject to the procedures. Persons classified as mentally deficient, feeble minded, and, in some instances, epileptic, are included within the scope of the statutes. Several states also have included certain sexual deviates and persons classified as habitual criminals. Such statutes ordinarily are said to be designed to prevent the transmission of hereditary defects to succeeding generations, but several statutes also have recognized the purpose of preventing procreation by individuals who would not be able to care for their offspring.

Although there have been many judicial decisions to the contrary, the U.S. Supreme Court in *Buck v. Bell*[55] specifically upheld the validity of such eugenic sterilization statutes provided that certain procedural safeguards are observed.

Several states have laws authorizing eugenic sterilization. The decision in *Wade v. Bethesda Hospital*[56] strongly suggests that in the absence of statutory authority, a state cannot order sterilization for eugenic purposes. At the minimum, eugenic sterilization statutes provide a grant of authority to public officials supervising state institutions for the mentally ill or prisons and to certain public health officials to conduct sterilizations; a requirement of personal notice to the person subject to sterilization and, if that person is unable to comprehend what is involved, notice to the person's legal representative, guardian, or nearest relative; a hearing by the board designated in the particular statute to determine the propriety of the prospective sterilization; at the hearing, evidence may be presented, and the patient must be present or represented by counsel or the nearest relative or guardian; and an opportunity to appeal the board's ruling to a court.

The procedural safeguards of notice, hearing, and the right to appeal must be present in sterilization statutes to fulfill the minimum constitutional requirements of due process. An Arkansas statute was found to be unconstitutional in that it did not provide for notice to the incompetent patient and opportunity to be heard, or for the patient's entitlement to legal counsel.[57]

Current statutes do not authorize castration and often specifically prohibit it. Most eugenic sterilization statutes provide for vasectomy or salpingectomy. This prohibition against castration, along with provisions granting immunity only to persons performing or assisting in a sterilization that conforms to the law, is an added safeguard for persons subject to sterilization. Civil or criminal liability for assault and battery may be imposed on one who castrates or sterilizes another without following the procedure required by law.

ARTIFICIAL INSEMINATION

Generally, *artificial insemination* is the injection of seminal fluid into a woman to induce pregnancy. The term also may include insemination that takes place outside of the woman's body, as with so-called test-tube babies. If the semen of the woman's husband is used to impregnate her, the technique is called *homologous artificial insemination*. If the semen comes from a donor other than the husband, the procedure is identified as *heterologous artificial insemination*.

The absence of answers to many questions concerning heterologous artificial insemination may have discouraged couples from seeking to use the procedure and physicians from performing it. Some of the questions concern the procedure itself; others concern the status of the offspring and the effect of the procedure on the marital relationship.

Consent

The Oklahoma heterologous artificial insemination statute specifies that husband and wife must consent to the procedure.[58] It is obvious that the wife's consent must be obtained; without it, the touching involved in the artificial insemination would constitute a battery. Besides the wife's consent, it is important to obtain the husband's consent to ensure against liability accruing if a court adopted the view that without the consent of the husband, heterologous artificial insemination was a wrong to the husband's interest, for which he could sustain a suit for damages.

The Oklahoma statute also deals with establishing proof of consent. It requires the consent to be in writing and to be executed and acknowledged by the physician performing the procedure and by the local judge who has jurisdiction over the adoption of children, as well as by the husband and wife.

In states without specific statutory requirements, medical personnel should attempt to avoid such potential liability by establishing the practice of obtaining the written consent of the couple requesting the heterologous artificial insemination procedure.

Confidentiality of the Procedure

Another problem that directly concerns medical personnel involved in heterologous artificial insemination birth is preserving confidentiality. This problem is met in the Oklahoma heterologous artificial insemination statute, which requires that the original copy of the consent be filed pursuant to the rules for the filing of adoption papers and is not to be made a matter of public record.[59]

WRONGFUL BIRTH, LIFE, AND CONCEPTION

There is substantial legal debate regarding the impact of an improperly performed sterilization. Suits have been brought on such theories as wrongful birth, wrongful life, and wrongful conception. Wrongful life suits are generally unsuccessful, primarily because of the court's unwillingness, for public policy reasons, to permit financial recovery for the "injury" of being born into the world.

However, some success has been achieved in litigation by the patient (and his or her spouse) who allegedly was sterilized and subsequently proved fertile. Damages have been awarded for the cost of the unsuccessful procedure; pain and suffering as a result of the pregnancy; the medical expense of the pregnancy; and the loss of comfort, companionship services, and consortium of the spouse. Again, as a matter of public policy, the courts have indicated that the joys and benefits of having the child outweigh the costs incurred in raising a child.

There have been many cases in recent years involving actions for wrongful birth, wrongful life, and wrongful conception. Such litigation originated with the California case in which a court found that a genetic testing laboratory can be held liable for damages from incorrectly reporting genetic tests, leading to the birth of a child with defects.[60] Injury caused by birth had not been previously actionable by law. The court of appeals held that medical laboratories engaged in genetic testing owe a duty to parents and their unborn child to use ordinary care in administering available tests for the purpose of providing information concerning potential genetic defects in the unborn. Damages in this case were awarded on the basis of the child's shortened life span.

Wrongful Birth

In a wrongful birth action, the plaintiffs claim that but for a breach of duty by the defendant(s) (e.g., improper sterilization), the child would not have been born. A wrongful birth claim can be brought by the parent(s) of a child born with genetic defects against a physician who or a laboratory that negligently fails to inform them, in a timely fashion, of an increased possibility that the mother will give birth to such a child, therefore precluding an informed decision as to whether to have the child.

Recovery for damages was permitted for wrongful birth but not wrongful life in *Smith v. Cote*.[61] The physician in this case was negligent because he failed to test in a timely fashion for the mother's exposure to rubella and to advise her of the potential for birth defects. She therefore was entitled to maintain a cause of action for wrongful birth. However, for compelling reasons of public policy, the mother would not be permitted to assert on the child's behalf a claim for damages on the basis of wrongful life.

In *Proffitt v. Bartolo*,[62] the parents of a handicapped child stated a cause of action for wrongful birth against a physician who allegedly failed to properly interpret a rubella test performed during the mother's first trimester of pregnancy, thereby precluding the option of abortion. The physician had a duty to advise the parents so that they would have an opportunity to exercise the option of an abortion. If it could be established that the physician breached such a duty and that the parents would have terminated the pregnancy, the necessary causal connection would be demonstrated, and the parents would be entitled to recover for their extraordinary costs of raising the handicapped child and for any emotional harm that they might have suffered as a result of their child's handicap.

The Alabama Supreme Court in *Keel v. Banach*[63] held that a cause of action for wrongful birth is recognized in Alabama, and compensable losses are any medical and hospital expenses incurred as a result of the physician's negligence, physical pain suffered by the mother, loss of consortium, and mental and emotional anguish suffered by the parents. The basic rule of tort compensation is that the plaintiffs should be placed in the position where they would have been without the defendant's negligence. A jury could conclude that the defendants, in failing to inform the mother of the possibility of giving birth to a child with multiple congenital deformities, directly deprived her and her husband of the option to accept or reject a parental relationship with the child and thus caused them to experience mental distress.

The Alabama Supreme Court said that it agreed with the Illinois Supreme Court, finding:

> [m]any courts have accepted wrongful birth as a cause of action on the theory that it is a logical and necessary extension of existing principles of

tort law. . . . Some courts have recognized the cause of action because of the expanding ability of medical technology to accurately detect and predict genetic or other congenital abnormalities before conception or birth. Imposing liability on individual physicians or other health care providers, these courts say, vindicates the societal interest in reducing and preventing the incidence of such defects. . . . Other courts have expressed concern that refusing to recognize this cause of action would frustrate the fundamental policies of tort law: to compensate the victim, to deter negligence, and to encourage due care. . . . The Alabama legislature passed a new Medical Liability Act in 1987, regarding medical negligence causes of action. Nowhere in that Act are wrongful birth cases excluded as they are in the laws passed in Missouri and Minnesota.[64]

The state of Georgia did not recognize a cause of action for wrongful birth filed by the parent of child born with Down syndrome in *Etkind v. Suarez.*[65] Throughout her pregnancy, Dr. Etkind was a patient of Dr. Suarez. After giving birth to a child with Down syndrome, she and her husband filed suit against Suarez and his partnership, asserting a wrongful birth claim. The claim, brought by the parents of an impaired child alleged that but for the treatment or advice provided by the defendant, the parents would have aborted the fetus. The trial court granted the defendants' motion for judgment on the pleadings. A cause of action for wrongful birth is not recognized in Georgia.

In a New Jersey case, *Canesi ex rel. v. Wilson,*[66] the New Jersey Supreme Court reviewed the dismissal of an action for wrongful birth on the claim of the parents that, had the mother been informed of the risk that a drug, Provera, which she had been taking before she learned that she was pregnant, might cause the fetus to be born with congenital anomalies, such as limb reduction, she would have decided to abort the fetus. It was alleged that the physicians failed to disclose the risks associated with the drug. The physicians argued that the informed consent doctrine requires that the plaintiffs establish that the drug in fact caused the birth anomalies. The court rejected the argument and distinguished the wrongful birth action from one based on informed consent:

In sum, the informed consent and wrongful birth causes of action are similar in that both require the physician to disclose those medically accepted risks that a reasonably prudent patient in the plaintiff's position would deem material to her decision. What is or is not a medically acceptable risk is informed by what the physician knows or ought to know of the patient's history and condition. These causes of action, however, have important differences. They encompass different compensa-

ble harms and measures of damages. In both causes of action, the plaintiff must prove that a reasonably prudent patient in her position, if apprised of all material risks, would have elected a different course of treatment or care. In an informed consent case, the plaintiff must additionally meet a two-pronged test for proximate causation: she must prove that the undisclosed risk actually materialized and that it was medically caused by the treatment. In a wrongful birth case, on the other hand, a plaintiff need not prove that the doctor's negligence was the medical cause of her child's birth defect. Rather, the test of proximate causation is satisfied by showing that an undisclosed fetal risk was material to a woman in her position; the risk materialized, was reasonably foreseeable and not remote in relation to the doctor's negligence; and, had plaintiff known of that risk, she would have terminated her pregnancy. The emotional distress and economic loss resulting from this lost opportunity to decide for herself whether or not to terminate the pregnancy constitute plaintiff's damages.[67]

In addressing the issue of proximate cause, the court noted:

. . . the nature of the wrongful birth does not depend on whether a defendant caused the injury or harm to the child. Rather, the appropriate inquiry was viewed as to whether the defendant's negligence was the proximate cause of the parent's loss of the option to make an informed and meaningful decision either to terminate the pregnancy or to give birth to a potentially defective child.

• • • •

The appropriate proximate cause question, therefore, is not whether the doctor's negligence caused the fetal defect; the congenital harm suffered by the child is not compensable. Rather the determination to be made is whether the doctor's inadequate disclosure deprived the parents of their deeply personal right to decide for themselves whether to give birth to a child who could possibly be afflicted with a physical abnormality. There is sufficient evidence in the record of this case to enable the jury to make that determination.[68]

With the increasing consolidation of hospital services and physician practices, a case could be made for finding a hospital liable for the physician's failure to obtain informed consent where the hospital actually owns or controls the physician's practice or where both the hospital and the physician's practice are owned or controlled by another corporation that sets policy for both the hospital and the physician's practice.

Wrongful Life

A wrongful life claim is brought by the parent(s) or child who claims to have suffered harm as a result of being born. The plaintiffs generally contend that the physician or laboratory negligently failed to inform the child's parents of the risk of bearing a genetically defective infant and hence prevented the parents' right to choose to avoid the birth.[69] Because there is no recognized legal right not to be born, wrongful life cases are generally not successful.

> [L]egal recognition that a disabled life is an injury would harm the interests of those most directly concerned, the handicapped. Disabled persons face obvious physical difficulties in conducting their lives. They also face subtle yet equally devastating handicaps in the attitudes and behavior of society, the law, and their own families and friends. Furthermore, society often views disabled persons as burdensome misfits. Recent legislation concerning employment, education, and building access reflects a slow change in these attitudes. This change evidences a growing public awareness that the handicapped can be valuable and productive members of society. To characterize the life of a disabled person as an injury would denigrate both this new awareness and the handicapped themselves.[70]

A cause of action for wrongful life was not cognizable under Kansas law in *Bruggeman v. Schimke*.[71] A child born with congenital birth defects was not entitled to recover damages on the theory that physicians had been negligent when, after a prior sibling was born with congenital anomalies, they mistakenly advised the parents that the first child's condition was not because of a known chromosomal or measurable biochemical disorder. A fundamental principle of law is that human life is valuable, precious, and worthy of protection. A legal right not to be born rather than to be alive with deformities cannot be recognized. The Kansas Supreme Court held that there was no recognized cause for wrongful life.

A wrongful life action was brought against the physicians in *Speck v. Finegold* on behalf of an infant born with defects.[72] The court held that regardless of whether the claim was based on wrongful life or otherwise, no legally cognizable cause of action was stated on behalf of the infant even though the defendants' actions of negligence were the proximate cause of her defective birth. The parents could recover pecuniary expenses that they had borne and would bear for care and treatment of their child and that resulted in the natural course of things from the commission of the tort. The tort in this case was the failure of the urologist to perform a vasectomy properly and the failure of the obstetrician/gynecologist to perform an abortion properly. Recovery for negligence was allowed because the plaintiff parents did set forth a duty owed to them by the physicians and breached by the physicians with resulting injuries to the plaintiffs. Claims for emotional disturbance and mental distress were denied.

In *Pitre v. Opelousas General Hospital*,[73] the parents of a child born with a congenital defect filed a malpractice suit seeking damages for themselves and their child, alleging that the surgeon had been negligent in performing a tubal ligation. The suit also claimed that the hospital and the physician failed to inform Pitre that the operation was unsuccessful. A pathology report revealed that the physician had severed fibromuscular tissue, rather than the fallopian tissue, during the surgical procedure. The parents were not informed of this finding. The mother became pregnant and gave birth to an albino child. The court of appeals dismissed the child's claim for wrongful life and struck all the parents' individual claims with the exception of expenses associated with the pregnancy and the husband's loss of consortium. The Louisiana Supreme Court held that the physician owed a duty to warn the parents regarding the failure of the tubal ligation, the physician did not have a duty to protect the child from the risk of albinism, and the parents were entitled to damages relating to the pregnancy and the husband's consortium. Special damages relating to the child's deformity were denied.

In *Kassama v. Magat*,[74] Kassama alleged that Dr. Magat failed to advise her of the results of an alpha-fetoprotein blood test that indicated a heightened possibility that her child might be afflicted with Down syndrome. Had she received that information, Kassama contends, she would have undergone an amniocentesis, which would have confirmed that prospect. Kassama claims, if that occurred, she would have chosen to terminate the pregnancy through an abortion.

The Supreme Court of Maryland decided that for purposes of tort law, an impaired life was not worse than nonlife, and, for that reason, life itself was not, and could not, be considered an injury. There was no evidence that the child was not deeply loved and cared for by her parents or that she did not return that love. Allowing a recovery of extraordinary life expenses on a theory of fairness that the doctor or his or her insurance company should pay not because the doctor caused the injury but because the child was born ignores the fundamental issue that people afflicted with Down syndrome can lead productive and meaningful lives. They can be educated, employed, and form friendships.

Wrongful birth is based on the premise that being born, and having to live, with the affliction is a disadvantage and thus a cognizable injury. The injury sued upon is the fact that the child was born; she bears the disability and will bear the expenses only because, but for the alleged negligence of Magat, her mother was unable to terminate the pregnancy and avert her birth. The issue here is whether Maryland law is prepared to recognize that kind of injury—the injury of life itself.

The child has not suffered any damage cognizable at law by being brought into existence. One of the most deeply held beliefs of society is that life, whether experienced with or without a major physical handicap, is more precious than nonlife. No one is perfect, and each person suffers from some ailments or defects, whether major or minor, which make impossible participation in all the activities life has to offer. Our lives are not thereby rendered less precious than those of others whose defects are less pervasive or less severe. Despite their handicaps, the Down syndrome child is able to love and be loved and to experience happiness and pleasure—emotions that are truly the essence of life and that are far more valuable than the suffering that may be endured.

The right to life and the principle that all are equal under the law are basic to our constitutional order. To presume to decide that a child's life is not worth living would be to forsake these ideals. To characterize the life of a disabled person as an injury would denigrate the handicapped themselves. Measuring the value of an impaired life as compared to nonexistence is a task that is beyond mortals.

Unless a judgment can be made on the basis of reason, rather than the emotion of any given case, that nonlife is preferable to impaired life—that the child-plaintiff would, in fact, have been better off had he or she never been born—there can be no injury, and, if there can be no injury, whether damages can or cannot be calculated becomes irrelevant.

The crucial question, a value judgment about life itself, is too deeply immersed in each person's own individual philosophy or theology to be subject to a reasoned and consistent community response in the form of a jury verdict.

The mother, in her capacity as guardian for her minor son, brought a wrongful life action on behalf of the child against a physician. It was alleged, that because the physician failed to adequately and timely diagnose the child's condition, the mother was denied the opportunity to decide whether to terminate the pregnancy while legally allowed to do so. The court, in deciding whether to render a verdict in the child's favor or what damages, if any, should be awarded, a jury would be faced with an imponderable question: Is a severely impaired life so much worse than no life at all that the child is entitled to damages? The civil justice system places inestimable faith in the ability of jurors to reach a fair and just result under the law, but even a jury collectively imbued with the wisdom of Solomon would be unable to weigh the fact of being born with a defective condition against the fact of not being born at all; in other words, nonexistence. It is simply beyond the human experience to analyze this position. The court declined to recognize a cause of action for wrongful life brought by or on behalf of a child born with a congenital defect. It was untenable to argue that a child who already had been born should have the chance to prove it would have been better if he had never have been born at all.[75]

Wrongful Conception or Pregnancy

A wrongful conception or pregnancy claim is based on damages sustained by the parents of an unexpected child based on an allegation that conception of the child is the result, for example, of a negligent sterilization procedure. Damages sought for a negligently performed sterilization might include

- pain and suffering associated with pregnancy and birth

- expenses of delivery

- lost wages

- father's loss of consortium

- damages for emotional or psychological pain

- suffering resulting from the presence of an additional family member in the household

- the cost and pain and suffering of a subsequent sterilization

- damages suffered by a child born with genetic defects

The most controversial item of damages claimed is that of raising a normal healthy child to adulthood. The mother in *Hartke v. McKelway*[76] had undergone sterilization for therapeutic reasons to avoid endangering her health from pregnancy. The woman became pregnant as a result of a failed sterilization. She delivered a healthy child without injury to herself. It was determined that "the jury could not rationally have found that the birth of this child was an injury to this plaintiff. Awarding child rearing expense would only give Hartke a windfall."[77]

However, the costs of raising a normal healthy child in *Jones v. Malinowski*[78] were recoverable. The plaintiff had three previous pregnancies. The first pregnancy resulted in a breech birth; the second child suffered brain damage; and the third child suffered from heart disease. For economic reasons, the plaintiff had undergone a bipolar tubal laparoscopy, which is a procedure that blocks both fallopian tubes by cauterization. The operating physician misidentified the left tube and cauterized the wrong structure, leaving the left tube intact. As a result of the negligent sterilization, Mrs. Malinowski became pregnant. The court of appeals held that the costs of raising a healthy child are recoverable and that the jury could offset these costs by the benefits derived by the parents from the child's aid, comfort, and society during the parents' life expectancy. The jury was instructed not to consider that the plaintiffs "might have aborted the child or placed the child out for adoption [since] . . . as a matter of personal conscience and choice parents may wish to keep an unplanned child."[79]

The cost of raising a healthy newborn child to adulthood was recoverable by the parents of the child conceived as a result of an unsuccessful sterilization by a physician employee at Lovelace Medical Center. The physician in *Lovelace Medical Center v. Mendez*[80] found and ligated only one of the patient's two fallopian tubes and then failed to inform the patient of the unsuccessful operation. The court held that:

> the Mendezes' interest in the financial security of their family was a legally protected interest which was invaded by Lovelace's negligent failure properly to perform Maria's sterilization operation (if proved at trial), and that this invasion was an injury entitling them to recover damages in the form of the reasonable expenses to raise Joseph to majority.[81]

Some states bar damage claims for emotional distress and the costs associated with the raising of healthy children but will permit recovery for damages related to negligent sterilizations. In *Butler v. Rolling Hills Hospital*,[82] the Pennsylvania Superior Court held that the patient stated a cause of action for the negligent performance of a laparoscopic tubal ligation. The patient was not, however, entitled to compensation for the costs of raising a normal healthy child. "In light of this Commonwealth's public policy, which recognizes the paramount importance of the family to society, we conclude that the benefits of joy, companionship, and affection which a normal, healthy child can provide must be deemed as a matter of law to outweigh the costs of raising that child."[83]

As the Court of Common Pleas of Lycoming County, Pennsylvania, in *Shaheen v. Knight*, stated:

> Many people would be willing to support this child were they given the right of custody and adoption, but according to plaintiff's statement, plaintiff does not want such. He wants to have the child and wants the doctor to support it. In our opinion, to allow such damages would be against public policy.[84]

Prevention of Wrongful Birth, Life, and Conception Lawsuits

The occurrence of an unplanned pregnancy is not necessarily the result of negligence on the part of a physician. Although slight, there is known to be a given failure rate of sterilizations. Physicians can prevent lawsuits by informing each patient both orally and through written consent as to the likelihood of an unsuccessful sterilization, as well as the inherent risks in the procedure.

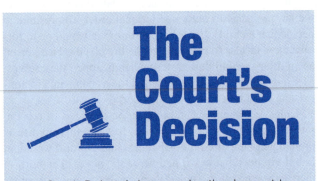

The Court's Decision

South Dakota's ban on abortion has yet to be heard by the Supreme Court. Sponsors of the bill want to force a reexamination of the ruling by the Supreme Court, which now includes two justices appointed by President George W. Bush.

CHAPTER REVIEW

1. *Abortion* is defined as the premature termination of a pregnancy, either spontaneous or induced. *Roe v. Wade* is the Supreme Court's ruling that, within certain guidelines, women are allowed to make decisions regarding how their pregnancies will end. According to *Roe v. Wade:*

   - during the first trimester, an abortion decision is between a woman and her physician

   - in the second trimester, the state may regulate the medical conditions under which an abortion is performed

   - a state can prohibit all abortions except those deemed necessary to protect maternal life or health during the third trimester—the final stage of pregnancy

2. States' and women's rights regarding reproductive decision have been further shaped and defined by a number of landmark rulings. In the 1992 ruling in the case of *Planned Parenthood v. Casey,* the Supreme Court nearly over-

turned *Roe v. Wade.* It did reject the trimester approach in favor of the Court evaluating the permissibility of state abortion rules based on whether they unduly burden a woman's ability to obtain an abortion. A rule is considered an undue burden if its purpose or effect is to place a substantial obstacle in the path of a woman seeking an abortion before the fetus is viable.

3. A *partial-birth abortion* is a late-term abortion that involves partial delivery of the baby prior to its being aborted. An Arkansas statute failed to prohibit this manner of abortion largely due to its broad coverage. The act was determined to be unconstitutional because it was unconstitutionally vague, imposed an undue burden on women seeking abortions, and did not adequately protect the health and lives of pregnant women.

4. In *Utah Women's Clinic, Inc. v. Leavitt,* the court determined that imposition of a 24-hour waiting period—except in the event of a medical emergency—does not impose an undue burden on the right to an abortion.

5. In *Doe v. Zimmerman,* the court declared unconstitutional the provisions of the Pennsylvania Abortion Control Act, which required that the written consent of the husband of a married woman be secured before the performance of an abortion. The court found that these provisions impermissibly permitted the husband to withhold his consent either because of his interest in the potential life of the fetus or for capricious reasons.

6. Individuals have a right to refuse to participate in abortions for reason of conscience or religious or moral conviction.

7. Several states have placed restrictions on abortions by reducing funding for the procedures. The Hyde Amendment, through which the U.S. Congress has limited the types of medically necessary abortions for which federal funds can be spent under the Medicaid program, opened the door to such provisions within states.

8. Physicians feel the effects of the abortion controversy. There are cases in which physicians have filed successful litigation regarding physical and mental injuries suffered as a result of the controversy.

9. *Sterilization* is defined as the termination of the ability to produce offspring.

10. A *vasectomy* is a surgical procedure performed on men in which the vas deferens is severed and tied to prevent the flow of seminal fluid into the urinary canal.

11. A *tubal ligation* is a surgical procedure performed on women in which the fallopian tubes are cut and tied. This prevents the passage of the ovum from the ovary to the uterus.

12. As long as proper consent is obtained and the procedure performed properly, elective sterilizations present few legal problems. A *therapeutic sterilization* is performed to preserve life or health. *Eugenic sterilization*—the involuntary sterilization of certain categories of persons—is often performed to prevent the transmission of hereditary defects and, in some states, is performed to prevent procreation by persons who would not be able to care for their offspring.

13. *Artificial insemination* most often takes the form of the injection of seminal fluid into a woman to induce pregnancy. *Homologous artificial insemination* is when the husband's semen is used in the procedure. *Heterologous artificial insemination* is when the semen is from a donor other than the husband.

14. *Wrongful birth* actions claim that, but for breach of duty by the defendant, a child would not have been born. *Wrongful life* suits—those in which a parent or child claims to have suffered harm as a result of being born—are generally unsuccessful. *Wrongful conception/pregnancy* actions claim that damages were sustained by parents of an unexpected child based on the allegation that the child's conception was the result of negligent sterilization procedures or a defective contraceptive device. Physicians can avoid liability in wrongful conception/pregnancy actions by obtaining oral and written consent that indicates that the physician has disclosed the inherent risks of the sterilization procedure.

REVIEW QUESTIONS

1. Discuss the legal and ethical issues involved in *Roe v. Wade.*
2. Do you agree that individual states should be able to place reasonable restrictions or waiting periods? Who should determine what is reasonable?
3. Should a married woman be allowed to abort without her husband's consent?
4. Give two arguments for and two arguments against partial-birth abortions.
5. Explain why you think *Roe v. Wade* is an example of legislating morality.
6. Do you agree that eugenic sterilization should be allowed? Why or why not?
7. Describe the distinctions among wrongful birth, wrongful life, and wrongful conception. Why is there such diversity in opinions from the different states?

WEB SITE RESOURCES

Center for Reproductive Rights	www.crlp.org
National Right to Life	www.nrlc.org
Pro-Life Action League	www.prolifeaction.org
Women's Reproductive Self-Determination	www.wordwiz72.com/choice.html

NOTES

1. WASHINGTON POST, February 23, 2006, at A01.

2. *Tragic: U.S. passed 47 million mark for abortions in 2005,* Michael Foust, Baptist Press, Jan 20, 2006. www.bpnews.net/bpnews.asp?ID =22488.

3. 410 U.S. 113 (1973).

4. *Id.* at 164.

5. *Id.*

6. *Id.*

7. *Id.*

8. *Planned Parenthood v. Casey,* 112 S. Ct. 2792 (1992).

9. 103 S. Ct. 2481 (1983).

10. 111 S. Ct. 1759 (1991).

11. 844 F. Supp. 1482 (D. Utah 1994).

12. 112 S. Ct. 2791 (1992).

13. 844 F. Supp. 1482 (D. Utah 1994) at 1494.

14. *Id.* at 1495.

15. 410 U.S. 179 (1973).

16. *Id.* at 198.

17. *Poe v. Gerstein,* 517 F.2d 787 (5th Cir. 1975).

18. 405 F. Supp. 534 (M.D. Pa.1975).

19. 486 U.S. 1308 (1988).

20. 428 U.S. 52 (1976).

21. 443 U.S. 622 (1979).

22. 101 S. Ct. 1164 (1981).

23. 515 So. 2d 1254 (Ala. Civ. App. 1987).

24. 107 F. Supp. 2d 1271 (2000).

25. 533 A.2d 523 (R.I. 1987).

26. 56 Fed. Reg. 22,762 (May 16, 1991).

27. 56 Fed. Reg. 22,762 (May 16, 1991).

28. 432 U.S. 438 (1977).

29. *Id.*

30. 432 U.S. 464 (1977).

31. 448 U.S. 297 (1980).

32. *Committee to Defend Reproductive Rights v. Myers,* 625 P.2d 779, 798 (Cal. 1981).

33. 56 P.3d 28 (Ariz. 2002).

34. 99 S. Ct. 675 (1979).

35. 492 U.S. 490 (1989).

36. 118 S. Ct. 1347 (1998).

37. 192 F.3d 794 (8th Cir. 1999).

38. *Planned Parenthood of Cent. N.J. v. Farmer,* 220 F.3d 127 (3d Cir. 2000).

39. 192 F.3d 1142 (8th Cir 1999), 120 S.Ct. 2597 (2000).

40. *Richmond Med. Ctr. For Women v. Hicks,* 409 F.3d 619 (C.A.4, Va. 2005).

41. www.crlp.org/pub_fac_ggrbush.html.

42. 515 F.2d 541 (8th Cir. 1975).

43. *Laws Protecting Pharmacist's Refusal,* National Constitutional Center, www.constitutioncenter.org/education/ForEducators/DiscussionStarters/ PharmacistConscienceLaws.shtml.

44. 565 N.Y.S.2d 833 (N.Y. App. Div. 1991).

45. *Forrester v. City of San Diego,* 25 F.3d 804 (9th Cir. 1994).

46. *Id.* at 807.

47. *NOW v. Operation Rescue,* 816 F. Supp. 729 (D. D.C. 1993).

48. *Id.* at 734.

49. ABORTION: A WORLD VIEW, SELF, Nov. 1992, at 54.

50. 774 P.2d 1171 (Wash. 1989).

51. 755 P.2d 678 (Okla. 1988).

52. 475 F.2d 701 (1st Cir. 1973).

53. 410 U.S. 113 (1973).

54. 410 U.S. 179 (1973).

55. 224 U.S. 200 (1927).

56. 337 F. Supp. 671 (E.D. Ohio 1971).

57. *McKinney v. McKinney,* 805 S.W.2d 66 (Ark. 1991).

58. Okla. Stat. Ann. 10, §§ 551–553.

59. Okla. Stat. Ann. 10, §§ 551–553.

60. 165 Cal. Rptr. 477 (Cal. Ct. App. 1980).

61. 513 A.2d 341 (N.H. 1986).

62. 412 N.W.2d 232 (Mich. Ct. App. 1987).

63. 624 So. 2d 1022 (Ala. 1993).

64. *Id.* at 1031.

65. 519 S.E.2d 210 (Ga. 1999).

66. 730 A.2d 806 (N.J. 1999).

67. *Id.* at 18.

68. *Id.*

69. *Smith v. Cote,* 513 A.2d 344 (N.H. 1986).

70. *Id.* at 353.

71. 718 P.2d 635 (Kan. 1986).

72. 66. 408 A.2d 496 (Pa. Super. Ct. 1979).

73. 530 So. 2d 1151 (La. 1988).

74. 136 Md. App. 38 (2002).

75. *Willis v. Wu,* No. 25915 (S.C. 2004).

76. 707 F.2d 1544 (D.C. Cir. 1983).

77. *Id.* at 1557.

78. 473 A.2d 429 (Md. 1984).

79. *Id.* at 431.

80. 805 P.2d 603 (N.M. 1991).

81. *Id.* at 612.

82. 582 A.2d 1384 (Pa. Super. Ct. 1990).

83. *Id.* at 1385.

84. 11 Pa. D. & C.2d 41, 46 (Lycoming Co. Ct. Com. Pl. 1957).

CHAPTER 15

Patient Rights and Responsibilities

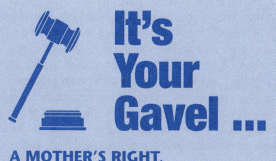

It's Your Gavel ...

A MOTHER'S RIGHT, A CHILD'S DEATH

Harrell, a Jehovah's Witness, was six months pregnant when physicians discovered a life-threatening blood condition that could deteriorate and place both her life and the life of the fetus in jeopardy. Because of religious beliefs, Harrell objected to a blood transfusion. After an emergency hearing, the court ruled that a blood transfusion could be given to Harrell if it was necessary to save the life of the fetus and that after the child was born, a blood transfusion could be given to the child if necessary to save the child's life. The Harrells appealed. The child was delivered by cesarean section and died two days later. No blood transfusion was given to Harrell or to the child. As a result, the hospital and the state claimed that the appeal of the trial court's order is moot. Because of the hospital's misunderstanding about its standing to bring such proceedings, the Florida District Court of Appeal addressed the issue as capable of repetition yet evading review.

The Florida Constitution guarantees that a competent person has the constitutional right to choose or refuse medical treatment. In cases where these rights are litigated, a party generally seeks to invoke the power of the state, through the exercise of the court's judicial power, either to enforce the patient's rights or to prevent the patient from exercising those rights. The state has a duty to ensure that a person's wishes regarding medical treatment are respected.

Harrell argued that the hospital should not have intervened in her private decision to refuse a blood transfusion. She claimed that the state never had been a party in this action, had not asserted any interest, and that the hospital had no authority to assume the state's responsibilities.[1]

WHAT IS YOUR VERDICT?

Every person possesses certain rights guaranteed by the Constitution of the United States and its amendments, including freedom of speech, religion, and association and the right not to be discriminated against on the grounds of race, creed, color, or national origin. The Supreme Court has interpreted the Constitution as also guaranteeing certain other rights not expressly mentioned, such as the right to privacy and self-determination and the right to accept or reject medical treatment. This chapter provides a brief overview of both the rights and responsibilities of all patients.

PATIENT SELF-DETERMINATION ACT

The continuing trend of consumer awareness, coupled with increased governmental regulations, makes it advisable for caregivers to understand the scope of patient rights and how to ensure them. The Patient Self-Determination Act of 1990 (PSDA),[2] for example, made a significant advance in the protection of the rights of patients to make decisions regarding their own health care. Health care organizations may no longer passively permit patients to exercise their rights but must protect and promote such rights. The PSDA provides that each individual has a right under state law (whether statutory or as recognized by the courts of the state) to make decisions concerning his or her medical care, including the right to accept or refuse medical or surgical treatment and the right to formulate advance directives.

PATIENT RIGHTS

Patients of the various states have certain rights and protections guaranteed by state and federal laws and regulations. Patients have a right to receive a clear explanation of tests, diagnoses, treatment options, prescribed medications, and prognosis; participate in health care decisions; understand treatment options; and discontinue or refuse treatment. It is recognized that a professional relationship between the physician and the patient is essential for the provision of proper medical care. The traditional physician/patient relationship takes on a new dimension when care is rendered within an organizational structure. Legal precedent has established that not only does the institution have responsibility to the patient, but that the patient also has responsibility to the institution.

Patients have the right to choose the medical care they wish to receive. As medical technology becomes more advanced, these decisions become increasingly difficult to decide. Should I have the surgery? Do I want to be maintained on a respirator? Frequently, these decisions involve not only medical questions, but moral and ethical dilemmas as well. What has the greater value, the length of life or the quality of life? What is the right choice for the patient? Although patients have a right to make their own care and treatment decisions, they often face conflicting religious and moral values. Often, it is difficult to make a choice when two roads may seem equally desirable.

Patient rights may be classified as either legal (those emanating from law) or human statements of desirable ethical principles (such as the right to health care or the right to be treated with human dignity). Both staff and patients should be aware and understand not only their own rights and responsibilities but also the rights and responsibilities of each other.

Right to Admission

At the time of admission, the patient should be informed in writing of his or her rights and responsibilities. If necessary, each patient has a right to have those rights explained.

Health care organizations must not discriminate by reason of race, creed, color, sex, religion, or national origin. Those that do discriminate violate constitutionally guaranteed rights. They also may be in violation of federal, state, and local laws. Discrimination in some states can be considered a misdemeanor and also may carry a civil penalty.

Most federal, state, and local programs specifically require, as a condition for receiving funds under such programs, an affirmative statement on the part of the organization that it will not discriminate. For example, the Medicare and Medicaid programs specifically require affirmative assurances by health care organizations that no discrimination will be practiced.

Federal and State Regulations

Discrimination in the admission of patients and segregation of patients on racial grounds are prohibited in any organization receiving federal financial assistance. Pursuant to Title VI of the Civil Rights Act of 1964, the guidelines of the Department of Health and Human Services (DHHS) prohibit the practice of racial discrimination by any organization or agency receiving money under any program supported by DHHS. This includes all providers of service receiving federal funds under Medicare legislation.

According to the Fourteenth Amendment to the Constitution, a state cannot act to deny any person equal protection of the laws. If a state or a political subdivision of a state, whether through its executive, judicial, or legislative branch, acts in such a way as to deny unfairly to any person the rights accorded to another, the amendment has been violated.

Government Facilities

Whether a person is entitled to admission to a particular governmental facility depends on the statute establishing that organization. Governmental hospitals, for example, are by definition creatures of some unit of government; their primary concern is service to the population within the jurisdiction of that unit. Military hospitals, for example, have been established to care for those persons who are active members of the military.

Although persons who are not within the statutory classes have no right of admission, hospitals and their employees owe a duty to extend reasonable care to those who present themselves for assistance and are in need of immediate attention. With respect to such persons, governmental hospitals are subject to the same rules that apply to private hospitals.

The patient in *Stoick v. Caro Community Hospital*[3] brought a medical malpractice action against a government physician in which she alleged that the physician determined that she was having a stroke and required hospitalization but that he refused to hospitalize her. The plaintiff's daughter-in-law called the defendant, Caro Family Physicians, P.C., where the patient had a 1:30 P.M. appointment. She was told to take the patient to the hospital. On arriving at the hospital, there was no physician available to see the patient, and a nurse directed her to Dr. Loo's clinic in the hospital. On examination, Loo found right-sided facial paralysis, weakness, dizziness, and an inability to talk. He told the patient that she was having a stroke and that immediate hospitalization was necessary. Loo refused to admit her because of a hospital policy that only the patient's family physician or treating physician could admit her. The plaintiff went to see her physician, Dr. Quines, who instructed her to go to the hospital immediately. He did not accompany her to the hospital. At the hospital she waited approximately one hour before another physician from the Caro Family Physicians arrived and admitted her. Loo claimed that he did not diagnose the patient as having a stroke and that there was no bad faith on his part.

The circuit court granted the physician's motion for summary judgment on the grounds of governmental immunity. The court of appeals reversed, holding that the plaintiff did plead sufficient facts constituting bad faith on the part of Loo. His failure to admit or otherwise treat the patient is a ministerial act for which governmental immunity does not apply and may be found by a jury to be negligence.

Right to Emergency Care

Patients have a right to receive emergency care in a hospital's emergency department. At the time of admission, each patient has the right to be informed in writing of his or her rights and responsibilities, including any explanations if needed.

Right to Bill of Rights

Patients have a right to receive a copy of their rights and responsibilities upon admission. Observance of a patient's rights will contribute to more effective patient care and greater satisfaction for patients, families, and caregivers. The patient has a right to make decisions regarding his or her medical care. Patients have a right to:

1. Receive an explanation of their rights.

2. Receive assistance in understanding their rights, including an interpreter.

3. Receive treatment without discrimination as to race, color, religion, sex, national origin, disability, sexual orientation, or source of payment.

4. Receive considerate and respectful care in a clean and safe environment free of unnecessary restraints.

5. Receive emergency care if needed.

6. Know the names, positions, and functions of any hospital staff involved in their care and refuse treatment, examination, or observation by them.

7. Receive complete information about their diagnosis, treatment, and prognosis.

8. Receive all the information they need to give informed consent for any proposed procedure or treatment, including the risks, benefits and alternatives to care or treatment.

9. They also have the right to designate an individual to give this consent if they are too ill to do so.

10. Discontinue care or refuse treatment.

11. Receive an explanation as to what can be expected if care is refused.

12. Refuse to consent or decline to participate in research.

13. Expect privacy while in the hospital and confidentiality of all information and records regarding their care.

14. Participate in all decisions about their treatment and discharge from the hospital.

15. Review and obtain a copy of their medical records.

16. Receive an itemized bill and explanation of all charges.

17. Complain, without fear of reprisal, about the care and services they are receiving.

18. Know the hospital's relationships with outside parties that may influence a patient's treatment and care. These relationships may be with educational institutions, insurers, and other health care providers.

19. Know about hospital resources, such as patient representatives or ethics committees, that can assist in resolving problems and questions about their hospital stay and care.

20. Be informed of any unanticipated outcomes or mistakes that may affect the patient's health status (e.g., administration of the wrong medication).

Right to Explanation of Rights

Patients have a right to receive an explanation of their rights and responsibilities. An organization's description of patient rights and responsibilities should be viewed as a document with legal significance whether or not the state in question has adopted a similar code. The rights of patients must be respected at all times. Each patient is an individual with unique health care needs. The patient has a right to make decisions regarding his or her medical care, including the decision to discontinue treatment, to the extent permitted by law.

Organization policy should provide that upon admission, each patient will be provided with a written statement of his or her rights, responsibilities, and a privacy notice. This statement includes the rights of the patient to make decisions regarding medical care and information regarding protected health information. Patients have a right to receive an explanation of the patient's bill of rights.

Right to Ask Questions

Patients have the right and should be encouraged to ask questions regarding their care ("I saw blood in my IV tubing. Is this OK? Is it infiltrating?" and "My wound dressing seems wet. Is this OK? Should the dressing be changed?"). Reducing medical errors requires that the patient actively participate in his or her care. Patients should not hesitate to ask for the following:

- Clarification of the caregiver's instructions.
- Interpretation of a caregiver's illegible handwriting.
- Instructions for medication usage (e.g., frequency, dosing, drug-drug, drug-food interactions, contraindications, side effects).
- Clarification of the physician's diet orders (e.g., "Does my iced tea contain sugar-free substitutes?").
- Explanation of the treatment plan.
- A copy of the organization's hand-washing policy.
- A description of the hospital's procedures to prevent wrong site surgery (e.g., the surgical site has been appropriately marked. If the site cannot be directly marked, have the surgeon draw an arrow pointing to the surgical site).
- The opportunity to provide the organization with a copy of any advance directives that may have been executed (e.g., living will).
- The right to appoint a surrogate decision maker should you become incapacitated.
- A second opinion.

Right to Know the Caregivers

Patients have a right to be informed of the names, qualifications, and positions of the caregivers who will be in charge of their care in the hospital. Patients have a right to know the functions of any hospital staff involved in their care and to refuse treatment, examination, or observation by any of them. These rights include:

- Patients should know who is treating them by name, discipline, and their role and responsibility in their care plan.
- Patients should know the names of all consulting physicians and hospital-designated caregivers.
- Caregivers should identify themselves to patients by name, discipline, specialty, and identification badge of the treatment team.

Right to Know of Third-Party Care Relationships

Patients have a right to know the hospital's relationships with outside parties that may influence their care and treatment. These relationships may be with educational institutions, insurers, and other health care caregivers.

Right to Participate in Care Decisions

Patients have a right to participate in all aspects of their care and should be encouraged to do so. They have a right to know their treatment options and to accept or refuse care.

Right to Informed Consent

Patients have a right to receive all the information necessary to make an informed decision prior to consenting to a proposed procedure or treatment. This information should include the possible risks and benefits of the procedure or treatment. The right to receive information from the physician includes information about the illness, the suggested course of treatment, the prospects of recovery in terms that can be understood, risks of treatment, benefits of treatment, alternative care options, and proof of consent.

Right to Have Special Needs Addressed

Patients have a right to an interpreter whenever possible. Patients who have physical or mental disabilities, or are hearing or vision impaired, have a right to special help, such as an interpreter.

Right to Sensitive and Compassionate Care

Patients have a right to be free from harassment, including verbal and physical abuse. They should receive considerate and respectful care given from competent caregivers who respect the patient's personal belief systems.

Right to a Timely Response to Care Needs

Patients have a right to have their care needs responded to within a reasonable time frame. Delay in responding to patient needs can put patients' lives at risk.

Right to Pain Management

Pain management is the process whereby caregivers work with the patient to develop a pain control treatment plan. Patients have a right to have a pain assessment and management of any pain identified. The process involves educating the patient as to the importance of pain management in the healing process. With current treatments, pain can often be prevented or at least be controlled.

Right to Refuse Treatment

Patients have a right to refuse treatment and be told what effect such a decision could have on his or her health. The responsibility of caregivers requires balancing risks and benefits. This balancing can lead to situations in which health care professionals view their obligations to a patient different from the patient's own assessment. The patient may refuse a certain procedure, for example, and forcing the patient to undergo an unwanted procedure would result in a failure to respect the patient's right of self-determination.

RIGHT TO REFUSE BLOOD TRANSFUSION

Citation: *Matter of Dubreuil*, 629 So. 2d 819 (Fla. 1993)

Facts

A patient was in the advanced stage of pregnancy when she was admitted through the emergency department of the hospital. At the time of her admission, she signed a standard consent form that included her agreement to have a blood transfusion if necessary. The next day she was going to have a cesarean section, but she would not consent to a blood transfusion because of her religious beliefs. During the course of the delivery, after she had lost a significant amount of blood, it was determined that she needed a transfusion to save her life, but she would not give her consent. Her estranged husband was contacted, and upon his arrival at the hospital gave his consent for the transfusion. After the first transfusion, physicians determined that she would need more blood, so they petitioned the circuit court for an emergency hearing to determine if they could give the transfusion in spite of the patient's lack of consent.

The trial court decided to allow the hospital to administer blood as they deemed necessary. The patient moved for a rehearing, and the circuit court denied it. The patient then sought review by the Florida Supreme Court, arguing that her federal and state constitutional rights of privacy, self-determination, and religious freedom had been denied.

Issue

Should a competent person have a right to refuse treatment? Did the patient's refusal of a blood transfusion constitute abandonment of her minor children, thus giving the state an interest that outweighed her constitutional rights of privacy and religion?

Holding

A competent person has a right to refuse treatment. Under Florida law, the state cannot intervene in a patient's right to refuse treatment if there is a surviving parent to care for minor children.

Reason

A competent person has the right to choose or refuse medical treatment, including all decisions relevant to his or her health. That right merges with the right to refuse a blood transfusion while exercising one's religious beliefs. A health care provider must comply with the patient's wishes unless supported by a court order to do otherwise. Here, the state interest was the protection of the children as innocent third parties. However, in this case there would have been no abandonment, because under Florida law, when there are two living parents, they share equally in the responsibilities of parenting. Had the patient died, her husband would have assumed the care of the children.

Discussion

1. What are the competing rights of the state and patient with regard to refusing blood transfusions because of the patient's religious beliefs?

2. Do you agree with the court's decision? Explain.

Right to Access Medical Records

The courts have taken the view that patients have a legally enforceable interest in the information contained in their medical records and, therefore, have a right to access their records. Some states have enacted legislation permitting patients access to their records. Patients may generally have access to review and/or obtain copies of their records, X-rays, and laboratory and diagnostic tests. Access to information includes that maintained or possessed by a health care organization and/or a health care practitioner who has treated or is treating a patient. Organizations and physicians can withhold records if it is determined that the information could reasonably be expected to cause substantial and identifiable harm to the patient (e.g., patients in psychiatric hospitals, institutions for the mentally disabled, or alcohol- and drug-treatment programs).

Right to Execute Advance Directives

Patients must be informed of their right to execute advance directives. The advance directives must be honored within the limits of the law and the organization's mission, philosophy, and capabilities.

Right to Designate a Decision Maker

Patients have a right to appoint a health care decision maker to make health care decisions when the patient becomes incapacitated or is unable to make decisions on his or her behalf.

Right to Privacy and Confidentiality

Patients have a right to expect that information regarding their care and treatment will be kept confidential. Information received by a caregiver in a confidential capacity relating to a patient's health should not be disclosed without the patient's consent. Confidentiality requires that the caregiver safeguard a patient's confidences within the constraints of law. An exception to the rule of confidentiality of patient communications is the implied right to make available to others involved in the patient's care the information necessary to that care.

The limitations of space and financial restraints make it difficult to continuously preserve a patient's right to privacy in many hospital settings (e.g., emergency departments). Nevertheless, health care organizations have a responsibility to provide for a reasonable amount of privacy for patients. For example, sign-in sheets are often used for appointments. The HIPAA Privacy Rule permits the incidental disclosures that may result from this practice. However, such incidental disclosures are only permitted when reasonable steps have been taken to minimize the release of confidential information. Sign-in sheets may not display medical information that is not necessary for sign-in purposes.

Disclosure may be made under compelling circumstances (e.g., suspected child abuse) to a person with a legitimate interest in the patient's health. The issues of confidentiality and privacy are both ethical and legal. Caregivers must safeguard each patient's right to privacy and the right to have information pertaining to his or her care to be kept confidential. Patients have a right to receive "Notice of Privacy Standards," a requirement under HIPAA.

Disclosures Permitted Without Authorization

The following list describes some of the ways a health care provider may disclose medical information about a patient without his or her written consent.

- Patient information (e.g., diagnoses, anesthesia history, surgical and other invasive procedures, drug allergies, medication usage, lab test results, and imaging studies) may be disclosed to other providers who may be caring for the patient in order to provide safe health care treatment.

- Disclosure of patient information to third-party payers so that providers can obtain payment for services rendered.

- Disclosure of patient information for health care operations.

- Disclosure of patient information as may be required by a law enforcement agency.

- Disclosure of patient information as may be required to avert a serious threat to public health or safety.

- Disclosure of patient information as required by military command authorities for their medical records.

- Disclosure of patient information to worker's compensation or similar programs for processing of claims.

- Disclosure of patient information to a coroner or medical examiner for purposes of identification.

Right to Limit Disclosures

Some of the individual rights a patient has regarding disclosure of access to his or her medical information are as follows:

- Right to request restrictions or limitations regarding information used or disclosed about one's treatment.

- Right to an accounting of nonstandard disclosures: The patient has a right to request a list of the disclosures made of information released regarding his or her care.

- Right to amend: If a patient believes that medical information regarding his or her care is incorrect or incomplete, he or she has a right to request that the information be corrected.

- Right to inspect and copy medical information that may be used to make decisions about one's care.

- Right to file a complaint with the provider, or the Secretary of the Department of Health and Human Services in Washington, DC, if one believes one's privacy rights have been violated.

- Right to a paper copy of a notice pertaining to the patient.

Right to Know of Restrictions on Rights

Any restrictions on a patient's visitors, mail, telephone, or other communications must be evaluated for their therapeutic effectiveness and fully explained to and agreed upon by the patient or patient representative.

Right to Discharge

Patients have a right to be discharged and not detained in a health care setting merely because of an inability to pay for services rendered. An unauthorized detention of this nature could subject the offending organization to charges of false imprisonment. Although patients have a right not to be held against their will, there are circumstances where reasonable detainment can be justified (e.g., a minor's release only to a parent or authorized guardian).

Discharge Orders

When discharging a patient, a physician should issue and sign all discharge orders. If there is no need for immediate care, the patient should be advised to seek follow-up care with his or her family physician.

Release from Hospital Contraindicated

The plaintiff in *Somoza v. St. Vincent's Hospital*[4] was admitted to the hospital during the 29th week of her pregnancy. She was admitted under the care of her private attending physician, defendant Dr. Svesko. She presented herself to the hospital with complaints of severe abdominal pain. Upon the plaintiff's admission to the hospital, Dr. Gutwein (a resident physician at the hospital) examined her. According to the notations she made on the plaintiff's chart, Gutwein independently formed the impression that the plaintiff might be suffering from either left pyelonephritis, premature labor, or polyhydramnios. Gutwein recorded a written plan and orders requiring that the plaintiff be hooked up to a fetal monitor. She also was to undergo a number of diagnostic tests, including a renal pelvic sonogram. The results of the sonogram were abnormal, and the radiologist recommended a follow-up sonogram. However, the attending physician did not order a follow-up. Despite the abnormal sonogram and various findings on the physical examinations, Svesko decided to release the plaintiff from the hospital because her pain had subsided. He orally conveyed this order to Gutwein. According to Gutwein, she did not formulate an opinion as to the correctness of the decision to discharge because she was of the opinion that it was not her place to make such a decision. Instead, pursuant to Svesko's instruction, on her early morning rounds, Gutwein simply signed an order discharging the plaintiff from the hospital. Four days later, the plaintiff returned to the hospital suffering severe pain and soon thereafter delivered twin girls. The twins were diagnosed as suffering from cerebral palsy resulting from their premature birth. The plaintiff brought a medical malpractice action against the hospital and Svesko arising out of the premature birth of the twins. The defendants filed a motion for summary judgment, and it was denied. The defendants appealed.

The New York State Supreme Court, Appellate Division, held that there were material issues of fact as to whether the mother's symptoms exhibited during her physical assessment contraindicated her release from the hospital and that ordinary prudence required further inquiry by the resident physician, Gutwein.

The plaintiffs presented an affidavit by expert witness Dr. Sherman, who stated that "the failure of the hospital staff to discharge without another physical examination, in my opinion, with a reasonable degree of medical certainty, is a departure from good and accepted medical practice. The resident clearly had an obligation to examine even a private patient in the face of a changing cervix and not just to discharge her pursuant to some attending physician's order."[5] A hospital whose staff carries out a physician's order may be held responsible where the hospital staff knows, or should know, that the orders are so clearly contraindicated by normal practice that ordinary prudence requires inquiry into the correctness of the orders. In this case, the plaintiff's release from the hospital was so clearly contraindicated by normal practice that ordinary prudence required further inquiry by Gutwein into the correctness of the discharge order.

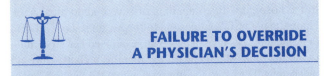

FAILURE TO OVERRIDE A PHYSICIAN'S DECISION

Citation: *Greer v. Bryant*, 621 A.2d 999 (Pa. Super. Ct. 1993)

Facts

While at the Philadelphia College of Osteopathic Medicine (PCOM) and under the care of her physician, Dr. Bryant, Greer was diagnosed with pre-eclampsia, a condition characterized by high blood pressure in the mother that poses a risk to the unborn child. On September 20, the patient suffered symptoms of fetal distress and was examined by the hospital's interns and residents. Tests ordered at the time of her visit revealed that the fetus was suffering from "decelerations," a periodic lowering of the heartbeat. Following her examination, Greer was instructed to return to the hospital on September 23. During that visit, it was noted that the fetus was experiencing "poor beat-to-beat variability." Greer was once again sent home with instructions to return to the hospital on September 27. However, on September 26, Greer, experiencing severe pains, called the hospital emergency department. She was told to wait until her scheduled appointment the following day. Her appointment was subsequently canceled because of weather. Upon the insistence of her sister, Greer went to the hospital on September 27, where she delivered her child. The infant, suffering from "severe meconium aspi-

ration" (inhalation by the fetus of its own fecal matter while in utero), died several days later.

The plaintiff alleged that the hospital, through its negligence, contributed to her child's death. Greer sued Bryant and PCOM separately. She alleged that based on the prenatal test results during her September 23 visit to PCOM, she should have been delivered on that date by Bryant. The plaintiff argued that even if the test results had been communicated to Bryant and he decided to send her home, the residents should have recognized the serious condition of the fetus and, if necessary, sought approval from their superiors to keep her at the hospital.

Bryant made an offer to settle, and the plaintiff accepted. The Court of Common Pleas, upon jury verdict, entered judgment for the mother, finding PCOM 41 percent liable to the plaintiff. PCOM appealed. The plaintiff's expert witness, Dr. Gabrielson, opined in her medical report that Greer should have been admitted and the child delivered despite the private physician's instructions to send her home.

Issue

Was Bryant properly notified that the fetus was suffering heart decelerations, and did the plaintiff's expert witness, Dr. Gabrielson, exceed her scope of opinion in her medical report by stating that the plaintiff should have been admitted and the child delivered despite the private physician's instructions to send her home?

Holding

The Pennsylvania Superior Court determined that the jury could find that the hospital's staff was negligent by not reporting the fetal distress of the unborn child to Bryant and that the plaintiff's expert witness did not exceed her scope of opinion in her medical report.

Reason

Although a resident and intern claimed that they had called Bryant, neither could testify as to the content of their conversation with him. Bryant testified that he did not recall receiving any telephone calls. He stated that if he had been aware of the decelerated heart rate, he would have ordered delivery of the child. "Since many of the critical events occurred on September 23, the jury could have determined that PCOM's employees' crucial nonfeasance occurred on that date . . . we must assume that the jury drew this inference." *Id.* at 1002.

Gabrielson, in three written reports and through oral testimony, testified that if the test results had not been reported to Bryant, such conduct, in her opinion, fell below the required standard of care. PCOM argued that this new "failure to override [Dr. Bryant's possible orders to send Rachel home] theory" was not contained in the reports and that they were unfairly surprised by the opinion. The superior court did not agree. The following is an excerpt from a report, which presents questioning of Gabrielson by the plaintiff's counsel:

3. Ms. Greer was sent to Osteopathic Hospital on three occasions for non-stress and contraction stress testing. On the second occasion . . . it was noted that the baby's heart rate showed poor variability . . . Could you explain the significance of this finding with regard to the health and well-being of the fetus?

A. The episode of bradycardia observed on September 20 was a very ominous sign and very suggestive of cord compression probably resulting from oligo-hydramnios. This would result in fetal distress with meconium passage and aspiration. It could result in sudden intra-uterine death.

4. Once the fetal distress was detected, did the hospital act appropriately by sending Ms. Greer home?

A. No.

5. What measures, if any, should have been taken to ensure the health and well-being of the fetus?

A. Ms. Greer should have been admitted and delivered. *Id.* at 1004.

The question of hospital negligence in sending the plaintiff home was within the fair scope of Gabrielson's oral testimony and written reports. "PCOM's decision to send Rachel home was contemplated and counsel should have anticipated that the 'failure to override theory' was looming." *Id.* at 1004.

Discussion

1. What steps should hospitals take when a patient is faced with life-threatening test results and the attending physician makes a determination to send the patient home?
2. What effect, if any, should such cases have upon the training of students and residents?
3. What action should a nurse take when faced with questionable actions by physicians and residents?
4. What policies and procedures should be in place to address similar issues in other patient care settings (emergency departments and ambulatory care centers)?

Right to Transfer

Patients have a right to be transferred when an admitting health care organization is unable to meet a patient's particular needs. This will at times necessitate the transfer of the patient to a facility that has the special services the patient requires. For this reason, it is important for each organization to execute transfer agreements with other health care organizations.

Health care organizations should have a written transfer agreement in effect with other organizations to help ensure the smooth transfer of patients from one facility to another when such is determined appropriate by the attending physician(s). Generally speaking, a transfer agreement is a written document that sets forth the terms and conditions under which a patient may be transferred to a facility that more appropriately provides the kind of care required by the patient. It also establishes procedures to admit patients of one facility to another when their condition warrants a transfer.

Transfer agreements should be written in compliance with and reflect the provisions of the many federal and state laws, regulations, and standards affecting health care organizations. The parties to a transfer agreement should be particularly aware of applicable federal and state regulations.

Patients also have a right to choose a receiving facility, whenever possible. The Medicaid patient in *Macleod v. Miller*[6] was entitled to an injunction preventing his involuntary transfer from the nursing home. The patient had not been accorded a pretransfer hearing as was required by applicable regulations. In addition, it was determined that the trauma of transfer might result in irreparable harm to the patient. The appeals court remanded the case to the trial court with directions to enter an order prohibiting the defendants from transferring the plaintiff pending exhaustion of his administrative remedies.

In another case, a 97-year-old resident in petitioned for review of a decision by the Department of Consumer and Regulatory Affairs to involuntarily discharge her from a community residence facility.[7] The resident had lived in the facility for eight years. The basis for the agency's decision was that the resident's discharge was essential to be in accordance with her prescribed level of care, pursuant to D.C. Code Annotated Section 32-1421(a). The only evidence presented by the facility was three medical certification forms completed by Dr. Choisser, the treating physician. Two forms indicated in an ambiguous check-off system that the resident required an intermediate level of care. This was contradicted by a letter written by Choisser that stated, "I see no reason why she should not continue to reside in Chevy Chase House with complete safety. . . . It is my opinion that a change in her residence, at this stage in her life, would prove harmful to her emotionally, and I strongly suggest that she be left as she is."[8] The court held that the need for the discharge was not proven by clear and convincing evidence.

Omnibus Budget Reconciliation Act of 1990

The Omnibus Budget Reconciliation Act of 1987 (OBRA 87) and 1990 was designed to reduce the federal budget deficit. The act sets mandatory minimum standards for nursing homes participating in the Medicare and Medicaid programs and addresses such areas as resident rights, quality of life, quality assurance, and facility practices.

Under the OBRA 87, nursing facilities must maintain or enhance the quality of life of each resident. Under OBRA 87, there is a comprehensive residents' bill of rights, including appeals of discharges and transfers; access and visitation rights; and admissions policy guaranteeing equal access to quality care.

Resident Suffers Indignities

Claims were made in *Henry v. West Monroe Guest House, Inc.*[9] that a nursing home resident suffered the indignities of having to lie in her own waste for extended periods of time.

This claim fell under the Nursing Home Resident's Bill of Rights (NHRBR) and not the Medical Malpractice Act (MMA). Although the nursing home asserted that the claim concerned decubitus ulcers and thus presentation to a medical review panel was necessary before filing suit in district court, changing a diaper is not considered medical treatment. A medical expert was not needed to establish whether a diaper was in need of a changing. Changing a diaper was something routinely performed by nurses' aides, and not under the direction of a physician. The resident would have suffered a loss of dignity for having dirty diapers, regardless of her residence in the nursing home. Under such analysis, the claims fell under the NHRBR, and not the MMA.

PATIENT RESPONSIBILITIES

The following description of patient responsibilities provides the reader with a sense of the ever-changing emphasis on patients' responsibilities from both an historical and contemporary perspective.

Historical Perspective

The following is an excerpt from Cornwall General Hospital's "Rules for Patients," which were posted in that hospital in 1897:

> 1. Patients on admission to the Hospital must have a bath, unless orders to the contrary are given by the Attending Medical Attendant.

> • • • •

> 6. Patients must be quiet and exemplary in their behaviour and conform strictly to the rules and regulations of the Hospital, and carry out all orders and prescriptions of the various officers of the establishment.

> • • • •

> 8. No male patient shall, under any pretense whatever, enter the apartments or wards for the females, nor shall a female patient enter the apartments or wards for males, without express orders from the Medical Attendant or Lady Superintendent.

> • • • •

> 10. Every patient shall retire to bed at 9 P.M. from First May to First November, and at 8 P.M. from November to May; and those who are able shall rise at 6 A.M. in the Summer and 7 A.M. in the Winter.

11. Such patients as are able, in the opinion of the physicians and surgeons, shall assist in nursing others, or in such services as the Lady Superintendent may require.

. . . .

13. Patients must not take away bottles, labels or appliances when leaving the Hospital.

14. No patients shall enter into the basement story, operating theater, or any of the officers' or attendants' rooms, except by permission of an officer of the Hospital.

. . . .

17. Any patient bringing spirituous liquors into the Hospital or the grounds, or found intoxicated, will be discharged.

18. Whenever patients misbehave or violate any of the standing rules of the Hospital, the Attending Physician may remove or discharge them, as provided by clauses 91 and 93 of Rules for Medical Staff.

Contemporary Perspective

A 1997 report to the president by the Advisory Commission on Consumer Protection and Quality in the Health Care Industry Consumer Responsibilities clearly describes patient responsibilities:

> In a health care system that protects consumers' rights, it is reasonable to expect and encourage consumers to assume reasonable responsibilities. Greater individual involvement by consumers in their care increases the likelihood of achieving the best outcomes and helps support a quality improvement, cost-conscious environment. Such responsibilities include[10]:
>
> - Take responsibility for maximizing healthy habits, such as exercising, not smoking, and eating a healthy diet.
>
> - Become involved in specific health care decisions.
>
> - Work collaboratively with health care providers in developing and carrying out agreed-upon treatment plans.
>
> - Disclose relevant information and clearly communicate wants and needs.

> - Use the health plan's internal complaint and appeal processes to address concerns that may arise.
>
> - Avoid knowingly spreading disease.
>
> - Recognize the reality of risks and limits of the science of medical care and the human fallibility of the health care professional.
>
> - Be aware of a health care provider's obligation to be reasonably efficient and equitable in providing care to other patients and the community.
>
> - Become knowledgeable about his or her health plan coverage and health plan options (when available) including all covered benefits, limitations, and exclusions, rules regarding use of network providers, coverage and referral rules, appropriate processes to secure additional information, and the process to appeal coverage decisions.
>
> - Show respect for other patients and health workers.
>
> - Make a good-faith effort to meet financial obligations.
>
> - Abide by administrative and operational procedures of health plans, health care providers, and government health benefit programs.
>
> - Report wrongdoing and fraud to appropriate resources or legal authorities.

Patient responsibilities also include:

- Providing caregivers with information relevant to medical complaints, symptoms, past illnesses, treatments, surgical procedures, hospitalizations, and medications. Information provided must be accurate, timely, and complete.

  - Patients must provide full disclosure of all information relevant to one's medical condition (the court of appeals in *Fall v. White*[11] affirmed the superior court's ruling that the patient had a duty to provide the physician with accurate and complete information and to follow the physician's instructions for further care or tests).

  - *Driving Against Medical Advice.* A patient had been sedated during the performance of a colonoscopy at a free-standing endoscopy center. He decided to drive himself home against medical advice; summary dismissal of claims against the clinic and a nurse with respect to fatal injuries that the patient received during a one-car collision was appropriate. The trial court correctly ruled that the nurse had no duty to prevent the patient from leaving its premises once she repeatedly warned the patient not to drive. The nurse was justified in relying upon the patient's false representations that he had a friend available to drive him home. She was not required to keep the patient in a gown in the recovery room once she learned the truth, and she was not required to use other options to prevent him from driving such as putting him in a taxi cab; putting him in a hotel; calling the police; admitting him to the hospital; personally driving him home; taking his keys away from him; or, physically restraining him. The center and the nurse owed no legal duty to the patient to do more than warn him that he should not drive. The center is not an insurer of its patients' safety. The patient acted recklessly in ignoring the advice he was given and suffered the consequences. The circuit court correctly found no duty to insure that no patient drives after the procedure.[12]

- Reporting unexpected changes in condition to caregivers

- Making it known whether one clearly understands the plan of care and course of treatment

- Following the treatment plan recommended (which may include following the instructions of nurses and allied health personnel)

- Following an organization's rules and regulations

- Refraining from the self-administration of medications not prescribed by the physician

- Accepting responsibility for the consequences of refusing treatment or not following instructions

- Being considerate of the rights of others, including health care personnel, in the control of noise, smoking, and limitation on number of visitors

- Being respectful of the property of others

- Recognizing the effect of lifestyle on one's health

- Keeping appointments (Patients have a responsibility to promptly notify caregivers whenever they are unable to keep a scheduled appoint-

ment. Failure to notify caregivers of a cancellation means longer delays for other patients who may already be finding it difficult to schedule appointments with specialists.)

- Speaking up and asking questions (Patients have a responsibility to ask questions and understand explanations. Such questions include those regarding medications, diet, and infection control-related issues.)

- Requesting a second opinion

- Describing the location and severity of pain

- With your surgeon, making sure that staff accurately mark the site of your surgical procedure to avoid confusion in the operating suite

- Making sure that the staff are aware of your preferences for care, including who your decision maker will be in the event that you become incapacitated

- Making sure that you understand caregiver instructions

RESPONSIBILITY TO DISCLOSE INFORMATION

Citation: *Oxford v. Upson County Hosp., Inc.,* 438 S.E.2d 171 (Ga. Ct. App. 1993)

Facts

Oxford brought a lawsuit against the Upson County Hospital and nurses claiming that their medical malpractice caused her injury from a fall in the hospital's bathroom. Oxford had been admitted to the hospital after having been diagnosed with gastroenteritis and dehydration. Nothing on her chart indicated that she had experienced dizziness. Testimony at the trial indicated that Oxford told her nurse that she had to go to the bathroom. Oxford did not inform the nurse that she felt dizzy. After the nurse escorted her to the bathroom, Oxford fainted while sitting on the toilet. As she fainted, she hit her head on the bathroom wall.

Two nurse experts testified that it is a patient's responsibility to communicate to the staff any symptoms the patient is experiencing. Oxford had told her physician prior to her hospitalization about feeling dizzy, but he had not related this information to the hospital's staff.

After a jury verdict for the hospital, Oxford appealed, arguing that the trial court's jury charges on causation, failure to exercise ordinary care, and comparative negligence were wrong.

Issue

Was there sufficient evidence to warrant the judge's charges to the jury?

Holding

The Georgia Court of Appeals affirmed the jury verdict and found that the judge's charges on the issues had been sufficient. The court followed its determination in *Carreker v. Harper,* 196 Ga. App. 658, 659, 396 S.E.2d 587 (1990), that when a patient fails to disclose all information related to her condition and fails to exercise ordinary care for her safety by seeking medical attention for her worsening condition, a charge of comparative negligence is applicable. In this case, the court did not require that Oxford diagnose herself, but she should have told the staff about her symptoms so that they could have treated her using their professional judgment.

Discussion

1. Do you agree with the appellate court's decision?
2. What precautions should the admitting physician and nurses take to help prevent similar injuries from occurring in the future? Explain.

PATIENT ADVOCACY

Because patients are often helpless and unable to speak for themselves, all caregivers, whether they are volunteers or paid staff, should consider themselves as patient advocates. Patient advocacy can be accomplished by caregivers providing care in their particular areas of responsibility and expertise.

Many states have established, by legislation, ombudsperson programs. Ombudspersons are responsible for the investigation of reports of resident abuse in nursing facilities. The primary impetus for the program came from the Nixon Administration, and gradually the program spread throughout the country. It was not until 1978 that the Older Americans Act Amendments (PUB. L. No. 95-478) mandated that every state have an ombudsperson program and that a certain amount of the Older Americans Act funds from Title III-B (the Social Services section) had to be allocated to the ombudsperson program.

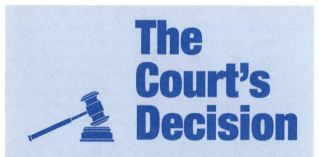

The Court's Decision

The Florida District Court of Appeal concluded that a health care provider must not be forced into the position of having to argue against the wishes of its own patient. Patients do not lose their right to make decisions affecting their lives when they enter a health care facility. A health care provider's function is to provide medical treatment in accordance with the patient's wishes and best interests, not supervening the wishes of a competent adult. A health care provider cannot act on behalf of the state to assert state interests. The Florida court found that when a health care provider, acting in good faith, follows the wishes of a competent and informed patient to refuse medical treatment, the health care provider is acting appropriately and cannot be subjected to civil or criminal liability.

CHAPTER REVIEW

1. The Patient Self-Determination Act of 1990 made a significant advance in the protection of a patient's right to make decisions regarding his health care. This act requires that health care organizations not only observe these rights, but also protect and promote them.

2. Each patient should be informed of his rights and responsibilities at the time of admission. If a patient does not understand his rights and responsibilities, they should be explained to the patient.

3. Patient rights include the right to admission; emergency care; ask questions; know the caregivers; know of third-party care relationships; participate in care decisions; have special needs addressed; sensitive and compassionate care; pain management; refuse treatment; access medical records; execute advance directives; designate a decision maker; privacy; know of restrictions on rights; discharge; and transfer.

4. Patients also have responsibilities. Patient responsibilities include maximizing healthy habits, such as exercising, not smoking, and eating healthy; being involved in health care decisions; working collaboratively with health care providers in developing treatment plans; disclosing relevant information and clearly communicating wants and needs; recognizing the risks and limits of medicine and the human fallibility of health care professionals; showing respect for other patients, caregivers, and visitors; making a good-faith effort to meet financial obligations; providing caregivers with relevant medical complaints, symptoms, past illnesses, treatments, and hospitalizations; making it known whether one clearly understands the plan of care and course of treatment; following the agreed-upon treatment plan; and speaking up and asking questions.

5. Caregivers should consider themselves patient advocates because of their position to help patients who are often helpless and unable to speak for themselves.

REVIEW QUESTIONS

1. Describe the significance of the Patient Self-Determination Act.
2. Describe the rights of patients as reviewed in this chapter.
3. Describe the responsibilities of patients as reviewed in this chapter.
4. Should a competent person have a right to refuse treatment?
5. Why do you think a patient's responsibilities are as important as his or her rights?
6. Should a hospital be able to assert whatever interest the state itself may have in seeking to compel an unwilling patient to undergo a routine, lifesaving medical procedure? Explain.
7. Discuss the importance of the patient's responsibility to communicate to the staff any symptoms he or she is experiencing.

WEB SITE RESOURCES

Home Care Provider & Patient Rights	www.nahc.org/Consumer/wamraap.html
Mental Health Patient Rights	www.athealth.com/Practitioner/Newsletter/FPN_3_11.html
Protect Your Healthcare	www.protectyourhealthcare.org
Patient Rights in New York	www.health.state.ny.us/
Patient Rights & Responsibilities	www.consumer.gov/qualityhealth/rights.htm

20 Tips to Help Prevent Medical Errors	www.ahrq.gov/consumer/20tips.htm
The California Patient's Guide	www.calpatientguide.org/
University of Michigan Hospitals' Patient Rights	www.med.umich.edu/1toolbar/visinfo/umh11.htm
Veterans—Patients Rights and Responsibilities	www.va.gov/healtheligibility/gettingcare/PatientRights.asp

NOTES

1. *Harrell v. St. Mary's Hosp., Inc.,* 678 So. 2d 455 (Fla. Dist. Ct. App. 1996).
2. 42 U.S.C. 1395cc(a)(1).
3. 421 N.W.2d 611 (Mich. Ct. App. 1988).
4. 596 N.Y.S.2d 789 (N.Y. App. Div. 1993).
5. *Id.* at 791.
6. 612 P.2d 1158 (Colo. Ct. App. 1980).
7. *Henson v. Department of Consumer and Regulatory Affairs,* 560 A.2d 543 (D.C. 1989).
8. *Id.* at 545.
9. 895 So.2d 680 (La. Ct. App. 2005).
10. *Consumer Bill of Rights and Responsibilities, Chapter Eight, Consumer Responsibilities,* President's Advisory Commission on Consumer Protection and Quality in the Health Care Industry, July 17, 1998. www.hcqualitycommission.gov/cborr/chap8.html.
11. 449 N.E.2d 628 (Ind. Ct. App. 1983).
12. *Young v. Gastro-Intestinal Center, Inc.,* No. 04-595 (Ark. 2005).

Acquired Immune Deficiency Syndrome

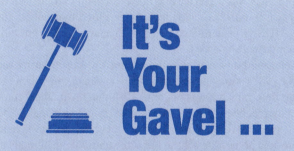

It's Your Gavel ...

AMERICA'S MOST FEARED DISEASE

The patient-plaintiff had a blood specimen drawn and sent to SmithKline Laboratories for testing for the human immunodeficiency virus (HIV). The laboratory informed the physician that his patient tested positive for HIV. On June 13, 1988, the patient was informed that he had acquired immune deficiency syndrome (AIDS). Not believing that his symptoms mimicked those of an individual with AIDS, the patient was retested for HIV. On three separate occasions (July 1, 1988; July 15, 1988; and July 22, 1988) involving two separate laboratories, he tested negative for the virus. In September 1990, the plaintiff later filed a lawsuit against his physician and SmithKline for the negligent interpretation and reporting of his blood samples as being HIV positive.

The circuit court ruled that the plaintiff stated a claim upon which relief could be granted in alleging that the defendants caused him to suffer major depression. The defendants appealed.[1]

WHAT IS YOUR VERDICT?

The AIDS epidemic is considered to be the deadliest epidemic in human history with the first case appearing in the literature in 1981.[2] AIDS, generally, is accepted as a syndrome—a collection of specific, life-threatening, opportunistic infections and manifestations that are the result of an underlying immune deficiency. AIDS is caused by the HIV, a highly contagious blood-borne virus, and is the most severe form of the HIV infection. It is a fatal disease that destroys the body's capacity to ward off bacteria and viruses that ordinarily would be fought off by a properly functioning immune system. Although there is no effective long-term treatment of the disease, indications are that proper management of the disease can improve the quality of life and delay progression of the disease. Internationally, AIDS is posing serious social, ethical, economic, and health problems.

SPREAD OF AIDS

AIDS is spread by direct contact with infected blood or body fluids, such as vaginal secretions, semen, and breast milk. At the present time, there is no evidence that the virus can be transmitted through food, water, or casual body contact; HIV does not survive well outside the body. Although there is presently no cure for AIDS, early diagnosis and treatment with new medications can help HIV-infected persons remain healthy for longer periods. High-risk groups include homosexual men, intravenous drug users, and those who require transfusions of blood and blood products, such as hemophiliacs.

Blood Transfusions

The administration of blood is considered to be a medical procedure. It results from the exercise of professional medical judgment that is composed of two parts: (1) diagnosis (the deciding for the need for blood); and (2) therapy (the actual administration of blood).

Suits often arise as a result of a person with AIDS claiming that he or she contracted the disease as a result of a transfusion of contaminated blood or blood products. In blood transfusion cases, the standards most commonly identified as having been violated concern blood testing and donor screening. An injured party generally must prove that a standard of care existed, that the defendant's conduct fell below the standard, and that this conduct was the proximate cause of the plaintiff's injury.

The most common occurrences that lead to lawsuits in the administration of blood involve

- transfusion of mismatched blood

- improper screening and transfusion of contaminated blood

- unnecessary administration of blood

- improper handling procedures (i.e., inadequate refrigeration and storage procedures)

In *Roberts v. Suburban Hospital Association,*[3] the Maryland Court of Special Appeals held that a blood transfusion constituted provision of a service (i.e., the rendering of health care rather than the sale of a product) and was subject to the exhaustion of Maryland's Health Claims Arbitration Act. The *Roberts* case involved the contraction of AIDS by a hemophiliac through the transfusion of contaminated blood. The court stated: "A transfusion is not just a sale of blood which the patient takes home in a package. The transfusion of the blood—the injecting of it into the patient's bloodstream—is what he really needs and pays for, and that involves the application of medical skill."[4]

The risk of HIV infection and AIDS through a blood transfusion has been reduced significantly through health history screening and blood donations testing. All blood donated in the United States has been tested for HIV antibodies since May 1985. Blood units that test positive for HIV are removed from the blood transfusion pool.

A summary dismissal against a hospital and the American Red Cross was ordered in *Kozup v. Georgetown University,*[5] in which it was alleged that the death of a premature infant was due to causes related to AIDS contracted through a blood transfusion given in January 1983, without the parent's informed consent. The case was dismissed on the basis that no reasonable jury would have found that the possibility of contracting AIDS from a blood transfusion in 1983 was a material risk. Dismissal also was justified on the basis that the transfusion was the only method of treating the child for a life-threatening condition.

A hemophiliac patient in *McKee v. Miles Laboratories*[6] contracted AIDS from a coagulation protein, which was provided by the defendants, and subsequently died. The defendants moved for summary judgment contending that at the time the plaintiff's decedent contracted AIDS, there were no tests that would have revealed the presence of the AIDS virus. The plaintiff argued that there was a genuine issue of material fact as to whether an alternative testing method was available when the decedent contracted AIDS in 1983. The district court held that the provision of blood and blood byproducts was a service and not a sale, and that the lack of any test to purify or screen blood or blood byproducts for the AIDS virus demonstrated that the supplier did not violate industry standards.

The methods available for testing for AIDS during the early 1980s were analyzed carefully in *Kozup,* in which the court determined it was not until 1984 that the medical community reached a consensus as to the proposition that AIDS was transmitted by blood. The district court in *McKee* held there was no need to rehash the same chronological medical history of AIDS that *Kozup* so methodically composed.

The plaintiff in McKee appealed the district court's decision to the U.S. Court of Appeals for the Sixth Circuit in *McKee v. Cutter Laboratories.*[7] The court of appeals upheld the district court's decision that the manufacturer was not negligent.

HIV TRANSMITTED TO PATIENT AND SPOUSE

Citation: *J.K. & Susie L. Wadley Research Inst. v. Beeson,* 835 S.W.2d 689 (Tex. Ct. App. 1992)

Facts

In January 1983, a blood center knew that blood from homosexual or bisexual males should not be accepted under any circumstances. The blood center's written policy provided that donors who volunteer that they are gay should not be permitted to donate blood.

On April 22, 1983, Kraus, a cardiologist, discovered that Mr. B, the patient, had severe blockage of two major arteries in his heart and recommended cardiac bypass surgery. During surgery, B received seven units of blood by transfusion. In May 1987, B had chest pain and trouble breathing. On June 5, 1987, B was hospitalized. Kraus consulted with two specialists in pulmonary medicine about the unusual pneumonia evident in X-rays of B's lungs. Because there was a possibility that the lung infection was secondary to AIDS, B was tested for HIV. Although B had not yet been formally diagnosed, physicians started him on therapy for AIDS.

B was formally diagnosed as HIV positive. His wife was then tested for HIV, and she learned that she was also HIV positive. On July 2, 1987, B expired. On April 21, 1989, the plaintiffs, Mrs. B and her son, filed suit against the blood center, alleging that her husband contracted HIV from the transfusion of a unit of blood donated at the blood center on April 19, 1983, by a donor identified at trial as Doe. The parties stipulated at trial that Doe was a sexually active homosexual male with multiple sex partners.

The plaintiffs contend that the blood center's negligence in testing and screening blood donors caused Mrs. B's contraction of HIV. At trial, the jury awarded the plaintiffs $800,000 in damages. The blood center filed an appeal arguing the evidence of causation was legally insufficient to support the jury verdict.

Issue

Did the evidence support a finding that the blood center's negligence was the proximate cause of B's contraction of HIV?

Holding

The Texas Court of Appeals held that the evidence supported a finding that the blood center's negligence in the collection of blood was the proximate cause of B's HIV infection.

Reason

The blood center, despite its knowledge about the dangers of HIV-contaminated blood, failed to reject

gay men, that the blood center's donor screening was inadequate, and that these omissions were substantial factors in causing Mr. and Mrs. B's HIV infections. The blood center's own technical director admitted that there was "strong evidence" that the blood accepted from Doe was contaminated with HIV. Another recipient of components of Doe's blood was diagnosed as HIV positive less than six months of Mr. B having been diagnosed as HIV positive.

Discussion

1. What precautions should the blood center have taken to prevent this unfortunate event?
2. What is meant by foreseeability as it relates to this case?

Sexual Transmission

Heterosexual relations are becoming a main conduit for the spread of AIDS. Heterosexual transmission is the predominant mode of infection and is increasing.

AIDS AND HEALTH CARE WORKERS

The ever-increasing likelihood that health care workers will come into contact with persons carrying the AIDS virus demands that health care workers comply with approved safety procedures. This is especially important for those who come into contact with blood and body fluids of HIV-infected persons.

SURGEON'S REFUSAL TO TREAT HIV PATIENT

The hospital's on-call surgeon in *Fiske v. U.S. Health Corp. of Southern Ohio*[8] had a duty to treat patients who came to the emergency room and required his services. The surgeon's alleged refusal to treat a patient allegedly because of his HIV-positive status constituted an act of omission that could provide the basis for an action in negligence. In view of the hospital's absolute duties to emergency room patients to provide competent medical care, it could be held vicariously liable for the negligence (both acts of commission and acts of omission) of the surgeon. Thus, notwithstanding the hospital's assertion the surgeon's refusal to treat the patient was a willful or intentional act that was outside the scope of his employment, the trial court was found to have improperly dismissed the patient's vicarious liability claim against the hospital.

SUSPENSION OF SURGICAL PRIVILEGES

An AIDS-infected surgeon in New Jersey was unable to recover on a discrimination claim when the hospital restricted his surgical privileges. In *Estate of Behringer v. Medical Center at Princeton,*[9] the New Jersey Superior Court held that the hospital acted properly in initially suspending a surgeon's surgical privileges, thereafter imposing a requirement of informed consent and ultimately barring the surgeon from performing surgery. The court held that in the context of informed consent, the risk of a surgical accident involving an AIDS-positive surgeon and implications thereof would be a legitimate concern to a surgical patient that would warrant disclosure of the risk. "The 'risk of harm' to the patient includes not only the actual transmission of HIV from the surgeon to patient but the risk of a surgical accident, i.e., a scalpel cut or needle stick, which may subject the patient to postsurgery HIV testing."[10]

CONFIDENTIALITY

Guidelines drafted by the Centers for Disease Control and Prevention (CDC) call for health care workers who perform exposure-prone procedures to undergo tests voluntarily to determine whether they are infected. The guidelines also recommend that patients be informed. Both health care workers and patients claim mandatory HIV testing violates their Fourth Amendment right to privacy. The dilemma is how to balance these rights against the rights of the public in general to be protected from a deadly disease.

State laws that protect the confidentiality of HIV-related information have been enacted. The unauthorized disclosure of confidential HIV-related information can subject an individual to civil and/or criminal penalties.

Information regarding a patient's diagnosis as being HIV positive must be kept confidential and should be shared with other health care professionals on a need-to-know basis. Each person has a right to privacy as to his or her personal affairs. The plaintiff surgeon, in the *Estate of Behringer v. Medical Center at Princeton,*[11] was entitled to recover damages from the hospital and its laboratory director for the unauthorized disclosure of his condition during his stay at the hospital. The hospital and the director breached their duty to maintain confidentiality of the surgeon's medical records by allowing placement of the patient's test results in his medical chart without limiting access to the chart, which

they knew was available to the entire hospital community. "The medical center breached its duty of confidentiality to the plaintiff, as a patient, when it failed to take reasonable precautions regarding the plaintiff's medical records to prevent the patient's AIDS diagnosis from becoming a matter of public knowledge."[12]

The hospital in *Tarrant County Hospital District v. Hughes*[13] was found to have properly disclosed the names and addresses of blood donors in a wrongful death action alleging that a patient contracted AIDS from a blood transfusion administered in the hospital. The physician-patient privilege expressed in the Texas Rules of Evidence did not apply to preclude such disclosure because the record did not reflect that any such relationship had been established. The disclosure was not an impermissible violation of the donors' right of privacy. The societal interest in maintaining an effective blood donor program did not override the plaintiff's right to receive such information. The order prohibited disclosure of the donors' names to third parties.

In *Doe v. University of Cincinnati,*[14] a patient who was infected with HIV-contaminated blood during surgery brought an action against a hospital and a blood bank. The trial court granted the patient's request to discover the identity of the blood donor, and the defendants appealed. The court of appeals held that the potential injury to a donor in revealing his identity outweighed the plaintiff's modest interest in learning of the donor's identity. A blood donor has a constitutional right to privacy not to be identified as a donor of blood that contains HIV. No test had been developed at the time of the plaintiff's blood transfusion in July 1984 to determine the existence of AIDS antibodies. By May 27, 1986, all donors donating blood through the defendant blood bank were tested for the presence of HIV antibodies. Patients who received blood from donors who tested positive were to be notified through their physicians. In this case, the plaintiff's family was notified because of his age and other disability.

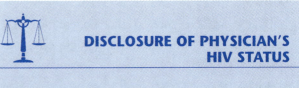

DISCLOSURE OF PHYSICIAN'S HIV STATUS

Citation: *Application of Milton S. Hershey Med. Ctr.,* 639 A.2d 159 (Pa. 1993)

Facts

The physician, John Doe, was a resident in obstetrics and gynecology (OB/GYN) at the medical center. In 1991, he cut his hand with a scalpel while he was assisting another physician. Because of the uncertainty that blood had been transferred from

Doe's hand wound to the patient through an open surgical incision, he agreed to have a blood test for HIV. His blood tested positive and he withdrew himself from participation in further surgical procedures. The medical center and Harrisburg Hospital, where Doe also participated in surgery, identified those patients who could be at risk. The medical center identified 279 patients, and Harrisburg identified 168 patients who fell into this category. Because hospital records did not identify those surgeries in which physicians may have accidentally cut themselves, the hospitals filed petitions in the Court of Common Pleas, alleging that there was, under the Confidentiality of HIV-Related Information Act [35 P.S. § 7608(a)(2)], a "compelling need" to disclose information regarding Doe's condition to those patients who conceivably could have been exposed to HIV. Doe argued that there was no compelling need to disclose the information and that he was entitled to confidentiality under the act.

The court issued an order for the selective release of information by: (1) providing the name of Doe to physicians and residents with whom he had participated in a surgical procedure or obstetrical care; (2) providing a letter to the patients at risk describing Doe as a resident in OB/GYN; and (3) setting forth the relevant period of such service. The physicians were prohibited under the HIV act from disclosing Doe's name. The superior court affirmed the decision of the trial court and Doe appealed.

Issue

Was there a need to release selective information regarding Doe's HIV-positive status as determined by the trial court?

Holding

The Pennsylvania Supreme Court held that a compelling need existed for at least a partial disclosure of the physician's HIV status.

Reason

There was no question that Doe's HIV-positive status fell within the HIV act's definition of confiden-

tial information. There were, however, exceptions within the HIV act that allowed for disclosure of the information. In this case, there was a compelling reason to allow disclosure of the information. All the medical experts who testified agreed that there was some risk of exposure and that some form of notice should be given to those patients at risk. Even the expert witness presented by Doe agreed that there was at least some conceivable risk of exposure and that giving a limited form of notice would not be unreasonable. Failure to notify patients at risk could result in the spread of the disease to other non-infected individuals through sexual contact and through exposure to other body fluids. Doe's name was not revealed to the patients, only the fact that a resident physician who participated in their care had tested HIV positive. "No principle is more deeply embedded in the law than that expressed in the maxim Salus populi suprema lex, . . . (the welfare of the people is the supreme law), and a more compelling and consistent application of that principle than the one presented would be quite difficult to conceive." *Id.* at 163.

Discussion

1. Do you agree that there was a need for a partial disclosure of the physician's HIV status?
2. If "the welfare of the people is the supreme law," did the court fall short of its responsibility by not allowing disclosure of the physician's name?
3. Why was it necessary to disclose Doe's full name to those physicians with whom he worked?

Health care professionals and others working with AIDS patients have a right to know when they are caring for patients with highly contagious diseases. There are times when the duty to disclose outweighs the rights of confidentiality. The U.S. Court of Appeals for the Tenth Circuit in *Dunn v. White*[15] declared there is no Fourth Amendment impediment to a state prison's policy of testing the blood of all inmates for HIV. Under the U.S. Supreme Court's drug-testing decisions, the proper analysis is to balance the prisoner's interest in being free from bodily intrusion inherent in a blood test against the prison's institutional rights in combating the disease. The U.S. Court of Appeals held that in or out of prison, a person has only a limited privacy interest in not having his or her blood tested. The court cited *Schmerber v. California*,[16] which rejected a Fourth Amendment challenge to the blood testing of a suspected drunken driver. Against the prisoner's minimal interest, prison authorities have a strong interest in controlling the spread of HIV.

Sexual Partners

A person has a right to know when his or her partner has tested positive for HIV. Physicians are expected to counsel an HIV-positive patient to notify his or her sexual or needle-sharing partners or to seek help in doing so from public health officials. If a patient refuses to do so, a physician may, without the patient's consent, notify a sexual partner known to be at risk of HIV infection. Some states have developed informational brochures and consent, release, and partner notification forms.

Patient's HIV Status Disclosed

A legal action was filed alleging that a physician had disclosed, in a worker's compensation report, the patient's HIV status to his employer without his consent. Learning of the employee's HIV disease, his supervisor and restaurant owner had agreed that the employee's HIV disease could pose a PR nightmare and that the employee would have to be discharged. The employee, Francies, was notified by mail that he had been replaced as general manager and would thereafter be considered an employee on unpaid leave without benefits. The employee's termination from his employment caused him to suffer physical, mental, and emotional distress. Evidence supported a finding of medical malpractice where the testimony of expert witnesses for both sides established that the standard of care was breached by the physician's disclosure of the patient's HIV status without his consent. The plaintiff-employee had a constitutionally protected interest in the privacy of his medical records, and his right to privacy.[17]

HIV Status Properly Disclosed to Employer

The trial court properly dismissed a claim for breach of medical confidentiality and unreasonable violation of privacy by an HIV-positive patient seeking damages from a consulting physician for disclosing his HIV status in a medical record that was forwarded to the employer. The patient, a veterinary assistant who had developed an infection after being bitten by a cat, sought treatment for a work-related injury. Thus, notwithstanding his assertion that KRS 214.\-181 conferred an absolute right to privacy with respect to his HIV

status, the matter was governed by provisions of the Kentucky Workers' Compensation Act, KRS 342.\-020\-(8) and 803 KAR 25:\-010, under which the patient was required to execute a release for medical information concerning his treatment for the work-related injury. Since the employer was required by law to pay the work-related medical bills, the very same law gave the employer the right to know the pertinent medical information.[18]

RIGHT TO TREATMENT

Some health care organizations are expressing in their ethics statements that HIV-infected patients have a right not to be discriminated against in the provision of treatment. The ethics committee of the American Academy of Dermatology, for example, states that "it is unethical for a physician to discriminate against a class or category of patients and to refuse the management of a patient because of medical risk, real or imagined."[19] Patients with HIV infection, therefore, should receive the same compassionate and competent care given to other patients.

MANDATORY TESTING

The U.S. District Court found that routine testing of firefighters and paramedics for the AIDS virus does not violate an individual's Fourth Amendment or constitutional privacy rights.[20] Because the tested employees are a high-risk group for contracting and transmitting HIV to the public, the city has a compelling interest and legal duty to protect the public from contracting the virus. Firefighters and paramedics are in a higher-risk category than hospital personnel because they work in a noncontrolled setting. *Skinner v. Railway Executives Association* confirmed "society's judgment that blood tests do not constitute an unduly extensive imposition on an individual's privacy and bodily integrity."[21] However, "mandatory testing by a governmental agency for the sole purpose of obtaining a baseline to determine whether an employee contracted AIDS on the job, and thereby to determine the validity of any future worker's compensation claim, is not valid. Mandatory AIDS testing of employees can be valid only if the group of employees involved is at risk of contracting or transmitting AIDS to the public."[22]

NEWS MEDIA AND CONFIDENTIALITY

The Pennsylvania Superior Court in *Stenger v. Lehigh Valley Hospital Center*[23] upheld the court of common pleas' order denying the petition of The Morning Call, Inc., which challenged a court order closing judicial proceedings to the press and public in a civil action against a hospital and physicians. A patient and her family had contracted AIDS after the patient received a blood transfusion. The access of the media to pretrial discovery proceedings in a civil action is subject to reasonable control by the court in which the action is pending. The protective order limiting public access to pretrial discovery material did not violate the newspaper's First Amendment rights. The discovery documents were not judicial records to which the newspaper had a common-law right of access. Good cause existed for nondisclosure of information about the intimate personal details of the plaintiffs' lives, disclosure of which would cause undue humiliation.

DISCRIMINATION

Discrimination against persons who have contracted the AIDS virus often is found to be in violation of their constitutional rights. The sufferings and hardships of those who have contracted the disease extend to family as well as friends. The infringements of those infected with HIV include discrimination in access to health care, education, employment, housing, insurance benefits, and military service. Those who believe that they have been discriminated against can contact their state's human rights commission.

Access to Health Care

The need for health care for AIDS patients continues to grow, particularly for those who are homeless or have no family support system. An AIDS survey conducted by mail in Oregon revealed that 79 percent of hospitals, 26 percent of skilled nursing facilities, and 69 percent of home health agencies responding had adequate resources to care for AIDS patients.[24] In response to the need for nursing home care, some health departments are encouraging the development of specialized HIV/AIDS nursing homes that will combine medical services and drug treatment for AIDS patients who have become infected through drug abuse.

With 40 million people around the world infected with AIDS, the Internet provides a wealth of information as to resources for care and treatment. The greatest challenge involves the nearly 90 percent of AIDS patients who live in resource-poor countries. As a result of poor access to health care, former President Bill Clinton made the battle against HIV/AIDS a focal point of his foundation's activities in global health security to reach the underserved populations.[25]

Education

A school's refusal to admit students with HIV generally is considered an unnecessary restriction on an individual's liberty. However, there are circumstances where it would be unreasonable to infer that Congress intended to force institutions to accept or readmit persons who pose a significant risk of harm to themselves or others. For example, in *Doe v. Washington University,*[26] the university disenrolled a dental student based on his positive HIV status: "the circumstance surrounding plaintiff's HIV status presented little alternative to those charged with evaluating plaintiff's ability to qualify as a dental student."[27]

Employment

AIDS-related employment issues are a two-sided coin: employment discrimination on one side and the refusal of employees to care for AIDS patients on the other. The growing consensus of case law indicates employment-related discrimination is unlawful. The California Court of Appeals, Second District, in *Raytheon v. Fair Employment & Housing Commission,*[28] determined an employee with AIDS who was admitted to and treated in a hospital was unlawfully denied his right to return to work after treatment in the hospital. The court held that AIDS is a protected physical handicap under California's Fair Employment and Housing Act and that the employer failed to prove its defense of protecting the health and safety of its other workers. The employer ignored the advice of county health officials and communicable disease authorities that there was no risk to other employees at the plant.

Employees who have contracted the AIDS virus and whose symptoms warrant should not be placed in positions that threaten the health and safety of patients and employees. The court in *School Board of Nassau County v. Airline* noted that "a person who poses a significant risk of communicating an infectious disease will not be otherwise qualified for his or her job if reasonable accommodations will not eliminate the risk."[29]

Situations may arise from time to time in which employees may refuse to treat AIDS patients. There are two basic approaches that can be taken in dealing with such problems. The most beneficial course of action for the employee and the institution would be to embark on a program of educating the staff. The alternative and less-desirable response to the problem may require that disciplinary steps be initiated against the employee. Such action could be justified on the basis that a health care organization has a right to manage its workforce by assigning staff in a responsible manner to carry out its mission of caring for the sick.

In the final analysis, many competing issues (e.g., humanitarian, legal, moral, ethical, and religious) pertain to the rights of patients and caregivers who have contracted the AIDS virus, as well as those who have not, and employers. As the search for answers continues, the debates and controversies will be heated. It is hoped that solutions that will meet the needs of those who have been infected with the

AIDS virus and those who are involved with providing health care to them will be forthcoming.

Insurance Benefits

In *Weaver v. Reagan*,[30] Medicaid recipients who were denied benefits for AZT (zidovudine, trade name Retrovir) treatments were found to be entitled to summary judgment in their class action suit to require Missouri's authorities to provide Medicaid coverage for the cost of AZT treatments. In this case, the U.S. Court of Appeals for the Eighth Circuit decided that states must provide Medicaid coverage for the drug AZT to HIV-infected individuals who are eligible for Medicaid and whose physicians had certified that AZT was a medically necessary treatment. The state argued that its reliance on the Food and Drug Administration's approval statement in limiting coverage for AZT treatments was a reasonable exercise of its discretion. The Eighth Circuit disagreed.

NEGLIGENCE

As noted in this section, there have been a variety of HIV- and AIDS-related lawsuits. Such suits, as described here, have involved the administration of blood and untimely diagnosis of AIDS.

Administration of Wrong Blood

The plaintiff, Mrs. Bordelon, in *Bordelon v. St. Francis Cabrini Hospital*,[31] was admitted to the hospital to undergo a hysterectomy. Prior to surgery, she provided the hospital with her own blood in case it was needed during surgery. During surgery, Bordelon did indeed need blood, but was administered donor blood other than her own. Bordelon filed a lawsuit claiming that the hospital's failure to provide her with her own blood resulted in her suffering mental distress. The hospital filed a peremptory exception claiming that there was no cause of action. The Ninth Judicial District Court dismissed the suit because the plaintiff did not allege that she suffered any physical injury.

On appeal by the plaintiff, the court of appeal held that the plaintiff did in fact state a cause of action for mental distress. It is well established in law that a claim for negligent infliction of emotional distress unaccompanied by physical injury is a viable claim of action. It is indisputable that HIV can be transmitted through blood transfusions even when the standard procedure for screening for the virus is in place. Bordelon's fear was easily associated with receiving someone else's blood, and therefore a conceivable consequence of the defendant's negligent act.[32] The hospital acquired a duty to ensure that Bordelon received her own blood when it accepted that as a condition of her hospitalization. It is undisputed that the hospital had a duty to administer the plaintiff's own blood. The hospital breached that duty by administering the wrong blood.

FAILURE TO MAKE A TIMELY DIAGNOSIS

Citation: *Doe v. McNulty*, 630 So. 2d 825 (La. Ct. App. 1993)

Facts

The plaintiff, Jane Doe, had been exposed to HIV as the result of sexual contact. The plaintiff consulted her defendant physicians but they failed to diagnose her condition as being positive for either HIV or AIDS. The disease weakened her immune system and she developed pneumonia and was admitted to a hospital. The patient was eventually diagnosed with AIDS. The patient's infectious disease expert, Dr. Hill, claimed that proper diagnosis prior to her acute episode would have provided greater opportunity for improved long-term treatment. The defendants admitted that they negligently failed to timely diagnose the patient's condition.

The defendants' expert witness, Dr. Lutz, testified from his review of the patient's medical record that the patient's diagnosis could not have been determined based on the symptoms as described in the record. Lutz never examined the patient and based his determination on the documentation contained in the medical record. Lutz did, however, agree that if the patient's immune system had not been totally destroyed, preventive treatment could have resulted in a longer life span.

The civil district court entered judgment on a jury verdict of $700,000 in general damages, which included pain and suffering, mental anguish, disability, and the loss of the enjoyment of life, and $314,000 for medical and special damages. The defendant appealed.

Issue

Did the defendant's failure to timely diagnose the plaintiff's condition shortened her life span?

Holding

The Louisiana Court of Appeal held that the evidence supported the jury's finding that the defendant failed to timely diagnose the plaintiff's condition.

Reason

The medical defendants agreed that they negligently failed to timely diagnose the patient's condition. The plaintiff's expert witness testified that within the "reasonable medical probability" standard and the "more-likely-than-not" standard, if the plaintiff had been properly diagnosed and treated no later than August 18, 1990, which was the date the medical defendants should have diagnosed and treated the patient, then she would have not contracted pneumonia. She would have worked, as well as lived, for another year.

Discussion

1. Discuss the importance of a thorough history and physical examination.
2. Discuss what steps should be taken to assure that a complete history and physical examination and plan of care (including all recommended treatments) are thorough and available in a readable format to those caregivers involved in a patient's care.

Patient Wrongly Notified She Had AIDS

A service member brought an action under the Federal Tort Claims Act in *Johnson v. United States*,[33] alleging that on or about October 8, 1986, Army physicians and medical personnel negligently and wrongly advised her that she had AIDS after she had donated blood to a public blood drive sponsored by the Walter Reed Hospital, which resulted in her having an unnecessary and unwanted abortion. In November 1986, prior to being notified of this error, the plaintiff discovered that she was pregnant. On November 21, 1986, physicians at Walter Reed Hospital advised the plaintiff that her child would most certainly be born with AIDS

and would not live beyond five years. The physicians indicated that under these circumstances it would be better for the plaintiff to have an abortion than to carry the child to term. As a result of this counseling, and for no other reason, the plaintiff had an abortion on December 4, 1986. It was not until February 3, 1987, nearly four months later, that a physician at Walter Reed Hospital told the plaintiff that there had been an error in the paperwork, and she did not have AIDS.

The United States moved to have the case dismissed on the grounds that the action was barred by the Feres doctrine. Under this doctrine, the United States is not liable under the Federal Tort Claims Act for injuries that arise out of or are in the course of activity incident to service. The district court held that the donation of blood was not incident to service, and, therefore, the Feres doctrine did not bar the action.

Serviceman Unknowingly Spreads AIDS to Family

The Feres doctrine did not bar a serviceman's claim in *C.R.S. v. United States*.[34] The serviceman had been infected with the AIDS virus during surgery performed on him while he was on active duty. He allegedly spread the virus to both his wife and daughter. The policy rationale for the Feres doctrine was not appropriate for barring the claims made in this case.

Insurance Company Fails to Disclose HIV Status

Unbeknownst to Wyoming residents Gary and Renna Pehle, husband and wife, they were infected with HIV at the time they applied for life insurance from the Farm Bureau Life Insurance Company in 1999. At the time of the application, Farm Bureau collected the initial premium and arranged for blood tests from the Pehles in furtherance of the application. Blood samples were forwarded for analysis to an independent laboratory, LabOne, which in turn reported the HIV status to the insurance company. On receipt of the information, Farm Bureau sent a notice of rejection to the Pehles and advised them that it would disclose the reason for their rejection to their physician if they so wished. No action was taken by the Pehles. Two years later, R.P. was diagnosed with AIDS and on inquiry she and her husband learned that Farm Bureau records showed the HIV infection at the time of the life insurance rejection. The Pehles sued, alleging that the defendants were negligent in failing to tell them they were HIV positive. A federal court, balancing all the interests involved as Wyoming law requires, concluded that if an insurance company, through independent investigation by it or a third party for purposes of determining policy eligibility, discovers that an applicant is infected with HIV, the company has a duty to disclose to the applicant information sufficient to cause a reasonable applicant to inquire further.[35]

CRIMINAL ACTIONS

On June 24, 1987, the defendant in *United States v. Moore*,[36] an inmate at the Federal Medical Center in Rochester, was convicted by a jury of assault and battery with a deadly or dangerous weapon. The indictment indicated that he had tested positive for the HIV antibody and later assaulted two federal correctional officers with his mouth and teeth. The defendant motioned the U.S. District Court for a judgment of acquittal and for a new trial. Evidence at trial showed that AIDS can be transmitted through body fluids such as blood and semen. The defendant had been informed that he had both the AIDS virus and the hepatitis antibody and that he potentially could transmit the diseases to other persons. He bit one officer on the leg twice, leaving a 4-inch saliva stain. He bit the second officer, leaving a mark that was visible five months later at trial. Expert testimony at trial indicated that any human bite can cause a serious infection and that blood is sometimes present in the mouth, particularly if an individual has ill-fitting teeth or gum problems. In the defendant's motion for a new trial, he claimed that the court erred in denying his requested Jury Instruction 12, which would have prohibited the officers' testimony as to medical instructions they were given to avoid infecting their families from being entered into evidence. The evidence was considered probative of the dangerousness of the bites inflicted by the defendant, and the probative value outweighed any prejudicial effect. The defendant's motions for a judgment of acquittal and a new trial were denied.

REPORTING REQUIREMENTS

AIDS is a reportable communicable disease in every state. Physicians and hospitals must report every case of AIDS—with the patient's name—to government public health authorities. Cases reported to local health authorities are also reported to the CDC, with the patients' names encoded by a system known as Soundex. CDC records come under the general confidentiality protections of the Federal Privacy Act of 1974. However, the statute permits disclosures to other federal agencies, under certain circumstances.

AIDS EMERGENCY ACT

AIDS has been reported in all 50 states. Because the incidence of HIV affects different localities of the United States disproportionately, the Senate and House of Representatives enacted the Ryan White Comprehensive AIDS Resources Emergency Act of 1990.[37] The purpose of the act is to:

> provide emergency assistance to localities that are disproportionately affected by the human immunodeficiency virus epidemic and to make financial assistance available to States and other public or private nonprofit entities to provide for the development, organization, coordination and operation of more effective and cost efficient systems for the delivery of essential services to individuals and families with the HIV disease.[38]

Under the HIV Care Grants section of the act, a state may use grant funds[39]

1. To establish and operate HIV care consortia within areas most affected by HIV disease that shall be designated to provide a comprehensive continuum of care to individuals and families with HIV disease.

2. To provide home- and community-based care services for individuals with HIV disease.

3. To provide assistance to ensure the continuity of health insurance coverage for individuals with HIV disease.

4. To provide treatments that have been determined to prolong life or prevent serious deterioration of health to individuals with HIV disease.

OCCUPATIONAL SAFETY AND HEALTH ACT

The Occupational Safety and Health Act (OSHA) requires that health care organizations implement strict procedures to protect employees against the virus that causes AIDS. OSHA requires strict adherence to guidelines developed by the CDC. Complaints investigated by OSHA can result in the issuance of fines for failure to comply with regulatory requirements.

AIDS EDUCATION

The ever-increasing likelihood that health care workers will come into contact with persons carrying HIV demands continuing development of and compliance with approved safety procedures. This is especially important for those who come into contact with blood and body fluids of HIV-infected persons. The CDC expanded its infection control guidelines and has urged hospitals to adopt universal precautions to protect their workers from exposure to patients' blood and other body fluids. Hospitals are following universal precautions in the handling of body fluids, which is the accepted standard for employee protection.

A wide variety of AIDS-related educational materials are available on the market. One of the most important sources of AIDS information is the CDC. The process of staff education in preparing to care for patients with AIDS is extremely

important and must include a training program on prevention and transmission in the work setting. Educational requirements specified by OSHA for health care employees include epidemiology, modes of transmission, preventive practices, and universal precautions. See the Center for AIDS Prevention Studies Web site for some helpful information: www.caps.ucsf.edu/siteindex.php.

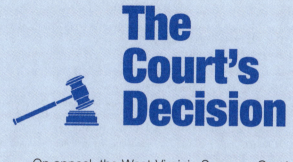

The Court's Decision

On appeal, the West Virginia Supreme Court of Appeals ruled that the plaintiff stated a claim for the negligent infliction of emotional distress. The supreme court found that, "Given the well known fact that AIDS had replaced cancer as the most feared disease in America and, as defendant SmithKline acknowledged, a diagnosis of AIDS is a death sentence, conventional wisdom mandates that fear of AIDS triggers genuine—not spurious—claims of emotional distress." *Id.* at 775.

CHAPTER REVIEW

1. *Acquired immune deficiency syndrome* (AIDS) is a fatal disease that destroys the body's ability to fight bacteria and viruses. AIDS is caused by the *human immunodeficiency virus* (HIV), and it is considered to be the deadliest epidemic in human history. HIV is spread through direct contact with infected blood or body fluids.
2. There have been cases in which a plaintiff has charged that he or she contracted AIDS as a result of the transfusion of contaminated blood or blood products. In such cases, the plaintiff must prove that there was a deviation from an established standard of care and that the deviation was the proximate cause of injury.
3. Historically, there have been conflicts centered on the CDC-issued guidelines that recommend regular HIV testing for health care workers who perform high-risk procedures and further recommend that patients be informed if their health care workers are infected. The argument has been made that mandatory HIV testing violates workers' and patients' rights to privacy. Information about a patient's HIV-positive status is to be distributed on only a need to-know basis.
4. Patients with HIV are entitled to the same level of treatment and compassion as all other patients. They have a right not to be discriminated against in the provision of treatment.
5. Because firefighters and paramedics are at high risk for contracting and transmitting HIV to the public, the U.S. District Court ruled that routine HIV/AIDS testing does not violate their Fourth Amendment or constitutional rights to privacy.
6. Although employment discrimination is unlawful, employers must try to achieve balance between protecting the rights of employees and the health and safety of patients and other employees.
7. Physicians and hospitals are required to report every case of AIDS because of its status as a communicable disease.
8. Employees are to be protected from HIV/AIDS under the Occupational Safety and Health Act.
9. The high rate of exposure to HIV/AIDS among health care workers requires that health care organizations comply with approved safety procedures. The CDC has expanded its infection control guidelines and has encouraged hospitals to adopt universal precautions to protect workers.

REVIEW QUESTIONS

1. Should a professional who refuses to treat an AIDS patient be suspended from an organization's staff?
2. Describe how AIDS patients are discriminated against.
3. Discuss the privacy and confidentiality issues of HIV-positive patients.
4. Should a hospital be permitted to publish the identity of AIDS patients in order to protect other patients and staff?
5. Is AIDS a reportable disease? Why?
6. Discuss what steps can be taken in the health care setting to help prevent the spread of AIDS.

NOTES

1. *Bramer v. Dotson,* 437 S.E.2d 775 (W. Va. 1993).
2. CANTWELL, Alan, *AIDS: The Mystery and the Solutions,* L.A. (1986), at 54.
3. 532 A.2d 1081 (Md. Ct. Spec. App. 1987).
4. *Id.* at 1088.
5. 663 F. Supp. 1048 (D.D.C. 1987).
6. 675 F. Supp. 1060 (D.C. Ky. 1987).
7. 866 F.2d 219 (6th Cir. 1989).
8. Case No. 04CA2942 (Ohio Ct. App. 2005).
9. 592 A.2d 1251 (N.J. Super. Ct. Law Div. 1991).
10. *Id.* at 1255.
11. 592 A.2d 1251 (N.J. Super. Ct. Law Div. 1991).
12. *Id.* at 1255.
13. 734 S.W.2d 675 (Tex. Ct. App. 1987).
14. 538 N.E.2d 419 (Ohio Ct. App. 1988).
15. No. 88-2194 (10th Cir. Aug. 1, 1989) (unpublished).
16. 384 U.S. 757 (1966).
17. *Francies v. Kapla,* 127 Cal.App.4th 1381, 26 Cal.Rptr.3d 501 (Cal. Ct. App. 2005).
18. *Meld v. Barnett,* 157 S.W.3d 596 (Ky. 2005).
19. ETHICS COMMITTEE OF THE AMERICAN ACADEMY OF DERMATOLOGY, *Ethics in Medical Practice,* 1992, at 6.

20. *Anonymous Fireman v. Willoughby,* No. C88-1182 (D.C. N. Ohio Dec. 31, 1991) (unpublished).
21. 489 U.S. 602, 625 (1989).
22. *Anonymous Fireman,* No. C88-1182.
23. 554 A.2d 954 (Pa. Super. Ct. 1989).
24. WHITE, C. M., & BERGER, M. C., *Response of Hospitals, Skilled Nursing Facilities, and Home Health Agencies in Oregon to AIDS: Reports of Nursing Executives,* 81(4) AM. J. PUB. HEALTH 495 (1991).
25. *HIV/AIDS Initiatives,* Clinton Foundation. www.clintonfoundation.org/aids-initiative2.htm.
26. 780 F. Supp. 628 (E.D. Mo. 1991).
27. *Id.* at 628.
28. No. B035809 (Cal. Ct. App. Aug. 7, 1989) (unpublished).
29. 107 S. Ct. 1131 (1987).
30. 886 F.2d 194 (8th Cir. 1989).
31. 640 So. 2d 476 (La. App. 3d Cir. 1994).
32. *Id.* at 479.
33. 735 F. Supp. 1 (D.D.C. 1990).
34. 761 F. Supp. 665 (D.C. Minn. 1991).
35. The plaintiffs in *Pehle v. Farm Bureau Life Insurance Company, Inc.*
36. No. Crim. 4-87-44 (D. Minn. Sept. 3, 1987) (unpublished).
37. *HIV/AIDS,* Rep. Henry Waxman. www.waxman.house.gov/issues/health/issues_health_HIV_legislation_sum_82_91.htm.
38. PUB. L. NO. 101-381, 1990 U.S. CODE CONG. & AD. NEWS (104 Stat.) 576.
39. *Id.* at 586.

Health Care Ethics

THE RIGHT TO CHOOSE:
A MINOR'S CONSENT

Abraham Cherrix was 16 years old when he was diagnosed in August 2005 with Hodgkin's disease. He was treated with chemotherapy. In February of 2006 he learned that chemotherapy had not cured his disease. Doctors recommended a higher dosage of chemotherapy combined with radiation and culminating in stem cell therapy. The treatment program offered Abraham less than a 50 percent chance of survival. Abraham and his family chose to pursue alternative treatment in Mexico. Cherrix's oncologist reported the family's decision to the Accomack County Department of Social Services (ACDSS). Cherrix's parents were accused of medical neglect by ACDSS. A judge granted the ACDSS temporary joint custody with the Cherrixes. The parents faced charges in the Juvenile and Domestic Court for parental neglect. The family obtained a stay from the Circuit Court.[1]

WHAT IS YOUR VERDICT?

The human struggle to survive and dreams of immortality have been instrumental in pushing humankind to develop means to prevent and cure illness. Advances in medicine and related technologies that have resulted from human creativity and ingenuity have given society the power to prolong life. However, the process of dying also can be prolonged. Those victims of long-term pain and suffering, as well as patients in vegetative states and irreversible comas, are the most directly affected. Rather than watching hopelessly as a disease destroys a person or as a body part malfunctions, causing death to a patient, physicians now can implant artificial body organs. Exotic machines and antibiotics are weapons in a physician's arsenal to help extend a patient's life. Such situations have generated vigorous debate. This chapter reviews a variety of ethical and legal issues that inevitably come as one approaches the end of life.

ETHICS

Ethics is that branch of philosophy that deals with values relating to human conduct with respect to the rightness and wrongness of actions and the goodness and badness of motives and ends. Ethics encompasses the decision-making process of determining the ultimate values and standards by which actions are judged. It involves how individuals decide to live, how they exist in harmony with the environment, and how they live with each other when so few have so much and so many have so little.

The scope of health care ethics encompasses numerous issues, including the right to choose or refuse treatment and the right to limit the suffering one will endure. The incredible advances in technology and the resulting capability to extend life beyond the point of what some may consider a reasonable quality of life have complicated the process of health care decision making. The scope of health care ethics is not limited to philosophical issues but embraces economic, medical, political, and legal dilemmas.

End-of-life issues continue to cause the most controversy and debate facing health care providers. Although it is well settled that competent terminally ill patients may refuse life-sustaining treatment, physician-assisted suicide remains a major point of contention. The competing concerns of privacy, morality, patient autonomy, legislation, and states' interests swirl around those involved in the decision-making process. The numerous ethical questions involve the entire life span, from the right to be born to the right to die. The following events are some of many that have had a significant impact on health care ethics.

1932   Tuskegee Study of Syphilis

1972   The Tuskegee study, involving African-American men, analyzed the natural progression of untreated syphilis. This study was conducted from 1932 through the early 1970s. The participants were not warned during the study that there was a cure for syphilis (i.e., penicillin). The Tuskegee syphilis study used disadvantaged, rural black men to investigate the untreated course of a disease. The selection of research subjects must be closely monitored to ensure that specific classes of individuals are not selected for research studies because of their easy availability, compromised position, or manipulability.

1946   Military Tribunal for War Crimes

In 1946, a military tribunal began criminal proceedings against 23 German physicians and administrators for war crimes and crimes against humanity. As a direct result of these proceedings, the Nuremberg Code was established, which made it clear that the voluntary and informed consent of human subjects is essential to research, and that benefits of research must outweigh risks to the human subjects involved.[2]

1949   Nuremberg Trials: International Code of Medical Ethics

This code was adopted following numerous experiments conducted by the Nazis on prisoners in concentration camps.

1954   First Kidney Transplant

The National Institutes of Health published guidelines on human experimentation. The transplantation of human organs has generated numerous ethical issues (e.g., the harvesting and selling of organs, who should have first access to freely donated human organs, how death is defined).

1960s   Cardiopulmonary Resuscitation

Prolonging life beyond what reasonably would be expected has generated numerous ongoing ethical dilemmas. Should limited resources, for example, be spent on those who have been determined to be in a comatose vegetative state with no hope of recovery?

1964   World Medical Association

In 1964, the World Medical Association established guidelines for medical doctors doing biomedical research involving human subjects.[3]

1968   Harvard Medical School Report on Brain Death Criteria

The Harvard Ad Hoc Committee on Brain Death published a report describing the characteristics of a permanently nonfunctioning brain, a condition it referred to as "irreversible coma," now known as *brain death*.

1971   Kennedy Institute of Ethics at Georgetown University

The Kennedy Institute of Ethics was established. It is the world's oldest and most comprehensive academic bioethics center. The institute and its library serve as a resource for those who research and study ethics, as well as those who debate and make public policy.[4]

1972   Informed Consent

The *Canterbury v. Spence*[5] case set the "reasonable-man" standard requiring informed consent for treatment. Patients must be informed of the risks, benefits, and alternatives associated with recommended treatments.

1974   National Research Act

This act created the National Commission for the Protection of Human Subjects of Biomedical and Behavioral Research.[6]

1976   Substitute Judgment Permitted

In *In the Matter of Karen Ann Quinlan*,[7] the Supreme Court of New Jersey rendered a unanimous decision providing for the appointment of Joseph Quinlan as personal guardian of his daughter, Karen.

First Living Will Statute

California enacted the first living will statute permitting a person to sign a declaration stating that, if there is no hope of recovery, no heroic measures need to be taken to prolong life. This provision is now available in every state.

1978   President's Commission for Study of Ethical Problems in Medicine

The duties of the commission include conducting studies of the ethical and legal requirements for informed consent to participate in research projects and the matter of defining death. . . .

1980   Hemlock Society Formed

The Hemlock Society, a nationally known organization advocating the right to die, was formed to advocate for physician-assisted dying for the terminally ill, mentally competent patient.

1983   First Durable Power of Attorney Statute

California passed the first durable power-of-attorney statute permitting an advance directive to be made describing the kind of health care that one would desire when facing death by designating an agent to act on the patient's behalf.

1990   Physician-Assisted Suicide

Jack Kevorkian, a physician, assisted terminally ill patients in suicide outside the boundaries of the law.

Patient Self-Determination Act

The Patient Self-Determination Act of 1990[8] was enacted to ensure that patients are informed of their rights to execute advance directives and accept or refuse medical care.

Feeding Tube Removed

The U.S. Supreme Court ruled that the parents of Nancy Cruzan, a 32-year-old woman who had been unconscious since a 1983 car accident, could have her feeding tube removed.[9]

Patient Rights Self-Determination Act

Congress passed the Patient Rights Self-Determination Act. The act requires federally funded health care organizations to explain to patients that they have a right to complete an advance directive.

1994   Oregon's Death with Dignity Act

Physician-assisted suicide became a legal medical option for terminally ill residents in the state of Oregon. The Oregon Death with Dignity Act allows terminally ill Oregon residents to obtain prescriptions from their physicians for self-administered, lethal medications.[10]

1996   The Health Insurance Portability and Accountability Act

The Health Insurance Portability and Accountability Act of 1996 (Public Law 104-191) was enacted to protect the privacy, confidentiality, and security of patient information.

14th Amendment

The Second and Ninth U.S. Circuit Courts of Appeals ruled that there is a constitutional right under the 14th Amendment for a terminally ill person to receive help from a physician in dying.

1998   Oregon voters reaffirm support for the Death with Dignity Act

1999   Kevorkian was convicted of second-degree murder.

2001   President's Council on Bioethics Established

The President's Council on Bioethics was created. The council is charged with advising the president on bioethical issues that may emerge as a consequence of advances in biomedical science and technology.[11]

Attorney General Challenges Physician Assisted Suicide Law

U.S. Attorney General John Ashcroft decides that physician-assisted suicide was a violation of the Federal Controlled Substance Act because it served no "legitimate medical purpose." In *State of Oregon v. Ashcroft,* CV 01-1647 (D. Oregon), the court allowed Oregon's law to remain in effect.

2002   U.S. District Court Upholds Oregon's Death with Dignity Act

U.S. District Court Judge Robert Jones upheld Oregon's Death with Dignity Act. Attorney General Aschroft appealed to the 9th U.S. Circuit Court of Appeals asking it to lift the U.S. district court's ruling.

2003   Human Genome Became Fully Sequenced

The human genome system became fully sequenced, allowing molecular genetics and medical research to accelerate at an unprecedented rate. The ethical implications of human genome research are as immense as the undertaking of the totality of the research that was conducted to map the human genome system (e.g., cloning of humans).

2004   U.S. Circuit Court of Appeals Upholds Oregon's Death with Dignity Act

On May 26, a three-judge panel of the 9th U.S. Circuit Court of Appeals voted two to one to uphold the Oregon lawsuit initiated in 2002. This blocked the attempt by the U.S. Justice Department, under Attorney General Ashcroft, to use the federal Controlled

Substances Act to prevent doctors in the state from prescribing drugs to assist the suicide of their patients. The Ashcroft directive interfered with Oregon's authority to regulate medical care within its borders and therefore altered the usual constitutional balance between state and the federal governments.[12]

2005 The 2nd edition to the 2005 *Human Cloning, Ethical Issues* publication is released by the United Nations Educational, Scientific, and Cultural Organization. (http://unesdoc.unesco.org/images/0013/001359/135928e.pdf).

2006 The Supreme Court blocked the Bush administration's attempt to punish doctors who help terminally ill patients die, protecting Oregon's one-of-a-kind assisted-suicide law.[13]

Morning-After Pill

The *morning-after pill* which is taken to prevent contraception was approved by the Food and Drug Administration on August 24, 2006, for use without a prescription. This decision has added another dimension to the on-going controversy between right-to-life and pro-choice advocates.

MORALITY

Morality is a code of conduct. It is a guide to behavior that all rational persons would put forward for governing their behavior. Morality describes a class of rules held by society to govern the conduct of its individual members. A moral dilemma occurs when moral ideas of right and wrong conflict.

Moral judgments are those judgments concerned with what an individual or group believes to be the right or proper behavior in a given situation. It involves assessing another person's moral character based on how he or she conforms to the moral convictions established by the individual and/or group. What is considered right varies from nation to nation, culture to culture, religion to religion, as well as from one person to the next. In other words, there is no universal morality.

When it is important that disagreements be settled, morality is often legislated. Law is distinguished from morality by having explicit rules and penalties, and officials who interpret the laws and apply the penalties. There is often considerable overlap in the conduct governed by morality and that governed by law. Laws are created to set boundaries for societal behavior. They are enforced to ensure that the expected behavior happens.[14]

VIRTUES AND VALUES

The term *virtue* is normally defined as some sort of moral excellence or beneficial quality. In traditional ethics, virtues are those characteristics that differentiate good people from bad people. Virtues, such as honesty and justice, are abstract moral principles. Properly understood, virtues serve as indispensable guides to our actions. However, they aren't ends in themselves; virtues are merely abstract means to concrete ends. The ends are values: the things in life that we aim to gain or keep. Most individuals have a tendency to focus on values and not virtues. Simply stated, most individuals find it difficult to make the connection between abstract principles (virtues) and that which has value. The relationship between means and ends, principles (virtues) and practice (values) is often difficult to grasp.

A *moral value* is the relative worth placed on some virtuous behavior. What has value to one person may not have value to another. A *value* is a standard of conduct. Values are used for judging the goodness or badness of some action. *Ethical values* imply standards of worth. They are the standards by which we measure the goodness in our lives. *Intrinsic value* is something that has value in and of itself. *Instrumental value* is something that helps to give value to something else (e.g., money is valuable for what it can buy).

All people make value judgments and make choices among alternatives. The values one so dearly proclaims may change as needs change. Values are the motivating power of a person's actions and are necessary to survival, both psychologically and physically.

SITUATIONAL ETHICS

A person's moral values and moral character can be compromised when faced with difficult choices. Why do good people behave differently in similar situations? Why do good people sometimes do bad things? The answer is fairly simple: One's moral character can sometimes change as circumstances change; thus the term situational ethics.

Situational ethics refers to a particular view of ethics, in which absolute standards are considered less important than the requirements of a particular situation. The standards used may, therefore, vary from one situation to another, and may even contradict one another. For example, a decision not to use extraordinary means to sustain the life of an unknown 84-year-old may result in a different decision if the 84-year-old is one's mother. To better understand this concept, consider the desire to live, and the extreme measures one will take in order to do so. Remember that *ethical decision making* is the process of determining the right thing to do in the event of a moral dilemma.

AUTONOMY

The principle of autonomy involves recognizing the right of a person to make one's own decisions. *Auto* comes from a

Greek word meaning "self" or the "individual." In this context, *autonomy* means recognizing an individual's right to make his or her own decisions about what is best for himself or herself. Autonomy is not an absolute principle, meaning that the autonomous actions of one person must not infringe upon the rights of another.

Respect for autonomy has been recognized in the 14th amendment to the Constitution of the United States. The law upholds an individual's right to make his or her own decisions about health care. A patient has the right to refuse to receive health care even if it is beneficial to saving his or her life. Patients can refuse treatment, refuse to take medications, refuse blood or blood by-products, and refuse invasive procedures regardless of the benefits that may be derived from them. They have a right to have their decisions followed by family members who may disagree simply because they are unable to let go.

What has been mandated by law has been reflected in bioethical thinking. Although patients have a right to make their own decisions, they also have a concomitant right to know the risks, benefits, and alternatives to recommended procedures.

Autonomous decision making can be affected by one's disabilities, mental status, maturity, or incapacity to make decisions. Although the principle of autonomy may be inapplicable in certain cases, one's autonomous wishes may be carried out through an advance directive and/or an appointed health care agent in the event of one's inability to make decisions.

Life or Death: The Right to Choose

Vega, a Jehovah's Witness, executed a release requesting that no blood or its derivatives be administered to her during her hospitalization. Vega's husband also signed the release. She delivered a healthy baby. Following the delivery, Vega bled heavily. Her obstetrician, Dr. Sood, recommended a dilation and curettage (D&C) to stop the bleeding. Although Vega agreed to permit Sood to perform the D&C, she refused to allow a blood transfusion.

Vega's condition continued to worsen. Eventually, when she was having difficulty breathing, her physicians placed her on a respirator in the intensive care unit. Because Sood and other physicians involved in Vega's care believed that it was essential that she receive blood in order to survive, the hospital filed a complaint requesting that the court issue an injunction that would permit the hospital to administer blood transfusions. The trial court convened an emergency hearing at the hospital. Although Vega's attorney, who was en route to the hospital, had not yet arrived, the court appointed Vega's husband as her guardian and began hearing testimony. Vega's physicians testified that, with reasonable medical certainty, she would die without blood transfusions. Her husband testified that, on the basis of his religious beliefs as a

Jehovah's Witness, he continued to support his wife's decision to refuse transfusions. The court, relying on the state's interests in preserving life and protecting innocent third parties, and noting that Vega's life could be saved by a blood transfusion, granted the hospital's request for an injunction permitting it to administer blood transfusions. Vega recovered and was discharged from the hospital.

Did the issuance of the injunction, followed by the administration of the blood transfusions, violate Vega's common law right of bodily self-determination?

The court determined that the hospital had no common-law right or obligation to thrust unwanted medical care on a patient who, having been sufficiently informed of the consequences, competently and clearly declined that care. The hospital's interests were sufficiently protected by Vega's informed choice, and neither it nor the trial court was entitled to override that choice. Vega's common-law right of bodily self-determination was entitled to respect and protection. The trial court improperly issued an injunction that permitted the hospital to administer blood transfusions to Vega.[15]

ORGANIZATIONAL ETHICS

The purpose of organizational ethics in the health care setting is to promote responsible behavior in the decision-making process. Recent interest in organizational ethics is, in part, the result of government regulations (e.g., Sarbanes-Oxley Act, EMTALA) and accrediting agencies (e.g., The Joint Commission) concerns that certain unethical practices continue to plague the industry. These practices include billing scams, inappropriate advertising and marketing, and patient care issues (e.g., inappropriate patient transfers based on ability to pay, transferring patients before they have been clinically stabilized).

Although most health care organizations have published their mission, vision, and values statements, policy and practice continue to be distant relatives. Commitment to organizational ethics must begin with the organization's leadership. If the culture for organizational change fails at this level, the trickle-down theory will not work.

PROFESSIONAL ETHICS

It is the direct caregivers who are frequently confronted with complex ethical dilemmas in the delivery of patient care. In response to ethical conflict, each professional's conduct should be governed by the code of ethics of one's profession, as well as by any other ethical policies, procedures, and guidelines deemed appropriate by the organization by which he or she is employed. The following cases illustrate ethical misconduct involving health professionals.

Nurse's Misconduct

The nurse in *Williams v. Bd. of Exam'rs for Prof. Nurses*[16] improperly, incompletely, or illegibly documented the delivery of nursing care and failed to adhere to established standards in the practice setting to safeguard patient care. Based on these findings, the hearing examiner determined that the nurse was guilty of conduct derogatory to the morals or standing of the profession of registered nursing. Pursuant to the provisions of West Virginia Code § 30-7-11 (1965) (Repl. Vol. 2002), the West Virginia Board of Examiners for Registered Professional Nurses has the power to deny, revoke, or suspend any license to practice registered professional nursing for upon proof that he or she is guilty of conduct derogatory to the morals or standing of the profession of registered nursing. Conduct that qualifies as derogatory to the morals or standing of the nursing profession includes improperly, incompletely, or illegibly documenting the delivery of nursing care, including but not limited to treatment or medication

The board proved that the nurse improperly, incompletely, or illegibly documented the delivery of nursing care and failed to adhere to established standards in the practice setting to safeguard patient care. The nurse falsified patient records or intentionally charted incorrectly. Upon its review of the board's action, the circuit court upheld the board's action. The order of the circuit court was affirmed by the appellate court. There was sufficient evidence to support a West Virginia Board of Medical Examiners one-year suspension of a nurse's license to practice nursing.

Psychologist's Sexual Misconduct

The defendant-psychologist in *Gilmore v. Board of Psychologist Examiners*[17] claimed that sexual improprieties with clients did not take place during treatment sessions. The board of psychologist examiners revoked the psychologist's license for sexual improprieties. The psychologist petitioned for judicial review. She argued that therapy had terminated before the sexual relationships began. The court of appeals held that evidence supported the board's conclusion that the psychologist violated an ethical standard in caring for her patients. When a psychologist's personal interests intrude into the practitioner-client relationship, the practitioner is obliged to recreate objectivity through a third party. The board's findings and conclusions indicated that the petitioner failed to maintain that objectivity.

Attorney's Misconduct

A minister was paid by an attorney to attend a hospital chaplain's course in furtherance of a plan by which the minister could gain access to the emergency areas of a hospital in order to solicit patients and their families for the purpose of aiding the attorney in gaining legal cases based on negligence and malpractice. The improper solicitations were a part of organized schemes that lasted for years with multiple offenses, including two different schemes which led to at least 22 improper solicitations. Disbarment was decided appropriate with respect to an attorney who hired an ordained minister as a paralegal.[18]

PATERNALISM

Those who believe they know what is best for another often make or influence decisions they consider in the best interests of that person. Paternalism can occur because of such things as one's age, cognitive ability, and/or level of dependency. *Medical paternalism* involves making choices for patients who are capable of making their own choices. Physicians are often in situations where they can influence a patient's health care decision simply by selectively telling the patient what he or she prefers based on personal beliefs. This directly violates patient autonomy. The problem of paternalism involves a conflict between principles of autonomy and beneficence, each of which is conceived by different parties as the overriding principle in cases of conflict.

ETHICS COMMITTEE

An *ethics committee* in the health care setting is a multidisciplinary committee that serves as a hospital resource to patients, families, and staff, offering an objective counsel when facing difficult health care issues and decisions. To be successful, an ethics committee must be structured to include a wide range of community leaders in positions of power, respect, and diversity (e.g., ethicists, health care professionals, clergy, lawyers, corporate leaders).

The function of an *ethics committee* is to analyze ethical dilemmas and to advise and educate health care providers, patients, and families. Its goal is to assist the patient and family, as appropriate, in coming to consensus with the options that best meet the patient's goal for care. The ethics committee enhances but does not replace the important patient/family-physician relationship, yet it affords support for decisions made within the relationship.

Ethics committees had their origins in the 1976 landmark *Quinlan* case,[19] where parents were granted permission by the New Jersey Supreme Court to remove their daughter, Karen, from a ventilator after she had been in a coma for a year. She died 10 years later at the age of 31, having been in a persistent vegetative state the entire time.

The *Quinlan* court looked to the prognosis committee to verify Karen's medical condition. It then factored in the committee's opinion with all other evidence to reach the decision to allow withdrawing her life-support equipment. To date, ethics committees do not have sole surrogate decision-making authority. However, they play an ever-expanding role in the development of policy and procedural guidelines to assist in resolving ethical dilemmas.

Committee Functions

The functions of ethics committees are multifaceted and include development of policy and procedure guidelines to assist in resolving ethical dilemmas; staff and community education; conflict resolution; case reviews, support, and consultation; and political advocacy. The degree to which an ethics committee serves each of these functions varies in different health care organizations.

Policy and Procedure Development

The ethics committee is a valuable resource for developing policies and procedures (e.g., committee structure, function, consultation process) to assist health care professionals in making difficult decisions.

Educational Role

The ethics committee typically provides education on current ethical concepts and issues to committee members, organization staff, and the community at large.

Consultative Role

The ethics committee often consults with caregivers, patients, and patient families to assist in making difficult treatment decisions. Always mindful of its basic orientation toward the patient's best interests, the committee provides options and suggestions for resolution of ethical conflict in actual cases. Consultation with an ethics committee is not mandatory, but it is conducted at the request of a physician, patient, family member, or other health care professional.

The ethics committee strives to provide viable alternatives that will lead to the optimal resolution of ethical dilemmas involving the continuing care of the patient. It is important to remember that an ethics committee functions in an advisory capacity and should not be considered a substitute proxy for the patient.

Requests for an ethics committee consultation often involve:

- clarification of issues regarding decision-making capacity, informed consent, and advanced directives

- do-not-resuscitate orders

- withdrawal of treatment

- assistance in conflict resolution

Consultations must be conducted in a timely manner. The ethics committee member initially contacted should consider these questions:

- Who requested the consultation?

- What is the issue?

- Is there a problem that needs referral to another service?

- What specifically is being requested of the ethics committee (e.g., conflict resolution between family members)?

If an issue is common and easily resolved, a designated member of the ethics committee should be able to consult on the case without the need for a full committee meeting. If the problem is unusual, problematic, delicate, or has important legal ramifications, a full committee meeting should be called.

Evaluation of a case consultation should take into consideration:

- the patient's current medical status, diagnosis, and prognosis

- benefits and burdens of recommended treatment, or alternative treatments

- effect of no treatment

- life expectancy, treated and untreated

- views of caregivers and consultants

- quality-of-life issues (e.g., pain and suffering)

Decisions concerning patient care must take into consideration the patient's:

- value system

- personal assessment of quality of life

- current expressed choices

- advance directives

- competency to make decisions

- ability to process information rationally to compare risks, benefits, and alternatives to treatment

- ability to articulate major factors in decisions and reasons for them

- ability to communicate

The patient must have all the information necessary to allow a reasonable person to make a prudent decision on his or her own behalf. The patient's choice must be voluntary and free from coercion by family, physicians, or others.

Family members must be identified and the following facts taken into consideration when making decisions:

- Do they understand the situation?

- Is there any conflict of interest?

- Are they in agreement with what is believed to be the patient's wishes?

- Does the patient have an advance directive?

- Has the patient appointed an agent?

- Are there any religious proscriptions?

- Are there any financial concerns?

- Are there any legal factors (applicable state statutes and case law)?

The ethical issues under review must be delineated as clearly as possible. Options must be clarified and questions answered, such as:

- Are recommendations consistent with appropriate medical goals for the patient under the circumstances?

- Are the recommendations consistent with the patient's preferences or best interests?

- Is there a conflict between the patient's preferences, best interests, and the medical indications, and how can it be resolved?

- Are recommendations consistent with ethical and legal principles?

When the ethics committee is engaged in the consulting process, its recommendations should be offered as suggestions, imposing no obligation for acceptance on the part of the patient, organization, its governing body, medical staff, attending physicians, or other persons. Exhibit 17–1 presents a suggested form for documenting an ethics committee consultation.

Political Advocacy: Expanding Role of the Ethics Committee

The role of an organization's ethics committee is evolving into more than a group of individuals who periodically gather together to meet regulatory requirements and review and address advance directives and end-of-life issues. The expanding role of the ethics committee involves addressing external issues that affect internal operations (e.g., managed care, malpractice insurance, complicated HIPAA regulations that increase legal and other financial costs burdening hospitals). Ethics committees need to periodically review their functions and redefine themselves.

As described here, ethics committees face a wide variety of ethical issues:

- Dilemma of blind trials: Who gets the placebo when the investigational drug looks promising?

- Informed consent: Are patients informed as to the benefits and risks of alternative care options?

- What is the physician's responsibility regarding informing the patient of his or her education, training, and skill in performing a procedure?

- What is the role of the ethics committee when the medical staff is reluctant or fails to take timely action, knowing that one of its members practices questionable medicine?

- Should a hospital's medical staff implement best-practice protocols or follow their own best judgment?

- To what extent should the organization participate in and/or support biomedical and genetic research?

- How does the ethics committee address confidentiality issues?

- To what extent should medical information be shared with the patient's family?

- What role should the ethics committee assume as it relates to HIPAA?

- To what extent should the scope of issues that the ethics committee addresses be controlled by the organization's leadership?

- What are the demarcation lines as to what information should be provided to the patient when mistakes are made relative to his or her care?

- What role should the ethics committee play as it relates to conflict resolution?

- Should the ethics committee involve itself in external matters; for example, reimbursement proposals that may negatively affect the hospital?

- How do local hospitals and emergency services transport personnel collaborate when addressing emergency transport needs? For example, knowing that one hospital may be better equipped and staffed to address certain care issues, to which hospital should the patient be taken? To which hospital should an ambulance transport a suspected stroke victim? To the closest hospital when both are in close proximity to one another? To the hospital with a well-trained, well-equipped stroke team or to a hospital without a stroke team?

The size of these listings is somewhat formidable. With this in mind, the ethics committee needs to periodically reevaluate its scope of activities and effectiveness in accomplishing stated goals.

Organizational politics may prevent an ethics committee from becoming involved in many of the issues just described. Although the committee's involvement is strictly advisory, its full value to an organization has yet to be realized.

The ethics committee is health care's sleeping giant. Because of its potential to bring about change, its mission must not be limited to end-of-life issues. Its vision must not be restricted to issues internal to the organization, but must include external matters that affect internal operations.

AUTONOMY AND REMOVAL OF LIFE SUPPORT

No right is held more sacred, or is more carefully guarded, by the common law, than the right of

Ethics Consultation

Date _____ Time _____ Caller _____

Reason for call _____ Action taken _____

Patient _____ Age _____ Medical record # _____

Consultation requested by _____ Relationship (e.g., caregiver or spouse) _____

Attending physician _____ Other physician _____

Patient participation in consultation: ☐ Yes   ☐ No

Does patient have decision-making capacity: ☐ Yes   ☐ No. Explain _____

Surrogate/legal guardian: ☐ Yes   ☐ No   If yes, name: _____

Phone # _____ Advanced directives (e.g., living will) _____

Advance directive: ☐ Yes   ☐ No   Describe: _____

Consultation participants:

☐ Family/relationship _____   ☐ Social worker _____

☐ Physician(s) _____   ☐ Patient advocate _____

☐ Nurse RNs _____   ☐ Chaplain or other religious leader _____

☐ Administrator _____   ☐ Other _____

☐ Ethics committee members:_____

_____

Medical Treatment/Care Information

Diagnosis _____ Prognosis _____

Course of illness _____

_____

Contacts with administrative/legal representative(s) _____

Treatment options _____

Treatment options available _____

Treatment options beneficial _____

Known patient wishes _____

Ethical issues/dilemmas _____

Legal issues _____

Additional information needed: ☐ Yes   ☐ No Explain _____

Other persons to contact for input _____

Consultative guidance _____

Guidance communicated _____

Consultation noted on medical record: ☐ Yes   ☐ No

Disposition _____

Form completed by _____ Date/time _____

Exhibit 17–1 Request for Ethics Committee Consultation

every individual to the possession and control of his own person, free from all restraint or interference of others, unless by clear and unquestioned authority of law.[20]

To analyze the important questions regarding whether life-support treatment can be withheld or withdrawn from an incompetent patient, it is necessary to consider first what rights a competent patient possesses. Both statutory law and case law have presented a diversity of policies and points of view. Some courts point to common law and the early case of *Schloendorff v. Society of New York Hospital*[21] wherein the eminent Justice Cardozo stated:

Every human being of adult years and sound mind has a right to determine what shall be done with his own body and a surgeon who performs an operation without his patient's consent commits an assault, for which he is liable in damages, except in cases of emergency where the patient is unconscious and where it is necessary to operate before consent can be obtained.[22]

This right of self-determination was emphasized in *In re Storar*[23] when the court announced that every human being of adult years and sound mind has the right to determine what shall be done with his or her own body. The *Storar* case was a departure from the New Jersey Supreme Court's rationale in the case of *In re Quinlan*. The *Quinlan* case was the first to significantly address the issue of whether euthanasia should be permitted when a patient is terminally ill. The *Quinlan* court, relying on *Roe v. Wade*,[24] announced that the constitutional right to privacy protects a patient's right to self-determination. The court noted that the right to privacy "is broad enough to encompass a patient's decision to decline medical treatment under certain circumstances, in much the same way as it is broad enough to encompass a woman's decision to terminate pregnancy under certain conditions."[25]

The *Quinlan* court, in reaching its decision, applied a test balancing the state's interest in preserving and maintaining the sanctity of human life against Karen's privacy interest. It decided that, especially in light of the prognosis (physicians determined that Karen Quinlan was in an irreversible coma), the state's interest did not justify interference with her right to refuse treatment. Thus, Karen Quinlan's father was appointed her legal guardian, and the respirator was shut off. Opponents of euthanasia argue that before the *Quinlan* decision, any form of euthanasia was defined as murder by the U.S. legal system. Although acts of euthanasia did take place, the law was applied selectively, and the possibility of criminal sanctions against active participants in euthanasia was enough to deter physicians from assisting a patient in committing euthanasia.

Despite intense criticism by legal and religious scholars, the *Quinlan* decision paved the way for courts to consider extending the right to decline treatment to incompetents as well. State courts recognize the right but differ on how this right is to be exercised.

In the same year as the *Quinlan* decision, the case of *Superintendent of Belchertown State School v. Saikewicz*[26] was decided. There, the court, using the balancing test enunciated in *Quinlan,* approved the recommendation of a court-appointed guardian that it would be in Saikewicz's best interests to end chemotherapy treatment. Saikewicz was a mentally retarded, 67-year-old patient suffering from leukemia. The court found from the evidence that the prognosis was grim, and even though a "normal person" would probably have chosen chemotherapy, it allowed Saikewicz to die without treatment to spare him the suffering.

Although the court also followed the reasoning of the *Quinlan* opinion in giving the right to an incompetent to refuse treatment, based on either the objective best-interests test or the subjective substituted-judgment test, which it favored because Mr. Saikewicz always had been incompetent, the court departed from *Quinlan* in a major way. It rejected the *Quinlan* approach of entrusting a decision concerning the continuance of artificial life support to the patient's guardian, family, attending physicians, and a hospital ethics committee. The *Saikewicz* court asserted that even though a judge might find the opinions of physicians, medical experts, or hospital ethics committees helpful in reaching a decision, there should be no requirement to seek out their advice. The court decided that questions of life and death with regard to an incompetent should be the responsibility of the courts, which would conduct detached but passionate investigations. The court took a "dim view of any attempt to shift the ultimate decision-making responsibility away from duly established courts of proper jurisdiction to any committee, panel, or group, ad hoc or permanent."[27]

This main point of difference between the *Saikewicz* and *Quinlan* cases marked the emergence of two different policies on the incompetent's right to refuse treatment. One line of cases has followed *Saikewicz* and supports court approval before physicians are allowed to withhold or withdraw life support. Advocates of this view argue that it makes more sense to leave the decision to an objective tribunal than to extend the right of a patient's privacy to a number of interested parties, as was done in *Quinlan*. They also attack the *Quinlan* method as being a privacy decision effectuated by popular vote.[28]

Six months after *Saikewicz,* the Massachusetts Appeals Court narrowed the need for court intervention in *In re Dinnerstein*[29] by finding that no-code orders are valid to prevent the use of artificial resuscitative measures on incompetent, terminally ill patients. The court was faced with the case of a 67-year-old woman who was suffering from Alzheimer's disease. It was determined that she was permanently comatose at the time of trial. Further, the court decided that *Saikewicz*-type judicial proceedings should take place only when medical treatment could offer a reasonable expectation of affecting a permanent or temporary cure of or relief from the illness.

The Massachusetts Supreme Judicial Court attempted to clarify its *Saikewicz* opinion with regard to court orders in *In re Spring*.[30] It held that such different factors as the patient's mental impairment and his or her medical prognosis with or without treatment must be considered before judicial approval is necessary to withdraw or withhold treatment from an incompetent patient. The problem in all three cases is that there is still no clear guidance as to exactly when the court's approval of the removal of life-support systems would be necessary. *Saikewicz* seemed to demand judicial approval in every case. *Spring,* however, in partially retreating from that view, stated that it did not have to articulate what combination of the factors it discussed, thus making prior court approval necessary.

The inconsistencies presented by the Massachusetts cases led many courts to follow the parameters set by *Quinlan,* requiring judicial intervention. In cases where physicians have certified the irreversible nature of a patient's loss of consciousness, a neurological team could certify the patient's hopeless neurological condition. Then a guardian would be free to take the legal steps necessary to remove life-support systems. The main reason for the appointment of a guardian is to ensure that incompetents, like all other patients, maintain their right to refuse treatment. Most holdings indicate that because a patient has the constitutional right of self-determination, those acting on the patient's behalf can exercise that right when rendering their best judgment concerning how the patient would assert the right. This substituted judgment doctrine could be argued on standing grounds, whereby a second party has the right to assert the constitutional rights of another when that second party's intervention is necessary to protect the other's constitutional rights. The guardian's decision is sound if based on the known desires of a patient who was competent immediately before becoming comatose.

Courts adhering to the *Quinlan* rationale have recognized that fact, and in 1984 the highest state court of Florida took the lead and accepted the living will as persuasive evidence of an incompetent's wishes. In *John F. Kennedy Memorial Hospital v. Bludworth*,[31] the Florida Supreme Court allowed an incompetent patient's wife to act as his guardian, and, in accordance with the terms of a living will he executed in 1975, she was told to substitute her judgment for that of her husband. She asked to have a respirator removed. The court declined the necessity of prior court approval, finding that the constitutional right to refuse treatment had been decided in *Satz v. Perlmutter*.[32] The court required the attending physician to certify that the patient was in a permanent vegetative state, with no reasonable chance for recovery, before a family member or guardian could request termination of extraordinary means of medical treatment.

In keeping with *Saikewicz,* the decision maker would attempt to ascertain the incompetent patient's actual interests and preferences. Court involvement would be mandated only to appoint a guardian in one of the following cases[33]:

- family members disagree as to the incompetent's wishes

- physicians disagree on the prognosis

- the patient's wishes cannot be known because he or she always has been incompetent

- evidence exists of wrongful motives or malpractice

- no family member can serve as a guardian

The decision in *John F. Kennedy Memorial Hospital v. Bludworth* increased the desire of the public, courts, and religious groups to know when a patient is considered to be legally dead and what type of treatment can be withheld or withdrawn. Most cases dealing with euthanasia speak of the necessity that a physician diagnose a patient as being either in a persistent vegetative state[34] or terminally ill.[35]

Traditionally, the definition of death adopted by the courts has been the *Black's Law Dictionary* definition: "ces-sation of respiration, heartbeat, and certain indications of central nervous system activity, such as respiration and pulsation."[36] At present, however, modern science has the capacity to sustain vegetative functions of those in irreversible comas. Machinery can sustain heartbeat and respiration even in the face of brain death. With thousands of patients existing in the twilight state of life at this time, every appellate court that has ruled on the question has recognized that the irreversible cessation of brain function constitutes death.

Ethicists who advocate the prohibition on taking action to shorten life agree that "where death is imminent and inevitable, it is permissible to forgo treatments that would only provide a precarious and painful prolongation of life, as long as the normal care due to the sick person in similar cases is not interrupted."[37]

Relying on the 1968 Harvard Criteria set forth by the Ad Hoc Committee of the Harvard Medical School To Examine the Definition of Brain Death, the American Medical Association in 1974 accepted that death occurs when there is "irreversible cessation of all brain functions including the brain stem."[38] Most states recognize brain death by statute or judicial decision. New York, for example, in *People v. Eulo,*[39] in rejecting the traditional cardiopulmonary definition of death, announced that the determination of brain death can be made according to acceptable medical standards. The court also repeated its holding in *In re Storar*[40] that clear and convincing evidence of a person's desire to decline extraordinary medical care may be honored, and that a third person may not exercise this judgment on behalf of a person who has not or cannot express the desire to decline treatment. Following the *Bludworth* logic, the court noted that health care professionals acting within these cases should not face liability.

The clear and convincing evidence standard was defined more succinctly by the New York Court of Appeals in *In re Westchester County Medical Center ex rel. O'Connor.*[41] There, the court determined that artificial nutrition could be withheld from O'Connor, a stroke victim who was unable to converse or feed herself. The court held that "nothing less than unequivocal proof of a patient's wishes will suffice when the decision to terminate life support is at issue."[42] The factors outlined by the court in determining the existence of clear and convincing evidence of a patient's intention to reject the prolongation of life by artificial means were the:

- persistence of statements regarding an individual's beliefs

- desirability of the commitment to those beliefs

- seriousness with which such statements were made

- inferences that may be drawn from the surrounding circumstances

The Missouri Supreme Court applied the *Westchester* ruling and held that the family of a woman who was in a persistent vegetative state since 1983 could not order physicians to remove artificial nutrition.[43] In 1983, Nancy Cruzan sustained injuries in a car accident, in which her car overturned, after which she was found face down in a ditch without respiratory or cardiac function. Although unconscious, her breathing and heartbeat were restored at the site of the accident. On examination at the hospital to which she was taken, a neurosurgeon diagnosed her as having suffered cerebral contusions and anoxia. It was estimated that she had been deprived of oxygen for 12 to 14 minutes. After remaining in a coma for three weeks, Cruzan went into an unconscious state. At first she was able to ingest some food orally. Thereafter, surgeons implanted a gastrostomy feeding and hydration tube, with the consent of her husband, to facilitate feeding her. She did not improve, and until December 1990, she lay in a Missouri state hospital in a persistent vegetative state that was determined to be irreversible, permanent, progressive, and ongoing. She was not dead, according to the accepted definition of death in Missouri, and physicians estimated that she could live in the vegetative state for an additional 30 years. Because of the prognosis, Cruzan's parents asked the hospital staff to cease all artificial nutrition and hydration procedures. The staff refused to comply with their wishes without court approval. The state trial court granted authorization for termination, finding that Cruzan had a fundamental right—grounded in both the state and federal constitutions—to refuse or direct the withdrawal of death-prolonging procedures. Testimony at trial from a former roommate of Cruzan indicated to the court that she had stated that if she were ever sick or injured, she would not want to live unless she could live halfway normally. The court interpreted that conversation, which had taken place when Cruzan was 25 years old, as meaning that she would not want to be forced to take nutrition and hydration while in a persistent vegetative state.

The case was appealed to the Missouri Supreme Court, which reversed the lower court decision. The court not only doubted that the doctrine of informed consent applied to the circumstances of the case, it moreover would not recognize a broad privacy right from the state constitution that would support the right of a person to refuse medical treatment in every circumstance. Because Missouri recognizes living wills, the court held that Cruzan's parents were not entitled to order the termination of her treatment, because "no person can assume that choice for an incompetent in the absence of the formalities required under Missouri's Living Will statutes or the clear and convincing, inherently reliable evidence absent here."[44] The court found that Cruzan's statements to her roommate did not rise to the level of clear and convincing evidence of her desire to end nutrition and hydration.

In June 1990, the U.S. Supreme Court heard oral arguments and held that[45]:

- The U.S. Constitution does not forbid Missouri from requiring that there be clear and convincing evidence of

an incompetent's wishes as to the withdrawal of life-sustaining treatment.

- The Missouri Supreme Court did not commit constitutional error in concluding that evidence adduced at trial did not amount to clear and convincing evidence of Cruzan's desire to cease hydration and nutrition.

- Due process did not require the state to accept the substituted judgment of close family members, absent substantial proof that their views reflected those of the patient.

In delivering the opinion of the Court, Justice William Rehnquist noted that although most state courts have applied the common-law right to informed consent or a combination of that right and a privacy right when allowing a right to refuse treatment, the Supreme Court analyzed the issues presented in the *Cruzan* case in terms of a 14th Amendment liberty interest, finding that a competent person has a constitutionally protected right grounded in the due-process clause to refuse lifesaving hydration and nutrition. Missouri provided for the incompetent by allowing a surrogate to act for the patient in choosing to withdraw hydration and treatment. Moreover, it put into place procedures to ensure that the surrogate's action conforms to the wishes expressed by the patient when he or she was competent. Although recognizing that Missouri had enacted a restrictive law, the Supreme Court held that right-to-die issues should be decided pursuant to state law, subject to a due-process liberty interest, and in keeping with state constitutional law. After the Supreme Court rendered its decision, the Cruzans returned to Missouri probate court, where on November 14, 1990, Judge Charles Teel authorized physicians to remove the feeding tubes from Cruzan. The judge determined that testimony presented to him early in November demonstrated clear and convincing evidence that Nancy would not have wanted to live in a persistent vegetative state. Several of her coworkers testified that she told them before her accident that she would not want to live like a vegetable. On December 26, 1990, two weeks after her feeding tubes were removed, Nancy Cruzan died.

Legislative Response

After the *Cruzan* decision, states began to rethink existing legislation and draft new legislation in the areas of living wills, durable powers of attorney, health care proxies, and surrogate decision making. Pennsylvania and Florida were two of the first states to react to the *Cruzan* decision. The new Pennsylvania law is applied to terminally ill or permanently unconscious patients. The statute, the Advance Directive for Health Care Act,[46] deals mainly with individuals who have prepared living wills. It includes in its definition of life-sustaining treatment the administration of hydration and nutrition by any means if it is stated in the individual's living will. The statute mandates that a copy of the living will be given to the physician to be effective. Further, the patient must be incompetent or permanently unconscious. If there is no evidence of the presence of a living will, the Pennsylvania probate codes allow an attorney-in-fact who was designated in a properly executed durable power of attorney document to give permission for "medical and surgical procedures to be utilized on an incompetent patient."[47]

The Supreme Court stated in *Cruzan* that only 15 percent of the population has signed a living will or other type of medical directive. In light of that, more states will have to address the problem of surrogate decision making for an incompetent. Legislation would not only have to include direction to consider evidence of an incompetent's wishes that had been expressed when he or she was competent, but should also include provisions for consideration and protection of an incompetent who never stated what he or she would want done if in a terminally ill or persistent vegetative state.

Unless there is some national uniformity in the legislation, patients and their families will shop for states that will allow them to have medical treatment terminated or withdrawn with as few legal hassles as possible. For example, on January 18, 1991, a Missouri probate court judge authorized a father to take his 20-year-old brain-damaged daughter, Christine Busalacchi, from the Missouri Rehabilitation Center to Minnesota for testing by a proeuthanasia physician, Dr. Cranford. Cranford, who practiced at the Hennepin County Medical Center, was the center of controversy in Minnesota. In January 1991, Pro Life Action Ministries demanded Cranford's resignation, claiming that he "desires to make Minnesota the killing fields for the disabled."[48] He, however, viewed himself as an advocate of patients' rights. Although the situation involving Cranford is resolved, it is clear that the main reason Busalacchi sought authorization to take his daughter to Minnesota is that he believed that he would have to deal with fewer legal impediments there to allow his daughter to die.

Because of the continuing litigation concerning the right-to-die issue, it is clear that the public must be educated about the necessity of expressing their wishes concerning medical treatment while they are competent. Uniformity with regard to the legal instruments available for demonstrating what a patient wants should be a common goal of legislators, courts, and the medical profession. If living wills, surrogates, and durable powers of attorney were to be enacted pursuant to national rather than individual state guidelines, the result should be a greater ease in resolving the myriad conflicting issues in this area. Some states have addressed the problem by statutorily providing for these instruments, thereby enabling individuals to have a say in the medical care they should receive if they become unable to speak for themselves.

Chief Justice Dore of the Washington Supreme Court voiced his opinion that a legislative response to right-to-die issues could be better addressed by the legislature.

The United States Supreme Court, in *Cruzan,* questioned whether a federally protected right to forgo nutrition and hydration existed. The *Cruzan* Court confronted the same philosophical issues that we face today and wisely recognized and deferred to the Legislature's superior policy-making abilities. As was the case in *Cruzan,* our legislature is far better equipped to evaluate this complex issue and should not have its power usurped by the court.[49]

Patient Self-Determination Act

The Patient Self-Determination Act of 1990 (PSDA) requires health care organizations to explain to patients their legal right to direct their own medical and nursing care as it corresponds to existing state law. A person's right to refuse medical treatment is not lost when the person's mental or physical status changes. When a person is no longer competent to exercise his or her right of self-determination, the right still exists but the decision must be legally delegated to a surrogate decision maker. The PSDA provides that patients have a right to formulate advance directives (e.g., living wills) and to make decisions regarding their health care. Self-determination includes the right to accept or refuse medical treatment. Health care providers (including hospitals, nursing homes, home health agencies, health maintenance organizations, and hospices) receiving federal funds under Medicare are required to comply with the regulations. Providers are not entitled to reimbursement under the Medicare program if they fail to meet PSDA requirements.

Each state is required under PSDA to provide a description of the law in the state regarding advance directives to providers, whether such directives are based on state statutes or judicial decisions. Providers must ensure that written policies and procedures with respect to all adult individuals regarding advance directives are established:

(A) to provide written information to each such individual concerning—

(i) an individual's rights under State law (whether statutory or as recognized by the courts of the State) to make decisions concerning such medical care, including the right to accept or refuse medical or surgical treatment and the right to formulate advance directives . . . and

(ii) the written policies of the provider or organization respecting the implementation of such rights;

(B) to document in the individual's medical record whether or not the individual has executed an advance directive;

(C) not to condition the provision of care or to otherwise discriminate against an individual based on whether or not the individual has executed an advance directive;

(D) to ensure compliance with requirements of State law (whether statutory or as recognized by the courts of the State) respecting advance directives at facilities of the provider or organization; and

(E) to provide (individually or with others) for education for staff and the community on issues concerning advance directives.[50]

Although the PSDA has been cheered as a major advancement in clarifying and nationally regulating this often obscure area of law and medicine, there are continuing problems and new issues that must be addressed.

EUTHANASIA

Originating from the Greek word *euthanatos,* euthanasia, meaning "good death" or "easy death," was accepted in situations in which people had what were considered to be incurable diseases. *Euthanasia* is defined broadly as "the mercy killing of the hopelessly ill, injured or incapacitated."[51] Any discussion of euthanasia obliges a person to confront humanity's greatest fear—death. The courts and legislatures have faced it and have made advances in setting forth guidelines to assist decision makers in this arena. However, much more must be accomplished. Society must be protected from the risks associated with permitting the removal of life-support systems. Society cannot allow the complex issues associated with this topic to be simplified to the point where it is accepted that life can be terminated based on subjective quality-of-life considerations. The legal system must ensure that the constitutional rights of the patient are maintained, while at the same time protect society's interests in preserving life, preventing suicide, and maintaining the integrity of the medical profession. In the final analysis, the boundaries of patient rights remain uncertain.

From its inception, euthanasia has evolved into an issue with competing legal, medical, and moral implications, which continue to generate debate, confusion, and conflict. Currently, there is a strong movement advocating death with dignity, which excludes machines, monitors, and tubes. Figures 17–1 and 17–2 illustrate and summarize the numerous ramifications of euthanasia discussed in this chapter.

In the late 1870s, writings on euthanasia began to appear, mainly in England and the United States. Although such works were written, for the most part, by lay authors, the public and the medical community began to consider the issues raised by euthanasia. Then defined as the act or practice of painlessly putting to death persons suffering from incurable conditions or diseases, it was considered to be a merciful release from incurable suffering. By the beginning of the twentieth century, however, there were still no clear answers or guidelines regarding the use of euthanasia. Unlike in prior centuries when society as a whole supported or rejected euthanasia, different segments of today's society apply distinct connotations to the word, generating further confusion. Some believe euthanasia is meant to allow a painless death when one suffers from an incurable disease, yet is not dying. Others, who remain in the majority, perceive euthanasia as an instrument to aid only dying people in ending their lives with as little suffering as possible.

Active euthanasia is commonly understood to be the intentional commission of an act, such as giving a patient a lethal drug that results in death. The act, if committed by the patient, is thought of as suicide. Moreover, because the patient cannot take his or her own life, any person who assists in the causing of the death could be subject to criminal sanction for aiding and abetting suicide.

Passive euthanasia occurs when life-saving treatment (such as a respirator) is withdrawn or withheld, allowing the patient diagnosed as terminal to die a natural death. Passive euthanasia is generally accepted pursuant to legislative acts and judicial decisions.[52] These decisions, however, generally are based on the facts of a particular case. Regardless of the definitional differences, though, in both active and passive euthanasia, the end result is the same.

The distinctions are important when considering the duty and the liability of a physician who must decide whether to continue or initiate treatment of a comatose or terminally ill patient. Physicians are obligated to use reasonable care to preserve health and to save lives, so unless fully protected by the law, they will be reluctant to abide by a patient's or family's wishes to terminate life-support devices.

Voluntary or Involuntary Euthanasia

Voluntary euthanasia occurs when the suffering incurable patient makes the decision to die. To be considered voluntary, the request or consent must be made by a legally competent adult and be based on material information concerning the possible ramifications and alternatives available. The term legally competent was addressed in a right-to-refuse-treatment case, *Lane v. Candura.*[53] The case involved a patient who twice refused to permit surgeons to amputate her leg to prevent gangrene from spreading. The patient's daughter sought to be appointed as a legal guardian to enable her to consent to her mother's surgery. The appellate court, finding no evidence indicating that Mrs. Lane was incapable of appreciating the nature and consequence of her decision, overturned the trial court's holding of incompetence. Even though Lane's decision ultimately would lead to her death, she was found to be competent, and thus was allowed to reject medical treatment.

Involuntary euthanasia occurs when a person other than the incurable makes the decision to terminate the life of an

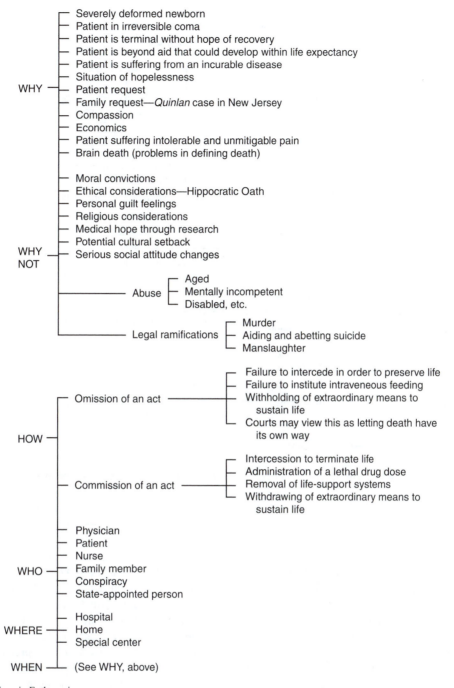

Figure 17–1 Considerations in Euthanasia

incompetent or an nonconsenting competent person's life. The patient's lack of consent could be due to mental impairment or comatose unconsciousness. Important value questions face courts grappling with making decisions regarding involuntary euthanasia:

- Who should decide to withhold or withdraw treatment?

- On what factors should the decision be based?

- Are there viable standards to guide the courts?

- Should criminal sanctions be imposed on a person assisting in ending a life?

- When does death occur?

Physician-Assisted Suicide

States have been confronted with the question of whether it is ever right for a physician to provide a patient with aid in

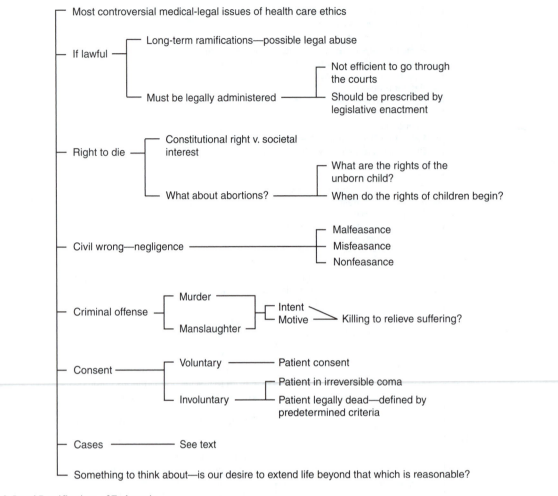

Figure 17–2 Legal Ramifications of Euthanasia

dying. On July 26, 1991, a Monroe County, New York, grand jury answered "yes" when it failed to indict Dr. Timothy Quill for giving a leukemia patient sleeping pills to enable her to take her own life. Dr. Quill wrote an article in the *New England Journal of Medicine* focusing on the suffering of terminally ill patients. He discussed how physicians could relieve an individual's suffering. He is not alone in his support of physician-assisted suicide. In the best-selling book, *The Final Exit,* Derek Humphry, executive director of the Hemlock Society, describes methods of self-assisted suicide for terminally ill people.

Dr. Jack Kevorkian of Michigan announced in October 1989 that he had developed a device that would end one's life quickly, painlessly, and humanely. The news of his invention was disconcerting due to fears that individuals would abuse the practice of euthanasia, which Kevorkian refers to as a medicide, despite any safeguards that are in place.

Kevorkian assisted Janice Adkins, a 54-year-old Alzheimer's disease patient, in committing suicide on June 4, 1990. In December 1990, he was charged with first-degree murder, but the charge was later dismissed because Michigan had no law against assisted suicide. He was ordered, however, not to help anyone else commit suicide or to give advice about it. On February 6, 1991, he violated the court order by giving advice about the preparation of a drug to a terminally ill cancer patient.[54] Additional murder charges were lodged against Kevorkian in October 1991, when he instructed two Michigan women in the use of his "suicide machine." In dismissing the charges against him on July 21, 1992, Oakland County Circuit Court Judge David Breck stated that some people with intractable pain cannot benefit from treatment. While emphasizing that Michigan has no law against assisting suicide, the judge also expressed his belief that physician-assisted suicide remains an alternative for patients experiencing "unmanageable pain."[55]

The Michigan House, however, approved legislation placing a temporary ban on assisted suicide on November 24, 1992. The Senate approved the temporary ban after Kevorkian assisted a sixth terminally ill patient to kill herself. On December 15, 1992, Michigan Governor John Engler signed the law just hours after two more women committed suicide with Kevorkian's aid.

The new law, which became effective on April 1, 1993, made assisting suicide a felony punishable by up to four years in prison and a $2,000 fine. Under the new law, assisted suicide was banned for 15 months. During this time period, a special commission studied assisted suicide and submitted its recommendations to the Michigan legislature for review and action. The new law apparently raised constitutional questions and was challenged by the Civil Liberties Union of Michigan because of the claim that it fails to recognize that the terminally ill have the right to end their lives painlessly and with dignity.

Kevorkian faced prosecution for murdering two people and for assisting in the suicides of three others. As a result, he appealed a Michigan Supreme Court ruling that found there is no right to assisted suicide.[56] The U.S. Supreme Court rejected Kevorkian's argument that assisted suicide is a constitutional right. The high court's decision allowed the state of Michigan to move forward and prosecute Kevorkian on the pending charges. At the time of the high court's ruling, Kevorkian had attended his twenty-second suicide, involving a retired clergyman, less than a month after he was left facing murder charges in Michigan.[57] In 1999, Kevorkian was convicted of second-degree murder and is presently serving a 10-year sentence in Michigan for performing and assisting in a patient's suicide.

Oregon's Death with Dignity Act of 1994

Ironically, Kevorkian is serving time in a Michigan prison for physician-assisted suicide, which became a legal medical option for the terminally ill residents of Oregon on October 27, 1997. The Oregon Death with Dignity Act[58] allows physicians to prescribe but not administer lethal drugs to the requester who must be terminally ill with fewer than six months to live. The patient must convince doctors that the decision is voluntary, sincere, and not based on being depressed. The waiting period is 15 days. The medication can only be given orally. Two physicians must examine the patient to confirm the diagnosis and prognosis. The patient must have made a witnessed request both orally and in writing. All prescriptions must be reported to the state health department.

Then, in June 1997, the U.S. Supreme Court, in two unanimous and separate decisions, ruled that the laws in Washington and New York prohibiting assisted suicide are constitutional—yet the U.S. Supreme Court also ruled that states can allow doctors to assist in the suicide of their terminally ill patients.

CRIMINALIZING ASSISTED SUICIDE

Citation: *Quill v. Vacco,* 117 S. Ct. 2293 (1997)

Facts

Drs. Quill, Klagsbrun, and Grossman challenged the constitutionality of two New York State statutes penalizing assisted suicide. The physicians contended that the statutes are invalid to the extent that they prohibit them from acceding to the requests of terminally ill, mentally competent patients for help in hastening death.

Ms. Doe, a 76-year-old retired physical education instructor, dying of thyroid cancer; Mr. Kingsley, a 48-year-old publishing executive, suffering from acquired immunodeficiency syndrome (AIDS); and Mr. Barth, a 28-year-old former fashion editor under treatment for AIDS, alleged they had been advised and understood that they were in the final stages of a terminal illness with no chance of recovery. Each sought to hasten death in a humane manner and for that purpose sought necessary medical assistance in the form of medications prescribed by their physicians, which were to be self-administered.

The physicians alleged that they were unable to exercise their professional judgment to prescribe the requested drugs and other plaintiffs alleged that they were unable to receive the requested drugs, because of the prohibitions contained in sections 125.15(3) and 120.30 of the New York Penal Law. Section 125.15 of the New York Penal Law provides in pertinent part: "A person is guilty of manslaughter in the second degree when . . . he intentionally . . . aids another person to commit suicide."

The physicians argued that the 14th Amendment guarantees the liberty of mentally competent, terminally ill adults with no chance of recovery to make decisions regarding the end of their lives. They argued that the 14th Amendment guarantees the liberty of physicians to practice medicine consistent with their best professional judgment, including using their skills to assist the decision of competent, terminally ill adults to hasten death by prescribing medications for patients to self-administer. The physicians claimed that relevant portions of the New York Penal Law deny patients and physicians equal protection of the law by taking from patients the right to choose to hasten death, while terminally ill persons whose treatment includes life support are able to exercise this choice by directing termination of such treatment.

The physicians requested judgment declaring the New York statutes constitutionally invalid and in violation of 42 U.S.C. § 1983 "as applied to physicians who assist mentally competent, terminally ill adults who choose to hasten inevitable death."

The U.S. District Court disagreed and concluded that the type of physician-assisted suicide at issue in this case does not involve a fundamental liberty interest protected by the Due Process clause of the 14th Amendment.

The U.S. Court of Appeals for the second circuit reversed the findings of the U.S. District Court, determining that New York law does not treat all competent persons equally in the final stages of fatal illness. It further held that the statutes were not rationally related to any legitimate state interest.

Issue

Do New York State statutes prohibiting assisted suicide violate the equal protection clause of the 14th Amendment?

Holding

The U.S. Supreme Court determined that New York's prohibition on assisted suicide does not violate the equal protection clause of the 14th Amendment.

Reason

The assisted suicide ban and the law permitting patients to refuse medical treatment do not conflict. There is a distinction between letting a patient die and making one die. In its decision, the Supreme Court determined that New York had valid reasons

for distinguishing between refusing treatment and assisting suicide. Those reasons included prohibiting intentional killing and preserving life; preventing suicide; maintaining the physician's role as his or her patient's healer; and protecting vulnerable people from indifference, prejudice, and psychological and financial pressure to end their lives.

Discussion

1. For what reasons did the U.S. Supreme Court find that New York's statute prohibiting assisted suicide did not violate the equal protection clause of the 14th Amendment?
2. Describe what the U.S. Supreme Court meant when it stated there is a difference between letting a person die and making a person die.

In the *Washington v. Glucksberg*[59] case, the Court held that assisted suicide is not a liberty protected by the Constitution's due-process clause. Although a majority of states now ban assisted suicide, these rulings do not affect the right of patients to refuse treatment. It is clear that this emotionally charged issue is not settled. Legislative, judicial, and public debates continue.

A Florida court ruled that a man dying of AIDS had a right to physician-assisted suicide under the privacy issues of the state's constitution. The court emphasized that the patient had to administer the lethal dose of medication, which was prescribed by his physician. Prosecutors were enjoined from bringing criminal charges against the physician.[60]

Caregivers must improve the variety of pain management alternatives to those who are dying, so that physician-assisted suicide does not become the answer to those who suffer. Society must learn to deal effectively with end-of-life issues. Thus far, progress is slow and inadequate.

ADVANCE DIRECTIVES

Under the PSDA, an *advance directive* is a written instruction, such as a living will or durable power of attorney for health care, recognized under state law (whether statutory or as recognized by the courts of the state) and relating to the provision of such care when the individual is incapacitated.

Advance directives allow the patient to state in advance the kinds of medical care that he or she considers acceptable or not acceptable. The patient can appoint an agent to make those decisions on his or her behalf. Patients should be asked at the time of admission to a health care facility if they have an advance directive. If a patient does not have an advance directive, the organization should provide the patient with information as to what an advance directive is and the opportunity to execute an advance directive. Every patient should clearly understand that an advance directive is a guideline for caregivers as to his or her wishes for what medical care he or she would and would not want to receive in the event he or she becomes incapacitated and unable to make decisions. This interaction should be documented in the patient's medical record. If the patient has an advance directive, a copy should be requested for insertion into the patient's record. If the patient does not have a copy of the advance directive with him or her, the substance thereof should be documented and flagged in the patient's medical record. Documentation should include the location of the advance directive, the name and telephone number of the designated health care agent, and any information that might be helpful in the immediate care situation (e.g., patient's desire for food and hydration). The purpose of such documentation should not be considered as a need to recreate a new directive, but should be considered as a desire to adhere to a patient's wishes in the event some untoward event occurs while waiting for a copy of the directive.

The patient can execute a new directive at any time if desired. Patient and family education should be provided as to the existence of the directive and its contents. The patient should be periodically queried as to whether he or she wishes to make any changes with regard to an advance directive.

Guardianship

Guardianship is a legal mechanism by which the court declares a person incompetent and appoints a guardian. The court transfers the responsibility for managing financial affairs, living arrangements, and medical care decisions to the guardian.

The right to refuse medical treatment on behalf of an incompetent person is not limited to legally appointed guardians but may be exercised by health care proxies or surrogates such as close family members or friends. When a patient has not expressed instructions concerning his or her future health care in the event of later incapacity but has merely delegated full responsibility to a proxy, designation of a proxy must have been made in writing.

When a person has been declared incompetent as a result of being in a persistent vegetative state and has left no advance directive, life-sustaining decisions become more complex. Since 1990, Terri Schiavo from Clearwater, Florida, had been in a persistent vegetative state after a heart attack cut off the supply of oxygen to her brain. Her husband Michael became her legal guardian and fought to have her feeding tube removed, which was against her parents' wishes. Michael argued that Terri had articulated her desire not to be kept alive by artificial means.

In an unprecedented move, on October 21, 2003, Gov. Jeb Bush signed an order based on a hastily passed law called Terri's Law, mandating the reinsertion of Ms. Schiavo's feeding tube, which had been removed six days earlier. Mr. Schiavo filed an appeal based upon a violation of his wife's right to privacy under the Florida Constitution, asserting that the law intruded upon the separation of powers. This case is the first time a governor and legislative branch of government have usurped not only the authority of the judiciary, but the rights of legal guardians to make decisions.

The law was narrowly tailored to fit Terri Schiavo's circumstances in which a patient has not left a living will, is in a persistent vegetative state, has had feeding tubes removed, and a family member challenges the removal.

Florida law Chapter 2003-418 was passed by the Florida legislature. It directly affected the patient, Theresa Schiavo, who had been in a persistent vegetative state since 1990. The act provided that the governor shall have authority to issue a one-time stay to prevent the withholding of nutrition and hydration from the patient. The act was determined to be unconstitutional as applied in the *Schiavo* case. The Supreme Court of Florida in *Schiavo* concluded:

> We recognize that the tragic circumstances underlying this case make it difficult to put emotions aside and focus solely on the legal issue presented. We are not insensitive to the struggle that all members of Theresa's family have endured since she fell unconscious in 1990. However, we are a nation of laws and we must govern our decisions by the rule of law and not by our own emotions. Our hearts can fully comprehend the grief so fully demonstrated by Theresa's family members on this record. But our hearts are not the law. What is in the Constitution always must prevail over emotion. Our oaths as judges require that this principle is our polestar, and it alone.

> As the Second District noted in one of the multiple appeals in this case, we "are called upon to make a collective, objective decision concerning a question of law. Each of us, however, has our own family, our own loved ones, our own children. . . . But in the end, this case is not about the aspirations that loving parents have for their children." . . . Schiavo IV, 851 So.2d at 186. Rather, as our decision today makes clear, this case is about maintaining the integrity of a constitutional system of government with three independent and coequal branches, none of which can either encroach upon the powers of another branch or improperly delegate its own responsibilities.

> The continuing vitality of our system of separation of powers precludes the other two branches

from nullifying the judicial branch's final orders. If the Legislature with the assent of the Governor can do what was attempted here, the judicial branch would be subordinated to the final directive of the other branches. Also subordinated would be the rights of individuals, including the well established privacy right to self determination. See *Browning,* 568 So.2d at 11–13. No court judgment could ever be considered truly final and no constitutional right truly secure, because the precedent of this case would hold to the contrary. Vested rights could be stripped away based on popular clamor. The essential core of what the Founding Fathers sought to change from their experience with English rule would be lost, especially their belief that our courts exist precisely to preserve the rights of individuals, even when doing so is contrary to popular will.

The trial court's decision regarding Theresa Schiavo was made in accordance with the procedures and protections set forth by the judicial branch and in accordance with the statutes passed by the Legislature in effect at that time. That decision is final and the Legislature's attempt to alter that final adjudication is unconstitutional as applied to Theresa Schiavo. Further, even if there had been no final judgment in this case, the Legislature provided the Governor constitutionally inadequate standards for the application of the legislative authority delegated in chapter 2003-418. Because chapter 2003-418 runs afoul of article II, section 3 of the Florida Constitution in both respects, we affirm the circuit court's final summary judgment.[61]

The US Supreme Court, on January 24, 2005, denied an appeal by Florida Governor Jeb Bush to overturn a decision by the Florida Supreme Court, which ruled Terri's Law unconstitutional.

SPOUSE'S RIGHT AS GUARDIAN QUESTIONED BY RELATIVES

Citation: *In re Martin,* 517 N.W.2d 749 (Mich. Ct. App. 1994)

Facts

Martin sustained debilitating injuries as the result of an automobile accident. His injuries left him totally paralyzed on the left side. He could communicate to a very minimal degree through head nods.

The trial court determined that Martin did not have nor would he ever have the ability to have the requisite capacity to make decisions regarding the withdrawal of life-support equipment. Evidence demonstrated that Martin's preference would have been to decline life-support equipment given his medical condition and prognosis. The trial court's decision was based on the following four-part test for determining whether a person has the requisite capacity to make a decision: Whether the person (1) has sufficient mind to reasonably understand the condition, (2) is capable of understanding the nature and effect of the treatment choices, (3) is aware of the consequences associated with those choices, and (4) is able to make an informed choice that is voluntary and not coerced. The trial court determined that the spouse was a suitable guardian for Martin.

Mrs. Martin petitioned to withdraw her husband's life support. Martin's mother and sister counterpetitioned to have Mrs. Martin removed as the patient's guardian.

Issue

Was there sufficient evidence to support a finding that: (1) the patient lacked capacity to make decisions regarding the removal of life-sustaining treatment; (2) the patient would have had a medical preference to decline life-sustaining treatment under circumstances; and (3) Mrs. Martin would be a suitable individual to represent her husband as to the withdrawal of life-sustaining medical treatment?

Holding

The Michigan Court of Appeals held there was sufficient evidence to support a finding that: (1) the patient lacked capacity to make decisions regarding the withholding or withdrawal of life-sustaining treatment; (2) the patient would have declined treatment under the circumstances such as those that occurred; and, (3) there was sufficient evidence to show that the patient's spouse was a suitable guardian.

Reason

The test for determining whether Martin had the requisite capacity to make a decision regarding the withholding or withdrawal of life-supporting medical treatment was clear and convincing. It was the general consensus of all of the experts that Martin's condition and cognitive level of functioning would not improve in the future.

Testimony from two of Martin's friends described statements made by him that he would never want to be maintained in a coma or in a vegetative state. In addition, Mrs. Martin described numerous statements made to her by Martin prior to the accident that he would not want to be maintained alive given the circumstances described here. The trial court found that Mrs. Martin was credible. The court of appeals found no reason to dispute the trial court's finding as to Mrs. Martin's credibility.

Contrary to allegations made by the patient's mother and sister, the evidence was clear that Mrs. Martin's testimony was credible. There was no evidence that Mrs. Martin had anything but her husband's best interest at heart. There were allegations, but no evidence, of financial considerations or pressure from another individual that would show that Mrs. Martin's testimony was influenced by other individuals.

Discussion

1. Knowing that the patient had some ability to interact with his environment, discuss the four-part test for determining the patient's ability to make a decision.
2. Do you agree with the court's decision? Explain.
3. Should the concern of the mother and sister have carried more weight in removing custody from Mrs. Martin?

Durable Power of Attorney

Power of attorney is a legal device that permits one individual, known as the "principal," to give to another person, called the "attorney-in-fact," the authority to act on his or her behalf. The attorney-in-fact is authorized to handle banking and real estate affairs, incur expenses, pay bills, and handle a wide variety of legal affairs for a specified period of time. The power of attorney may continue indefinitely during the lifetime of the principal as long as that person is competent and capable of granting power of attorney. If the principal becomes comatose or mentally incompetent, the power of attorney automatically expires, just as it would if the principal dies.

Because a *power of attorney* is limited by the competency of the principal, some states have authorized a special legal device for the principal to express intent concerning the durability of the power of attorney, to allow it to survive disability or incompetency. The durable power of attorney is more general in scope, and the patient does not have to be in imminent danger of death as is necessary in a living will situation. Although it need not delineate desired medical treatment specifically, it must indicate the identity of the principal's attorney-in-fact and that the principal has communicated his or her health care wishes to the attorney-in-fact. Although the laws vary from state to state, all 50 states and the District of Columbia have durable power of attorney statutes. This legal device is an important alternative to guardianship, conservatorship, or trusteeship. Because a durable power of attorney places a considerable amount of power in the hands of the attorney-in-fact, the power of attorney should be drawn up by an attorney in the state in which the client resides.

Health Care Proxy

A *health care proxy* is a legal document that allows a person to appoint a health care agent to make treatment decisions in the event he or she becomes incapacitated and is unable to make decisions. The agent must be made aware of the patient's wishes regarding nutrition and hydration in order to be allowed to make a decision concerning withholding or withdrawing them. In contrast to a living will, a health care proxy does not require a person to know about and consider in advance all situations and decisions that could arise. Rather, the appointed agent would know about and interpret the expressed wishes of the patient and then make decisions about the medical care and treatment to be administered or refused. The *Cruzan* decision indicates that the Supreme Court views advance directives as clear and convincing evidence of a patient's wishes regarding life-sustaining treatment.

Although most of the statutes fail to cover incompetents, cases such as *Quinlan* and *Saikewicz* created a constitutionally protected obligation to terminate the incurable incompetent's life when guardians use the doctrine of substituted judgment. Further, some states provide for proxy consent in the form of durable power-of-attorney statutes. Generally, these involve the designation of an agent to speak on the incompetent incurable's behalf. They represent a combination of the intimate wishes of the patient and the medical recommendations of the physicians.

Oral declarations are accepted only after the patient has been declared terminally ill. Moreover, the declarant bears the responsibility of informing the physician to ensure that the document becomes a part of the medical record. California statute provides that the document be reexecuted after five years. Other statutes differ in the length of time of effectiveness. Most states allow the document to be effective until revoked by the individual. To revoke, the patient must sign and date a new writing, personally destroy the first document, direct another to destroy the first document in his or her presence, or orally state to the physician an intent to revoke. The effect of the directive varies among jurisdictions. However, there is unanimity in the promulgation of regulations that specifically authorize health care personnel to honor the directives without fear of incurring liability. The highest court of New York in *In re Eichner*[62] complied with the request of a guardian to withdraw life-support systems from an 83-year-old brain-damaged priest. The court reached its result by finding the patient's previously expressed wishes to be determinative.

Before exercising an incompetent patient's right to forgo medical treatment, the surrogate decision maker must satisfy the following conditions:

- The surrogate must be satisfied that the patient executed a document (e.g., Durable Power of Attorney for Health Care and Health Care Proxy) knowingly, willingly, and without undue influence, and that the evidence of the patient's oral declaration is reliable.

- The patient must not have reasonable probability of recovering competency so that the patient could exercise the right.

- The surrogate must take care to ensure that any limitations or conditions expressed either orally or in written declarations have been considered carefully and satisfied.

Health Care Surrogate Act: No Duty Imposed on Hospital

The Health Care Surrogate Act did not impose a duty on a health care provider, such as the hospital in this case, to inquire into the availability of a surrogate decision maker until after the attending physician has made a written determination under the act that the patient lacked decisional capacity. Because no such determination was made in *Collins v. Lake Forest Hospital,* the hospital owed no duty to inquire, and the trial court properly dismissed the plaintiffs' complaint.[63]

Determining Incapacity

Before declaring an individual incapacitated, the attending physician must find with a reasonable degree of medical certainty that the patient lacks capacity. A notation should be placed in the patient's medical record describing the cause, nature, extent, and probable duration of incapacity. Before withholding or withdrawing life-sustaining treatment, a second physician must confirm the incapacity determination and make an appropriate entry on the medical record before honoring any new decisions by a health care agent.

Agent's Rights

A health care agent's rights are no greater than those of a competent patient. However, the agent's rights are limited to any specific instructions included in the proxy document. An agent's decisions take priority over any other person except the patient. The agent has the right to consent or refuse to consent to any service or treatment, routine or otherwise; to refuse life-sustaining treatment; and to access all of the patient's medical information to make informed decisions. The agent must make decisions based on the patient's moral and religious beliefs. If a patient's wishes are not known, decisions must be based on a good-faith judgment of what the patient would have wanted.

Living Will

A *living will,* also referred to in many states as a *directive* or *declaration,* is the instrument or legal document that describes those treatments an individual wishes or does not wish to receive should he or she become incapacitated and unable to make medical decisions. Typically, a living will allows a person, when competent, to inform caregivers in writing of his or her wishes with regard to withholding and withdrawing life-supporting treatment, including nutrition and hydration. The living will is helpful to health care professionals because it provides guidance about a patient's wishes for treatment, provides legally valid instructions about treatment, and protects the patient's rights and the provider that honors them.

The living will should be signed and dated by two witnesses who are not blood relatives or beneficiaries of property. A living will should be discussed with the patient's physician, and a signed copy should be placed in the patient's medical record. A copy also should be given to the individual designated to make decisions in the event the patient is unable to do so. A person who executes a living will when healthy and mentally competent cannot predict how he or she will feel at the time of a terminal illness. Therefore, it should be updated regularly so that it accurately reflects a patient's wishes. The written instructions become effective when a patient is either in a terminal condition, permanently unconscious, or suffering irreversible brain damage.

Living Will Declaration Upheld

The plaintiff/sister (Oris Pettis) was not entitled to enjoin her brother and sister from implementing the living will in which their mother, Doris Smith, directed the withdrawal of life-sustaining medical procedures in the event she should have a terminal and irreversible condition.

Smith, an 89-year-old resident, suffered a debilitating stroke in March 2004. Although she survived, she no longer has any significant brain function. Dr. Maran examined the resident and assessed her condition as being in a vegetative state with no chance of improvement. After consideration of their mother's condition, Steve Smith and Dianne Braddock indicated that the hospital should stop providing their mother nutrition through the gastric feeding tube that had been inserted. Mr. Smith and Mrs. Braddock informed Dr. El-Malah, her treating physician, that their mother had executed living wills in March 2001. Drs. Maran and El-Malah signed the form, attesting that the resident would die whether or not life-sustaining procedures are utilized, and that the application of such procedures would serve only to prolong artificially the dying process.

The resident's declarations specifically prohibit her daughters from making decisions about life-sustaining procedures pursuant to La. R.S. 40:1299.58.1, et seq. The second section, captioned "Declaration of living will for terminal illness pursuant to La. R.S. 40:1299.58.1," declares:

> I willfully and voluntarily make known my desire that my dying shall not be artificially prolonged under the circumstances set forth below and do hereby declare:
>
> If at any time I should be diagnosed as having incurable injury, disease, or illness certified to be a terminal and irreversible condition by two physicians who have personally examined me, one of whom shall be my attending physician, and the physicians have determined that my death will occur whether or not life-sustaining procedures are utilized and where the application of life-sustaining procedures would serve only to prolong artificially the dying process; I direct that such procedures be withheld or withdrawn and that I be permitted to die naturally with only the administration of medication or the performance of any medical procedure deemed necessary to provide me with comfort care.
>
> In the absence of my ability to give directions regarding the use of such life-sustaining procedures, it is my intention that this declaration shall be honored by my family and physician(s) as the final expression of my legal right to refuse medical or surgical treatment and accept the consequences of such refusal. I understand the full import of this declaration and appointment of my Attorney in Fact and I am emotionally and mentally competent to make this declaration.[64]

PATIENT'S OBLIGATION TO MAKE MEDICAL WISHES KNOWN

Patients have an obligation to make medical preferences known to the treating physician. Any glimmer of uncertainty as to a patient's desires in an emergency situation should be resolved in favor of preserving life.

The patient in *Matter of Hughes*[65] signed a standard hospital form entitled "Refusal to Permit Blood Transfusion." There was no indication on the form that the consequences of her refusal had been explained to her in the context of the elective surgical procedure she was about to undergo. The form should have contained an unequivocal statement that under any and all circumstances, blood is not to be used and an acknowledgment that the consequences of the refusal were fully explained. The form should have fully released the physician, all medical personnel, and the hospital from liability should complications have arisen from the failure to administer blood, thereby resolving any doubt as to the physician's responsibility to his patient. If Hughes would have refused to sign such a form, her physician could then decide whether to continue with Hughes's treatment or aid her in finding a physician who would carry out her wishes.

The court emphasized that this case arose in the context of elective surgery. This was not an emergency situation in which the physician and patient did not have time to fully discuss the potential risks, benefits, and alternatives of the planned surgery and the conflict arising over the patient's religious beliefs. Patients have an obligation to make medical preferences known to the treating physician, including the course to follow, if life-threatening complications should arise. This protects the patient's right to freedom of religion and self-determination. In addition, it is helpful to the hospital when faced with the dilemma of trying to preserve life whenever possible and honoring the patient's wishes to forgo sustaining treatment.

FUTILITY OF TREATMENT

> . . . *When we finally know we are dying,*
> *And all other sentient beings are dying with us,*
> *We start to have a burning, almost heartbreaking*
> *sense of the fragility and preciousness of each*
> *moment and each being, and from this can grow a*
> *deep, clear, limitless compassion for all beings.*

> Sogyal Rinpoche

Futility of treatment, as it relates to medical care, occurs when the physician recognizes that the effect of treatment will be of no benefit to the patient. Morally, a physician has a duty to inform the patient when there is little likelihood of success. The determination as to futility of medical care is a scientific decision.

After a diagnosis has been made that a person is terminally ill with no hope of recovery and is in a chronic vegetative state with no possibility of attaining cognitive function, a state generally has no compelling interest in maintaining life. The decision to forgo or terminate life-support measures is, at this point, simply a decision that the dying process will not be artificially extended. Although the state has an interest in the prolongation of life, it has no interest in the prolongation of dying, and although there is a moral and ethical decision to be made to end the process, that decision can be made only by the surrogate. The decision whether to end the dying process is a personal decision for family members or those who bear a legal responsibility for the patient.

A determination as to the futility of medical care is a decision that must be made by a physician. Even if death is not imminent but a patient's coma is irreversible beyond doubt and there are adequate safeguards to confirm the accuracy of the diagnosis with the concurrence of those responsible for the patient's care, it is not unethical to discontinue all means of life-prolonging medical treatment.

WITHDRAWAL OF TREATMENT

Withdrawal of treatment is a decision not to initiate treatment or medical interventions for the patient. When death is imminent and cannot be prevented by available treatment, it is morally permissible to withhold treatment that can yield only a precarious prolongation of life that may involve a great burden for the patient or family. Palliative care should be encouraged in end-of-life situations.

Withdrawal of treatment should be considered when: (1) the patient is in a terminal condition and there is a reasonable expectation of imminent death of the patient; (2) the patient is in a noncognitive state with no reasonable possibility of regaining cognitive function, and/or (3) restoration of cardiac function will last for a brief period.

Theologians and ethicists have long recognized a distinction between ordinary and extraordinary medical care. The theological distinction is based on the belief that life is a gift from God that should not be destroyed deliberately by humans. Therefore, extraordinary therapies that extend life by imposing grave burdens on the patient and family are not required. A patient, however, has an ethical and moral obligation to accept ordinary or life-sustaining treatment. Although the courts have accepted decisions to withhold or withdraw extraordinary care, especially the respirator, from those who are comatose or in a persistent vegetative state with no pos-

sibility of emerging, they have been unwilling until now to discontinue feeding, which they have considered ordinary care.

In 1985, the New Jersey Supreme Court heard the case of *In re Claire C. Conroy*.[66] The case involved an 84-year-old nursing home patient whose nephew petitioned the court for authority to remove the nasogastric tube that was feeding her. The court held that life-sustaining treatment, including nasogastric feeding, could be withheld or withdrawn from incompetent nursing home patients who will, according to physicians, die within one year, in three specific circumstances[67]:

1. When it is clear that the particular patient would have refused the treatment under the circumstances involved (the subjective test)
2. When there is some indication of the patient's wishes (but he or she has not "unequivocally expressed" his or her desires before becoming incompetent) and the treatment "would only prolong suffering" (the limited objective test)
3. When there is no evidence at all of the patient's wishes, but the treatment "clearly and markedly outweighs the benefits the patient derives from life" (the pure objective test based on pain)

The court also found tubal feeding to be a medical treatment, and as such, it is as intrusive as other life-sustaining measures. If physicians follow the *Quinlan/Conroy* standards and decide to end medical treatment of a patient, the duty to continue treatment ceases. Thus, the termination of treatment becomes a lawful act.

Although *Conroy* presents case-specific guidelines, there is concern that the opinion will have far-reaching repercussions. There is fear that decisions to discontinue treatment will not be based on the balancing-of-interests test, but rather that a quality-of-life test.

Advocates of the right to life fear that the right to die for the elderly and handicapped will become a duty to die.[68] In both the *Saikewicz* and *Spring* cases, age was a determining factor weighing against life-sustaining treatment.

The American Medical Association on March 17, 1986, changed its code of ethics on comas,[69] allowing physicians to withhold food, water, and medical treatment from patients in irreversible comas or persistent vegetative states with no hope of recovery—even if death is not imminent.[70] Although physicians can consider the wishes of the patient and family or the legal representatives, they cannot cause death intentionally. The wording is permissive, so those physicians who feel uncomfortable withdrawing food and water may refrain from doing so. The AMA's decision does not comfort those who fear abuse or a mistake in euthanasia decisions nor does it have any legal value as such.

On April 23, 1986, the New Jersey Superior Court ruled that the husband of severely brain-damaged Nancy Jobes could order the removal of her life-sustaining feeding tube, which would ultimately cause the 31-year-old comatose patient, who had been in a vegetative state in a hospice for six years, to starve to death.[71] Dr. Fred Plum created and defined the term persistent vegetative state as one in which:

> . . . the body functions entirely in terms of its internal controls. It maintains temperature. It maintains digestive activity. It maintains heart beat and pulmonary ventilation. It maintains reflex activity of muscles and nerves for low-level conditioned responses. But there is no behavioral evidence of either self-awareness or awareness of the surroundings in a learned manner.[72]

Medical experts testified that the patient could, under optimal conditions, live another 30 years. Relieving the nursing home officials from performing the act on one of its residents, the court ruled that the patient could be taken home to die (with the removal to be supervised by a physician and medical care to be provided to the patient at home).

The court's decision applied "the principles enunciated in *Quinlan* and . . . *Conroy*" and the "ruling by the American Medical Association's Council on Judicial Affairs that the provision of food and water is, under certain circumstances, a medical treatment like any other and may be discontinued when the physician and family of the patient feel it is no longer benefiting the patient."[73]

The Illinois Supreme Court in *In re Estate of Longeway*,[74] agreed with the logic of the *Jobes* decision and other sister state rulings regarding the characterization of artificial nutrition and hydration as medical treatment. The Illinois court found that the authorized guardian of a terminally ill patient in an irreversible coma or persistent vegetative state has a common-law right to refuse artificial nutrition and hydration. The court found that there must be clear and convincing evidence that the refusal is consistent with the patient's interest. The court also required the concurrence of the patient's attending physician and two other physicians. Court intervention is also necessary to guard against the possibility that greed may taint the judgment of the surrogate decision maker.

Also, Elizabeth Bouvia, a mentally competent cerebral palsy victim, won her struggle to have feeding tubes removed even though she was not terminally ill.[75] The California Court of Appeals announced on April 16, 1986, that she could go home to die. The court found that Bouvia's decision to let nature take its course did not amount to a choice to commit suicide with people aiding and abetting it. The court stated that it is not "illegal or immoral to prefer a natural, albeit sooner, death than a drugged life attached to a mechanical device."[76] The court's finding that it was a moral and philosophic question, not a legal or medical one, leaves one wondering if the courts are opening the door to permitting legal starvation to be used by those who are not terminally ill but who do wish to commit suicide.

Although there may be a duty to provide life-sustaining equipment in the immediate aftermath of cardiopulmonary arrest, there is no duty to continue its use once it has become futile and ineffective to do so in the opinion of qualified medical personnel. Two physicians in *Barber v. Superior Court*[77] were charged with the crimes of murder and conspiracy to commit murder. The charges were based on their acceding to requests of the patient's family to discontinue life-support equipment and intravenous tubes. The patient suffered a cardiopulmonary arrest in the recovery room after surgery. A team of physicians and nurses revived the patient and placed him on life-support equipment. The patient suffered severe brain damage that placed him in a comatose and vegetative state, from which, according to tests and examinations by other specialists, he was unlikely to recover. The patient, on the written request of the family, was taken off life-support equipment. The patient's family (his wife and eight children) made the decision together after consultation with the physicians. Evidence had been presented that the patient, before his incapacitation, had expressed to his wife that he would not want to be kept alive by machine or become another Karen Ann Quinlan. There was no evidence indicating that the family was motivated in their decision by anything other than love and concern for the dignity of their loved one. The patient continued to breathe on his own. Showing no signs of improvement, the physicians again discussed the patient's poor prognosis with the family. The intravenous lines were removed, and the patient died sometime thereafter. A criminal complaint was filed against the two physicians. The California Court of Appeals held that the physicians' omission to continue treatment, although intentional and with knowledge that the patient would die, was not an unlawful failure to perform a legal duty.

DO-NOT-RESUSCITATE ORDERS

Do-not-resuscitate (DNR) orders, given by a physician, indicate that in the event of a cardiac or respiratory arrest, no resuscitative measures should be used to revive the patient. A DNR order is an extremely difficult decision to make for both the patient and family. It is generally made when one's quality of life has been so diminished that heroic rescue methods are no longer in the patient's best interests.

DNR orders must be in writing, signed, and dated by the physician. Appropriate consents must be obtained from the patient or his or her health care agent. Many states have acknowledged the validity of DNR orders in cases involving terminally ill patients in which the patients' families make no objections to such orders.

DNR orders must comply with statutory requirements, be of short duration, and be reviewed periodically to determine whether the patient's condition or other circumstances (e.g., change of mind by the patient or family) surrounding the no-code[78] orders have changed. Presently, it is generally accepted that if a patient is competent, a DNR order is considered to be the same as other medical decisions in which a patient may choose to reject life-sustaining treatment. In the case of an incompetent, absent any advance written directives, the best interests of the patient must be considered. In *Payne v. Marion General Hospital,*[79] the Indiana Court of Appeals overturned a lower court decision in favor of a physician. The physician issued a no-code status on Mr. Payne despite evidence given by a nurse that up to a few minutes before his death Payne could communicate. The physician determined that Payne was incompetent, thereby rendering him unable to give informed consent to treatment. Because Payne left no written directives, the physician relied on one of Payne's relatives who asked for the DNR order. The court found that there was evidence that Payne was not incompetent and should have been consulted before a DNR order was given. Further, the court reviewed testimony that one year earlier Payne had suffered and recovered from the same type of symptoms, leading to the conclusion that there was a possibility that he could have survived if resuscitation had continued. There was no DNR policy in place at the hospital to assist the physician in making his decision. To avoid this type of problem, health care providers should adopt policies with respect to the issuance of no-code orders.

AUTOPSY

Autopsies, or postmortem examinations, are conducted to ascertain the cause of a person's death, which, in turn, may resolve several legal issues. An autopsy may reveal whether death was the result of criminal activity, whether the cause of death was one for which payment must be made in accordance with an insurance contract, whether the death is compensable under workers' compensation and occupational disease acts, or whether death was the result of a specific act or a culmination of several acts. Aside from providing answers to these specific questions, the information gained from autopsies adds to medical knowledge. As such, medical schools have an interest in autopsies for educational purposes.

In those instances when the death of a patient is the result of criminal activity or unusual or suspicious circumstances, the patient's death must be reported to the medical examiner. Deaths resulting from natural causes within 24 hours of admission to a hospital do not need to be reported as long as the patient was in the hospital at the time of death and as long as an appropriate physician signs the death certificate and records the cause of death.

Deaths that occur during a surgical procedure are generally reportable events to the medical examiner. If an autopsy for medical evaluation is desired by the hospital, consent must be obtained from the next of kin. An unauthorized autopsy may disturb persons whose religious beliefs prohibit such a procedure as well as those persons who have a general aversion to the procedure. When autopsies are performed without statutory authorization and without the consent of the decedent, the surviving spouse, or an appropriate relative, liability may be imposed.

Damages awarded in cases of liability through interference with the rights of a surviving spouse or near relative with regard to the body of a decedent are based on the emotional and mental suffering that results from such interference. For damages to be awarded, the conduct of the alleged wrongdoer must be sufficiently disturbing to a person of ordinary sensibilities as to cause emotional harm. Cases involving the wrongful handling of dead bodies may be classified into four groups: (1) mutilation of a body, (2) unauthorized autopsy, (3) wrongful detention, and (4) unauthorized use or publication of photographs taken after death.

To limit lawsuits regarding the disposition of dead bodies, appropriate handling and release procedures should be established. Legal counsel should review such procedures. Interfering with rights to a body can result in liability. For example, in the case of *Lott v. State,*[80] two bodies were mistagged. The body of a person of the Roman Catholic faith was prepared for Orthodox Jewish burial, and the person of the Orthodox Jewish faith was prepared for Roman Catholic burial. This negligent conduct interfered with burial plans and caused mental anguish, for which liability was imposed.

Autopsy Consent Statutes

Recognizing both the need for information that can be secured only through the performance of a substantial volume of autopsies and the valid interests of relatives and friends of the decedent, most states have enacted statutes dealing with autopsy consent. Such legislation seems intended to have a twofold effect: first, to protect the rights of the decedent's relatives, and second, to guide those performing autopsies in establishing procedures for consent to autopsy. Most autopsy consent statutes establish an order for obtaining consent to autopsy based on the degree of family relationship.

Authorization by the Decedent

Most autopsy consent statutes provide that persons may authorize an autopsy prior to death. Ordinarily such consent must be in writing. There may be legal as well as practical problems in obtaining authorization for an autopsy from a patient before death if the state does not statutorily provide for such authorization.

In states where there is neither an autopsy consent statute nor a statute permitting donation that may be construed to include autopsy, it is unwise to rely exclusively on the authorization of a decedent to perform an autopsy. This is especially true when relatives of the deceased who assume custody of the body for burial object to an autopsy.

Although the courts have upheld the wishes of the deceased with respect to the place of internment or the manner of disposition of the remains (i.e., by burial or cremation), it is possible that the courts will not afford the same weight to the decedent's wishes concerning an autopsy. In such instances, compelling reasons presented by certain next of kin of the decedent, especially the surviving spouse, may prevail over the wishes of the decedent.

Authorization by Person Other Than the Decedent

Generally, the primary right to custody of a deceased person belongs to the surviving spouse. When there is no spouse, the right passes (in the absence of statutes furnishing a preference order of responsibility for burial and consent for autopsy) to the adult children of the deceased, parents, adult brothers and sisters, grandparents, uncles and aunts, and finally cousins. A court may find that a surviving spouse's unwillingness to assume responsibility for burial is sufficient to permit the right to custody of the body to devolve on a relative who is willing to assume such responsibility.

In *Callsen v. Cheltenham York Nursing Home,*[81] the relatives of the decedent, Mrs. Callsen, sued the defendants regarding the transfer of her body to a teaching hospital for dissection purposes. The defendants claimed immunity from liability under good-faith provisions of the Uniform Anatomical Gift Act. An amended complaint named 22 separate defendants. The complaint recited that Callsen was the mother of the plaintiffs and that prior to her death she resided at the Cheltenham York Nursing Home. The nursing home maintained records of family and friends who visited her. On May 27, 1990, the nursing home transferred Callsen (who expired on or about June 9, 1990) to the Einstein Medical Center. The medical center was notified that there was no family information for Callsen. Plaintiffs allege that the medical center made no further efforts to contact family members or friends.

The plaintiffs also alleged in their amended complaint that, following Callsen's death, no efforts were made to locate and notify family members regarding the transfer of the decedent's remains. The family did not discover her whereabouts until about 10 days after her death, and by that time the body had been partially dissected. The plaintiffs also claim that the defendants were negligent in failing to follow the statutory procedures for disposition of a deceased person's remains and that their conduct was grossly negligent and outrageous. The common pleas court sustained preliminary objections and dismissed the complaint, and an appeal was taken. The question arises as to whether or not there were triable issues of fact with regard to making appropriate efforts to locate the patient's family.

The commonwealth court held that there were triable issues of fact as to whether appropriate efforts to locate the patient's family had been made. Although the nursing facility had access to the names of family members, the nursing facility agreement did not record their names. One of the facility's nurses reported to Einstein Medical Center that there was no family information for the decedent. The complaint does not disclose what efforts, if any, were made to locate the relatives or to notify any of them as to the proposed disposition of the decedent's remains. The court held that the ultimate decision as to the presence or absence of the exercise of good faith by any of the three parties must await the filing of further pleadings, the completion of any necessary discovery, and possible motions for summary judgment.

Scope and Extent of Consent

Legal issues may arise as a result of an autopsy even if consent has been obtained from the person authorized by law to grant such consent. If autopsy procedures go beyond the limits imposed by the consent or if the consent to an autopsy is obtained by fraud or without the formal requisites, liability may be incurred. It is a fundamental principle that a person who has the right to refuse permission for the performance of an act also has the right to place limitations or conditions on consent.

It is especially important that the hospital and its personnel adhere to any limitations or conditions placed on the permission to autopsy; if such limitations are exceeded, the physician or the hospital has no defense on the ground of emergency or medical necessity.

Although consent to autopsy also may encompass authorization for removal of body parts for examination, a separate question may arise concerning disposal of tissues and organs on completion of the examination: May the hospital and its personnel dispose of such material in a routine manner or use it for the hospital's own purposes, or must the hospital return the tissue and organs to the body before burial? In *Hendriksen v. Roosevelt Hospital,*[82] permission had been granted for a complete autopsy, including an examination of the central nervous system by a scalp incision. Yet the court held that liability might be imposed on the hospital if the jury found that the hospital retained parts of the body. Pursuant to a New York statute requiring the authorization of the next of kin, consent was given for dissection; however, the court held that this statute should be construed narrowly and that special consent would have to be obtained to retain the internal organs of the decedent.

Consent given with the understanding that organs and tissue could be removed and retained for examination would seem to authorize the hospital to dispose of such materials in a suitable manner or to use them after the autopsy. However, the *Hendriksen* decision raises doubts on this matter.

When the party giving consent expressly stipulates that parts severed from the body are to be returned to the body for burial, conduct deviating from this provision may result in liability. Also, it would appear that consent to autopsy does not include authorization to mutilate or disfigure the body. Therefore, when autopsy involves the removal of exterior body parts and the physical appearance of the body cannot be restored without return of such parts, the hospital may be subject to liability for exceeding the scope of the authorization if the removed parts are not returned. In general, hospitals should periodically review protocols for obtaining consent, limitations placed on an autopsy, and the disposition of body parts.

Fraudulently Obtained Consent

It is a long-accepted principle that consent obtained through fraud or material misrepresentation is not binding and that the person whose consent is so obtained stands in the same position as if no consent had been given. This principle can apply to autopsies when facts are misrepresented to the person who has the right to consent to induce his or her consent. If a physician or a hospital employee states, as fact, something known to be untrue to gain consent, the autopsy would be unauthorized, and liability might follow.

Determination of Death

The time of a patient's death must be determined by a physician in attendance at the donor's death, or a physician certifying death, who shall not be a member of the team of physicians engaged in the transplantation procedure.

Consideration of legal duties regarding the use, handling, and disposition of dead bodies cannot be divorced from the legal questions involved in determining when death occurs. In many contexts, such as deciding rights to the property of the deceased person, the determination of death does not involve the hospital or its personnel. However, when permission has been granted for use of a patient's body or organs for the benefit of another or science in general, determination of the point of death becomes critical. New technology, specifically medical advancement in artificially sustaining life and transplanting vital organs, raises both legal and moral questions regarding the viability of the traditional methods of determining death.

Unclaimed Dead Bodies

Persons entitled to possession of a dead body must arrange for release of the body for transfer to an undertaker for final disposal. The body of a deceased person imposes a duty on a health care facility to make reasonable efforts to give notice to persons entitled to claim the body. When there are no known relatives or friends of the family who can be contacted by the facility to claim the body, the facility has a responsibility to dispose of the body in accordance with law. Most states have statutes providing for the disposal of such bodies.

Most states have statutes providing for the disposal of unclaimed bodies by delivery to institutions for educational and scientific purposes. The public official in charge of the body has a duty to notify the government agency of the presence of the body. The agency then arranges for the transfer of the body in accordance with the statute. If no such agency exists under the statute, the health care facility or a public official may be authorized to allow a medical school or other institution or person, designated by the statute as an eligible recipient of unclaimed dead bodies, to remove the body for scientific use. For public health reasons, the statutes usually do not permit distribution of the bodies of persons who have died from contagious diseases.

Although most statutes explicitly require notification of relatives and set time limits for holding the body to allow relatives an opportunity to claim it, strict compliance with the statutory provisions is often impossible because of the very nature of the problems that arise in the handling of dead bodies and in the required procedures themselves. An example of such a provision is the requirement that relatives be notified immediately on death and that the body be held for 24 hours subject to claim by a relative or friend. The procedure of locating and notifying relatives may consume the greater part of the 24-hour period after death. If relatives who are willing to claim the body are located, the body should be held for a reasonable time to allow them to arrange custody for burial.

ORGAN DONATIONS

Federal regulations require that hospitals have, and implement, written protocols regarding the organization's organ procurement. The regulations impose specific notification duties, as well as other requirements concerning informing families of potential donors. It encourages discretion and sensitivity in dealing with the families and in educating hospital staff on a variety of issues involved with donation matters, in order to facilitate timely donation and transplantation.

Developments in medical science have enabled physicians to take tissue from persons immediately after death and use it to replace or rehabilitate diseased or damaged organs or other parts of living persons. Success rates have increased because of improved patient selection, improved clinical and operative skills, and the development of immunosuppressant drugs to aid in decreasing the incidence of tissue rejection. Progress in this field of medicine has created the problem of obtaining a sufficient supply of replacement body parts. Fear that people would buy and sell organs led to enactment of the National Organ Procurement Act in 1984, making it illegal to buy or sell organs. Throughout the country, there are tissue banks and other facilities for the storage and preservation of organs and tissue that can be used for transplantation and for other therapeutic services.

The ever-increasing success of organ transplants and the demand for organ tissue require the close scrutiny of each case, making sure that established procedures have been followed in the care and disposal of all body parts. Section 1138, Title XI, of the Omnibus Budget Reconciliation Act of 1986 requires hospitals to establish organ procurement protocols or face a loss of Medicare and Medicaid funding. Physicians, nurses, and other paramedical personnel assigned with this responsibility often are confronted with several legal issues. Liability can be limited by complying with applicable regulations. Organs and tissues to be stored and preserved for future use must be removed almost immediately after death. Therefore, it is imperative that an agreement or arrangement for obtaining organs and tissue from a body be completed before death, or very soon after death, to enable physicians to remove and store the tissue promptly.

The Uniform Anatomical Gift Act drafted by the Commission on Uniform State Laws has been enacted by all 50 states and has many detailed provisions that apply to a wide variety of issues raised in connection with the making, acceptance, and use of anatomic gifts. The act allows a person to make a decision to donate organs at the time of death and allows potential donors to carry an anatomical donor card. State statutes regarding donation usually permit the donor to execute the gift during his or her lifetime. Virtually all states have based their enactments on the Uniform Anatomical Gift Act, but it should be recognized that in some states there are deviations from this act or laws dealing with donation.

Individuals who are of sound mind and 18 years of age or older are permitted to dispose of their own bodies or body parts by will or other written instrument for medical or dental education, research, advancement of medical or dental science, therapy, or transplantation. Among those eligible to receive such donations are any licensed, accredited, or approved hospitals; accredited medical or dental schools; surgeons or physicians; tissue banks; or specified individuals who need the donation for therapy or transplantation. The statute provides that when only a part of the body is donated, custody of the remaining parts of the body shall be transferred to the next of kin promptly after removal of the donated part.

A donation by will becomes effective immediately on the death of the testator, without probate, and the gift is valid and effective to the extent that it has been acted on in good faith. This is true even if the will is not probated or is declared invalid for testimonial purposes.

Failure to Obtain Consent

Although failure to obtain consent for removal of body tissue can give rise to a lawsuit, not all such claims are successful. In *Nicoletta v. Rochester Eye & Human Parts Bank,*[83] the father of a deceased patient brought an action against a hospital for alleged emotional injuries resulting from the removal of his son's eyes for donation after a fatal motorcycle accident. The hospital was immune from liability under the provisions of the Uniform Anatomical Gift Act because the hospital had neither actual nor constructive knowledge that the woman who had authorized the donation was not the decedent's wife. The hospital was entitled to the immunity afforded by the "good-faith" provisions of Section 4306(3) of the act in which its agents made reasonable inquiry as to the status of the purported wife, who resided with the decedent for 10 years and was the mother of their two children. The hospital had no reason to believe that any irregularity existed. The father, who was present at the time his son was brought to the emergency department, failed to object to any organ donation and failed to challenge the authority of the purported wife to sign the emergency department authorization.

RESEARCH AND EXPERIMENTATION

The science of medicine, by the very nature of the object that it studies, the human body, is often prevented from making progress through direct experimentation. It must resort to necessary tests in laboratories and on animals, whose reactions are similar to humans—but most of all, it advances through observation of functions of the body in health and in disease. It is natural that much of this laboratory experimentation and clinical observation should be done in the hospital. To increase the possibility of advancement by observation, clinical records must be accurate and complete in every case, no matter how trivial, and they should be preserved in such a manner as to be available for the study of similar cases. New remedies of all kinds should be tried under conditions that favor accurate observation. Laboratories should be available under the direction of physicians, and results of examinations should be carefully compiled and studied. Systematized research is possible only when directed by a physician with a scientific specialty, and it is rare not to find one such individual working in every hospital.

In 1964, the World Medical Association developed the Declaration of Helsinki that contains ethical principles that provide guidance to physicians and other participants in medical research involving human subjects. The declaration includes medical research that involves readily identifiable human material or identifiable data. The declaration contains strict guidelines for protecting the life, health, and privacy of the human subject.

The Nuremberg Code and the Declaration of Helsinki provided guidelines for the development of federal regulations for medical research and the protection of human subjects in the United States. Federal regulations control federal grants that apply to experiments involving new drugs, new medical devices, stem cell research and human cloning, or new medical procedures. Generally, a combination of federal and state guidelines and regulations ensures proper supervision and control over experimentation that involves human subjects. For example, federal regulations require hospital-based researchers to obtain the approval of an institutional review board prior to conducting clinical trials. This board functions to review proposed research studies and conduct follow-up reviews on a regular basis.

Federal and state regulations impose several other requirements on experiments involving human subjects. Institutions conducting medical research on human subjects must

- Disclose fully the inherent risks to the patient.
- Make a proper determination that the patient is competent to consent.
- Identify treatment alternatives.
- Obtain written consent from the patient.

Institutional Review Board

Each organization conducting medical research should have a mechanism in place for approving and overseeing the use of investigational protocols. This is often accomplished through the establishment of an institutional review board (IRB). The IRB should include community representation. The IRB is responsible for reviewing, monitoring, and approving clinical protocols for investigations of drugs and medical devices involving human subjects. The IRB is responsible for ensuring that the rights of each individual are protected and that all research is conducted within appropriate state and federal guidelines (e.g., FDA guidelines).

Medical Research: Duty to Warn

About 5,000 patients at the Michael Reese Hospital and Medical Center, located in Chicago, were treated with X-ray therapy for benign conditions of the head and neck from 1930 to 1960. Among them was Joel Blaz, who received this treatment for infected tonsils and adenoids.

In 1974, Michael Reese set up a thyroid follow-up project to conduct research among those who had been subjected to the X-ray therapy. In 1975, Blaz was notified by mail that he was at increased risk of developing thyroid tumors because of the treatment. In 1976, someone associated with the program gave him similar information by phone and invited him to return to Michael Reese for evaluation and treatment at his own expense, which he declined to do.

Dr. Schneider was put in charge of the program in 1977. In 1979, Schneider and Michael Reese submitted a research proposal to the National Institutes of Health stating that a study based on the program showed evidence of a connection between X-ray treatments of the sort administered to Blaz and various sorts of tumors, including thyroid and neural. In 1981, Blaz received but did not complete or return a questionnaire attached to a letter from Schneider in connection with the program. The purpose of the questionnaire was to investigate the long-term health implications of childhood radiation treatments and to determine the possible associated risks. It did not say anything about strong evidence of a connection between the treatments and any tumors. In 1996, after developing neural tumors, Blaz sued Michael Reese's successor, Galen Hospital, and Dr. Schneider, alleging that they failed to notify and warn him of their findings that he might be at greater risk of neural tumors in a way that might have permitted their earlier detection and removal or other treatment.

The court here found that the harm alleged, neural and other tumors, would here be reasonably foreseeable as a likely consequence of a failure to warn, and was, in fact, foreseen by Schneider. A reasonable physician could foresee that if someone were warned of "strong evidence" of a connection between treatments to which he had been subjected and tumors, he would probably seek diagnosis or treatment to perhaps avoid these tumors; and if he were not warned, he probably would not seek diagnosis or treatment, increasing the likelihood that he would suffer from such tumors.[84]

Informed Consent

Written consent should be obtained from each patient who agrees to participate in a clinical trial. Consent should include the risks, benefits, and alternatives to the proposed treatment protocol. The consent form should be signed, witnessed, and dated. The consent form must not contain any coercive or exculpatory language through which the patient is forced to waive his or her legal rights, including the release of the investigator, sponsor, or organization from liability for negligent conduct.

The necessity of informed consent cannot be overemphasized. In *Friter v. Iolab Corp.*,[85] the hospital contracted with the FDA to participate in a clinical study involving the implantation of experimental intraocular lenses. They were so experimental that they had not yet obtained FDA approval. Hence, the FDA promulgated regulations requiring the hospital to obtain informed consent, using a very detailed, five-page consent form, setting forth with particularity the possibility of the existence of unknown risks, because the lenses were still being tested. The court held in this case that the failure to obtain informed consent is actionable.

Federal regulations require that the nature of experimental drugs and possible adverse consequences must be explained to the patient. Failure to obtain consent for the administration of experimental drugs can give rise to a lawsuit. The district court in *Blanton v. United States*[86] held that when a new drug of unknown effectiveness was administered to a patient at a Navy medical center, despite the availability of other drugs of known effectiveness, the hospital violated the accepted medical standards and its duty of due care, so that in the absence of the patient's consent to the experiment, the United States was liable for the resulting injury.

Food and Drug Administration

The Food and Drug Administration (FDA), under enormous criticism over the years because of the red tape involved in the approval of new drugs, issued rules to speed up the approval process. The rules permit the use of experimental drugs outside a controlled clinical trial if the drugs are used to treat a life-threatening condition. In *Abigail Alliance for Better Access to Developmental Drugs v. Eschenbach,* the U.S. Court of Appeals for the District of Columbia ruled that terminally ill patients have a "fundamental right" protected by the U.S. Constitution to access to experimental drugs that have not yet been fully approved by the FDA. The appeals court ruled that once FDA has determined, after Phase I trials, that a potentially life-saving new drug is sufficiently safe for expanded human trials, terminally ill patients have a constitutional right to seek treatment with the drug if no other FDA-approved drugs are available. The court said that if FDA wishes to prevent such patients from gaining access to investigational drugs that have completed Phase I trials, it bears the burden of demonstrating that its restrictions are "narrowly tailored" to serve a compelling governmental interest.[87]

Nursing Facilities

The Centers for Medicare and Medicaid Services' review process includes a review of the rights of any nursing facility residents participating in experimental research. Surveyors will review the records of residents identified as participating in a clinical research study. They will determine whether informed consent forms have been executed properly. The form will be reviewed to determine whether all known risks have been identified. Appropriate questions may be directed to both the staff and residents or the residents' guardians.

Possible questions to ask staff include[88]:

- Is the facility participating in any experimental research?

- If yes, what residents are involved? (Interview a sample of these residents.)

Residents or guardians may be asked questions such as[89]:

- Are you participating in the study?

- Was this explained to you well enough so that you understand what the study is about and any risks that might be involved?

Patients participating in research studies should fully understand the implications of their participation. Health care organizations involved in research studies should have appropriate protocols in place that protect the rights of patients. Consent forms should describe both the risks and benefits involved in the research activity.

The Court's Decision

The Accomack Virginia Circuit Court Judge cleared Abraham's parents of all charges of medical neglect and allowed Abraham to pursue alternative treatment under a doctor of the family's choice. Abraham will be monitored by a board-certified oncologist who is experienced in alternative cancer treatment. The family will provide the court updates on Abraham's care every three months until he's cured or turns 18. The question to be asked in this case includes: Whose body is it, anyway? Did the state go too far? The judge must have thought so.

The judge agreed to allow me to see an oncologist of my choice! My alternative treatments WILL continue. He also ruled that my parents were not guilty of medical neglect, and social services no longer has any jurisdiction over my case! Free, happy, and ready to live, that's me!"[90]

CHAPTER REVIEW

1. *Ethics* is that branch of philosophy that deals with values related to human conduct in regard to right and wrong actions, good and bad motives, and ends. In relation to health care, ethics includes not only philosophical, but also economic, medical, political, and legal dilemmas.

2. *Morality* is a code of conduct. It is a guide to behavior that all rational persons would put forward for governing their behavior. Morality describes a class of rules held by society to govern the conduct of its individual members. A *moral dilemma* occurs when ideas of right and wrong conflict. *Moral judgments* are those judgments concerned with what an individual or group believes to be the right or proper behavior in a given situation.

3. A *virtue* is normally defined as some sort of moral excellence or beneficial quality. A moral value is the relative worth placed on some virtuous behavior. A *value* is a standard of conduct. Values are used for judging the goodness or badness of some action. Ethical values imply standards of worth. They are the standards by which we measure the goodness in our lives. *Intrinsic value* is something that has value in and of itself. *Instrumental value* is something that helps to give value to something else (e.g., money is valuable for what it can buy).

4. *Situational ethics* refers to a particular view of ethics, in which absolute standards are considered less important than the requirements of a particular situation.

5. *Autonomy* involves recognizing the right of a person to make one's own decisions. Autonomy is not an absolute principle, meaning that the autonomous actions of one person must not infringe upon the rights of another.

6. *Medical paternalism* involves making choices for patients who are capable of making their own choices. This directly violates patient autonomy.

7. Health care ethics committees are designed to educate and advise health care providers, patients, and families and to analyze ethical dilemmas. Such a committee serves as a hospital resource designed to offer objective counsel. The committee performs functions such as developing policy and procedure guidelines to assist in resolving ethical dilemmas, educating staff and community, resolving conflicts, reviewing cases, offering support and consultation, and offering political advocacy.

8. When there exists an element of uncertainty regarding a patient's wishes in an emergency situation, the situation should be resolved in a way that favors the preservation of life.

9. Euthanasia is the mercy killing of the hopelessly ill, injured, or incapacitated. The debate over euthanasia is complex, and the legal system must maintain a balance between ensuring that the patient's constitutional rights are protected and protecting society's interests in preserving life, preventing suicide, and maintaining the integrity of the medical profession.

   - *Active euthanasia* is the intentional commission of an act that will result in death.

   - *Passive euthanasia* involves the withdrawal or withholding of life-saving treatment.

10. The invention of machinery that can sustain heartbeat and respiration has called into question the idea of what constitutes death. By statute, most states recognize brain death.

11. Because of the debate surrounding right-to-die issues, patients should be counseled to make decisions regarding their wishes while they are competent. Living wills, designation of surrogates, health care proxies, and powers of attorney are legal steps that allow patients to express their wishes.

12. According to the Patient Self-Determination Act of 1990, health care organizations have a responsibility to explain to patients, staff, and families that patients have legal rights to direct their medical and nursing care as it corresponds to existing state law. This includes right-to-die directives.

13. Health care proxies do not require that a person know about and consider in advance every situation and decision that could arise. Instead, the appointed agent would have to interpret the patient's wishes based on the information given at the time that the patient is incapacitated and unable to make decisions. A living will provides specific instructions as to a patient's wishes, such as a desire not to be maintained on a respirator.

14. Dr. Jack Kevorkian is probably the most famous figure in the debate surrounding assisted suicide. The Supreme Court ruled that there exists no constitutional right to assisted suicide, and this decision allowed the state of Michigan to prosecute him for helping patients commit suicide.

15. Do-not-resuscitate orders are given by physicians and indicate that, in the event of a cardiac or respiratory arrest, no resuscitative measures should be used to revive the patient. These orders must be in writing and must be signed and dated by the physician.

16. The Oregon Death with Dignity Act allows terminally ill Oregon residents to obtain prescriptions from their physicians for self-administered, lethal medications.

17. Autopsies are postmortem examinations conducted to ascertain the cause of death. Most states have enacted autopsy consent statutes that establish an order to obtain consent to autopsy based on the degree of family relationship.

18. The Uniform Anatomical Gift Act allows a person to make a decision to donate organs at the time of death.

19. In most states, a combination of federal and state guidelines and regulations ensures the proper supervision and control over experimentation involving human subjects. An organization's institutional review board is responsible for reviewing, monitoring, and approving clinical investigations of drugs and medical devices that involve human subjects. Written consent must be obtained from patients participating in clinical investigations.

REVIEW QUESTIONS

1. Discuss how one caregiver's beliefs can be in conflict with another when making end-of-life decisions. Consider the topics discussed on morality, virtues, situational ethics, autonomy, and medical paternalism when framing your answer.

2. Discuss the ever-expanding role of ethics committees, including internal operational issues and external influences that affect internal operations.

3. What are the differences between allowing a patient to die and physician-assisted suicide?

4. Examine the statement: "The inherent risk is that society's faith in doctors as healers would become subverted if doctors participate in physician-assisted suicide."

5. Constitutionally, what gives patients the right to self-determination?

6. Explain why you think the *Schiavo* case is or is not an example of legislating morality.

WEB SITE RESOURCES

Advance Directives	www.mindspring.com/~scottr/will.html
Bioethics	www.bioethics.net
Biotech and Health Care Ethics	www.scu.edu/ethics/practicing/focusareas/medical/
Center for Bioethics in Human Society	www.cbhd.org/
National Advisory Board on Health Care Ethics	www.etene.org/e/index.shtml
National Center for Biotechnology Information	www.ncbi.nlm.nih.gov/
Questia-Medical Ethics	www.questia.com/Index.jsp?CRID=medical_ethics&OFFID=se1
TransWeb	www.transweb.org

NOTES

1. *My Journey,* Abraham Cherrix's Home Page, http://www.abrahamsjourney.com/theHOMEpage.html.

2. *Protection and Use of Human Subjects in Research,* Eastern University of Michigan, www.rcr.emich.edu/module1/a_7part1.html.

3. WMA History, *The Golden Years in Medical Ethics,* The World Medical Association, www.wma.net/e/history/index.htm.

4. *The Kennedy Institute of Ethics,* Georgetown University. www.georgetown.edu/research/kie/site/index.htm.

5. 464 F.2d 772 (D.C. Cir. 1972).

6. The National Commission for the Protection of Human Subjects of Biomedical and Behavioral Research, *The Belmont Report, Ethical Principles and Guidelines for the Protection of Human Subjects of Research.* www.hhs.gov/ohrp/humansubjects/guidance/belmont.htm.

7. *In re Quinlan,* 355 A.2d 647 (N.J. 1976).

8. 42 U.S.C. 1395cc(a)(1).

9. *Cruzan v. Director of the Mo. Dep't of Health,* 497 U.S. 261 (1990).

10. Oregon Revised Statutes, Chapter 127—Powers of Attorney; Advance Directives for Health Care; Declarations for Mental Health Treatment; Death with Dignity, 2005 Edition. http://landru.leg.state.or.us/ors/127.html.

11. Advising the President on ethical issues related to advances in biomedical science and technology, The President's Council on Bioethics, www.bioethics.gov/.

12. *State of Oregon v. Ashcroft,* No. 02-35587 (C.A. 9, Ore. 2004).

13. *Gonzales v. Oregon,* 04-623.

14. *The Definition of Morality,* Stanford Encyclopedia of Philosophy, 2005, http://plato.stanford.edu/entries/morality-definition/.

15. *Stamford Hosp. v. Vega,* 674 A.2d 821 (Conn. Super. Ct. 1996).

16. No. 31328 (W.Va. 2004).

17. 725 P.2d 400 (Or. Ct. App. 1986).

18. *Florida Bar v. Barrett,* No. SC03-375 (Fla. 2005).

19. *In re Quinlan, Supra note* 7.

20. *Union Pac. Ry. Co. v. Botsford,* 141 U.S. 250, 251 (1891).

21. 105 N.E. 92, 93 (N.Y. 1914).

22. *Id.*

23. 438 N.Y.S.2d 266, 272 (N.Y. 1981).

24. 410 U.S. 113 (1973).

25. *Quinlan,* 355 A.2d at 663 (N.J. 1976).

26. 370 N.E.2d 417 (Mass. 1977).

27. *Id.* at 434.

28. GELFORD, *Euthanasia and the Terminally Ill Patient,* 63 NEB. L. REV. 741, 747 (1984).

29. 380 N.E.2d 134 (Mass. 1978).

30. 405 N.E.2d 115 (Mass. 1980).

31. 452 So. 2d 925 (Fla. 1984).

32. 362 So. 2d 160 (Fla. Dist. Ct. App. 1978).

33. *John F. Kennedy Mem'l Hosp. v. Bludworth,* 452 So. 2d 921, 925 (Fla. 1984) (citing *In re Welfare of Colyer,* 660 P.2d 738 (Wash. 1983), in which the court found prior court approval to be "unresponsive and cumbersome").

34. *Severns v. Wilmington Med. Ctr.,* 425 A.2d 156 (Del. Ch. 1980) (incompetent's right to refuse medical treatment may be expressed through a guardian when the patient is in a chronic vegetative state); *Leach v. Akron Gen. Med. Ctr.,* 426 N.E.2d 809 (Ohio Com. Pl. 1980) (right to privacy includes right of terminally ill patient in a vegetative state to determine his or her own course of treatment).

35. *Satz v. Perlmutter,* 379 So. 2d 359 (Fla. 1980) (constitutional right to privacy supports decision of competent adult suffering from a terminal illness to refuse extraordinary treatment); *Superintendent of Belchertown State Sch. v. Saikewicz,* 370 N.E.2d 417 (Mass. 1977) (right to refuse medical treatment for terminal illness extends to incompetent patients).

36. *Schmitt v. Pierce,* 344 S.W.2d 120 (Mo. 1961).

37. CONNERY, *Prolonging Life: The Duty and Its Limits, Moral Responsibility in Prolonging Life's Decisions,* in TO TREAT OR NOT TO TREAT 25 (1984).

38. *Statement of Medical Opinion Re: "Brain Death,"* A.M.A. HOUSE OF DELEGATES RES. (June 1974).

39. 482 N.Y.S.2d 436 (1984).

40. 438 N.Y.S.2d 266 (1981).

41. 534 N.E.2d 886 (N.Y. 1988).

42. *Id.* at 891.

43. *Cruzan v. Harman,* 760 S.W.2d 408 (Mo. 1988).

44. *Id.* at 425.

45. *Cruzan v. Director of the Mo. Dep't of Health,* 497 U.S. 261 (1990).

46. Pa. S.646, Amendment A3506, Printer's No. 689, Oct. 1, 1990.

47. 20 PA. CONS. STAT. ANN. § 5602(a)(9) (1988).

48. *Hospital Wants to Let Wife Die,* NEWSDAY, Jan. 11, 1991, at 13.

49. *Farnam v. Crista Ministries,* 807 P.2d 830, 849 (Wash. 1991).

50. 42 U.S.C. § 1395cc (1992).

51. J. PODGERS, *Matters of Life and Death,* A.B.A.J. May 1992, at 60.

52. *In re Estate of Brooks,* 205 N.E.2d 435 (Ill. 1965); *Superintendent of Belchertown State Sch. v. Saikewicz,* 370 N.E.2d 417 (Mass. 1977); *In re Quinlan,* 355 A.2d 647 (N.J. 1976).

53. 376 N.E.2d 1232 (Mass. App. Ct. 1979).

54. *Dr. Death at Work,* NEWSDAY, Feb. 7, 1991, at 12.

55. *Kevorkian Charges Dropped,* NEWSDAY, July 22, 1992, at 4.

56. *Hobbins v. Attorney Gen. of Mich.,* No. 94-1473 (Mich. 1994); *Kevorkian v. Michigan,* No. 94-1490 (Mich. 1994).

57. *22nd Death for "Dr. Death,"* USA TODAY, May 9, 1995, at 2A.

58. *Or. Rev. Stat. Sects. 127.800-.897*

59. 117 S. Ct. 2258 (1997).

60. *McIver v. Krischer,* No. CL-96-1504-AF (Jan. 31, 1997) (stay issued February 11, 1997).

61. *Bush v. Schiavo,* No. SC04-925 (Fla. App. 2004).

62. 420 N.E.2d 64 (N.Y. 1981).

63. *Collins v. Lake Forest Hospital,* 821 N.E.2d 316, 213 Ill.2d 234, 290 Ill. Dec. 265 (Ill. 2004).

64. *Pettis v. Smith,* 880 So.2d 145 (La. Ct. App. 2004).

65. 611 A.2d 1148 (N.J. Super Ct. 1992).

66. 486 A.2d 1209 (N.J. Sup. Ct. 1985).

67. *Id.*

68. U.S. CONGRESS, OFF. OF TECHNOLOGY ASSESSMENT, PUB. NO. OTA-BA306, *Life-Sustaining Technologies and the Elderly* 48 (1987).

69. *John F. Kennedy Mem'l Hosp. v. Bludworth,* 452 So. 2d 921, 925 (Fla. 1984) (citing *In re Welfare of Colyer,* 660 P.2d 738 (Wash. 1983), in which the court found prior court approval to be "unresponsive and cumbersome").

70. *AMA Changes Code of Ethics on Comas,* NEWSDAY, Mar. 17, 1986, at 2.

71. *In re Jobes,* 529 A.2d 434 (N.J. 1987).

72. *Id.* at 438.

73. *Man Wins Right to Let Wife Die,* NEWSDAY, Apr. 24, 1986, at 3.

74. 549 N.E.2d 292 (Ill. 1989).

75. *Bouvia v. Superior Court (Glenchur),* 225 Cal. Rptr. 297 (Cal. Ct. App. 1986).

76. *Id.* at 306.

77. 147 Cal. App. 3d 1006 (Cal. Ct. App. 1983).

78. *John F. Kennedy Mem'l Hosp. v. Bludworth,* 452 So. 2d 921, 925 (Fla. 1984) (citing *In re Welfare of Colyer,* 660 P.2d 738 (Wash. 1983), in which the court found prior court approval to be "unresponsive and cumbersome").

79. 549 N.E.2d 1043 (Ind. Ct. App. 1990).

80. 225 N.Y.S.2d 434 (N.Y. Ct. Cl. 1962).

81. 624 A.2d 663 (Pa. Comm. Ct. 1993).

82. 297 F. Supp. 1142 (S.D.N.Y. 1969).

83. 519 N.Y.S.2d 928 (N.Y. Sup. Ct. 1987).

84. *Blaz v. Michael Reese Hosp. Found.,* 74 F. Supp. 2d 803 (D.C. Ill. 1999).

85. 607 A.2d 1111 (1992).

86. 428 F. Supp. 360 (D.D.C. 1977).

87. *Abigail Alliance for Better Access to Developmental Drugs v. Eschenbach,* Washington Legal Foundation, www.wlf.org/Litigating/casedetail.asp?detail=266.

88. 2 C.F.R. § 488.115 (1989).

89. *Id.*

90. Cherrix, *supra note* 1.

Professional Liability Insurance

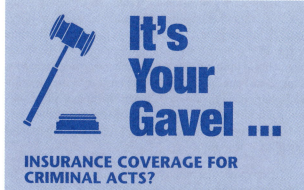

It's Your Gavel ...

INSURANCE COVERAGE FOR CRIMINAL ACTS?

A physician was convicted for the sexual assault of a minor. He was then sued in federal court for civil damages. An insurer had issued medical malpractice policies to the physician. Under the policies, the insurer agreed to pay on behalf of the insured all sums that the insured became legally obligated to pay as damages because of bodily injury or personal injury resulting from rendering or failing to render, during the policy period, professional services by the insured. The policies contained an express exclusion barring liability of the insurer for any acts of the insured arising out of the performance of a criminal act.

Does sexual assault constitute rendering professional services within the coverage provisions of the physician's insurance policy? Should a malpractice insurer be required to indemnify a physician for liability resulting from the sexual assault of a minor?[1]

WHAT IS YOUR VERDICT?

I never was ruined but twice—once when I gained a lawsuit, and once when I lost one.

Francois Marie de Voltaire (1694–1778)

This chapter introduces the reader to some of the basic concepts related to liability insurance. The purpose of liability insurance is to spread the risk of economic loss among members of a group who share common risks. For example, an obstetrician would share risk with other obstetricians. As risks increase, premiums increase to cover associated risks. The premiums are placed in a shared risk fund from which funds are drawn to cover the costs of lawsuits. As high awards are paid out of the fund, there is a danger that patients will have a more difficult time to find physicians willing to accept them as patients. Some physicians, because of skyrocketing malpractice premiums, find it to costly to maintain a private practice. As a result, they often limit their practice to less costly procedures or, to those that have able practices.

Medical malpractice insurance, as in all insurance, is subject to the cyclical nature of the insurance market. Problems intrinsic in malpractice insurance include the uncertainty of the U.S. legal system, the effects of inflation on ultimate claim values, emerging technology, and new treatments.

THE INSURANCE POLICY

Insurance is a contract that creates legal obligations on the part of both the insured and the insurer. It is a contract in which the insurer agrees to assume certain risks of the insured for consideration or payment of a premium. Under the terms of the contract, also known as the *insurance policy,* the insurer promises to pay a specific amount of money if a specified event takes place. An insurance policy contains three necessary elements:

1. identification of the risk covered

2. the specific amount payable

3. the specified occurrence

Insurance companies are required by the laws of the different states to issue only policies that contain certain mandated provisions and to maintain certain financial reserves to guarantee to policyholders that their expectations will be met when coverage is needed. The basic underlying concept of insurance is the spreading of risk. By writing coverage for a large enough pool of individuals, the company has determined actuarially that a certain number of claims will arise within that pool, and if the premium structure has been established correctly and the prediction of claims made accurately, the company ought to be able to meet those claims and return a profit to its shareholders.

Risk Categories

A *risk* is the possibility that a loss will occur. The main function of insurance is to provide security against this loss. Insurance does not prevent or hinder the occurrence of the loss, but it does compensate for the damages.

An insured individual may be exposed to three categories of risk: (1) property loss or damage, (2) personal injury or loss of life, and (3) incurring legal liability. *Property risk* is the possibility that an insured's property may be damaged or destroyed by fire, flood, tornado, hurricane, or other catastrophe. *Personal risk* is the possibility that the insured may be injured in an accident or may become ill; the possibility of death is a personal risk covered in the typical life insurance plan. *Legal liability risk* is the possibility that the insured may become legally liable to pay money damages to another and includes accident and professional liability insurance.

Insurance Polices

Insurance policies include *occurrence policies,* which cover all incidents that arise during a policy year, regardless of when they are reported to the insurer; and *claims-made policies,* which cover only those claims made or reported during the policy year. *Tail coverage policies* provide for

an uninterrupted extension of an insurance policy period. *Umbrella policies* cover awards over the amount provided in the basic policy coverage. The dollar amount of coverage is specified in the policy dollar.

LIABILITY OF THE PROFESSIONAL

An individual who provides professional services to another person may be legally responsible for any harm the person suffers as a result of negligence. Many professionals protect themselves from their exposure to a legal loss by acquiring a professional liability insurance policy.

All Professionals Need Insurance

All health care professionals should carry liability insurance. Even though a hospital, for example, as an employer can be held liable for the acts of its employees under the doctrine of *respondeat superior,* the employee can be financially liable to the employer for his or her own negligent acts. From a cost-benefit standpoint, the answer to the question "Do I really need insurance?" is yes. Insurance premiums for allied health professionals are relatively reasonable.

Malpractice insurance coverage is especially important if a caregiver is working:

- as a volunteer at a clinic or health fair not sponsored by his or her employer

- as an independent contractor providing a service in a patient's home

- for an independent agency or registry

- for an organization that is covered by an insurance policy that has an exclusionary provision by which the insurance company disclaims liability for malpractice actions brought against the insured organization

If a private agency has inadequate insurance coverage, there is always a possibility that recovery will be sought against a nurse's estate.

There are disadvantages to nurses obtaining malpractice insurance. First, acquisition of malpractice coverage by nurses could encourage naming nurses as defendants in malpractice suits. Second, an increase in complaints against nurses could cause a rise in insurance premiums, eventually placing the cost of malpractice insurance outside their financial means.

A nurse's insurance policy was primary with respect to the first $100,000 of a settlement that resulted from a malpractice action against the nurse in *American Nurses Association v. Passaic General Hospital.*[2] The National Fire Insurance Company had issued an insurance policy covering the contractual obligation of the American Nurses Association to its members. The New Jersey Supreme Court held that the judgment against the nurse in excess of $100,000 was properly apportioned equally between the hospital's liability insurer and the association's liability insurer.

The court in *Jones v. Medox, Inc.*[3] held that only the nurse's insurance carrier, Globe Insurance, was liable for injuries sustained by the plaintiff while at Doctors Hospital; these injuries resulted from an injection administered by the nurse. Medox, Inc., a corporation providing temporary medical personnel to Doctors Hospital, employed Ms. Jones. After settlement of the claim against the nurse, the hospital, and the nurse's employer, the nurse and her insurer brought an action against Doctors Hospital, Medox, Inc., and their insurers. The trial court granted summary judgment in favor of the hospital and its insurer and dismissed the claim against Medox, Inc., and its insurer.

Private-Duty Nurse

A private-duty nurse is not considered an employee but rather is engaged by the patient (or the patient's family) to provide services to that patient. As such, the nurse should obtain personal coverage. The patient engaging the nurse would be well advised to ask about the availability of such coverage, as would the institution in which the nurse is providing professional care for that patient.

Even though a patient employs a special-duty nurse, an organization can be liable for damages resulting from a nurse's negligent conduct. The existence of an employer-employee relationship, which determines the applicability of *respondeat superior,* is a matter to be determined by the jury.

An organization also can be liable for damages awarded in a malpractice action if a nurse and his or her registry have inadequate insurance to cover a jury award. In such instances, an organization then would have a right to seek recovery from the nurse and the registry.

Students

The potential for liability is not limited to licensed professionals. Students engaged in learning a profession who engage in activities involving the care and treatment of others face potential liability for their acts. For this reason, these individuals often obtain personal insurance coverage or assure themselves of such coverage through the organization in which they are employed or the institution in which they are enrolled to obtain their education.

THE INSURANCE AGREEMENT

Health care organizations, nurses, physicians, and other health care practitioners who are covered by an insurance policy must recognize the rights and duties inherent in the policy. The professional being insured should be able to identify the risks that are covered, the amount of coverage, and the conditions of the contract.

Although the policies of different insurance companies may vary, the standard policy usually provides that the insurance company will pay on behalf of the insured all sums that the insured shall become legally obligated to pay as damages because of injury arising out of malpractice error or mistake in rendering or failing to render professional services. A standard liability insurance policy has five distinct parts:

1. insurance agreement

2. defense and settlement

3. policy period

4. amount payable

5. conditions of the policy

The insurer, under the terms of the policy, has a legal obligation to pay the sum that has been agreed to or determined by a court, up to the policy limit, including legal fees. Under a professional liability policy, the professional is protected from damages arising from rendering or failing to render professional services. Thus, a professional who performs a negligent act resulting in legal liability or who fails to perform a necessary act (thereby incurring damages) is personally protected from paying an injured party. The insurer makes payment of damages to the injured party.

Defense and Settlement

In the defense and settlement portion of the insurance policy, the insured and the insurance company agree that the company will defend any lawsuit against the insured arising from performance or nonperformance of professional services. The insurance company is delegated the power to effect a settlement of any claims as it deems necessary. In a professional liability policy, the duty of the insurer under this clause is limited to the defense of lawsuits against the insured that are a consequence of professional services.

The insurance company fulfills its obligation to provide a defense by engaging the services of an attorney on behalf of the insured. The obligation of the attorney is to the insured directly, because the insured is the attorney's client. Here is, to some extent, a divided loyalty because the attorney looks to the insurance company to obtain business. Nevertheless, the attorney-client relationship exists between only the attorney and the insured, and the insured has the right to expect the attorney to fulfill the requirements of such a relationship.

If an insurance company has established the right to obtain a settlement of any claim prior to trial, the company's only obligation is to act reasonably and not to the detriment of the insured.

Policy Period

The period of the policy is stated in the insurance contract. Under an *occurrence policy,* the contract provides protection only for claims that occur during the time frame within which the policy is stated to be in effect. Any incident that occurs before or after the policy period would not be covered under the insuring agreement. Occurrence policies provide coverage for all claims that may arise out of a policy period. The actual reporting time has no bearing on the validity of the claim, so long as it is filed before the applicable statute of limitations tolls. Although the reporting time has no bearing on the validity of the claim from the standpoint of coverage under the policy, the conditions of the policy will require notice within a specified time. Failure to provide such notice could void the insurer's obligation under the policy if it can be demonstrated that the carrier's position was compromised as a result of filing an untimely claim or report.

A *claims-made policy* provides coverage for only those claims instituted during the policy period. Notice of a claim is required during the policy period. Failure to give notice of a claim to the insurer in a claims-made policy until after the policy expires can result in denial by the insurance company to cover the claim.

Coverage: The Amount Payable

The amount to be paid by an insurer is determined by the amount of damages incurred by the injured party. The insurance company and the injured party may negotiate a settlement prior to or during trial. Some states have provisions mandating that consent of the court must be obtained prior to the settlement of a negligence claim on behalf of a minor.

In any event, the insurance company will pay the injured party no more than the maximum limit stated in the insurance policy. The insured professional must personally pay any damages that exceed the policy limits. For example, under a policy with a maximum coverage of $1 million for each claim and $3 million for aggregate claims (the total amount payable to all injured parties), the insured must pay any amount over $1 million on each individual claim and any amount over $3 million in a policy period.

Punitive Damages

A claim for punitive damages awarded in a malpractice suit was submitted to an insurance carrier for payment but was subsequently denied by the carrier.[4] The insurance carrier cited Florida public policy, which prohibits coverage of punitive damage awards.

Uninsured Claims

An insurer has no duty to defend or provide coverage for intentional torts. Contracts insuring against loss from intentional wrongs are generally void as being against public policy.

Intentional Torts

An action was brought by a comprehensive liability insurer for declaratory judgment as to its duty to defend the insured in civil actions alleging slander, interference with business relations, and violations of the federal antitrust laws in *St. Paul Insurance Co. v. Talladega Nursing Home.*[5] The federal district court ruled for the insurer, and the nursing facility appealed. The Fifth Circuit held that the insurer has no duty to defend or provide coverage for alleged intentional torts. Under Alabama law, all contracts insuring against loss from intentional wrongs are void as being against public policy.

Sexual Assault

Sexual assault does not constitute rendering professional services within the coverage provisions of insurance policies. As a result, malpractice insurers are not required to indemnify the insured for liability resulting from the sexual assault. The Medical Protective Company, in *R.W. v. Schrein,*[6] a physician's professional liability insurer, sought a judgment determining that it had no duty to defend or indemnify the physician with respect to five former patients who claimed that they were sexually abused during examination and treatment. The Supreme Court of Nebraska held that there is no clearly articulated public policy that would permit or require the court to disregard the fact that the physician's acts did not fall within the coverage provided. The physician's liability to the appellants was not based on the provision or failure to provide professional services.

There was no duty by the malpractice insurer in *Sanzi v. Shetty*[7] to defend the pediatric neurologist who allegedly sexually abused a patient for a period of eight years, beginning when she was just 14 years old. It was asserted that such abuse led to the patient's suicide approximately 12 years after the neurologist ended his relationship with the patient. It was alleged that the neurologist had deceived the patient's parents into believing that it would be beneficial to the patient to spend Saturdays working in his office, where he allegedly sexually abused the patient during regular medical visits and on the purported Saturday workdays. A hearing justice found that the malpractice insurer had no duty to defend or indemnify the neurologist. The state supreme court held that because the claim against the doctor did not allege injury arising from the rendering or failure to render professional services, it was not covered by the policy. The only connection between the doctor's acts and his profession was that the sexual abuse of the deceased occurred at his office while she worked there. Because the alleged sexual abuse carried with it an inferred intent to harm, there was no accidental nature to the resulting injuries. Consequently, the insurer was relieved from its duty to defend or indemnify the insured physician.

Conditions of an Insurance Policy

Each insurance policy contains a number of important conditions. Failure to comply with these conditions may cause forfeiture of the policy and nonpayment of claims against it. Generally, insurance policies contain the following conditions:

- *notice of occurrence*—When the insured becomes aware that an injury has occurred as a result of acts covered under the contract, the insured must notify the insurance company promptly. The form of notice may be either oral or written, as specified in the policy.

- *notice of claim*—Whenever the insured receives notice that a claim or suit is being instituted, prompt notice must be sent by the insured to the insurance company. This provides the insurance company with an opportunity to investigate the facts of a case. The policy will specify what papers are to be forwarded to the company. The mere failure to advise in a timely manner may be in and of itself a breach of the insurance contract, entitling the insurer to decline coverage. It may not matter that the insurer has in no way been prejudiced by the late notification. The mere fact that the insured failed to carry out obligations under the policy may be sufficient to permit the insurer to avoid its obligations. When the insurer has refused to honor a claim because of late notice and the insured wishes to challenge such refusal, an action can be brought, asking a court to determine the reasonableness of the insurer's position.

- *assistance of the insured*—The insured must cooperate with the insurance company and render any assistance necessary to reach a settlement.

- *other insurance*—If the insured has pertinent insurance policies with other insurance companies, the insured must notify the insurance company so that each company may pay the appropriate amount of the claim.

- *assignment*—The protections contracted for by the insured may not be transferred unless the insurance company grants permission. Because the insurance company was aware of the risks the insured would encounter before the policy was issued, the company will endeavor to avoid protecting persons other than the policyholder.

- *subrogation*—This is the right of a person who pays another's debt to be substituted for all rights in relation to the debt. When an insurance company makes a payment for the insured under the terms of the policy, the company becomes the beneficiary of all the rights of recovery the insured has against any other persons who also may have been negligent. For example, if several nurses were found liable for negligence arising from the same occurrence and the insurance company for one nurse pays the entire claim, the company will be entitled to the rights of that nurse and may collect a proportionate share of the claim from the other nurses.

- *changes*—The insured cannot make changes in the policy without the written consent of the insurance company. Thus, an agent of the insurance company ordinarily cannot modify or remove any condition of the liability contract. Only the insurance company, by written authorization, may permit a condition to be altered or removed.

- *cancellation*—A cancellation clause spells out the conditions and procedures necessary for the insured or the insurer to cancel the liability policy. Written notice usually is required. The insured person's failure to comply with any terms of the policy can result in cancellation and possible nonpayment of a claim by the insurance company. As a legal contract, failure to meet the terms and conditions of an insurance policy can result in a breach of contract and voidance of coverage.

MEDICAL LIABILITY INSURANCE

The fundamental tenets of insurance law and their application to the typical liability insurance policy are pertinent to the provisions of medical professional liability insurance as applied to individuals and institutions. Professional liability policies vary in the broadness, the exclusions from coverage, and the interpretations a company places on the language of the contract.

There are three medical professional liability classes:

1. individuals including (but not limited to) physicians, surgeons, dentists, nurses, osteopaths, chiropractors, opticians, physiotherapists, optometrists, and different types of medical technicians (This category may include medical laboratories and blood banks.)

2. health care institutions, such as hospitals, extended-care facilities, homes for the aged, institutions for the mentally ill, and other health care facilities where bed and board are provided for patients or residents

3. outpatient facilities and clinics where there are no regular bed or board facilities (These institutions may be related to industrial or commercial enterprises; however, they are to be distinguished from facilities operated by

dentists or physicians, which usually are covered under individual professional liability contracts.)

The insuring clause usually will provide for payment on behalf of the insured if an injury arises from either of the following:

- malpractice, error, or mistake in rendering or failing to render professional services in the practice of the insured's profession during the policy period

- acts or omissions on the part of the insured during the policy period as a member of a formal accreditation or similar professional board or committee of a health care facility or a professional society

Although injury is not limited to bodily injury or property damage, it must result from malpractice, error, mistake, or failure to perform acts that should have been performed.

The most common risks covered by medical professional liability insurance are

- negligence

- assault and battery as a result of failing to obtain consent to a medical or surgical procedure

- libel and slander

- invasion of privacy for betrayal of professional confidences

Coverage may vary from company to company, but standards of policy coverage generally are followed. Rates will differ for individuals by profession and specialty and by type of health care facility (e.g., nursing facility and hospital).

SELF-INSURANCE

Exorbitant malpractice insurance premiums often have produced situations in which the premium cost of insurance has approached and, on occasion, reached the face amount of the policy. Because of the extremely high cost of maintaining such insurance, some institutions have sought alternatives to this conventional means of protecting against medical malpractice. One alternative is self-insurance. When a health care facility self-insures its malpractice risks, it no longer purchases a policy of malpractice insurance but instead periodically sets aside a certain amount of its own funds as a reserve against malpractice losses and expenses. An institution that self-insures generally retains the services of a self-insurance consulting firm and of an actuary to determine the proper level of funding that the institution should maintain.

A self-insurance program need not involve the elimination of insurance coverage in its entirety. A health care organization may find it prudent to purchase excess cover-

age whereby the organization self-insures the first agreed-on dollar amount of risk and the insurance carrier insures the balance. For example, in a typical program the organization may self-insure the first $1 million of professional liability risk per year. Because most claims will be disposed of within such limitation, the cost of excess insurance may be quite reasonable.

Before a corporation makes a decision to self-insure, not only must it determine the economic aspects of such a decision and the necessary funding levels to maintain an adequate reserve for future claims, but it also must determine whether there are any legal impediments to such a program. A corporation that has obtained funding from governmental sources or that has issued bonds or other obligations containing certain covenants may find itself unable to self-insure because of these prior commitments. Health care organizations should consult legal counsel to review appropriate and applicable documentation before making the self-insurance decision.

TRUSTEE COVERAGE

Trustees should be covered by liability insurance just as physicians and other health care professionals. Such coverage is generally provided for by the organization. Such coverage is helpful in attracting qualified board members. Before an insurer writing a trustee policy (generally known as directors' and officers' liability insurance) will respond to defend or pay a claim on behalf of a trustee, it must be shown that the trustee acted in good faith and within the scope of his or her responsibilities. Ordinarily, coverage would not be afforded when a trustee is accused of acting improperly in his or her relationship with the corporation. Also, insurance coverage for officers' and directors' liability generally excludes as a covered event the failure to obtain other necessary insurance for the institution (e.g., fire insurance).

Insurance coverage for officers and directors of a corporation should include indemnification, to the extent possible by law, for all liabilities and expenses including:

- counsel fees and expenses that are reasonably incurred as the result of any legal proceeding stemming from lawsuits that might arise in connection with an officer's or director's position with the corporation

- funds paid in satisfaction of judgments

- fines and penalties

- coverage that extends to actions taken while in office or thereafter, by reason of being or having been a director or officer of the corporation, excepting when the officer or director has not acted in good faith or in the reasonable belief that an officer's or director's action was not in the best interest of the corporation

MANDATED MEDICAL STAFF INSURANCE COVERAGE

Physicians often are required by health care organizations to carry their own malpractice insurance. Physicians who fail to maintain such coverage can be suspended from a hospital's medical staff. A federal district court in *Pollack v. Methodist Hospital*[8] ruled that a hospital has the legal right to suspend a staff physician for failing to comply with its requirement that physicians carry medical malpractice insurance coverage. The decision resulted from a suit brought against a hospital by a physician whose staff privileges were suspended because he failed to comply with a newly adopted hospital requirement that all staff physicians provide proof of malpractice coverage of at least $1 million. The court rejected the physician's charges that the requirement violated his civil rights and antitrust laws.

As held in *Wilkinson v. Madera Community Hospital,*[9] a health care organization can require its medical staff to show evidence of professional liability insurance. The physician in this case was refused reappointment because he failed to maintain malpractice insurance with a recognized insurance company as required by the hospital.

INVESTIGATION AND SETTLEMENT OF CLAIMS

An injured party may request settlement of a claim prior to instituting legal action. As a first step toward settlement of a claim, the insurance carrier may have an investigator interview a claimant regarding the details of the alleged occurrence that led to the injury. After an investigation, the insurance company may agree to a settlement if liability is questionable and the risks of proceeding to trial are too great. Should settlement negotiations fail, an attorney may be employed by the injured party to negotiate a settlement. If the attorney fails to obtain a settlement, either the claim can be dropped or legal action commenced.

Once a claim is settled, a general release, signed by the plaintiff, surrenders the right of action against the defendant. If the claimant is married, a general release also should be obtained from the spouse because there may be a cause of action due to loss of the injured spouse's services (e.g., companionship). A parent's release surrenders only a parental claim. Approval of a court may be necessary to release a child's claim. A release by a minor, in some instances, may be repudiated by the minor upon reaching majority. A general release can be voided if the releasee:

- is intoxicated, under the influence of drugs, in shock, or in extreme pain that prevents sufficient understanding of a general release and therefore prevents or voids its execution

- does not understand the language of the release

- has not had the opportunity to obtain appropriate legal consultation

- has been the victim of mental or physical duress

- has executed the release as a result of misrepresentation or fraud

- is mentally incompetent and cannot give a valid release (In this instance, a court-appointed guardian is required to execute a release on behalf of a mental incompetent, and a court must pass on the terms of any settlement.)

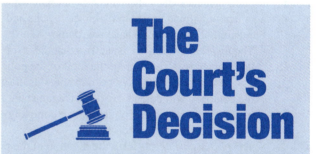

The Court's Decision

Sexual assault did not constitute rendering professional services within coverage provisions of the physician's insurance policy. The New Mexico Supreme Court held that the malpractice insurer was not required to indemnify a physician for liability resulting from the sexual assault of a minor. The physician's conviction was admitted into evidence not to prove negligence but to prove that the physician's misconduct constituted criminal acts within exclusions of liability policies.

CHAPTER REVIEW

1. As with all insurance, medical malpractice insurance is affected by the cyclical nature of the insurance market. Specific issues that affect malpractice insurance are the changing legal system, inflation's effects on claim values, new technology, and new treatments.

2. *Insurance* is a contract in which the company providing the insurance agrees to assume some of the risks of the insured party for consideration or the payment of a premium. There are three primary components of an insurance policy:
   - identification of the covered risks
   - specification of the amounts payable
   - specification of the occurrence

3. By creating a large pool of individuals, an insurance company can balance its risk—the possibility that loss will occur—enough that it should be able to both cover claims and return a profit to shareholders.

4. There are three primary categories of risk:
   - The possibility that the insured's property may be damaged or destroyed by catastrophe is *property risk.*
   - *Personal risk* is the possibility that the insured will be injured in an accident or will become seriously ill.
   - *Legal liability* is the possibility that the insured will be found legally liable to pay damages to another.

5. *Occurrence policies* cover all accidents during a policy year, regardless of when they are reported, while *claims-made policies* cover claims made or reported during the policy year, no matter when they occurred.

6. Nurses may want to obtain malpractice insurance because even though their employers can be held responsible for negligence, nurses also can be held liable for their own negligence. However, drawbacks include the encouragement of naming nurses in malpractice suits and a concurrent rise in insurance premiums.

7. Standard liability policies have five parts:
   - The *insurance agreement* specifies that the insurer has a legal obligation to pay any sum that has been agreed or determined by a court, up to the limit of the policy, including legal fees.
   - The *defense and settlement* portion contains the agreement between the insured and the insurance company that the company will defend any lawsuit against the insured that arises from the performance or nonperformance of professional services. The insurance company also obtains the power to enact a settlement of any claims it deems necessary or appropriate.
   - The *policy period* sets forth the duration of the policy period and the circumstances under which claims will be processed.
   - The policy also details *coverage,* or the maximum amount that the insurance company will pay an injured party.
   - The policy will include several *conditions.* If the insured does not comply with these conditions, forfeiture of the policy and nonpayment of claims against it could result.

8. Most medical professional liability insurance covers risks such as negligence; assault and battery that result from failing to obtain consent to a medical or surgical procedure; libel and slander; and invasion of privacy for betrayal of professional confidences.

9. *Self-insurance* is a practice in which a health care organization periodically sets aside a certain amount of money to cover malpractice losses and expenses. These organizations often seek the advice of self-insurance consulting firms and actuaries to estimate the proper level of funding for these expenses.

10. When a claim is settled, the plaintiff signs a *general release,* which states that the plaintiff surrenders the right of action against the defendant.

REVIEW QUESTIONS

1. Describe the conditions of an insurance policy as described in this chapter.
2. Under what circumstances should a health care professional be self-insured?
3. Should a health care provider who has been sued lose staff privileges? Discuss your answer.
4. Why do insurance carriers require "timely" notice of a claim?

NOTES

1. *New Mexico Physicians Mut. Liab. Co. v. LaMure,* 860 P.2d 734 (N.M. 1993).
2. 484 A.2d 670 (N.J. 1984).
3. 430 A.2d 488 (D.C. 1981).
4. *American Nursing Ctr.-Greenbrook v. Heckler,* 592 F. Supp. 1311, 1312 (D.D.C. 1984).
5. 606 F.2d 631 (5th Cir. 1979).
6. 263 Neb. 708, 642 N.W.2d 505 (2002).
7. 864 A.2d 614 (R.I. 2005).
8. 392 F. Supp. 393 (E.D. La. 1975).
9. 192 Cal. Rptr. 593 (Cal. Ct. App. 1983).

Labor Relations

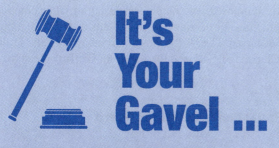

It's Your Gavel ...

UNFAIR LABOR PRACTICES

Ms. Welton attended a union organization meeting on July 5. At a hearing before an administrative law judge (ALJ), she testified that the day after the meeting her supervisor asked whether she or anyone from the dietary department attended the meeting. Welton's supervisor denied having any conversation with Welton about the union meeting. The National Labor Relations Board (NLRB) found that the questioning of Welton constituted unlawful interrogation.

Mr. Hopkins worked as a janitor for the nursing facility. He also attended the meeting on July 5. He testified that his supervisor approached him at work and questioned him as to whether any of the nurses or aides harassed him about the union. The board credited Hopkins's and Welton's version of the events, noting that they had nothing to gain by fabricating their testimony.

On July 18, the facility circulated a memorandum to all employees that stated: "This is to advise that the NLRB has tentatively set a hearing on Wednesday, July 25th, to decide who can vote in a union election. Our position is that supervisors, RNs, and LPNs cannot vote. We will keep you advised."

On July 19, the facility held a mandatory meeting for all nurses and supervisors. The facility's administrator, Mr. Wimer; the facility's attorney, Mr. Yocum; and the chief executive officer, Mr. Colby, told the nurses that, in the facility's opinion, nurses could not vote in the upcoming election but must remain loyal to the facility. When asked by Sands, a union supporter, what he meant by loyalty, Yocum replied that all nurses were prohibited from engaging in union activities. When asked by Sands why the facility opposed the union, Yocum responded, "Well, for one thing, they cost too . . . much money. . . . Do you think those dues come out of thin air?"

The board concluded that the facility, through Yocum, violated the National Labor Relations Act (NLRA) by telling nurses present at the meeting that they could not vote in the upcoming union election or participate in union activities, and that such activities could subject them to dismissal.[1]

WHAT IS YOUR VERDICT?

The relationships between employees and employers are regulated by both state and federal laws. Health care organizations are not exempt from the impact of these laws and therefore are required to take into account such matters as employment practices (wages, hours, and working conditions), union activity, workers' compensation laws, occupational safety and health laws, and employment discrimination laws.

Federal or state regulation generally pervades all areas of employer-employee relationships. The most significant piece of federal legislation dealing with labor relations is the NLRA. Although federal laws generally take precedence over state laws when there is a conflict between the state and the federal laws, state laws are applicable and must be considered, especially when state regulations are more rigid than federal legislation. This chapter provides an overview of those laws affecting the health care industry.

U.S. DEPARTMENT OF LABOR

The U.S. Department of Labor is a department within the executive branch of government. The secretary of labor advises the president on labor policies and issues. The functions of the department of labor are to foster, promote, and develop the welfare of wage earners, to improve working conditions, and to advance opportunities for profitable employment. In carrying out this mission, the department administers a variety of federal labor laws guaranteeing workers' rights to safe and healthful working conditions, a minimum hourly wage and overtime pay, freedom from employment discrimination, unemployment insurance, and workers' compensation. As the department seeks to assist all Americans who need and want to work, special efforts are made to meet the unique job market problems of older workers, youths, minority group members, women, the handicapped, and other groups. Within the department of labor are various agencies responsible for carrying out the purpose of the department (e.g., Occupational Safety and Health Administration).

UNIONS AND HEALTH CARE ORGANIZATIONS

Through the mid-1930s, union organizational activity in the health care industry was minimal, and it continued that way with relatively slow growth until the late 1950s. Union activity has been successful most often in those geographic areas in which unions have been active in other industries.

Many labor organizations attempt to become the recognized collective bargaining representatives for employees in health care settings. Craft unions devote their primary organizing efforts to skilled employees, such as carpenters and electricians, and industrial unions and unions of governmental employees seek to represent large groups of unskilled or semiskilled employees. Professional and occupational associations, such as state nurses' associations, historically known for their social and academic efforts, have involved themselves in collective bargaining for their professions. To the extent that the professional organizations seek goals directly concerned with wages, hours, and other employment conditions and engage in bargaining on behalf of employees, they perform the functions of labor unions.

NATIONAL LABOR RELATIONS ACT

The National Labor Relations Act (NLRA)[2] was enacted by Congress in July 1935 to govern the labor-management relations of business firms engaged in interstate commerce. The act is generally known as the Wagner Act, after Senator Robert R. Wagner of New York. The act defines certain conduct of employers and employees as unfair labor practices and provides for hearings on complaints that such practices have occurred. The NLRA was modified by the Taft-Hartley amendments of 1947 and the Landrum-Griffin amendments of 1959.

National Labor Relations Board

The National Labor Relations Board (NLRB), which is entrusted with enforcing and administering the NLRA, has jurisdiction over matters involving proprietary and not-for-profit health care organizations. The NLRB is an agency, independent of the department of labor, that is responsible for preventing and remedying unfair labor practices by employers and labor organizations or their agents. The NLRB conducts secret ballot elections among employees in appropriate collective bargaining units to determine whether they desire to be represented by a labor organization and among employees under union-shop agreements to determine whether they wish to revoke their union's authority. The general counsel of the NLRB has final authority to investigate charges of unfair labor practices, issue complaints, and prosecute such complaints before the NLRB. There are regional directors, under the direction of the general counsel, who are responsible for processing representation, unfair labor practice, and jurisdictional dispute cases.

The NLRB's basic method of operation is to investigate claims or complaints of unfair practices submitted by the employer or employees, or both. The board reviews the claim to determine whether there have been unfair labor practices and recommends a remedy. Most questions submitted to the board involve claims by employees that their rights of self-organization or of choosing their collective bargaining representative have been interfered with by the employer. Employers also may submit complaints to the NLRB (e.g., when two unions are seeking recognition and one of them intimidates employees by making allegations that a sweetheart relationship exists between the employer and the competing union in an effort to disrupt the certification process).

An exemption for governmental institutions was included in the 1935 enactment of the NLRA, and charitable health care institutions were exempted in 1947 by the Taft-Hartley Act amendments to the NLRA. However, a July 1974 amendment to the NLRA extended coverage to employees of nonprofit health care organizations that previously had been exempted from its provisions. In the words of the amendment, a health care facility is "any hospital, convalescent hospital, health maintenance organization, health clinic, nursing home, extended care facility, or other institution devoted to the care of the sick, infirm or aged."[3]

The amendment also enacted unique, special provisions for employees of health care organizations who oppose unionization on legitimate religious grounds. These provisions allow a member of such an organization to make periodic contributions to one of three nonreligious charitable funds selected jointly by the labor organization and the employing institution rather than paying periodic union dues and initiation fees. If the collective bargaining agreement does not specify an acceptable fund, the employee may select a tax-exempt charity.

Elections

The NLRA sets out the procedures by which employees may select a union as their collective bargaining representative to negotiate with health care organizations over employment and contract matters. A health care organization may choose to recognize and deal with the union without resorting to the formal NLRA procedure. If the formal process is adhered to, the employees vote on union representation in an election held under NLRB supervision.

The NLRA provides that the representative, having been selected by a majority of employees in a bargaining unit, is the exclusive bargaining agent for all employees in the unit. The scope of the bargaining unit is often the subject of dispute, for its boundaries may determine the outcome of the election, the employee representative's bargaining power, and the level of labor relations stability.

When the parties cannot agree on the appropriate unit for bargaining, the NLRB has broad discretion to decide the issue—however, the NLRB's discretion is limited to determining appropriate units for only those employees who are classified as professional, supervisory, clerical, technical, or service and maintenance employees when they are included in units outside their particular category. This is the case unless there has been a self-determination election in which the members of a certain group vote, as a class, to be included within the larger bargaining unit. For example, nurses and other professional employees can be excluded from a bargaining unit composed of service and maintenance employ-

ees unless the professionals are first given the opportunity to choose separate representation and reject it. Supervisory nurses also have been held entitled to a bargaining unit separate from the unit composed of general-duty nurses.

Although the NLRA does not require employee representatives to be selected by any particular procedure, the act provides for the NLRB to conduct representation elections by secret ballot. The NLRB may conduct such an election when a petition for certification has been filed by an employee, a group of employees, an individual, a labor union acting on the employees' behalf, or an employer. When the petition is filed, the NLRB must investigate and direct an election if it has reasonable cause to believe a question of representation exists. Any party to an election who believes that certain conduct created an atmosphere that interfered with free choice may file objections with the NLRB.

Unfair Labor Practices

The NLRA prohibits health care organizations from engaging in certain conduct classified as employer unfair labor practices. For example, discriminating against an employee for holding union membership is not permitted. The NLRA stipulates that the employer must bargain in good faith with representatives of the employees; failure to do so constitutes an unfair labor practice. The NLRB may order the employer to fulfill the duty to bargain.

If the employer dominates or controls the employees' union or interferes with and supports one of two competing unions, the employer is committing an unfair labor practice. Such employer support of a competing union is illustrated clearly in a situation in which two unions are competing for members in the same facility, as well as for recognition as the employees' bargaining organization. If the organization permits one of the unions to use its facilities for its organizational activities but denies the use of the facilities to the other union, an unfair labor practice is committed. Financial assistance to one of the competing unions also constitutes an unfair labor practice.

The NLRA places duties on labor organizations and prohibits certain employee activities that are considered unfair labor practices. Coercion of employees by the union constitutes an unfair labor practice; such activities as mass picketing, assaulting nonstrikers, and following groups of nonstrikers away from the immediate area of the facility plainly constitute coercion and can be ordered stopped by the NLRB. Breach of a collective bargaining contract by the labor union is another example of an unfair labor practice.

NORRIS-LAGUARDIA ACT

Congress enacted the Norris-LaGuardia Act[4] to limit the power of federal courts to issue injunctions in cases involving or growing out of labor disputes. The act's strict standards must be met before such injunctions can be issued. Essentially, a federal court may not apply restraints in a labor dispute until after the case is heard in open court and the finding is that unlawful acts will be committed unless restrained and that substantial and irreparable injury to the complainant's property will follow.[5]

The Norris-LaGuardia Act is aimed at reducing the number of injunctions granted to restrain strikes and picketing. An additional piece of legislation designating procedures limiting strikes in health care institutions is the 1974 amendment to the NLRA. This amendment sets out special procedures for handling labor disputes that develop from collective bargaining at the termination of an existing agreement or during negotiations for an initial contract between a health care institution and its employees. The procedures were designed to ensure that the needs of patients would be met during any work stoppage (strike) or labor dispute in such an institution.

The amendment provides for creating a board of inquiry if a dispute threatens to interrupt health care in a particular community. The board is appointed by the director of the Federal Mediation and Conciliation Service (FMCS) within 30 days after notification of either party's intention to terminate a labor contract. The board then has 15 days in which to investigate and report its findings and recommendations in writing. After the report is filed with the FMCS, both parties are expected to maintain the status quo for an additional 15 days.

The board's findings provide a framework for arbitrators' decisions, while recognizing both the community's need for continuous health services and the good-faith intentions of labor organizations to avoid a work stoppage whenever possible and to accept arbitration when negotiations reach an impasse.

The amendment also mandates certain notice requirements by labor groups in health care institutions: (1) the institution must be given 90 days' notice before a collective bargaining agreement expires, and (2) the FMCS is entitled to 60 days' notice. Previously, only 60 days' notice to the employer and 30 days' notice to the FMCS were required. However, if the bargaining agreement is the initial contract between the parties, only 30 days' notice need be given to the FMCS.

More significantly, 10 days' notice is required in advance of any strike, picketing, or other concerted refusal to work, regardless of the source of the dispute. This allows the NLRB to determine the legality of a strike before it occurs and also gives health care institutions ample time to ensure the continuity of patient care. At the same time, any attempt to use this period to undermine the bargaining relationship is implicitly forbidden.

The 10-day notice may be concurrent with the final 10 days of the expiration notice. Any employee violation of these provisions amounts to an unfair labor practice and automatically may result in the discharge of the employee. Also, injunctive relief may be available from the courts if circumstances warrant.

In summary, the amendment's provisions are designed to ensure that every possible approach to a peaceful settlement is explored fully before a strike is called.

LABOR-MANAGEMENT REPORTING AND DISCLOSURE ACT

The Labor-Management Reporting and Disclosure Act of 1959[6] places controls on labor unions and the relationships between unions and their members. Also, it requires that employers report payments and loans made to officials or other representatives of labor organizations or any promises to make such payments or loans. Expenditures made to influence or restrict the way employees exercise their rights to organize and bargain collectively are illegal unless the employer discloses them. Agreements with labor consultants, under which such persons undertake to interfere with certain employee rights, also must be disclosed.

Reports required under the act must be filed with the secretary of labor and are then made public. Both charitable and proprietary health care organizations that make such payments or enter into such agreements must file reports. Penalties for failing to make the required reports or for making false reports include fines up to $10,000 and imprisonment for one year.

FAIR LABOR STANDARDS ACT

The Fair Labor Standards Act (FLSA)[7] of 1938 established a national minimum wage, guaranteed time and one half for overtime, and maximum hours of employment and prohibited most employment for minors. The FLSA is administered by the Wage & Hour Division of the U.S. Department of Labor, which conducts audits and workplace inspections. The FLSA provides for direct federal actions by employees and offers substantial financial incentives for private litigants and their counsel.

Employees of all governmental, charitable, and proprietary health care organizations are covered by the FLSA. Employers must conform to the minimum wage and overtime pay provisions. However, bona fide executive, administrative, and professional employees are exempted from the wage and hour provisions.

The law permits employers to enter into agreements with employees, establishing a work period of 14 consecutive days as an alternative to the usual 7-day week. If the alternative period is chosen, the employer must pay the overtime rate only for hours worked in excess of 80 hours during the 14-day period. The alternative 14-day work period does not relieve a facility from paying overtime for hours worked in excess of 8 hours in any one day even if no more than 80 hours are worked during the period.

CIVIL RIGHTS ACT

Title VII of the Civil Rights Act of 1964, as amended by the Equal Employment Opportunity Act of 1972,[8] prohibits private employers and state and local governments from discrimination in employment in any business on the basis of race, color, religion, sex, or national origin. The act prohibits harassment based on one's affiliation (e.g., religion), physical and cultural traits and clothing (e.g., skin color, headscarf), perception (e.g., due to national origin: he is from Pakistan and must, therefore be a terrorist), and association (e.g., discrimination based on association with an individual or organization). The federal antidiscrimination law provides that it is unlawful for most public and private employers to discriminate against, fail or refuse to hire, or to discharge any individual, with respect to his or her compensation, terms, conditions, or privileges of employment because of such individual's race, color, religion, sex (including pregnancy), or national origin.

Title VII also prohibits retaliation against employees who oppose such unlawful discrimination. The Equal Employment Commission (EEOC) enforces Title VII. The EEOC investigates, mediates, and sometimes files lawsuits on behalf of employees. Title VII also provides that an individual can bring a private lawsuit.

An exception to prohibited employment practices may be permitted when religion, sex, or national origin is a bona fide occupational qualification necessary to the operation of a particular business or enterprise.

This act does not apply to a religious corporation (e.g., hospitals), association, educational institution, or society with respect to the employment of individuals of a particular religion to perform work connected with the carrying on by such corporation, association, educational institution, or society of its activities.

Many states have enacted protective laws with respect to the employment of women. The EEOC guidelines on sex discrimination make it clear that state laws limiting the employment of women in certain occupations are superseded by Title VII and are no defense against a charge of sex discrimination.

OCCUPATIONAL SAFETY AND HEALTH ACT

OSHA's mission is to assure the safety and health of America's workers by setting and enforcing standards; providing training, outreach, and education; establishing partnerships; and encouraging continual improvement in workplace safety and health.[9]

Congress enacted the Occupational Safety and Health Act of 1970[10] (OSHA) to establish administrative machinery for the development and enforcement of standards for occupational health and safety. The legislation was enacted based on congressional findings that personal injuries and illnesses arising out of work situations impose a substantial burden on and are substantial hindrances to interstate commerce in terms of lost production, wage loss, medical expenses, and disability compensation payments. Congress declared that its purpose and policy were to ensure, so far as possible, every working man and woman in the nation safe and healthful working conditions and to preserve human resources by doing the following:

1. encouraging employers and employees in their efforts to reduce the number of occupational safety and health hazards at their places of employment, and stimulating employers and employees to institute new and to perfect existing programs for providing safe and healthful working conditions;

2. providing that employers and employees have separate but dependent responsibilities and rights with respect to achieving safe and healthful working conditions;

3. authorizing the Secretary of Labor to set mandatory occupational safety and health standards applicable to businesses affecting interstate commerce, and by creating an Occupational and Health Review Commission for carrying out adjudicatory functions under the Act;

4. building upon advances already made through employer and employee initiative for providing safe and healthful working conditions;

5. providing for research in the field of occupational safety and health, including the psychological factors involved, and by developing innovative methods, techniques, and approaches for dealing with occupational safety and health problems;

6. exploring ways to discover latent diseases, establishing causal connections between diseases and work in environmental conditions, and conducting other research relating to health problems, in recognition of the fact that occupational health standards present problems often different from those involved in occupational safety;

7. providing medical criteria that will assure, insofar as practicable, that no employee will suffer diminished health, functional capacity, or life expectancy as a result of his or her work experience;

8. providing for training programs to increase the number and competence of personnel engaged in the field of occupational safety and health;

9. providing for the development and promulgation of occupational safety and health standards;

10. providing an effective enforcement program that shall include a prohibition against giving advance notice of any inspection and sanctions for any individual violating this prohibition;

11. encouraging the States to assume the fullest responsibility for the administration and enforcement of their occupational safety and health laws by providing grants to the States to assist in identifying their needs and responsibilities in the area of occupational safety and health, to develop plans in accordance with the provisions of this Act, to improve the administration and enforcement of state occupational safety and health laws, and conducting experimental and demonstration projects in connection therewith;

12. providing for appropriate reporting procedures with respect to occupational safety and health, which procedures will help achieve the objectives of this Act and accurately describe the nature of the occupational safety and health problem;

13. encouraging joint labor-management efforts to reduce injuries and disease arising out of employment.[11]

The employer must comply with the occupational and health standards under the act and employees must follow the rules, regulations, and orders issued under the act that are applicable to their actions and conduct on the job. The duties of employers and employees under the act are as follows:

a. Each employer—

1. shall furnish to each of his employees employment and a place of employment which is free from recognized hazards that are causing or are likely to cause death or serious physical harm to his employees;

2. shall comply with occupational safety and health standards promulgated under this Act.

b. Each employee shall comply with occupational safety and health standards and all rules, regulations, and orders pursuant to this Act which are applicable to his own actions and conduct.[12]

Promulgation and Enforcement of OSHA Standards

OSHA develops and promulgates occupational safety and health standards for the workplace. It develops and issues regulations, conducts investigations and inspections to determine the status of compliance, and issues citations and proposes penalties for noncompliance. Inspections are conducted without advance notice.

Employers are responsible for becoming familiar with standards applicable to their businesses and for ensuring that employees have and use personal protective equipment when required for safety. Employees must comply with all rules and regulations that are applicable to their work environment. Where OSHA has not promulgated specific standards, the employer is responsible for following the act's general duty clause. The general-duty clause states that each employer must furnish a place of employment that is free from recognized hazards that are causing or likely to cause death or serious physical harm.

Recordkeeping

Employers of 11 or more employees are required to maintain records of occupational injuries and illnesses. The purpose of maintaining records is to permit the Bureau of Labor Statistics to help define high-hazard industries and to inform employees of the status of their employer's record.

Education

Employers are responsible for keeping employees informed about OSHA and about the various safety and health matters with which they are involved. OSHA requires that employers post certain material at a prominent location in the workplace (e.g., a job safety and health protection workplace poster informing employees of their rights and responsibilities under the act).

Infectious Body Fluids

OSHA issued standards on December 2, 1991, that are to be followed by employers to protect employees from bloodborne infections. Universal precautions are mandatory, and employees who are likely to be exposed to body fluids must be provided with protective clothing (e.g., masks, gowns, and gloves). In addition, postexposure testing must be available to employees who have been exposed to body fluids.

Employee Complaints

Employees should inform their supervisors if they suspect or detect a dangerous situation in the workplace. Employers are expected to address reported hazards in the workplace. Employees or their representatives have the right to file complaints with an OSHA office and request a survey when they believe that conditions in the workplace are unsafe or unhealthy. If a violation of the act is found at the time of a survey, the employer may receive a citation stating a time frame within which the violation must be corrected.

State Regulation

The states have statutes charging employers with the duty to furnish employees with a safe working environment. The city and county in which a health care facility is located also may prescribe rules regarding the health and safety of employees. Many communities have enacted sanitary and health codes that require certain standards.

Legal Liability

From a liability point of view, an employer can be held legally liable for damages suffered by employees through exposure to dangerous conditions that are in violation of OSHA standards. Proof of an employee's exposure to non-compliant conditions is generally necessary to find an employer liable.

REHABILITATION ACT

The essential purpose of the Rehabilitation Act of 1973[13] provides protection to handicapped people from discrimination. The law basically is administered by the Department of Health and Human Services (DHHS), which derives its jurisdiction from the fact that health care organizations participate in such federal programs as Medicare, Medicaid, and Hill-Burton. The law therefore is applied to both public and private organizations, because both participate in these programs.

Section 503 of the act applies to government contractors whose contracts exceed $2,500 in value. Section 504, which applies to employers who are recipients of federal financial assistance, states, "[n]o . . . qualified handicapped individual in the United States . . . shall solely by reason of his handicap, be excluded from participation in, be denied the benefits of, or be subjected to discrimination under any program as actively receiving federal financial assistance." Section 504 applies to virtually every area of personnel administration, including recruitment, advertising, processing of applications, promotions, rates of pay, fringe benefits, and job assignments.

Since July 1977, all institutions receiving federal financial assistance from DHHS have been required to file assurances of compliance forms. Each employer must designate an individual to coordinate compliance efforts. A grievance procedure should be in place to address employee com-plaints alleging violation of the regulation. All employment decisions must be made without regard to physical or mental handicaps that are not disqualifying (e.g., an employer is not obligated to employ a person with a highly contagious disease that can be easily transmitted to others).

Employers receiving federal funds are required to perform a self-evaluation as to their compliance with Section 504 of the Rehabilitation Act of 1973. If discriminatory practices are identified through the self-evaluation process, remedial steps are to be taken to eliminate the effects of any discrimination. Records of the evaluation are to be maintained on file for at least three years after the review for public inspection.[14]

Jobs should not be purposely designed so as to eliminate the hiring of disabled persons. Employers, however, are not required to change the essential elements of a job in order to create a position for a disabled person. The Iowa Supreme Court, in *Schlitzer v. U of I Hosp and Clinics*,[15] decided that an employer is not required to create a vacancy or a job for a disabled person. The court found that a nurse's 20-pound lifting restriction, due to a car accident, limited her ability to lift, thus making the demands of her job incompatible with her physical disability. The law does not require that an employer change the essential elements of a job in order to meet a claimant's disability. In this case, the job required that the nurse be able to work with severely disabled persons. The 20-pound limitation, in this case, was an impossible hurdle to overcome.

FAMILY AND MEDICAL LEAVE ACT

The Family and Medical Leave Act of 1993 (FMLA) was enacted to grant temporary medical leave to employees under certain circumstances. The act provides that covered employers must grant an eligible employee up to a total of 12 workweeks of unpaid leave during any 12-month period for one or more of the following reasons: the birth and care of an employee's child; placement of an adopted or foster child with the employee; for the care of an immediate family member (spouse, child, or parent) with a serious health condition; or inability to work because of a serious health condition. It is illegal to terminate health insurance coverage for an employee on FMLA leave. Following an FMLA leave, the employee's job—or an equivalent job with equivalent pay, benefits, and other terms and conditions of employment—must be restored.

STATE LABOR LAWS

The federal labor enactments serve as a pattern for many state labor laws that comprise the second labor regulation system touching health care organizations. State labor acts vary from state to state. Therefore, it is important that each institution familiarize itself not only with federal regulations but also with state regulations affecting labor relations within the institution.

Because the NLRA excludes from coverage health care organizations operated by the state or its political subdivisions, regulation of labor-management relations in these organizations is left to state law. Unless the constitution in such a state guarantees the right of employees to organize and imposes the duty of collective bargaining on the employer, health care organizations do not have to bargain collectively with their employees. However, in states that do have labor relations acts, the obligation of an organization to bargain collectively with its employees is determined by the applicable statute.

State laws vary considerably in their coverage, and often employees of state and local governmental organizations are covered by separate public employee legislation. Some of these statutes cover both state and local employees, whereas others cover only state or only local employees.

Some of the states that have labor relations acts granting employees the right to organize, join unions, and bargain collectively have specifically prohibited strikes and lockouts and have provided for compulsory arbitration whenever a collective bargaining contract cannot otherwise be executed amicably. Anti-injunction statutes would not forbid injunctions to restrain violations of these statutory provisions.

The doctrine of federal preemption, as applied to labor relations, displaces the states' jurisdiction to regulate an activity that is arguably an unfair labor practice within the meaning of the NLRA. Nonetheless, the U.S. Supreme Court has ruled that states can still regulate labor relations activity that also falls within the jurisdiction of the NLRB when deeply rooted local feelings and responsibility are affected.

Union Security Contracts and Right-to-Work Laws

Labor organizations frequently seek to enter union security contracts with employers. Such contracts are of two types: (1) the closed-shop contract, which provides that only members of a particular union may be hired, and (2) the union-shop contract, which makes continued employment dependent on membership in the union, although the employee need not have been a union member when applying for the job.

Many states have made such contracts unlawful. Statutes forbidding such agreements generally are called *right-to-work laws* on the theory that they protect everyone's right to work even if a person refuses to join a union. Several state statutes or court decisions purport to restrict union security contracts or specify procedures to be completed before such agreements may be made.

Wage and Hour Laws

When state minimum wage standards are higher than federal standards, the state's standards are applicable.

Child Labor Acts

Many states prohibit the employment of minors younger than a specified age and restrict the employment of other minors. Child labor legislation commonly requires that working papers be secured before a child may be hired, forbids the employment of minors at night, and prohibits minors from operating certain types of dangerous machinery.

This kind of legislation rarely exempts charitable institutions, although some exceptions may be made with respect to the hours when student nurses may work.

Workers' Compensation

Workers' compensation is a program by which an employee can receive certain wage benefits because of work-related injuries. An employee who is injured while performing job-related duties is generally eligible for workers' compensation. Workers' compensation programs are administered by the states.

State legislatures have recognized that it is difficult and expensive for employees to recover from their employers and therefore have enacted workers' compensation laws. Employers are required to provide workers' compensation as a benefit. Workers' compensation laws give the employee a legal way to receive compensation for injuries on the job. The acts do not require the employee to prove that the injury was the result of the employer's negligence. Workers' compensation laws are based on the employer-employee relationship and not on the theory of negligence.

The scope of workers' compensation varies widely. Some states limit an employee's compensation to the amount recoverable by the workers' compensation law, and further lawsuits against the employer are barred. Other states permit employees to choose whether to accept the compensation provided by law or to institute a lawsuit against the employer. Some acts go farther and provide a system of insurance that may be under the supervision of state or private insurers.

Physical Injury

The courts have been somewhat liberal in allowing workers' compensation benefits to be paid to employees injured while on duty, even when challenged by the employer under seemingly justifiable circumstances. The employee, for example, in *Fondulac Nursing Home v. Industrial Commission*[16] was found to be entitled to workers' compensation despite orders that she was not to lift patients because of a back injury. When a patient was being transferred from her wheelchair to her bed and began to fall, the nurse attempted to prevent the fall, injuring herself. The nurse acted within her scope of employment by attempting to prevent the fall to her own detriment and her employer's best interests by protecting the patient from injury.

Job Stress

Workers' compensation has been awarded for depression related to job stress. In *Elwood v. SAIF*,[17] a registered nurse filed a workers' compensation claim for an occupational disease based on depression. The referee and the workers' compensation board affirmed the insurer's denial of the claim and the claimant sought judicial review. The questions that needed to be answered to determine job stress were:

- What were the "real" events and conditions of plaintiff's employment?

- Were those real events and conditions capable of producing stress when viewed objectively, even though an average worker might not have responded adversely to them?

- Did the plaintiff suffer a mental disorder?

- Were the real stressful events and conditions the major contributing cause of plaintiff's mental disorder?

The record established that many events and conditions of her employment, including her termination, were real and capable of producing stress when viewed objectively. The claimant's treating physician advised her that she was suffering from anxiety, depression, and stress and advised her to seek a psychiatric evaluation. The court held that the claimant established that her condition was compensable.

Influenza Vaccination

A hospital employee's reaction to an influenza vaccination given by an emergency department employee while he or she is on duty most likely will be a compensable injury under workers' compensation. A housekeeping employee in *Monette v. Manatee Memorial Hospital*[18] suffered a serious reaction to the influenza vaccination administered to her while on duty and was entitled to workers' compensation.

LIMITATIONS ON NUMBER OF BARGAINING UNITS

A major area of concern for health care institutions is the number of bargaining units allowed in any one institution.

Rules and regulations issued on April 21, 1989, by the NLRB allow up to eight collective bargaining units in health care organizations as opposed to the three normally allowed before the regulations. The American Hospital Association brought an action to enjoin the NLRB from enforcing the newly promulgated regulation recognizing up to eight bargaining units in *American Hospital Association v. NLRB*.[19] A federal district court enjoined enforcement of the rule. The NLRB and intervening unions appealed. The U.S. Court of Appeals for the Seventh Circuit held that the rule was not arbitrary and was within the authority of the NLRB. No rule is necessary to confer the rights already conferred by statute entitling guards and professional employees to form separate bargaining units.

In making unit determinations, the NLRB is required to strike a balance among the competing interests of unions, employees (whose interests are not always compatible to those of unions), employers, and the broader public. The statute can be read to suggest that the tilt should be in favor of unions and toward relatively many, rather than relatively few, units.

This balancing act is not spelled out in the statute, thus requiring an NLRB decision. The decision is particularly difficult and delicate in the health care industry because the workforce of a hospital, nursing home, or rehabilitation center tends to be small and heterogeneous.

On appeal, the U.S. Supreme Court, on April 23, 1991, by unanimous decision, upheld an NLRB rule allowing hospital workers to form up to eight separate bargaining units, including those for physicians, registered nurses, other professionals, technical employees, clerical employees, skilled maintenance employees, other nonprofessional employees, and security guards.[20]

LABOR RIGHTS

Rights and responsibilities run concurrently. Employee rights include such things as:

- the right to organize and bargain collectively

- the right to solicit and distribute union information during nonworking hours (i.e., mealtimes and coffee breaks)

- the right to picket (Picketing is the act of patrolling, by one or more persons, of a place related to a labor dispute. It varies in purpose and form. It may be conducted by employees or nonemployees and, like strikes, some picketing may be legislatively or judicially disapproved and subject to regulation.)

- the right to strike (A strike may be defined as the collective quitting of work by employees as a means of inducing the employer to assent to employee demands. Employees possess the right to strike, although this right is not absolute and is subject to limited exercise. The 1974 amendments to the NLRA have added requirements with respect to strikes and picketing in an attempt to reduce the interruption of health care services. The NLRB is urged to give top priority to settling labor-management disputes resulting in the loss of health care personnel or medical services.)

Employees granted these rights have the concomitant responsibility to perform their work duties properly. A nursing home housekeeper, for example, was terminated properly after repeated oral and written reprimands concerning her improper cleaning of rooms in *Ford v. Patin*.[21] Her substandard performance, despite repeated warnings, evidenced willful and wanton disregard of her employer's interest and constituted misconduct within purview of Section 23:1601(2) of the Louisiana Revised Statutes Annotated.

MANAGEMENT RIGHTS

As with labor, management also has certain rights and responsibilities. Specific management rights are reviewed here.

Right to Receive Strike Notice

Management has a right to a 10-day advance notice of a bargaining unit's intent to strike.

Right to Hire Replacement Workers

Although management may not discharge employees in retaliation for union activity, concomitant with the employees' right to strike is management's right to hire replacement workers in the event of a strike. The nursing home in *Charlesgate Nursing Center v. State of Rhode Island*[22] brought an action against the state, seeking a determination that a state statute prohibiting strike-affected employers from using the services of a third party to recruit replacement workers during a strike was unconstitutional. Employees of the nursing home went on strike June 2, 1988, and Charlesgate hired temporary replacement workers to provide continued services for its patients. The temporary employees were hired through employment agencies. The actions of Charlesgate and the agencies violated Sections 28-10-10 and 28-10-12 of the General Laws of Rhode Island (1956) (1986 Reenactment), which read:

> 28-10-10. Recruitment prohibited—It shall be unlawful for any person, partnership, agency, firm or corporation, or officer or agent thereof, to know-

ingly recruit, procure, supply or refer any person who offers him or herself for employment in the place of an employee involved in a labor strike or lockout in which such person, partnership, agency, firm, or corporation is not directly interested.

> 28-10-12. Agency for procurement—It shall be unlawful for any person, partnership, firm or corporation, or officer or agent thereof, involved in a labor strike or lockout to contract or arrange with any other person, partnership, agency, firm or corporation to recruit, procure, supply, or refer persons who offer themselves for employment in the place of employees involved in a labor strike or lockout for employment in place of employees involved in such labor strike or lockout.

Citing these statutes, the labor unions involved in the strike notified nursing pools throughout the state that it was unlawful to provide Charlesgate with replacement workers. At the same time, the unions urged the city of Providence and the Rhode Island attorney general to prosecute Charlesgate, at which time Charlesgate filed its suit claiming that the Rhode Island statutes were unconstitutional.

Although the strike was settled, the federal district court held that the statute was unconstitutional because it prohibited activity that Congress had intended to leave open to strike-affected employers as a peaceful weapon of economic self-help.

Right to Restrict Union Activity to Prescribed Areas

Management has the right to reasonably restrict union organizers to certain locations in the health care facility and to certain time periods to avoid interference with facility operations.

Right to Prohibit Union Activity During Working Hours

Management has the right to prohibit union activities during employee working hours.

Right to Prohibit Supervisors from Participating in Union Activity

Management has the right to prohibit supervisors from engaging in union organizational activity. A nursing supervisor brought a lawsuit for wrongful discharge against a nursing facility and its director of nursing. She was dismissed for her activities in attempting to form an organization to represent the nurses. The circuit court granted summary judgment for the defendants and the appeals court affirmed. On review, the Wisconsin Supreme Court held in *Arena v. Lincoln Lutheran of Racine*[23] that after the NLRB had determined that the nurse in this case was a supervisor rather than an employee within the meaning of the NLRA, federal labor law preempted the state court from determining whether the nurse's discharge for engaging in concerted activities was wrongful under Wisconsin law. Employees who are supervisors as defined in the NLRA are treated differently than professional employees. The definition of the term supervisor found in Section 2(11) provides: "The term 'supervisor' means any individual having authority, in the interest of the employer, to hire, transfer, suspend, lay off, recall, promote, discharge, assign, reward, or discipline other employees, or responsibly to direct them, or to adjust their grievances, or effectively to recommend such action, if in connection with the foregoing the exercise of such authority is not merely a routine or clerical nature, but requires the use of independent judgment."

The petitioner alleged in her complaint that she had become concerned with certain policies that included nurses being treated in an arbitrary manner. The petitioner held a meeting outside of Racine with the nurses to discuss their concerns and the possibility of forming an association to represent the collective interests of the nurses. The NLRA did not protect the nursing supervisor because she was a supervisor rather than an employee. Congress excluded supervisors from protection afforded rank-and-file employees engaged in concerted activity for their mutual benefit to assure management of the undivided loyalty of its supervisory personnel by making sure that no employer would have to retain as its agent one who is obligated to a union.

Seven RNs at a small, 72-bed nursing home were found not to function as supervisors and were, therefore, eligible for a separate bargaining unit in *NLRB v. Res-Care, Inc.*[24] Although the nurses had the authority to assign nurses' aides, their exercise of this authority was merely routine and did not require independent judgment. The nurses were not shown to have any authority to hire, discipline, and/or fire any of the nursing aides. Such authority, if present, would have indicated some sort of supervisory status. Allowing seven nurses to form their own collective bargaining unit rather than merging them into a unit consisting of nurses' aides and other workers was not found to be improper nor was it an undue proliferation of bargaining units at the facility.

Certification of 17 RNs as an employee-bargaining unit in *NLRB v. American Medical Services*[25] was shown to be improper. The nursing home contended that a very low ratio of supervisors to employees would occur if the NLRB's decision was upheld. Substantial evidence had been presented to the court showing that the nurses exercised substantial supervisory powers, including the authority to issue work assignments and discipline employees.

The Taft-Hartley Act as applied in this case illustrates the importance of balancing the rights of both employees and employers.

> Taft-Hartley applied some brakes, so that the balance of power between companies and unions would not shift wholly to the union side. The exclusion of supervisors is one of the brakes. If supervisors were free to join or form unions and enjoy the broad protection of the Act for concerted activity, see Sec. 7, 29 U.S.C. Sec. 157, the impact of a strike would be greatly amplified because the company would not be able to use its supervisory personnel to replace strikers. More important, the company with or without a strike could lose control of its work force to the unions, since the very people in the company who controlled hiring, discipline, assignments, and other dimensions of the employment relationship might be subject to control by the same union as the employees they were supposed to be controlling on the employer's behalf.[26]

EQUAL EMPLOYMENT OPPORTUNITY— AFFIRMATIVE ACTION PLAN

Health care organizations are required to comply with all applicable DHHS regulations "including but not limited to those pertaining to nondiscrimination on the basis of race, color, or national origin (45 C.F.R. part 80), nondiscrimination on the basis of handicap (45 C.F.R. part 84), nondiscrimination on the basis of age (45 C.F.R. part 91), protection of human subjects of research (45 C.F.R. part 46), and fraud and abuse (42 C.F.R. part 455). Although these regulations are not in themselves considered requirements under this part, their violation may result in the termination or suspension of or the refusal to grant or continue payment with federal funds."[27] To comply with the spirit of these regulations and Executive Order 11246, health care organizations should have an equal employment opportunity or affirmative action plan in place.

An affirmative action program includes such things as the collection and analysis of data on the race and sex of all applicants for employment, as well as a statement in the personnel policy/procedure manuals and employee handbooks that would read, for example, "Health Care Facility, Inc., is an equal opportunity/affirmative action employer and does not discriminate on the basis of race, color, religion, sex, national origin, age, handicap, or veteran status."

PATIENT RIGHTS DURING LABOR DISPUTES

Patient rights take precedence over employee and management rights when a patient's right to privacy or well-being is in jeopardy due to labor disputes.

INJUNCTIONS

An injunction is an order by a court directing that a certain act be performed or not performed. Persons who fail to comply with court orders are said to be in contempt of court. The earliest use of injunctions in labor relations was by employers to stop strikes or picketing by employees. Today, the general rule limits the availability of injunctive relief to halt work stoppages. The federal government and many states have enacted anti-injunction acts. These acts restrict the power of the courts to limit injunctions in labor disputes by setting strictly defined standards that must be met before injunctions can be granted to restrain activities such as strikes and picketing.

ADMINISTERING A COLLECTIVE BARGAINING AGREEMENT

Once a collective bargaining agreement has been negotiated in good faith, it should be administered with care and good faith as well. The first-line supervisors are responsible for administering the agreement at the grassroots level. They should familiarize themselves with the provisions of the agreement. Educational programs should be provided by the organization. Special emphasis should be placed on the use of corrective discipline, as provided under the contract, and on how to respond to grievances. The organization's management, through its human relations department, maintains the ultimate responsibility in the facility for the fair and effective administration of its union contract(s).

Maintaining propitious records of all grievances, grievance meetings, and grievance resolutions is the responsibility of supervisors and management. Regardless of whether a grievance is meritorious and settled by management or whether it is spurious and therefore denied, clear and complete records should be maintained. The ability to document resolutions of particular problems, as well as management's approach to grievances, is especially important if arbitration is required to settle a grievance.

Arbitration procedures are set in motion when the union files a demand for arbitration either with the employer or with the arbitration agency named in the contract. The arbitration hearing is a relatively informal proceeding at which labor and management frequently choose to be represented by counsel. The arbitrator's decision is binding on both parties.

The arbitrator's decision can be upset by showing any of the following:

- The arbitrator has clearly exceeded his or her authority under the collective bargaining agreement.

- The decision is the product of fraud or duress.

- The arbitrator has been guilty of impropriety.

- The award violates the law or requires a violation of the law.

DISCRIMINATION IN THE WORKPLACE

Discrimination in the workplace comes in many forms and in numerous ways and each has its own little twist of facts: You are either too old or too young for the job; you are either overqualified or underqualified. There are laws prohibiting discrimination against any individual because of his or her race, color, religion, sex, or national origin, or to classify or refer for employment any individual on the basis of his or her race, color, religion, sex, or national origin. Unfortunately, prohibition and practice do not always match up. A variety of cases are presented in this section that describe but a few of the various forms of discrimination prohibited by law.

Age Discrimination

The Age Discrimination in Employment Act of 1967 (ADEA)[28] prohibits age-based employment discrimination against persons 40 years of age or older. The purpose of this law is to promote employment of older persons on the basis of their ability without regard to their age. The law prohibits arbitrary age discrimination in hiring, discharge, pay, term, conditions, or privileges of employment. The ADEA covers private employers with 20 or more employees, state and local governments, employment agencies, and most labor unions. The Age Discrimination and Claims Assistance Amendment of 1990 extends the suit filing period for ADEA charges meeting certain criteria. There are strict time frames in which charges of age discrimination must be filed.

According to the U.S. Supreme Court in *Texas Department of Community Affairs v. Burdine,* a prima facie case of age discrimination requires that evidence sufficient to support a finding for the complainant must establish all of the following:[29]

- The complainant is in a protected age group.

- The complainant is qualified for his or her job.

- The complainant was discharged.

- The discharge occurred in circumstances that give rise to the inference of age discrimination.

A prima facie case of age discrimination was not established in *Pena v. Brattleboro Retreat*,[30] in which a 63-year-old female administrator of a psychiatric nursing facility alleged that she was dismissed as administrator so that a younger administrator could take over her position. The evidence established that the younger assistant administrator, a woman in her early 30s, had been hired at the suggestion of the administrator so that she could eventually take over the position of administrator on the administrator's retirement. A federal district court found in favor of the administrator on jury verdict, and an appeal was taken. The Second Circuit held that the former administrator failed to prove either explicit or constructive discharge. A *constructive discharge* occurs when the employer, rather than acting directly, deliberately makes an employee's working conditions so intolerable that the employee is forced into an involuntary resignation.

> The Retreat's treatment of Mrs. Pena cannot be described as intolerable. Mrs. Pena was simply asked to train her successor for a year and a half, rather than the six months she herself envisioned. This was no more than a change in job responsibilities based on a reasonable business decision on the part of the Retreat. Mrs. Pena was faced with no loss of pay or change in title.[31]

The retreat claimed that Mrs. Pena resigned on her own because of her inability to adjust to the retreat's business decisions. The Age Discrimination in Employment Act does not protect employees who resign in protest against business decisions.

Disability

The Americans with Disabilities Act of 1990 (ADA) was enacted by Congress to prohibit employers from discriminating against job applicants and employees on the basis of disability.[32] It applies to employers with 15 or more employees working for 20 or more weeks during a calendar year. The ADA protects employees who are qualified individuals with disabilities capable of performing the essential functions of the job in question with or without reasonable accommodation, from discrimination by the employer.

The number of disabled Americans is increasing as the population grows older. Society tends to isolate and segregate individuals with disabilities. Despite some improvements, discrimination against individuals with disabilities continues to be a serious and pervasive social problem. Discrimination continues in such crucial areas as employment, housing, public accommodations, education, transportation, and health services. Unlike individuals who have experienced discrimination on the basis of race, color, sex, national origin, religion, or age, those who have been disabled have had no legal recourse to redress such discrimination. Individuals with disabilities continually encounter different forms of discrimination, including outright intentional exclusion; the discriminatory effects of architectural, transportation, and communication barriers; the failure to make modifications to existing organizations and practices; exclusionary qualification standards and criteria; segregation; and relegation to lesser services, programs, activities, benefits, jobs, or other opportunities.

Census data, national polls, and other studies have documented that people with disabilities, as a group, occupy an inferior status in society. The nation's proper goals regarding individuals with disabilities are to ensure equality of opportunity, full participation, independent living, and economic self-sufficiency for such individuals.

The ADA prohibits job discrimination in hiring, promotion, or other provisions of employment against qualified individuals with disabilities by private employers, state and local governments, employment agencies, and labor unions. On July 26, 1991, the EEOC issued final regulations implementing Title 1 of the ADA. The purpose of the ADA is to[33]

- Provide a clear and comprehensive national mandate for the elimination of discrimination against individuals with disabilities.

- Provide clear, strong, consistent, enforceable standards addressing discrimination against individuals with disabilities.

- Ensure that the federal government plays a central role in enforcing the standards established in the Act on behalf of individuals with disabilities.

- Invoke the sweep of congressional authority, including the power to enforce the Fourteenth Amendment and to regulate commerce to address the main areas of discrimination faced day to day by people with disabilities.

The general rule of discrimination under Title I of the act provides that "no covered entity shall discriminate against a qualified individual with a disability because of the disability of such individual in regard to job application procedures, the hiring, advancement, or discharge of employees, employee compensation, job training, and other terms, conditions, and privileges of employment."[34]

A defense to a charge of discrimination under the act would require showing that the screening out of a specific disability was job related and consistent with business necessity, and that performance cannot be accomplished by reasonable accommodation.

Disability Requires Reasonable Accommodation

The appellee-Alley in *Alley v. Charleston Area Med. Ctr., Inc.*[35] worked for CAMC for over 17 years and suffered from epilepsy and asthma, with the asthma becoming increasingly aggravated by on-the-job exposure to certain chemicals. Alley requested a 12-week family medical leave of absence, which the hospital approved, with the agreement that the leave could be taken intermittently as needed. Alley began seeing Dr. Douglas with CAMC Physician Health Group for treatment of her asthma and epilepsy.

Alley's physician wrote a letter explaining her physical conditions and requested that Alley be allowed to work in an outpatient setting and not be exposed to people with multiple infections. Although Alley presented her request for accommodation to various CAMC supervisory personnel and to employee health services at the hospital, she was told that no accommodation would be made. The employee health services physician, Dr. Ranadive, met with Alley for five minutes. He did not perform any tests. Ranadive called the physician who had the written request and summarily concluded that there was no medical reason why Alley could not continue her employment and that CAMC would not accommodate her.

Alley was eventually terminated and she filed suit against CAMC in the circuit court alleging that she had been subjected to retaliatory discharge based on physical and mental impairment. Alley claimed that CAMC refused to make reasonable accommodations for her known impairments and that this was a violation of the West Virginia Human Rights Act and CAMC, with knowledge of Alley's asthma, exposed her to substances that exacerbated her condition.

The jury returned a verdict in favor of Alley, awarding of $325,000 in damages. On appeal, the court determined that the evidence was sufficient for a jury to find that Alley was a qualified person with a disability and that CAMC was aware of her disability and that a reasonable accommodation could have been made. The jury award was fair, considering all of the evidence and the instructions it received. The trial court did not abuse its discretion in refusing to grant a new trial.

National Origin

The Immigration Reform and Control Act of 1986, 1990, and 1996 (IRCA) prohibits most employers from discriminating against employees or applicants because of national origin or U.S. citizenship status, with respect to hiring, referral, or discharge. The act establishes penalties for employers who knowingly hire illegal aliens. Determining the legality of the employee's status is the employer's responsibility.

> A 1999 settlement with *Woodbine Healthcare Center* resolving allegations that the defendant recruited Filipino nurses with promises of hiring them as registered nurses in the United States, but instead placed them in nurse assistant positions at substantially lower pay, or in registered nurse assignments at reduced pay. EEOC also

claimed that the employer harassed the victims with threats of deportation when they complained. EEOC obtained relief of $2.1 million for sixty-five class members.[36]

Pay Discrimination

The Equal Pay Act (1963)[37] is an amendment to the Fair Labor Standards Act prohibiting any discrimination in the payment of wages for men and women performing substantially equal work under similar conditions. The EPA is applicable everywhere that the minimum wage law is applicable and is enforced by the EEOC. The EPA, simply stated, requires that employees who perform equal work receive equal pay. There are situations in which wages may be unequal as long as they are based on factors other than sex, such as in the case of a formalized seniority system or a system that objectively measures earnings by the quantity or quality of production.

The EPA of 1963 and Title VII of the Civil Rights Act of 1964 were violated when a female nurse's aide was paid less than male orderlies were paid for similar work in *Odomes v. Nucare, Inc.*[38] The nursing facility argued that the orderlies performed heavy lifting chores and provided a form of security for the mostly all-female shift. Testimony of the orderlies for Odomes indicated that the orderlies did little or nothing more than the nurse's aides. The security aspects of an orderly's job were at best his presence on the shift and his periodic checking of the facility's premises. The facility argued that the orderlies were involved in a training program that justified higher pay. The court considered this an "illusory post event justification for unequal pay for equal work."[39]

The Supreme Court stated in *Corning Glass Works v. Brennan* that Congress's purpose in enacting the Equal Pay Act was to remedy what was perceived to be a serious and endemic problem of employment discrimination in private industry. The wage structure of many segments of American industry has been based on an ancient outmoded belief that a man, because of his role in society, should be paid more than a woman even though his ideas are the same.[40]

Pregnancy Discrimination

The Pregnancy Discrimination Act is an amendment to Title VII of the Civil Rights Act of 1964. Discrimination on the basis of pregnancy, childbirth, or related medical conditions constitutes unlawful sex discrimination under Title VII. Women affected by pregnancy or related conditions must be treated in the same manner as other applicants or employees with similar abilities or limitations by, for example, providing modified tasks, alternative assignments, disability leave, or leave without pay. The X-ray technician in *Hayes v. Shelby Memorial Hospital*[41] brought an employment discrimination action against the hospital. The technician had been fired by the hospital when it learned that she was pregnant. The federal district court found that the hospital had violated the Pregnancy Discrimination Act. In affirming the lower court's decision, the appellate court held that the hospital failed to consider less-discriminatory alternatives to firing the technician.

Race Discrimination

Discharge of an employee on the basis of racial bias is actionable under state and federal laws. Title VII of the Civil Rights Act of 1964 "requires the elimination of artificial, arbitrary, and unnecessary barriers to employment that operate invidiously to discriminate on the basis of race."[42] An at-will employee's claim of racially motivated retaliatory discharge for filing a discrimination complaint can be actionable in tort as a violation of public policy.

The Civil Service Commission was found to have acted improperly in suspending a black licensed practical nurse as a result of a physical altercation with a white coworker in *Theodore v. Department of Health & Human Services.*[43] The white nurse had been accidentally struck by a crib being pushed by the black nurse. Evidence at trial supported the black nurse's contentions that she apologized for the accident. The white nurse struck the first blow and spoke inflammatory slurs. The black nurse's reaction had been defensive. The facts revealed no grounds for suspension or disciplinary action against the black nurse.

The Bethany Methodist Corporation's medical and skilled nursing care facility terminated a black certified nursing assistant because of its determination that she abused a patient on four separate occasions in *Billups v. Methodist Hospital of Chicago.*[44] The appellate court upheld a lower court order entering a summary judgment in favor of the defendant. The plaintiff did not offer traditional forms of indirect evidence to prove racial discrimination, such as statistics or evidence of comparable situations. There was no evidence in the record suggesting that Bethany terminated black employees more frequently for physically abusing a patient, while retaining nonblack employees.

In *Buckley Nursing Home v. Massachusetts Commission against Discrimination,*[45] Young, a black applicant for a nurse's aide position, filed a complaint alleging racial discrimination. Young responded to a newspaper advertisement for a nurse's aide position, filing her application on March 1, 1974, and was interviewed by the acting supervisor of nursing. The applicant called to inquire about the position on several occasions and eventually was told that the position had been filled. The advertisement ran again in the newspaper, and the applicant again called in response to the adver-

tisement. Young was told that her application was on file and that she would be called as needed. The facility hired four full-time and one part-time nurse's aides for the evening shift between March 1, 1974, and July 1, 1974.

On the upper right hand corner of Young's application, there is a handwritten notation "no openings," even though during the relevant time periods there were openings and other persons were hired for the evening shift. That notation does not appear on any other application, and none of Buckley's witnesses could identify who wrote it or when it appeared.

Despite testimony to the contrary, the commission found that Buckley had entered discussion about Young's race and had decided not to hire her on that basis. The commission thus concluded that Buckley's reason for not hiring Young (that she was not the best qualified applicant for the job) was a pretext, and that she would have been hired but for her race.

The commission awarded Young $6,986 plus interest for lost wages and $2,000 for emotional distress. Besides the monetary award to Young, the nursing facility had been instructed by the commission to develop a minority recruitment program. On appeal by the facility, the trial court upheld the commission's decision. On further appeal, the appeals court held that the evidence was sufficient to support a reasonable inference that the nursing facility's rejection of the applicant occurred after consideration of her race.

Religious Discrimination

Discrimination based on religion is valuing a person or group lower because of their religion, or treating someone differently because of what they do or don't believe. While many religious and secular authorities tend to stress that religion is something personal, the highly social nature of most religions makes conflicts between religious groups, and thus discrimination, still very probable. Reasonable accommodations should be made for an employee's religious beliefs.

Sex Discrimination

In *Jones v. Hinds General Hospital,*[46] a prima facie case of sex discrimination was established by evidence showing that a hospital laid off female nursing assistants while retaining male orderlies who performed the necessary functions. The court, however, held that Title VII of the Civil Rights Act was not violated by the hospital's use of gender as a basis for laying off employees. Gender was a bona fide occupational qualification for orderlies because a substantial number of male patients objected to the performance of catheterizations and surgical preparation by female assistants.

SEXUAL HARASSMENT HISTORICAL PERSPECTIVE

1964 The Civil Rights Act of 1964 was enacted, prohibiting job discrimination on the basis of sex.

1975 The first reported sexual harassment decision, in which two women claimed that they had suffered repeated verbal and physical advances by a supervisor, was rendered. The court ruled that the Civil Rights Act of 1964 did not cover such claims.

1977 A federal appeals court ruled that sexual harassment is discrimination under the Civil Rights Act of 1964, when a woman alleged that her position was abolished because she refused a supervisor's sexual advances.

1980 The Equal Employment Opportunity Commission (EEOC) issued landmark sexual harassment guidelines that prohibit unwelcomed sexual advances or requests that are made as a condition of employment. The guidelines also prohibit conduct that creates a hostile work environment.

1986 The U.S. Supreme Court upheld the validity of EEOC guidelines in those instances when harassment creates an abusive or hostile work environment.

1991 A Florida district court ruled that nude pin-ups in the workplace can constitute harassment. A California federal appeals court ruled that a hostile work environment should be evaluated from a reasonable woman standard and not a reasonable person standard.

1993 The U.S. Supreme Court held that a hostile work environment need not be psychologically injurious but only perceived as abusive.

Section 703 of Title VII and the EEOC defines sexual harassment in employment as unwelcome sexual advances, requests for sexual favors, and other verbal or physical conduct of a sexual nature when this conduct: explicitly or implicitly affects an individual's employment; unreasonably interferes with an individual's work performance; or creates an intimidating, hostile, or offensive work environment.

Sexual conduct becomes unlawful only when it is unwelcome by the victim. The victim must not have solicited or invited the actions and must have considered the conduct undesirable or offensive. To determine if the victim may have solicited or encouraged the claimed sexual harassment, a court may assess the victim's sexual aggressiveness or consistent use of sexually oriented language in the work environment. Of course, indications of an employee's sexually aggressive nature will not necessarily negate a claim of sexual harassment, just as voluntary participation in sexual conduct by the victim will not necessarily negate the claim. An employee may participate in sexual conduct for fear of repercussions, thus each claim must be examined individually to determine whether the particular conduct complained of was unwelcome.

Unwelcome sexual conduct becomes harassment when it creates a working environment that is unreasonably intimidating or offensive. A reasonable person must find the work environment offensive, and the complaining employee must have perceived the conduct as offensive.

When sexual conduct is determined to be unwelcome, the court must evaluate its level of interference with the employee's job, and whether the harassment created a hostile work environment. The court will consider the type of harassment (verbal, physical, or both), as well as the frequency of the harassment. A hostile work environment usually requires a pattern of conduct that has a repetitive effect. An isolated incident of physical advance is more likely to constitute a hostile environment (such as unwanted touching of the intimate body parts) than would a single case of verbal advance. In the same respect, sexual flirtation or vulgar language will not often constitute a hostile work environment as readily as would pervasive and continuous proliferation of pornography and demeaning comments.

An employer may be held liable for harassment inflicted by a supervisor, which results in a tangible employment action, or a significant change in the victim's employment status. Such tangible employment action may fall under categories such as: hiring, firing, promotion, demotion, undesirable reassignment, decision causing a significant change in benefits, compensation decisions, and work assignment. The victim of sexual harassment as well as the harasser may be a man or woman. The harasser can be the victim's supervisor, an agent of the employer, a supervisor in another area, a co-worker, or a non-employee. The victim does not have to be the person harassed but could be anyone affected by the offensive conduct. Unlawful sexual harassment may occur without economic injury.

An employee who claims harassment based upon a hostile work environment must demonstrate that the conduct complained of was sufficiently severe and/or pervasive to alter the conditions of employment and create a work environment that would qualify as hostile or abusive to employees because of their sex. An employer, however, will not always be held liable for sexual harassment that occurs in the workplace if the employer can prove: (1) it had in place an anti-harassment policy with an effective complaint procedure; (2) it promptly took action to prevent and correct any harassment; and (3) that the employee unreasonably failed to avoid further harm by complaining to management. If the harassment is committed by a non-supervisor, the lower courts have held that the employer will only be liable if it knew or should have known about the conduct and failed to take appropriate corrective action.

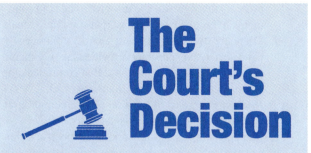

The Court's Decision

The U.S. Court of Appeals for the Seventh Circuit found that the employer's interrogation of nursing facility employees about a union meeting constituted an unfair labor practice. On the record as a whole, substantial evidence supported the board's conclusions that the questioning of Welton and Hopkins amounted to unlawful interrogation.

CHAPTER REVIEW

1. The National Labor Relations Act (NLRA) of 1935 is the most significant federal legislation concerning labor relations. It defines unfair labor practices and provides for hearings on complaints regarding such practices.
2. The National Labor Relations Board (NLRB) is responsible for administering and enforcing the NLRA. The board reviews claims submitted by employers or employees, determines whether unfair labor practices have taken place, and suggests a remedy.
3. The NLRA includes procedures through which employees can choose a union as a collective bargaining representative to negotiate employment and contract concerns with their employer.
4. The Norris-LaGuardia Act was enacted by Congress to limit the power of the federal courts to issue injunctions in cases that involve or have grown out of labor disputes. It is aimed specifically at reducing the number of injunctions granted to restrain strikes and picketing. In 1974, an amendment designating procedures that limit strikes in health care organizations was added to the NLRA. Among other provisions, this amendment requires that 10 days' notice of a strike be given. This allows the NLRB to determine the legality of the strike and gives the organization time to put in place provisions that will protect the level of patient care.
5. Title VII of the Civil Rights Act of 1964, as amended by the Equal Employment Opportunity Act of 1972, prohibits discrimination in employment in any business on the basis of race, color, religion, sex, or national origin. The act prohibits harassment based on one's affiliation (e.g., religion), physical and cultural traits, and clothing.
6. The Fair Labor Standards Act (FLSA) established minimum wages and maximum hours of employment. The Equal Pay Act, essentially an amendment to the FLSA, prohibits sex discrimination in the payment of wages. Further, the Equal Employment Opportunity Act of 1972 prohibits private employers, as well as state and local governments, from discriminating based on age, race, color, religion, sex, or national origin. An act that further addresses age discrimination is the Age Discrimination in Employment Act of 1967.
7. The Occupational Safety and Health Act of 1970 was enacted by Congress to ensure, to the extent possible, that every working man and woman in the country have safe and healthful working conditions and to preserve human resources. Employers are required to provide a place of employment that is without recognized hazards that cause or are likely to cause death or serious physical harm. For health care organizations, the city and county in which a facility is located may prescribe additional rules regarding the health and safety of employees.
8. The Rehabilitation Act of 1973 provides protection from discrimination to handicapped employees and is applied to both public and private organizations. The Americans with Disabilities Act of 1990 is legislation that further

protects the rights of the disabled. The act prohibits job discrimination in hiring, promotion, and other requirements of employment against qualified individuals with disabilities.

9. There are two kinds of union security contracts:
   (1) *Closed-shop contracts* provide that only members of a particular union may be hired.
   (2) *Union-shop contracts* hold that continued employment is dependent on membership in the union. A majority
   of states hold such contracts unlawful.

10. *Workers' compensation* is a reimbursement program for employees with work-related injuries. These programs are
    administered on a state-by-state basis.

11. Management has certain important, specific rights, including the right to hire replacement workers in the event of
    a strike and the right to prohibit supervisors from participating in organized union activity.

12. Most health care organizations have an equal employment opportunity or affirmative action plan. Affirmative
    action programs include the collection and analysis of data on the race and sex of all applicants for employment
    and a nondiscrimination statement in personal policy/procedure manuals and employee handbooks.

13. An *injunction* is an order by a court that instructs that a certain act be performed or not performed. Today, the rule
    limits the availability of injunctive relief to halt work stoppages. Anti-injunction acts restrict the courts' power to
    limit injunctions in labor disputes.

14. *Arbitration* procedures begin when a union files a demand for arbitration either with the employer or with the
    arbitration agency named in the contract. The decision of the arbitrator is binding on both parties.

15. Discrimination in the workplace comes in many forms and in numerous ways, each having its own little twist of
    facts. Discrimination is prohibited by law and may involve race, color, religion, sex, national origin, disability,
    pregnancy, and so forth.

REVIEW QUESTIONS

1. Provide a general overview of the NLRA.
2. Using the hospital as a setting, give two examples of what would violate the NLRA.
3. How do patients' rights come into play during a strike by nurses?
4. What is the purpose of OSHA?
5. Why was the Norris-LaGuardia Act enacted by Congress?
6. Where is the Equal Pay Act applicable? What is the purpose of the EPA?
7. Discuss the various ways in which discrimination can occur in the workplace.

WEB SITE RESOURCES

Industrial and Labor Relations Review	www.ilr.cornell.edu/ilrreview/
Labor Management Relations	www1.opm.gov/cplmr/index.asp
National Labor Relations Board	www.nlrb.gov/
Occupational Safety and Health Administration	www.osha.gov/
U.S. Code: Labor Management Relations	www4.law.cornell.edu/uscode/29/ch7.html
U.S. Department of Labor	www.dol.gov/

NOTES

1. *NLRB v. Shelby Mem'l Hosp. Ass'n,* 1 F.3d 550 (7th Cir. 1993).

2. 29 U.S.C. § 151.

3. NLRA § 2 (14) (1974).

4. Norris-LaGuardia Act 29 U.S.C. ch. 6 (1932).

5. *United States v. Hutcheson,* 312 U.S. 219 (1941).

6. Labor-Management Reporting and Disclosure Act of 1959, Pub. L. No. 86-257 (29 U.S.C. ch. 11).

7. Fair Labor Standards Act of 1938, 29 U.S.C. ch. 8.

8. Equal Employment Opportunity Act of 1972, 42 U.S.C. § 2000e et seq.

9. OSHA's Mission, Occupational Safety and Health Administration, U.S. Department of Labor, http://www.osha.gov/oshinfo/mission.html.

10. Occupational Safety and Health Act of 1970, 29 U.S.C. § 651.

11. PUB. L. NO. 91-596, § 2, 84 Stat. 1590 (Dec. 29, 1970); see also 29 U.S.C.A. § 651 (1990).

12. *Id.* at § 5, 84 Stat. 1593; *Id.* at § 654.

13. Rehabilitation Act of 1973, 29 U.S.C. ch. 14.

14. 45 C.F.R. § 4.6[c].

15. 641 N.W.2d 525 (Iowa 2002).

16. 460 N.E.2d 751 (Ill. 1984).

17. 676 P.2d 922 (Or. Ct. App. 1984).

18. 579 So. 2d 195 (Fla. Dist. Ct. App. 1991).

19. 899 F.2d 651 (7th Cir. 1990).

20. SUPREME COURT UPHOLDS NLRB BARGAINING-UNIT RULE, A.H.A. NEWS, Apr. 29, 1991, at 1.

21. 534 So. 2d 1003 (La. Ct. App. 1988).

22. 723 F. Supp. 859 (D.R.I. 1989).

23. 437 N.W.2d 538 (Wis. 1989).

24. 705 F.2d 1461 (7th Cir. 1983).

25. *NLRB v. American Medical Services, Inc.,* 705 F.2d 1472, 1474-75 (7th Cir. 1983).

26. *NLRB v. Res-Care, Inc.,* 705 F.2d 1461, 1465 (7th Cir.1983).

27. 42 C.F.R. § 483.75 (1989).

28. Age Discrimination in Employment Act of 1967, 29 U.S.C. ch. 14, as amended.

29. 450 U.S. 248, 253 (1981).

30. 702 F.2d 322 (2d Cir. 1983).

31. *Id.* at 325.

32. Americans with Disabilities Act of 1990, PUB. L. NO. 101-336, 104 Stat. 327 (July 26, 1990).

33. *Id.* at 329.

34. *Id.* at 331–332.

35. No. 31591 (W.Va. 2004).

36. *Furthering the Protections Against Workplace Discrimination and Harassment,* EEOC 35th. Anniversary, www.eeoc.gov/abouteeoc/35th/1990s/furthering.html.

37. Equal Pay Act of 1963, 29 U.S.C. ch. 8.

38. 653 F.2d 246 (6th Cir. 1981).

39. *Id.* at 247.

40. 417 U.S. 188, 195 (1974).

41. 726 F.2d 1543 (11th Cir. 1984).

42. *Griggs v. Duke Power Co.,* 401 U.S. 424 (1971).

43. 515 So. 2d 454 (La. Ct. App. 1987).

44. 922 F.2d 1300 (7th Cir. 1991).

45. 478 N.E.2d 1292 (Mass. App. Ct. 1985).

46. 666 F. Supp. 933 (D. Miss. 1987).

Employment, Discipline, and Discharge

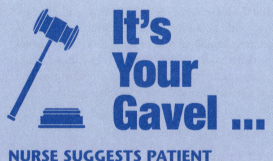

It's Your Gavel ...

NURSE SUGGESTS PATIENT CHANGE PHYSICIAN

The patient began losing weight and having hallucinations. A nurse documented the patient's difficulties and attempted on several occasions to call the patient's physician, however, the physician failed to return the nurse's calls. Because of the patient's deteriorating condition, the family contacted the nurse. After the nurse advised the patient's family as to her concerns, a member of the patient's family asked her what they should do. The nurse advised that she would reconsider their choice of physicians. The nurse was terminated by the nursing facility because she advised the patient's family to consider changing physicians.

The nurse brought a lawsuit for wrongful discharge in violation of public policy. The complaint was dismissed by a trial court and the nurse appealed.

The language in the Nursing Practice Act (NPA) of North Carolina and regulations of the board of nursing describes the practice of nursing as assessing a patient's health, which entails a responsibility to communicate, counsel, and provide accurate guidance to clients and their families. The nurse's comments that resulted in her termination were made in fulfillment of these responsibilities.

The defendant asserted that the NPA and the wording of the nursing board regulations relied on by the nurse did not express a policy prohibiting the discharge and that, in any event, the nurse had no duty to advise the patient's family.

The North Carolina Court of Appeals gave considerable attention to language in the NPA and the regulations that recognized nursing to include teaching and counseling about a patient's health care and of providing information to patients and their families, including making referrals to appropriate resources.[1]

WHAT IS YOUR VERDICT?

Man never fastened one end of a chain around the neck of his brother that God did not fasten the other end round the neck of the oppressor.

Lamartine (1790–1869)

Fairly balancing the rights of the employee and the needs of the organization is an extremely complex objective. This chapter provides some direction in this balancing act.

For the health care worker, an unexpected termination may mean a significant setback in career progression, financial hardship, and loss of self-esteem. For the organization and its community, a termination means a lack of stability in the management structure and possible disruption and realignment of services provided. A growing consensus is that high turnover rates are unhealthy and provide a disservice to an industry already plagued with cost constraints and other pressures.

Wrongful discharge claims are difficult, time consuming, and often mean expensive lawsuits to defend. Employers who experience favorable court decisions in wrongful discharge claims often have unfavorable repercussions because of bad press and the negative effects a discharge has on employee morale.

EMPLOYMENT AT WILL

An at will prerogative without limits could be suffered only in an anarchy, and there not for long; it certainly cannot be suffered in a society such as ours without weakening the bond of counter balancing rights and obligations that holds such societies together.

Sides v. Duke Hospital[2]

The common-law employment-at-will doctrine provides that employment is at the will of either the employer or the employee, and that employment may be terminated by the employer or the employee at any time for any or no reason, unless there is a contract in place that specifies the terms and duration of employment. Historically, termination of employees for any reason was widely accepted. However, contemporary thinking does not support this concept.

In recent years the rule that employment for an indefinite term is terminable by the employer whenever and for whatever cause he chooses without incurring liability has been the subject of

considerable scholarly debate, and judicial and legislative modification. Consequently, there has been a growing trend toward a restricted application of the at-will employment rule whereby the right of an employer to discharge an at-will employee without cause is limited by either public policy considerations or an implied covenant of good faith and fair dealing.[3]

In *Sides v. Duke Hospital,* the North Carolina Court of Appeals found it to be an

obvious and indisputable fact that in a civilized state where reciprocal legal rights and duties abound, the words "at will" can never mean "without limit or qualification," as so much of the discussion and the briefs of the defendants imply; for in such a state the rights of each person are necessarily and inherently limited by the rights of others and the interests of the public. An at will prerogative without limits could be suffered only in an anarchy, and there not for long, it certainly cannot be suffered in a society such as ours without weakening the bond of counter balancing rights and obligations that holds such societies together.

• • • •

If we are to have law, those who so act against the public interest must be held accountable for the harm inflicted thereby; to accord them civil immunity would incongruously reward their lawlessness at the unjust expense of their innocent victims.[4]

The concept of the employment-at-will doctrine is embroiled in a combination of legislative enactments and judicial decisions. Some states have a tendency to be more employer oriented, such as New York, whereas others, such as California, emerge as being much more forward thinking and in harmony with the constitutional rights of the employee.

The employment-at-will common law doctrine is not truly applicable in today's society and many courts have recognized this fact. In the last century, the common law developed in a laissez-faire climate that encouraged industrial growth and improved the right of an employer to control his own business, including the right to fire without cause an employee at will. . . . The twentieth century has witnessed significant changes in socioeconomic values that have led to reassessment of the common law rule. Businesses have evolved from small- and medium-size firms to gigantic corporations in which ownership is separate from management. Formerly there was a clear delineation between employers, who frequently were owners of their own businesses, and employees. The employer in the old sense has been replaced by a superior in the corporate hierarchy who is himself an employee.[5]

As discussed here, exceptions to the employment-at-will doctrine involve contractual relationships, public policy issues, defamation, retaliatory discharge, and fairness. It would seem that the doctrine has little applicability in modern society.

PUBLIC POLICY ISSUES

The public policy exception to the employment-at-will doctrine provides that employees may not be terminated for reasons that are contrary to public policy. Public policy originates with legislative enactments that prohibit, for example, the discharge of employees on the basis of disability, age, race, color, religion, sex, national origin, pregnancy, filing of safety violation complaints with various agencies (e.g., the Occupational Safety and Health Administration), or union membership. Any attempt to limit, segregate, or classify employees in any way that would tend to deprive any individual of employment opportunities on these bases is contrary to public policy.

Public policy also can arise as a result of judicial decisions that address those issues not covered by statutes, rules, and regulations. "[I]t can be said that public policy concerns what is right and just and what affects the citizens of the state collectively. It is to be found in the state's constitution and statutes and, when they are silent, in its judicial decisions."[6]

In those instances in which state and federal laws are silent, not all courts concur with the use of judicial decisions as a means for determining public policy. A California court determined that a public policy exception to the at-will employment doctrine must be based on constitutional or statutory provisions rather than judicial policy making.[7]

Reporting Patient Abuse

An employer may not discharge an employee for fulfilling societal obligations or in those instances in which the employer acts with a socially undesirable motive.[8] A tort claim for wrongful discharge was stated in *McQuary v. Air Convalescent Home*[9] by allegations that the plaintiff was discharged wrongfully from her position at the nursing facility in retaliation for threatening to report to state authorities instances of alleged patient mistreatment. Such mistreatment purportedly involved violation of a patient's rights under the Nursing Home Patient's Bill of Rights. To

prevail, the discharged employee was not required to prove that patient abuse actually had occurred but only that she acted in good faith.

> This conclusion is consistent with established Oregon law. Statutes which protect employees against retaliation do not require that the alleged violation which the employee claims be ultimately proved. See, e.g., ORS 652.355 (protects an employee who merely consults an attorney or agency about a wage claim); ORS 654.062(5) (protects any employee who makes a complaint under the Oregon Safe Employment Act); ORS 659.030(1)(f) (prohibits discrimination against an employee who filed a civil rights complaint); ORS 633.120(3) (prohibits discrimination against an employee for filing an unfair labor practices complaint). We have, in fact, upheld awards for retaliation despite holding that the original complaint did not show discrimination.

• • • •

> Similar considerations of public policy lead to our conclusion that an employee who reports a violation of a nursing home patient's statutory rights in good faith should be protected from discharge for that action.[10]

This case, which had been dismissed in the lower court, was reversed and remanded for trial.

Whistle-Blowing

A whistle-blower is one who reveals wrongdoing in the organization to a public entity or someone in authority. This often occurs when one believes that the public interest overrides the interest of the organization and can involve illegal or fraudulent activities. A whistle-blower provides information he or she reasonably believes evidences violation of any law, rule or regulation; gross mismanagement; a gross waste of funds; an abuse of authority; a substantial and specific danger to public health; and/or a substantial and specific danger to public safety.[11]

> [A]ccording to the public policy exception, an employer may not rely on the at-will doctrine as a basis for escaping liability for discharging an employee because of the doing of, or the refusing to do, such an act. Moreover, statutes in several jurisdictions protect an employee from an employer's retaliation for engaging in certain types of protected activities, such as whistleblowing.[12]

Whistle-Blower Suit Untimely

The plaintiffs were critical care nurses in an intensive care unit. Beginning in 1998 and continuing through May 1999, they began to complain to their supervisors about deficient patient care. Because of subsequent disciplinary action taken by their supervisors, the plaintiffs retained counsel to file a whistle-blower action pursuant to section 448.103, which authorizes an aggrieved employee who has been the object of retaliation to institute a civil action in a court within two years of discovering the alleged retaliatory personnel action or within four years after the personnel action was taken, whichever comes first. The Florida District Court of Appeal determined that the trial court erred by allowing the nurses to pursue their claim after the statute of limitations period expired. The final judgment awarding the nurses damages and attorney fees was reversed.[13]

PAVING HER WAY TO HEAVEN

Citation: *Kirk v. Mercy Hosp. Tri-County,* 851 S.W.2d 617 (Mo. Ct. App. 1993)

Facts

The nurse-plaintiff was employed as a charge nurse with supervisory duties. A short time after one of her patients had been admitted to the hospital, the charge nurse determined the patient was suffering from toxic shock syndrome. Knowing that death would result if left untreated, the charge nurse assumed the physician would order antibiotics. After a period of time passed without having received such orders, the charge nurse discussed the patient's condition with the nursing director. She was informed by the director to document, report the facts, and stay out of it.

The charge nurse discussed the patient's condition and lack of orders with the chief of staff. Although the chief of staff took appropriate steps to treat the patient, the patient died. After the nursing director was informed by a member of the patient's family that the charge nurse offered to obtain the medical records and was later told that the charge

nurse was heard to say that the physician was paving the patient's way to heaven, the charge nurse was terminated.

After her termination, the charge nurse received a service letter from the hospital that directed her to refrain from making any further false statements about the hospital and its staff.

The trial court entered a summary judgment for the defendant-hospital, stating that there were no triable issues of fact, and there was no public policy exception to the charge nurse's at-will termination. The court could not find any law or regulation prohibiting the hospital from discharging her as a nurse. The nurse appealed.

Issue

Was there a public policy exception to the Missouri employment-at-will doctrine?

Holding

The Missouri Court of Appeals reversed the granting of summary judgment and remanded the case for trial, holding that the Nursing Practice Act (NPA) provided a clear mandate of public policy that nurses had a duty to provide the best possible care to patients.

Reason

Public policy clearly mandates that a nurse has an obligation to serve the best interests of patients. Therefore, if the plaintiff refused to follow her supervisor's orders to stay out of a case where the patient was dying from a lack of proper medical treatment, there would be no grounds for her discharge under the public policy exception to the employment-at-will doctrine. Pursuant to the NPA, the plaintiff risked discipline if she ignored improper treatment of the patient. Her persistence in attempting to get the proper treatment for the patient was her absolute duty. The hospital could not lawfully require that she stay out of a case that would have obvious injurious consequences to the patient. Public policy, as defined in case law, holds that no one can lawfully do that which tends to be injurious to the public or against the public good.

Discussion

1. Explain how a public policy would be analyzed and then determined to apply in an employment-at-will case.

2. What was the public policy mandate in this case?

INTERFERENCE WITH EMPLOYMENT ACTIVITIES

Liability for discrimination is not limited strictly to employer-employee relationships, but can be applied in situations in which discriminatory practices can affect the ability of a nonemployee to obtain a job with a third party. This occurred in *Pardazi v. Cullman Medical Center,*[14] in which the court held that the physician stated a claim for relief under Title VII of the Civil Rights Act of 1964, based on the allegation that the hospital's denial of staff privileges interfered with his employment relationship with a third party. Dr. Pardazi, a medical practitioner, entered into an employment contract with an Alabama corporation that required Pardazi to become a staff member of the defendant hospital. Pardazi argued that the hospital's discriminatory practices in denying his appointment denied him the right of an attorney at rehearing, extended his observation period from four months to one year (a deviation from the medical staff bylaws), and interfered with his employment opportunities. The lower court's summary judgment for the hospital was reversed and the case remanded.

DEFAMATION ACTIONS

Dismissal was ordered properly for claims of wrongful termination and defamation in *Eli v. Griggs County Hospital & Nursing Home,*[15] in which a nurse's aide was terminated on the basis of an incident in the hospital dining room. In the presence of patients and visitors, she cursed her supervisor and complained that personnel were working short staffed. Given the nature of her employment and the high standard of care that persons reasonably expected from a nursing care facility, such behavior justified her termination on a charge of reported breach of patient-specific and facility-specific information. No defamation resulted from the entry of such charges in the aide's personnel file because the record established that the charges were true.

RETALIATORY DISCHARGE

There is a tendency for some people in positions of power to abuse that power through threats, abuse, intimidation, and retaliatory discharge, all of which are cause for legal action. Employees who become the targets of a vindictive supervisor often have difficulty proving a bad-faith motive. In an effort to reduce the probability of wrongful discharge, some states, such as Connecticut,[16] Maine,[17] Michigan,[18] and Montana,[19] have enacted legislation that protects employees from terminations found to be arbitrary and capricious. The Montana Supreme Court upheld state legislation that protects workers against arbitrary discharge, while at the same time limits the damages they can win.

Employees have brought claims alleging abusive discharge in violation of public policy. This type of action is usually found to be sound in tort, and thus in certain circumstances punitive damages have been awarded. The burden of proof for establishing some hidden motive for discharge from employment rests on discharged employees.

The National Labor Relations Act and other labor legislation illustrate the governmental policy of preventing employers from using the right of discharge as a means of oppression. . . . Consistent with this policy, many states have recognized the need to protect employees who are not parties to a collective bargaining agreement or other contract from abusive practices by the employer. . . . Those states have recognized a common law cause of action for employees-at-will who were discharged for reasons that were in some way "wrongful." The courts in those jurisdictions have taken various approaches: some recognizing the action in tort, some in contract.[20]

The court in *Khanna v. Microdata Corp.*[21] held that substantial evidence supported a finding that the employer fired the employee in bad-faith retaliation for bringing a lawsuit against the employer, thus violating an implied covenant of good faith and fair dealing.

Under the traditional common-law rule, codified in section 2922 of the [California] Labor Code, an employment contract of indefinite duration is in general terminable at the will of either party. During the past several decades, however, judicial authorities in California and throughout the United States have established the rule that, under both common law and the statute, an employer does not enjoy an absolute or totally unfettered right to discharge even an at-will employee.[22]

In *Shores v. Senior Manor Nursing Center,*[23] a formerly employed nurse's assistant brought an action against the nursing facility for retaliatory discharge. The circuit court dismissed the complaint for failure of the plaintiff to state a cause of action. On appeal, the appellate court held that the allegation of the former employee that she was discharged in retaliation for reporting to the nursing home administrator that the charge nurse was performing her nursing functions improperly, which allegedly violated the Nursing Home Care Reform Act, stated a cause of action for retaliatory discharge. The circuit court was reversed, and the case was remanded for further proceedings.

Dismissal of an employee shortly after a request for a grievance hearing regarding a salary discrepancy with another employee can raise an issue of liability for retaliatory discharge. The physician in *Jones v. Westside-Urban Health Center*[24] was found to have established a prima facie case of retaliatory discharge in which the record indicated that he had been fired from the hospital five days after his request for a grievance hearing on an alleged salary discrepancy.

RETALIATORY DISCHARGE AND EMOTIONAL DISTRESS

Citation: *Dalby v. Sisters of Providence,* 865 P.2d 391 (Or. Ct. App. 1993)

Facts

Dalby, a pharmacy technician, alleged that she was discharged for reporting to her supervisor on several occasions that there were inaccuracies in the drug inventory and that recordkeeping regarding these inaccuracies was in violation of Oregon administrative rules. Dalby alleged that rather than comply with the regulations, her supervisor retaliated against her because of her insistence that her employer comply with the rules.

Retaliatory actions against Dalby included accusations of stealing cocaine from the hospital's drug inventory. Dalby learned that the sheriff's department had been asked to arrest her for stealing the cocaine. The sheriff's department refused to make the arrest. Dalby also alleged that her supervisor refused to talk to her except for job-related purposes and that hospital attendance policies were rigidly applied against her. As a result of the defendant's actions, Dalby resigned her position.

Dalby's former employer argued that the allegations did not demonstrate constructive discharge by deliberately creating difficult working conditions with the intention of forcing the employee to leave employment, and that the employee left employment because of the working conditions.

The circuit court dismissed Dalby's claim, and she appealed.

Issue

Did the plaintiff state a cause of action for wrongful discharge and emotional distress?

Holding

The Oregon Court of Appeals, assuming the plaintiff's allegation to be true, reversed and remanded the case for trial, holding that the pharmacy technician stated a cause of action for wrongful discharge and intentional infliction of emotional distress.

Reason

Dalby made a good-faith report as to the hospital's noncompliance with the drug inventory and recordkeeping requirements required under Oregon regulations. Her report fulfilled an important societal obligation. An employer may not discharge an employee for making such reports. The conduct of the employer, including false accusations that she had taken cocaine, gave rise to an action for the infliction of emotional distress.

Discussion

1. Regardless of the final disposition of this case by the trial court, what issues remain open for review by management and the governing body?
2. Discuss the meaning of constructive discharge.

FAIRNESS: THE ULTIMATE TEST

"Is it fair?" is the ultimate question that a supervisor must ask when considering a termination. In general, bad faith and inexplicable terminations are subject to the scrutiny of the courts. Some courts and legislative enactments have overturned the view that employers have total discretion to terminate workers who are not otherwise protected by collective bargaining agreements or civil service regulations. Montana legislation grants every employee the right to sue the employer for wrongful discharge. The mere fact that an employment contract is terminable at will does not give the employer an absolute right to terminate it in all cases. The court in *Cleary v. American Airlines*[25] held that the longevity of the employee's services, together with the express policy of the employer, operated as a form of estoppel, precluding any discharge of the employee by the employer without good cause, and thus, the employee stated a cause of action for wrongful discharge.

There is an implied covenant of good faith and fair dealing in every contract that neither party will do anything that will injure the right of the other to receive benefits from the agreement. An employee in *Pugh v. See's Candies*[26] was found to have shown a prima facie case of wrongful termination in violation of an implied promise that the employer would not act arbitrarily in dealing with the employee. The employer's right to terminate an employee is not absolute. It is limited by fundamental principles of public policy and by expressed or implied terms of agreement between the employer and the employee.

Procedural issues are as important as issues of discrimination. In *Renny v. Port Huron Hospital,*[27] the Michigan Supreme Court found, as did the jury, that the employee's discharge hearing was not final and binding because it did not comport with elementary fairness. The court found that there was sufficient evidence for the jury to find that the employee had not been discharged for just cause. The existence of a just-cause contract is a question of fact for the jury when the employer establishes written policies and procedures and does not expressly retain the right to terminate an employee at will. That the hospital followed the grievance procedure with the plaintiff is evidence that a just cause contract existed on which the plaintiff relied.

The employee handbook provided for a grievance board as a fair way to resolve work-related complaints and problems. This was not a mandatory procedure to which the hospital's employees had to submit. The employee was not bound by the grievance board's determination that her discharge was proper, because evidence supported a finding that she was not given adequate notice of who the witnesses against her would be. She was not permitted to be present when the witnesses testified, and she was not given the right to present certain evidence.

There was sufficient evidence for the jury to conclude that the plaintiff had suffered damages. Evidence presented indicated that her subsequent professional employment did not equal her earnings before discharge and that she experienced increased expenses because of the loss of her health insurance as well as other financial losses that she suffered as a result of her discharge.

An employee who believes that he or she has been unfairly discharged will most likely seek access to the following information in defense of his or her claim:

- minutes of pertinent meetings

- written reports, typed or handwritten

- personnel file

- tapes

- letters, cards, and handwritten notes written on the employee's behalf from the public

- personnel handbook

- personnel and departmental policies and procedures books

- oral testimony from fellow employees and supervisors

Employers must document carefully and fairly any disciplinary proceedings that might be subject to discovery by a disgruntled employee; failure to do so could place the organization or supervisor at a disadvantage should a complaint reach the courts.

UNEMPLOYMENT COMPENSATION

Fair dealing in termination also should include fair dealing with the terminated employee who files for unemployment benefits. In *Mankato Lutheran Home v. Miller,*[28] a nursing assistant was found not to be disqualified from receiving unemployment benefits because of a single episode of profanity directed toward her supervisor while she was ill, frustrated, and, in part, provoked by actions of her supervisor. The nursing assistant had no prior record of misconduct in five years of employment; however, her illness and frustration at having to work after she repeatedly indicated that she was not feeling well increased over the course of several hours until she exploded emotionally. She had asked her supervisor, Ms. Darkow, if she could go home but was refused because of the probability of being unable to replace her in the middle of a shift.

> At about 5:30 A.M. Darkow entered a patient's room where Miller was helping a resident get dressed. When she asked how Miller was feeling, Miller became upset and said, "What the . . . do you care, you don't think I'm sick anyway. I could drop over dead and still have to do these . . . people." Darkow retorted that Miller should not have come to work if she was so sick, and Miller yelled back, "I never had this . . . pain until I came to this . . . hole."[29]

Although the assistant's outburst was directed toward her supervisor, one of two residents in the room who heard the incident was upset by it. The episode in this case did not represent a disregard for the employer's interests or of the nursing assistant's duties and responsibilities.

Denial of unemployment insurance benefits on the ground that a nursing assistant's employment was terminated due to misconduct was proper where the assistant admitted that he had become involved in an argument with a registered nurse over the use of a copy machine. Although the nursing assistant maintained that the nurse threatened him by stating that she was going to get him, the nurse indicated that the nursing assistant threatened her by telling her to watch her back and car. The conflicting account of the incident presented an issue of credibility for the Unemployment Insurance Appeal Board to resolve, and threatening conduct toward a coworker was misconduct disqualifying one from receiving unemployment insurance benefits.[30]

Fair dealing does not always imply that every discharged employee should be entitled to unemployment benefits. For example, in *Forbis v. Wesleyan Nursing Home,*[31] unemployment compensation was denied because of an employee's discharge resulting from theft of a patient's clock. The theft constituted willful and wanton disregard for the nursing home's interests. The Employment Security Commission on its investigation made the following findings of fact: the claimant was discharged for theft of patient property; the patient accused the claimant of taking the patient's clock; and, upon being confronted with the patient's accusation, the claimant produced the missing clock from her pocket and admitted taking it.[32]

In another case, a nursing assistant was properly denied unemployment benefits as a result of being terminated for poor work attendance, even though her most recent absence had been excused.[33] The employee's record indicated that the center had shown great tolerance in allowing the employee to continue employment for as long as it did.

Voluntary termination because of a change in working conditions will not necessarily make an employee eligible for unemployment benefits. In *Montclair Nursing Home v. Wills,*[34] a licensed practical nurse was found not to be eligible for unemployment benefits when she resigned after reassignment to a night shift. Voluntary termination because of a change in working hours was not considered sufficient cause to grant unemployment benefits, absent an "improper" purpose or motive in the change in the employee's work hours.

TERMINATION

A decision to terminate an employee should be reviewed carefully by a member of management familiar with the issues of wrongful discharge. Oral counseling, written counseling, written counseling with suspension, and written counseling with termination are the textbook responses to disciplinary action and discharge. Whatever form of discipline is used, it should be designed to produce a more effective and productive employee.

The employer's right to terminate an employee is not absolute. It is limited by fundamental principles of public policy and by express or implied terms of agreement between the employer and the employee.

> Formulating a standard for substantive fairness in employee dismissal law requires accommodating a number of different interests already afforded legal recognition. The legal interest of employees to be protected against certain types of unfair and injurious action . . . are at the core of any employee dismissal proposal. Arrayed against these interests are employer and societal interests in effective management of organizations, which require that employees not be shielded from the consequences of their poor performance or misconduct, and that supervisors not be deterred from exercising their managerial responsibilities by the inconvenience of litigating employees' claims.[35]

Before termination of an employee, the employer should ask, was the termination:

- a violation of public policy

- a violation of any policy or procedure outlined in an administrative manual, the employee handbook, the human resource department's policies and procedures, or any other health care facility policies and procedures or regulations

- retaliatory in nature (e.g., refusal to perform an illegal act or a questioning of a management practice)

- arbitrary and capricious

- discriminatory on the basis of age, disability, race, creed, color, religion, gender, national origin, or marital status

- a violation of any contract, oral or written

- consistent with the reasons for discharge

- discriminatory against the employee for filing a lawsuit

- fixed before any appeal actions can be taken

- an interference with an employee's rights as secured by the laws or Constitution of the United States (e.g., right to freedom of speech)

Employment Disclaimers

A *disclaimer* is the denial of a right that is imputed to a person or that is alleged to belong to him or her. Although a disclaimer is often a successful defense for employers in wrongful discharge cases, it should not be considered a license to discharge at will and at the whim of the supervisor in an arbitrary and capricious manner.

Employers can help prevent successful lawsuits for wrongful discharge that are based on the premise that an employee handbook or departmental policy and procedure manual is an implied contract by incorporating disclaimers in published manuals, such as that described in *Battaglia v. Sisters of Charity Hospital*,[36] in which a personnel manual could not be interpreted to limit the hospital's power to terminate an at-will employee. Language in the manual indicated that the personnel manual was not a contract; that it could be modified, amended, or supplemented; and that the hospital retained the right to make all necessary management decisions for the delivery of patient care services and the selection, direction, compensation, and retention of employees.

Handbooks that do not contain disclaimers can alter an employee's at-will status. An appeals court in *Trusty v. Big Sandy Health Care Center*[37] noted that the handbook did not contain any disclaimer or any other language that employment was at will. The court held that there was sufficient evidence to establish that the handbook had altered the employee's at-will status and determined that the employee could bring a wrongful discharge suit.

Disclaimers must be clear to the employee. The court in *Harvet v. Unity Medical Center*[38] held in a wrongful discharge suit that the hospital's employee handbook was sufficiently definite to form an employment contract.

> Unity's handbook contained detailed provisions on conduct and procedures for discipline. As the trial court observed, "there can be no question that [respondent's] handbook provisions are sufficiently definite to form a contract." The handbook represents much more than Unity's general statement of policy. Moreover, the terms of the handbook were sufficiently definite to allow a fact finder to determine whether there had been a breach.

• • • •

> Respondent contends the handbook contained the following reservations on the part of the employer indicating it was not being offered as a contract: "Exceptions to any personnel policy or procedure may be permitted on a documented form showing of good and sufficient cause."

• • • •

> In the present case the trial court correctly found, "the clause does not clearly tell employees that the handbook is not part of an employment contract."[39]

The employer's disclaimers were considered clear in *Simonson v. Meader Distribution Co.*,[40] in which an employee filed a breach of contract suit alleging a dismissal was outside company-adopted disciplinary guidelines. The court held that the company could and did reserve the discretion to discipline employees outside adopted guidelines. The policy manual contained the following three specific reservations of management discretion[41]:

1. Management reserves the right to make any changes at any time by adding to, deleting, or changing any existing policy.

2. The rules set out below are as complete as we can reasonably make them. However, they are not necessarily all-inclusive, because circumstances that we have not anticipated may arise. Some currently unanticipated circumstances may warrant the application of discipline, including discharge.

3. Management may vary from the above policies if, in its opinion, the circumstances require.

Health care organizations can be successful when confronted with wrongful discharge suits based on breach of contract by placing similar language in their personnel manuals.

Job Description

The job description is not intended to be an employment contract, nor does it dissolve the at-will employment relationship. It is a record of the basic purpose, typical level of authority, typical source of action, and representative function or duties of the job. It is designed to provide management and others with a clear understanding of the level of the job and its working relationships, skills, and requirements in relation to other jobs.

Termination for Cause

A termination-for-cause-only clause in an employment contract is binding. An employment contract in *Eales v. Tanana*[42] that provided that an employee hired up to retirement age could be terminated only for cause was upheld by the court.

Violation of No-Smoking Policy

Unemployment compensation was properly denied a nursing assistant for breach of a no-smoking rule in *Selan v. Commonwealth Unemployment Compensation Board of Review*.[43] The nursing facility's personnel handbook clearly provided that smoking was allowed only in specified areas. The handbook provided that employees must refrain from smoking in offices, resident areas, elevators, corridors, or any area where it might be hazardous.

The nursing home assistant admitted that she was smoking but argued that she did not break the facility's smoking rules. The court disagreed. Evidence was sufficient to show that the employee knowingly violated Methodist Home's rule by smoking in a patient's bathroom. Deliberate violation of a reasonable employer rule, without due cause, constitutes willful misconduct warranting disqualification for unemployment compensation.

Termination and Financial Necessity

No breach of employment contract occurred in *Wilde v. Houlton Regional Hospital*[44] when, because of financial difficulties, a hospital terminated the employment of two nurses, a ward clerk, and a dietary supervisor. Even if the employees were correct in contending that their indefinite contracts of employment had been modified by virtue of a dismissal for cause provision in the employee's handbook and by management's oral assurances that they were permanent, full-time employees whose jobs were secure so long as they performed satisfactorily, the employees' discharge for financial or other legitimate business reasons did not offend the employment contracts as thus modified. A private employer had an essential business prerogative to adjust its workforce as market forces and business necessity required, and the layoffs in question violated no compelling public policy.

> [T]he appellants have failed to set forth specific facts showing that they were discharged for any reasons other than financial difficulties and overstaffing. The record does not suggest, for example, that financial difficulties were a pretext for discharges that were actually motivated by Houlton Regional's bad faith or retaliatory purpose.[45]

Termination and Hostile Attitude

The chief X-ray technician in *Paros v. Hoemako Hospital*[46] was dismissed because of a chronic argumentative and hostile attitude inconsistent with the performance of supervisory duties. The trial court entered a summary judgment in favor of the hospital and the administrator. On appeal, the appeals court held that the discharge was properly based on good cause and precluded recovery for breach of contract and wrongful discharge.

Termination and Improper Billing Practices

The hospital in *Jagust v. Brookhaven Memorial Association*[47] was found to have properly dismissed a staff physician

from his administrative position as director of the hospital's family practice residency program without a hearing. The hospital learned that the physician had engaged in improper billing practices by submitting bills for services that he never rendered. The physician was an employee at will as far as his administrative position was concerned. Neither the hospital's administrative procedure manual nor the employee handbook stated that the employee was subject to discharge for cause. Procedural protection was provided in the medical staff bylaws; however, the bylaws pertained to medical staff privileges and not administrative positions.

Termination and Poor Work Performance

In *Yerry v. Ulster County*,[48] a nurse's aide had been terminated from a county infirmary for misconduct. Among other things, she failed to report, in a timely manner, bumping and injuring a resident's leg, failed to feed a resident properly as ordered by the resident's physician, and, on another occasion, fed a resident food that burned the resident's mouth. The court held that eyewitness testimony and believable hearsay were sufficient to sustain the findings of the hearings officer who recommended her termination.

> As to the imposition of discipline, when petitioner's serious performance deficiencies are considered in light of her experience and the grave responsibility her work demanded in caring for helpless and dependent patients, the court found that the penalty imposed was not disproportionate to the offenses. She showed an insensitivity and a lack of ability that made her unsuitable for the work and this constituted a danger to the well-being of the infirmary's elderly residents.[49]

The plaintiff in *Silinzy v. Visiting Nurse Association*[50] brought an action claiming racial discrimination and retaliatory discharge. The court granted a motion for summary judgment by the defendant-employer. The district court held that the plaintiff failed to establish a prima facie case of racial discrimination and retaliatory discharge. The plaintiff's poor job performance was the reason for her discharge. The defendant was found to have produced ample evidence that the plaintiff was not performing her job adequately. Numerous complaints regarding her negative attitude and poor job performance, from a variety of sources, were documented.

Termination and Alcoholism

Discharge of an employee because of alcoholism is not necessarily a discriminatory practice. The hospital's discharge of a staff physician for alcoholism in *Soentgen v. Quain & Ramstad Clinic*[51] was found not to be a discriminatory practice. The physician had been discharged on a bona fide occupational qualification reasonably necessary for a physician.

Termination and Damages

An employee who is wrongly discharged may maintain a cause of action in contract or tort, or both. In a tort action for wrongful discharge, the court can award punitive damages. This remedy is not available under the law of contract.

A California Supreme Court decision that prohibits plaintiffs from seeking punitive and emotional distress damages from former employers in wrongful dismissal cases applies retroactively to thousands of cases pending in that state's courts. In *Newman v. Emerson Radio Corp.,*[52] the court, by a 4–3 vote, decided that its December 29 decision in *Foley v. Interactive Data Corp.*[53] applies to all wrongful dismissal cases pending as of January 30. The California Supreme Court held in Foley that a wrongful discharge claim asserting a breach of an implied covenant of good faith and fair dealing may give rise to contract, but not tort, damages. As a result of this ruling, punitive damages will not ordinarily be available to wrongfully discharged plaintiffs.

The Montana Supreme Court held that a Montana statute that limits the damages recoverable in wrongful discharge suits to four years' wages and benefits does not violate the state constitution.[54] According to the court, the state constitution's guarantee of full legal redress affords the plaintiff, a former nursing home administrator, only a right to judicial access to obtain remedies, not a fundamental right to full redress. The statute abolishes common-law causes of action for discharge and creates a statutory action. It is the first of its kind in the nation. Punitive damages are available only on clear and convincing evidence that the employer acted with actual malice or committed actual fraud.

EFFECTIVE HIRING PRACTICES

The best way for the human resources manager to prevent negligent hiring litigation for the employer is to become familiar with the risks and avoid hiring workers who are likely to become problematic employees. The organization should:

- Develop clear policies and procedures on hiring, disciplining, and terminating employees.

- Include appropriate language in the organization's policies and procedures reserving the right to add, delete, and/or revise the same.

- Develop an application that realistically determines an applicant's qualifications before hiring.

- Take appropriate precautions to prevent the hiring of those who might be a hazard to others.

- Review each applicant's background and past work behavior.

- Become familiar with any state laws that might be applicable when hiring an individual with a past criminal record.

- Develop a two-tiered interview system for screening applicants. (The interviews should be conducted first by an appropriately trained member of the human resources department and then by the supervisor of the service to which the applicant is applying.)

- Solicit references with the applicant's permission using a release form, and follow up with a telephone call for further information.

- Provide an employee handbook and present a job description to each new employee. (Signed documentation should be maintained in the employee's personnel folder indicating that the employee received, read, and understood the employee handbook and job description.)

- Develop constructive performance evaluations that reinforce good behavior and provide instruction in those areas needing improvement. (The performance evaluation should include a written statement regarding the employee's performance.)

- Develop a progressive disciplinary action policy.

- Provide in-service education programs for supervisors on such subjects as interviewing techniques, evaluations, and discipline. (Various colleges, universities, and consultants provide in-service education programs for employers.)

- Be mindful of the importance of developing appropriate employment contract language.

Employee References

Mark Passmore believes that a bruise on his mother was the result of an assault by Parke County's maintenance supervisor, Richardson. He sued Parke County and Richardson's former employer, Lee Alan Bryant Nursing Care Facilities, Inc. It was asserted that the former employer wrongly gave Richardson a favorable recommendation and thus should be liable for the injury.

Richardson was a maintenance worker at Lee Alan. Bratcher, Lee Alan's residential supervisor of psychiatric patients, received several reports from residents alleging misconduct between Richardson and some female residents. These were not formal complaints, but Bratcher looked into the matter and was unable to verify them. Bratcher informed the facility administrator, but never conducted a formal investigation.

Parke County sent Lee Alan a preprinted request for reference form. Lee Alan administrator Hein completed the form by indicating Richardson would be eligible for rehire. Hein checked boxes on the reference form indicating that Richardson had generally performed his job adequately. Richardson's direct supervisors stated they never heard accusations that Richardson was ever sexually involved with a Lee Alan resident while he was employed. Parke County subsequently closed and reopened as Parke County Residential Care Center.

The Parke Circuit Court granted summary judgment in favor of Lee Alan. The court of appeals affirmed, stating that Indiana does not recognize conscious or negligent misrepresentation.

Passmore asked the court to hold that a regulated nursing facility owes a duty to third persons not to misrepresent material facts that describe qualifications and character of a former employee. The facts, however, before the trial court on summary judgment did not reflect that Lee Alan had any substantial information indicating that Richardson committed sexual misconduct with residents at Lee Alan when Hein completed the reference form. Bratcher had been unable to substantiate what she had heard about Richardson. This may

have constituted negligence, but could not be considered purposeful misrepresentation.

Declaring employers liable for negligence in providing employment references will lead universally to employer reluctance to provide any information other than name, rank, and serial number. A legal policy that discourages providing assessments to subsequent employers will not make for safer nursing homes. It was appropriate to grant judgment to Lee Alan on Passmore's claim of negligent misrepresentation.[55]

CLEAR COMMUNICATIONS

Employers must communicate clearly to prospective employees that their employment is at will and can be terminated at any time by either the employer or the employee. During the course of employment, handbooks and personnel manuals must provide fair and unambiguous standards for employee discipline and termination.

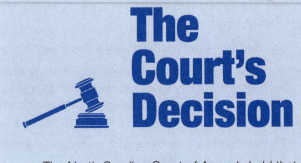

The Court's Decision

The North Carolina Court of Appeals held that the nurse stated a claim for wrongful discharge in violation of public policy. Termination for fulfilling one's responsibilities as a practicing nurse in North Carolina violates state public policy, and, in this case, was a factual question for the jury to decide. Although there may be a right to terminate at-will employment for no reason, or for an arbitrary or irrational reason, there can be no right to terminate such employment for an unlawful reason or purpose that contravenes public policy.

CHAPTER REVIEW

1. *Employment at will* is a doctrine by which employment can be terminated at any time by either the employee or employer. Exceptions to this doctrine include employment contracts, as well as issues involving public policy.
2. *Public policy* prohibits the termination of an employee based on factors such as disability, age, race, color, religion, sex, national origin, pregnancy, filing safety violation complaints with various agencies, or membership in a union. Public policy also can result from judicial decisions that address issues not covered by statutes, rules, and regulations.
3. A *whistle-blower* is one who reveals wrongdoing in the organization to a public entity or someone in authority. This often occurs when one believes that the public interest overrides the interest of the organization and can involve illegal or fraudulent activities.
4. Employees who believe that they have suffered *retaliatory discharge* are entitled to bring legal action against their former employer. The burden of proof, however, lies with the discharged employee.
5. The fact that an employment contract is terminable at will does not, in all cases, allow an employer the absolute right to terminate the contract. Many bad-faith and inexplicable terminations are subject to the scrutiny of the courts.

6. Employers are required to deal fairly with terminated employees who file for unemployment benefits.
7. The denial of a right that is alleged to belong to a person is a *disclaimer.*
8. Termination of employees for financial or other legitimate business reasons does not constitute a breach of employment contract.
9. Employers can reduce exposure to liability for wrongful discharge by establishing and maintaining effective hiring practices.

REVIEW QUESTIONS

1. Discuss the employment at-will doctrine.
2. Is the employment-at-will doctrine appropriate in today's society? Discuss your answer.
3. What are the pros and cons of the employment-at-will doctrine?
4. What are the public policy exceptions to the employment-at-will doctrine?
5. Discuss what questions an employer (supervisor) should consider before terminating an employee.
6. Discuss what actions an employer can take in order to help reduce the necessity for discharging an employee.

NOTES

1. *Deerman v. Beverly Cal. Corp.,* 518 S.E.2d 804 (N.C. App. 1999).
2. 328 S.E.2d 818 (N.C. Ct. App. 1985).
3. 44 A.L.R. 4th 1136 (1986).
4. *Sides v. Duke Hosp.,* 328 S.E.2d 818 (N.C. Ct. App. 1985).
5. *Pierce v. Ortho Pharm. Corp.,* 417 A.2d 505, 509 (N.J. 1980).
6. *Palmateer v. International Harvester Co.,* 421 N.E.2d 876, 878 (Ill. 1981).
7. *Gantt v. Sentry Ins.,* 824 P.2d 680, 687–688 (Cal. 1992).
8. *Delaney v. Taco Time Int'l,* 681 P.2d 114 (Or. 1984). This case involved an employer found liable by the Oregon Supreme Court for the wrongful discharge of an at-will employee who was discharged for fulfilling a societal obligation because he refused to sign a false and arguably tortious statement that cast aspersions on the work habits and moral behavior of a former employee.
9. 684 P.2d 21 (Or. Ct. App. 1984).
10. *Id.* at 24.
11. *Whistleblowing,* U.S. Office of Special Counsel, http://www.osc.gov/documents/pubs/post_wb.htm
12. Annotation, 99 A.L.R. Fed. 775.
13. *HCA Health Services of Florida, Inc. v. Hillman,* No. 2D03-1534 (Fla. Dist. Ct. App. 2004).
14. 838 F.2d 1155 (11th Cir. 1988).
15. 385 N.W.2d 99 (N.D. 1986).
16. Conn. Gen. Stat. Ann. § 31-51m(a) (West 1987).
17. Me. Rev. Stat. Ann. 26, §§ 831–840 (West 1987).
18. Mich. Comp. Laws Ann. §§ 15.361-369 (West 1981).
19. Mont. Code Ann. § 39-2-901 (1987).
20. *Pierce v. Ortho Pharm. Corp.,* 417 A.2d 505, 509 (N.J. 1980).
21. 215 Cal. Rptr. 860 (Cal. Ct. App. 1985).
22. *Id.* at 865.
23. 518 N.E.2d 471 (Ill. App. Ct. 1988).
24. 760 F. Supp. 1575 (D.C. Ga. 1991).
25. 168 Cal. Rptr. 722 (Cal. Ct. App. 1980).
26. 171 Cal. Rptr. 917 (Cal. Ct. App. 1981).
27. 398 N.W.2d 327 (Mich. 1986).
28. 358 N.W.2d 96 (Minn. Ct. App. 1984).
29. *Id.* at 98.
30. *Perkins v. Commissioner of Labor,* 16 A.D.3d 756, 790 N.Y.S.2d 313 (N.Y. 2005).
31. 325 S.E.2d 651 (N.C. Ct. App. 1985).
32. *Id.* at 652.
33. *Love v. Heritage House Convalescent Ctr.,* 463 N.E.2d 478 (Ind. Ct. App. 1983).
34. 371 N.W.2d 121 (Neb. 1985).
35. H. H. Perritt, Employee Dismissal Law and Practice 354 (1984).
36. 508 N.Y.S.2d 802 (N.Y. App. Div. 1986).
37. No. 89-CA-2272-MR (Ky. Ct. App. Mar. 22, 1991).
38. 428 N.W.2d 574 (Minn. Ct. App. 1988).
39. *Id.* at 577.
40. 413 N.W.2d 146 (Minn. Ct. App. 1987).
41. *Id.* at 147.
42. 663 P.2d 958 (Alaska 1983).
43. 415 A.2d 139 (Pa. Commw. Ct. 1980).
44. 537 A.2d 1137 (Me. 1987).
45. *Id.* at 1138.
46. 681 P.2d 918 (Ariz. Ct. App. 1984).
47. 541 N.Y.S.2d 41 (N.Y. Ct. App. Div. 1989).
48. 512 N.Y.S.2d 592 (N.Y. App. Div. 1987).
49. *Id.* at 593.
50. 777 F. Supp. 1484 (E.D. Mo. 1991).
51. 467 N.W.2d 73 (N.D. 1991).
52. 772 P.2d 1059 (Cal. 1989).
53. 765 P.2d 373 (Cal. 1988).
54. *Meech v. Hillhaven W., Inc.,* 776 P.2d 488 (Mont. 1989).
55. *Passmore v. Multi-Management Svcs., Inc.,* 810 N.E.2d 1022 (Ind. 2004).

CHAPTER 21

Managed Care and Organizational Restructuring

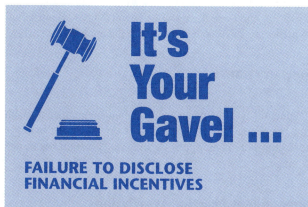

It's Your Gavel ...

FAILURE TO DISCLOSE FINANCIAL INCENTIVES

The patient in *Shea v. Esensten* died after suffering a heart attack. Although the patient had recently visited his primary-care physician and presented symptoms of cardiac problems, including a family history of cardiac trouble, the physician did not refer the patient to a cardiologist. The patient's widow sued the HMO for failing to disclose the financial incentive system it provided to its physicians to minimize referrals to specialists.[1]

WHAT IS YOUR VERDICT?

Health care has come a long way from the days when, answering a knock at the front door, you were met by a genuine, black leather bag–carrying, independent-practicing family physician. The physician knew you and every member of your family and, most likely, delivered you, as well as your mother and father. The only charge for a home visit may have been your mother's home-baked apple pie. This scene has changed dramatically over the years. The health care setting is a bombardment of mergers, buyouts, upsizing and downsizing, health maintenance organizations (HMOs), cost controls, regulations, and regulators monitoring regulators.

Managed care organizations (MCOs) represent a major shift away from the domination of the fee-for-service system toward networks of providers supplying a full range of services. Managed care is the process of structuring or restructuring the health care system in terms of financing, purchasing, delivering, measuring, and documenting a broad range of health care services and products. Managed care is nothing new to the U.S. health care delivery system; it has been around in some form for decades.

The relationships that are being restructured are those among employers, physicians, a wide variety of health care organizations, payers, and consumers. The two major and objected-to constraints of MCOs are their (1) limitations on the choice of providers by the consumer and (2) requirements for prior authorization in order to obtain services. As reviewed in this chapter, managed care comes in a variety of packages.

COMMON MODELS OF MANAGED CARE ORGANIZATIONS

There are a wide variety of managed care models that integrate financing and management with the delivery of health care services to an enrolled population. The following sections describe some of the common models.

Health Maintenance Organizations

HMOs are organized health care systems that are responsible for both the financing and the delivery of a broad range of comprehensive health services to an enrolled population. They are the most highly regulated form of MCOs. HMOs act both as insurer and provider of health care services. They charge employers a fixed premium for each subscriber. An independent practice association (IPA)-model HMO provides medical care to its subscribers through contracts it establishes with independent physicians. In a staff-model HMO, the physicians would normally be full-time employees of the HMO. Individuals who subscribe to an HMO are often limited to the panel of physicians who have contracted with the HMO to provide services to its subscribers.

Preferred Provider Organizations

Preferred provider organizations (PPOs) are entities through which employer health benefit plans and health insurance carriers contract to purchase health care services for covered beneficiaries from a selected group of participating providers. Most states have specific PPO laws that directly regulate such entities. Common characteristics of PPOs include

- select provider panel
- negotiated payment rates
- rapid payment terms
- utilization management (programs to control the utilization and cost)
- consumer choice (allow covered beneficiaries to use non-PPO providers for an additional out-of-pocket charge [point-of-service option])

In PPOs, a payer, such as an insurance company, provides incentives to its enrollees to obtain medical care from a panel of providers with whom the payer has contracted a discounted rate.

Exclusive Provider Organizations

Exclusive provider organizations (EPOs) limit their beneficiaries to participating providers for any health care services. EPOs use a gatekeeper approach to authorize nonprimary care services. The primary difference between an HMO and an EPO is that the former is regulated under HMO laws and regulations, whereas the latter is regulated under insurance laws and regulations. Characteristics of EPOs include:

- Primary care physicians are reimbursed through capitation payments or other performance-based reimbursement methods.
- Primary care physicians act as gatekeepers.

Point-of-Service Plans

Point-of-service (POS) plans use primary care physicians as gatekeepers to coordinate and control medical care. Subscribers covered under POS plans may decide whether to use HMO benefits or indemnity-style benefits for each instance of care. In other words, the member is allowed to make a coverage choice at the POS. A patient who chooses a provider outside the plan is responsible for higher copayments.

Experience-Rated HMOs

Under experience-rated benefit options, an HMO receives monthly premium payments much as it would under traditional premium-based plans. Typically, to arrive at a final premium rate, there is a settlement process in which the employer is credited with some portion, or all of the actual utilization and cost of its group. Then refunds or additional payments are calculated and made to the appropriate party.

Specialty HMOs

Specialty HMOs provide limited components of health care coverage. Dental HMOs, for example, have become more common as an option to indemnity dental insurance coverage.

Independent Practice Associations

An independent practice association (IPA) is a legal entity composed of physicians organized for the purpose of negotiating contracts to provide physician services. For example, an IPA might contract with an HMO or a physician-hospital organization (PHO). The physicians maintain their own practices and do not share services, such as claims, billing, scheduling, accounting, and so forth.

Group Practice

A physician group that has only one or a small number of service delivery locations is a group practice. It is completely integrated economically, sharing costs and revenues. Group practices often are either specialty or primary-care dominated.

Group Practice Without Walls

A group practice without walls is a physician organization formed for the purpose of sharing some administrative and management costs while continuing to practice at their own locations rather than at a centralized location.

Physician Hospital Organizations

A PHO is a legal entity consisting of a joint venture of physicians and a hospital. It is formed to facilitate managed care contracting, to improve cost management and services, and to create new health care resources in the community.

Medical Foundations

In a medical foundation, the foundation employs or contracts with physicians to provide care to the foundation's patients.

Management Service Organizations

A management service organization (MSO) is an entity that provides administrative and management services to physicians. The organization performs services, such as practice management, marketing, managed care contracting, accounting, billing, and personnel management. The MSO can be hospital affiliated, a hospital-physician joint venture, physician owned, or investor owned.

Vertically Integrated Delivery System

A vertically integrated delivery system (IDS) is any organization or group of affiliated organizations that provides physician and hospital services to patients. The goal of hospital-physician integration is to provide a full range of services to patients. A vertically IDS achieves this goal, providing services ranging from primary outpatient care to tertiary inpatient care. More elaborate systems provide additional services, such as home health care, long-term care, rehabilitation, and mental health care.

HORIZONTAL CONSOLIDATIONS

A horizontal merger involves similar or identical businesses at the same level of the market. There is no single qualitative or quantitative factor from which it can be determined whether such a group merger is permissible. Recognizing a congressional intent to preserve competition by preventing undue market concentration, the courts have focused primarily on the possibility that consolidation will substantially lessen competition.

FEDERALLY QUALIFIED HMOs

Many HMOs are federally qualified. Federal qualification, which is entirely voluntary, requires HMOs to meet federal standards for legal and organizational status, financial viability, marketing, and health service delivery systems, as delineated in the federal HMO act and its implementing regulations. The disadvantage of federal qualification—beyond the fees involved—is that a federally qualified HMO has less flexibility in its benefits package and in developing premium rates.

The standards for federal qualification were introduced in 1973, when Congress enacted Title XIII of the Public Health Service Act, commonly known as the HMO Act.[2] This law was intended to foster the growth of HMOs, which were considered to be a cost-effective method of health care delivery.

The law was amended in 1976 to ease some of the restrictions on open enrollment, community rating, and medical staffing. It was amended again in 1978 on financial disclosure and in 1981 for solvency protection. In 1986, certain HMO grant and loan programs were abolished.[3]

The most dramatic amendments, however, occurred in 1988. They permitted federally qualified HMOs to provide up to 10 percent of their physician services through non-HMO–affiliated physicians and authorized reasonable deductibles for those services. They also repealed the dual choice requirement, effective in 1995; broadened the definition of restrictive state laws; required disclosure of rate-making methods and data; addressed nondiscrimination in the financing of employee plans; deleted the requirement that one third of the policy-making body be composed of HMO members; and repealed the requirement that the policy-making body include equitable representation from underserved communities.

Federally qualified HMOs must provide or arrange for basic health services for their members as needed and without limitation as to time, cost, frequency, extent, or kind of services actually provided. Basic health services include

- physician services, including consultant and referral services by a physician

- inpatient and outpatient services, including short-term rehabilitation services and physical therapy

- medically necessary emergency health services

- 20 outpatient visits per member per year for short-term, evaluative, or crisis intervention mental health services

- medical treatment and referral services

- diagnostic laboratory and diagnostic and therapeutic radiology services

- home health services
- preventive health services, including immunizations and well-child care from birth

STATE LAWS

Most states have enacted comprehensive HMO laws which are often based on the National Association of Insurance Commissioners' Model HMO Act. State laws generally specify what type of entities can apply for a certificate of authority to operate an HMO. Typically, the state insurance department is the primary regulatory body.

Generally, state HMO laws require that an application for a certificate of authority be accompanied by a description of the proposed marketing plan that the regulator must approve. HMO laws generally specify that a schedule of charges and amendments must be filed and approved by the commissioner.

The majority of state HMO laws require that the provision of basic health services include emergency care, inpatient care, physician care, and outpatient care. State HMO laws contain several provisions designed to protect enrollees in the event that the HMO becomes insolvent. These include deposit, capital, reserve, and net worth requirements. State laws pertaining to HMOs generally require that

- The HMO cannot cancel or refuse to renew an enrollee solely because of the individual's health.

- If an individual terminates employment or membership in a group, that person must be permitted to convert to a direct-payment basis.

- Grievance procedures must be in place.

State HMO laws usually condition issuance of a certificate of authority on the submission and approval of a quality assurance program.

CASE MANAGEMENT FIRMS

Case management firms assist employers and insurers in managing catastrophic cases. They identify cases that will become catastrophic, negotiate services and reimbursement with providers who can treat the patient's condition, develop a treatment protocol for the patient, and monitor the treatment.

THIRD-PARTY ADMINISTRATORS

A third-party administrator (TPA) is a firm that provides services for employers and associations that have group insurance policies. The TPA acts as a liaison between the employer and the insurer. The TPA performs administrative activities, such as claims processing, certifying eligibility, and a preparation of reports required by the staff.

UTILIZATION REVIEW

Utilization review (UR) is a process whereby a third-party payer evaluates the medical necessity of a course of treatment. Managed care organizations use a utilization review process to compare a patient's request for care with what treatment doctors commonly practice in similar medical circumstances. Medical care is considered necessary when it is needed to prevent, diagnose, and treat a patient's medical condition. Generally, UR is performed prospectively, concurrently, or retrospectively.

- *Prospective review:* The payer determines whether to pay for treatment before the treatment is initiated. If the review reveals that the treatment is not medically necessary, the payer then indicates its decision not to pay for the medical care.

- *Concurrent review:* This review is performed during the course of treatment. Concurrent review entails monitoring whether medical care continues to be appropriate and necessary. If it is not, the payer will discontinue payment for additional care.

- *Retrospective review:* This type of review is performed after treatment has been completed. If the review indicates that medical care was not necessary, the insurer can deny the claim.

Most insurance companies and MCOs rely on prospective and concurrent UR to determine if care is necessary, as well as what level of care is appropriate. Utilization review has become an accepted and essential part of cost containment.

Case management is an increasingly important aspect of utilization management. It involves identifying at an early stage those patients who can be treated more cost effectively in an alternative setting or at a lower level of care without negatively affecting the quality of care. Case management usually is employed in catastrophic or high-cost cases.

Utilization Management Firms

Utilization management firms perform utilization management activities for managed care entities, insurers, or employers. Mental health and dental care are two common types of such firms. In recent years, the regulation of utilization by private review agents or utilization review organizations (UROs) has increased dramatically.

Just as health care entities have a corporate duty to select and monitor physicians carefully, they also have a duty to carefully select the URO with which they contract. That duty entails investigating the URO before contracting with it to ensure that its procedures are adequate and its personnel are qualified to perform UR activities.

Negligent UR Decisions

MCOs that perform UR may be found liable for undesirable patient outcomes because of defects or failures in the UR process or because of a negligent UR decision. The first reported case involving liability for UR was *Wickline v. State of California.*[4] In that case, the court stated that a third-party payer of health care services can be held legally accountable when medically inappropriate decisions result from defects in the design or implementation of cost-containment mechanisms. Liability in the UR process can arise from several sources, including failure to gather information adequately before making a decision as to medical necessity, failure to initiate a meaningful dialogue between UR personnel and the treating physician, failure to inform members of their right to appeal an adverse UR decision, and failure to issue a timely UR decision.

LIABILITY FOR NONPARTICIPATING PHYSICIANS

MCOs may be liable for the medical malpractice of non-employee participating physicians under an ostensible or apparent agency theory if (1) the patient reasonably views the entity rather than the individual physician as the source of care, and (2) the entity engages in conduct that leads the patient reasonably to believe that the source of care is the entity or that the physician is an employee of the entity.

The doctrine of corporate negligence clearly applies to staff-model HMOs in which the HMO employs the physicians and provides the facility within which they offer care. If an HMO employs physicians, such as in a staff-model HMO, the HMO can be held liable for the negligence of its employees under the doctrine of respondeat superior.

EMPLOYEE RETIREMENT INCOME SECURITY ACT

Congress enacted the Employee Retirement Income Security Act of 1974 (ERISA). It was designed to ensure that employee welfare and benefit plans conform to a uniform body of benefits law. ERISA sets minimum standards for most voluntarily established pension and health plans in private industry to provide protection for individuals in these plans. ERISA requires plans to provide participants with plan information including important information about plan features and funding; provides fiduciary responsibilities for those who manage and control plan assets; requires plans to establish a grievance and appeals process for participants to get benefits from their plans; and gives participants the right to sue for benefits and breaches of fiduciary duty.

The law does not, however, regulate the contents of the welfare benefit plans. For example, it does not mandate that specific benefits be provided to beneficiaries. To qualify as an employee benefit plan, the plan must be maintained by an employer or employee organization for the benefit of its employees. ERISA requires that every plan (1) describe procedures for the allocation of responsibilities for its operation and administration and (2) specify the basis on which payments are made to and from the plan.

The Consolidated Omnibus Budget Reconciliation Act (COBRA) included an amendment that expanded benefits, providing some workers and their families with the right to continue their health coverage for a limited time under certain circumstances, such as the loss of a job. Another amendment to ERISA is contained in the Health Insurance Portability and Accountability Act (HIPAA), which provides protection for employees and their families who have preexisting medical conditions or might otherwise suffer discrimination in health coverage based on factors that relate to an individual's health. In general, ERISA does not cover group health plans established or maintained by governmental entities, churches for their employees, or plans that are maintained solely to comply with applicable workers compensation, unemployment, or disability laws.

Although ERISA preempts state law affecting employee benefit plans, the following case illustrates that there are circumstances under which ERISA will not preempt state law. Ms. Moran in *Rush Prudential HMO, Inc. v. Moran*[5] sought treatment from Dr. LaMarre, her primary physician under her HMO plan (Rush Prudential HMO, Inc.), because of numbness, pain, and decreased mobility in her right shoulder. During a series of physiotherapy treatments under LaMarre, Moran obtained the name of an out-of-network physician, Dr. Terzis, and submitted a request to Rush for a referral to consult with this physician. Her request was denied. Moran had the consult anyway and was diagnosed with plexopathy and thoriac outlet syndrome. Terzis recommended a more involved and expensive surgery. Two plan physicians recommended a less-complicated surgery. LaMarre formally asked Rush to approve Terzis' recommended surgery. Rush denied approval of the surgery. Moran made a written demand to Rush seeking its compliance with the Illinois Health Maintenance Organization Act, Section 4-10, which requires HMOs to provide an independent physician review when a patient's primary care physician disagrees with an HMO about the medical necessity of a proposed treatment. Moran eventually decided to undergo the surgery with Terzis at her own expense. She later submitted the bill to Rush and sought a court order requiring Rush to comply with Section 4-10. Rush moved the case to a federal court citing the statute's conflict with ERISA.

The district court agreed with Rush that ERISA preempted Moran's claims and granted summary judgment to Rush. The case eventually reached the U.S. Supreme Court, which upheld Section 4-10 of the Illinois HMO Act which provides a mechanism whereby insured patients can enforce their rights under insurance plans.

REDUCING EXPOSURE TO LIABILITY

Employers, managed care entities, and providers can reduce liability exposure by complying with all formalities, considering contracting through the plan itself, and defining clearly discretionary responsibilities. Employers should seek and employ competent advisers. A managed contract should be developed between the employer and the selected fiduciary. The contract should ensure that

- The fiduciary is responsible for monitoring its discretionary authority.

- The fiduciary is committed to supplying the employer with data on the various aspects of its performance.

- Proper indemnities are negotiated on behalf of the employer and its employees.

- Hold-harmless clauses are provided for employees for payment for services rendered.

- Financial disclosures are made as appropriate.

- Sufficient reinsurance, fiduciary insurance, and liability insurance are maintained, and proof is supplied to the employer.

- Confidentiality agreements are established and observed.

- Quality-assurance programs are maintained.

- Claims and appeal procedures are available and assurances are given as to the program's operation and improvement.

- A description of the fiduciary's utilization control mechanism, methods for preadmission review of elective procedures, continuous stay review procedures, systems for retrospective review of ancillary services provided, retrospective review of surgical procedures, quality assurance programs, and mechanisms for denial of coverage or charges, as well as the method used for dispute resolution is provided.

HEALTH CARE QUALITY IMPROVEMENT ACT OF 1986

The Health Care Quality Improvement Act of 1986 (HCQIA) was enacted in part as a response to numerous antitrust suits against participants in peer-review and credentialing activities. Congress passed the act to encourage continued participation in these activities. The purpose of the HCQIA is to provide those persons giving information to professional review bodies and those assisting in review activities limited immunity from damages that may arise as a result of adverse decisions that affect a physician's medical staff privileges. The immunity does not extend to civil rights litigation or suits filed by the United States or an attorney general of a state.

In 1989, the Ethics in Patient Referral Act (frequently referred to as the Stark bill for its author, Rep. Fortney [Pete] Stark [D-Cal.]) was enacted as part of the Omnibus Budget Reconciliation Act of 1989. Effective January 1, 1992, the act prohibits physicians who have ownership interest or compensation arrangements with a clinical laboratory from referring Medicare patients to that laboratory. The law also requires all Medicare providers to report the names and provider numbers of all physicians or their immediate relatives with ownership interests in the provider entity prior to October 1, 1991. Failure to comply with the disclosure requirements exposes providers to a civil monetary penalty of up to $10,000 per day.

MANAGED CARE AND LEGAL ACTIONS

The following cases describe but a few of the many legal actions involving managed care.

Insurer and Tort-Feasor

The plaintiff in *Karsten v. Kaiser Foundation Health Plan*[6] brought a legal action against her HMO for malpractice. The plaintiff alleged that Kaiser's negligent care caused her to deliver a premature stillborn fetus. Although Kaiser denied any wrongdoing, the jury awarded the plaintiff $210,000 in damages. At trial, the plaintiff introduced hospital bills incurred as a result of the incident in question. Kaiser had paid these bills prior to trial. Although Kaiser agreed that, based on its contract with the plaintiff, it was required to pay these bills regardless of fault, Kaiser objected to the medical bills as part of the plaintiff's compensatory damages because they had already been paid by Kaiser.

The issue under Virginia law was: Does the collateral source rule allow the plaintiff to recover compensatory damages for medical bills previously satisfied by her HMO?

The U.S. District Court held that, under Virginia law, the collateral source rule allows a member to receive from the HMO compensatory damages for medical bills that the HMO previously paid under the HMO contract, when the HMO was also liable to the plaintiff as a tort-feasor. The court focused on the nature of each payment Kaiser was being asked to make. The first payment made by Kaiser was for the plaintiff's medical bills. The defendant made this payment in its capacity as the plaintiff's insurer. The defendant was then being asked to pay these same medical expenses as compensatory damages. Even though the defendant was being asked to pay the same damages twice, it is patent that the nature of the two payments is different.

Open Enrollment

Federal HMO regulations require federally qualified HMOs to hold an open enrollment period of not less than 30 days per year, during which the HMO must accept individual applicants for coverage regardless of their health status. Not all state HMO laws require open enrollment periods.

Emergency Care

HMOs can refuse benefit coverage to patients if they determine retrospectively that a patient's condition did not require emergency department care. Of course, hindsight is 20/20. Determining whether one's chest pains are because of diet or a coronary condition requires expensive testing. To refuse a patient care before determining the etiology of a patient's condition could be financially disastrous to an organization. In addition, federal law prohibits hospital emergency departments from turning away patients seeking emergency care. Unfortunately, retrospective denial places the burden on the provider to seek reimbursement from the patient if the insurer denies the charges.

Benefit Denials

The California Supreme Court has ruled that insurers must inform beneficiaries of their right to contest a benefit denial. The court, in *Davis v. Blue Cross of N. California*,[7] held that the insurer breached its duty of good faith and fair dealing by failing to adequately apprise an insured of his rights under the policy's arbitration clause.

The insured in *Katskee v. Blue Cross/Blue Shield*[8] brought action against the health insurer for breach of contract. In January 1990, on recommendation of her gynecologist, Dr. Roffman, the appellant consulted with Dr. Lynch regarding her family's history of breast and ovarian cancer, and particularly her health in relation to such a history. After examining the appellant and investigating her family's medical history, Lynch diagnosed her as suffering from a genetic condition known as breast-ovarian carcinoma syndrome. Lynch then recommended that the appellant have a total abdominal hysterectomy and bilateral salpingo-oophorectomy. Roffman concurred with Lynch's diagnosis and agreed that

the recommended surgery was the most medically appropriate treatment available.

Initially, Blue Cross/Blue Shield sent a letter to the appellant and indicated that it might pay for the surgery. Two weeks before surgery, Dr. Mason, the chief medical officer for Blue Cross/Blue Shield, wrote to the appellant and stated that Blue Cross/Blue Shield would not cover the cost of the surgery. Nonetheless, the appellant had the surgery. She filed an action for breach of contract, seeking to recover $6,022.57 in costs associated with the surgery. Blue Cross/Blue Shield filed a motion for summary judgment. The district court granted the motion. It found that there was no genuine issue of material fact and that the policy did not cover the appellant's surgery. Specifically, the court stated that

1. The appellant did not suffer from cancer, and although her high-risk condition warranted the surgery, it was not covered by the policy.

2. The appellant did not have a bodily illness or disease that was covered by the policy.

3. Under the terms of the policy, Blue Cross/Blue Shield reserved the right to determine what is medically necessary.

The appellant filed a notice of appeal to the Nebraska Court of Appeals contending that the district court erred in finding that no genuine issue of material fact existed and in granting summary judgment in favor of appellee. Blue Cross/Blue Shield denied coverage because it concluded that appellant's condition did not constitute an illness, and thus the treatment she received was not medically necessary.

An insurance policy is to be construed, as any other contract, to give effect to the parties' intentions at the time the contract was made. The issue was whether the insured's breast-ovarian carcinoma syndrome was an illness, defined as a bodily disorder or disease within meaning of the health insurance policy.

The Nebraska Supreme Court held that the insured's breast-ovarian carcinoma syndrome was an illness within meaning of the health insurance policy, notwithstanding the insurer's contention that the syndrome was merely predisposition to cancer. The court found that whether a policy is ambiguous is a matter of law for the court to determine. A general principle of construction, which the courts apply to ambiguous insurance policies, holds that an ambiguous policy will be construed in favor of the insured. The language used in the policy at issue in the present case was not reasonably susceptible to differing interpretations, and thus not ambiguous. The issue then becomes whether appellant's condition— breast-ovarian carcinoma syndrome—constituted an illness.

Blue Cross/Blue Shield argued that the appellant did not suffer from an illness because she did not have cancer. Blue Cross/Blue Shield characterized the appellant's condition only as a predisposition to an illness. The record on summary judgment included the depositions of Lynch, Roffman, and Mason. According to Lynch's testimony, some forms of cancer occur on a hereditary basis. Breast and ovarian cancer are such forms of cancer. Women diagnosed with the syndrome have at least a 50 percent chance of developing breast and/or ovarian cancer, whereas unaffected women have only a 1.4 percent risk of developing breast or ovarian cancer. Generally, by the time ovarian cancer is capable of being detected, it has already developed to an advanced stage, making treatment relatively unsuccessful. Lynch and Roffman agreed that the standard of care for treating women with breast-ovarian carcinoma syndrome ordinarily involves surveillance methods. However, for women at an inordinately high risk for ovarian cancer, such as the appellant, the standard of care may require radical surgery that involves the removal of the uterus, ovaries, and fallopian tubes. Blue Cross/Blue Shield did not provide any evidence disputing the premise that the origin of this condition is in the genetic makeup of the individual and that in its natural development it is likely to produce devastating results.

The medical evidence regarding the nature of breast-ovarian carcinoma syndrome persuaded the court that the appellant suffered from a bodily disorder or disease and, thus, suffered from an illness as defined by the insurance policy. Blue Cross/Blue Shield was, therefore, not entitled to judgment as a matter of law.

False and Misleading Statements

The plaintiff in *Drolet v. Healthsource, Inc.*[9] was a beneficiary of a health care plan administered by her employer, the Mitre Corporation. The plaintiff brought a class-action complaint alleging that Healthsource New Hampshire, Inc., and its parent corporation, Healthsource, Inc., are liable under ERISA for several materially false and misleading statements that Healthsource New Hampshire, Inc. allegedly made to the plan's beneficiaries.

The benefits provided by the plan require a member to choose a primary-care physician to be responsible for providing the member with routine medical care and coordinating the member's specialty care referrals. In defining the term primary-care physician, the agreement emphasized that the physician has a contractual relationship with Healthsource, which does not interfere with the exercise of the physician's independent medical judgment. The plaintiff contended that the physician-patient relationship is compromised by various undisclosed financial incentives that are provided to the plan's physicians to reduce expenditures on specialty care services. Among these incentives, the plaintiff alleged, are referral funds that permit a physician to earn up to 33 percent in additional income by minimizing the use of specialty services such as diagnostic tests, referrals, and hospitalizations. The plaintiff argued that the company breached the fiduciary duty it allegedly owed to Mitre plan's participants and beneficiaries under ERISA.

The duty to disclose material information is the core of a fiduciary's responsibility. Therefore, if Healthsource New Hampshire made material misrepresentations in the group subscriber agreement and other plan documents, it can be enjoined under ERISA to prevent further breaches of its fiduciary duty. Regulations do not authorize Healthsource New Hampshire, as a fiduciary, from making misrepresentations to beneficiaries.

Price Fixing

Price fixing is considered a per se violation of the antitrust laws. Price fixing occurs when two or more competitors come together to decide on a price that will be charged for services or goods. The per se rule applies to restraints in trade that are so inimical to competition and so unjustified that they are presumed to be unreasonable and, therefore, are illegal. Examinations of per se violations include price fixing, horizontal market allocation, tying, and group boycotts.

The provider-controlled MCO is at significant antitrust risk when setting provider reimbursement and bargaining with payers. There is a danger that provider-controlled organizations will be viewed as a horizontal conspiracy between competitors that acts as a mechanism for price fixing.

Even without organizational control, providers may have practical control of the plan. The Federal Trade Commission (FTC) has identified the following factors as indicative of control[10]:

- power to vote on plan reimbursement or coverage proposals

- representation on, or selection of, key plan policy-making committees

- delegated authority, including veto or approval power over plan policies

- power to appoint or approve plan management

- financing of plan operations

- interlocking directors, officers, or executives

- absence of other strong interest groups in the governing body

One of the leading cases involving price fixing is *Maricopa County Medical Society v. Arizona University,*[11] a U.S. Supreme Court case that involved the exercise of provider control over the level of physician reimbursement. Because the physicians had no financial stake in the success of the plan, the Supreme Court found that the maximum fee schedule set by the physicians constituted illegal price fixing.

In *Maine v. Alliance Healthcare, Inc.,*[12] an entity composed of four hospitals and their affiliated physician groups was formed to contract with managed care plans. The state attorney general charged that the entity was engaged in price fixing because it allegedly forced HMOs to pay physicians on a fee-for-service basis instead of a capitation basis. In the resulting consent decree, the entity agreed to cease collectively negotiating prices for its members. In *Hassan v. Independent Practice Assoc.*, the court found that a capitated IPA arrangement was appropriate when[13]:

- Physicians shared the risk of loss through acceptance of capitation payments.

- The plan did not dictate what participating physicians could charge to nonplan patients, including those belonging to competing health carriers.

- The plan constituted a new product, namely, guaranteed comprehensive physician services, for a prepaid premium different from fee-for-services.

In this context, the court held that the maximum reimbursement rates established by the IPA were lawful as a necessary part of the joint venture's integration of resources.

Market Power

Whenever an MCO possesses significant market power or deals with a group that has significant market power, antitrust implications should be considered. To determine market power, it is necessary first to identify the market in which the entity exercises power. For antitrust purposes, the relevant market has two components: (1) a product component and (2) a geographic component.

Product Market

The relevant product market involves the product or service at issue and all substantially acceptable substitutes for it. The relevant product market for MCOs is the market for health care financing. Broadly defined, this market includes traditional insurers, HMOs, PPOs, IPAs, and so on, and their subscriber members.

Market power results from the ability to cut back the market's total supply and then raise prices because of consumer demand for the product. Generally, the market in health care financing is competitive because the customers can switch companies readily, new suppliers can enter the market quickly, and existing suppliers can expand their sales rapidly.

Geographic Market

The relevant geographic market is the market area in which the seller operates, and to which the purchaser can practically turn for supplies. The primary factors that courts have examined to determine the geographic scope of the market for hospital services are

- patient flow statistics

- location of physicians who admit patients

- determinations of health planners

- public perception

Provider Exclusion

Providers who are excluded from managed care systems may bring group boycott charges alleging that the exclusion constitutes an illegal restraint of trade. Traditionally, group boycotts have been considered inherently anticompetitive and, therefore, characterized as per se violations of the Sherman Act.[14] In *Northwest Wholesale Stationers, Inc. v. Pacific Stationery and Printing Co.*, the U.S. Supreme Court identified three characteristics as indicative of per se illegal boycotts[15]:

1. The boycott cuts off access to a supply, facility, or market necessary to enable the victim firm to compete.

2. The defendant possesses a dominant market position.

3. The practices are not justified by plausible arguments as enhancing overall efficiency or competition.

Essentially, competitors who agree with each other not to deal with a supplier or distributor if it continues to serve a competitor whom they seek to injure is in violation of the Sherman Act.

Antitrust and Market Share

Competition between HMOs can bring about market share actions in antitrust. For example, in *U.S. Healthcare, Inc. v. Healthsource, Inc.*,[16] several HMOs—U.S. Healthcare, Inc., U.S. Healthcare of Massachusetts, Inc., and U.S. Healthcare of New Hampshire, Inc. (collectively U.S. Healthcare)— brought an action against Healthsource, Inc. (also an HMO) alleging that an exclusive dealing clause in Healthsource's service agreements with physicians violated antitrust laws. Both sides are engaged in providing medical services through HMOs in New Hampshire.

Healthsource, founded in 1985, an IPA-model HMO, was the first HMO established in New Hampshire. Aware that other HMOs were considering marketing in New Hampshire, Healthsource, in order to maintain its market share, offered its panel of physicians greater compensation if they agreed to an exclusive contract. Healthsource's new agreement provided the following optional paragraph:

> 11.01 Exclusive Services of Physicians. Physician agrees during the term of this agreement not to serve as a participating physician for any other HMO plan; this shall not, however, prevent

Physician from providing professional courtesy coverage arrangements for brief periods of time or emergency services to members of other HMO plans.[17]

U.S. Healthcare entered the New Hampshire market by applying for and obtaining a license on February 21, 1991, to market its HMO in New Hampshire. U.S. Healthcare claimed a per se violation of the Sherman Antitrust Act, in that the exclusivity clause consisted of a group boycott.

The U.S. Court of Appeals held that the exclusive dealing clause in Healthsource's service agreements with physicians did not give rise to a per se violation of the Sherman Antitrust Act. The court found that there was no evidence of a horizontal agreement among Healthsource's physicians. The exclusivity agreement challenged by U.S. Healthcare was vertical in form. It is "clear that a purely vertical arrangement, by which (for example) a supplier or dealer makes an arrangement, exclusively to supply or serve a manufacturer, is not a group boycott. Were the law otherwise, every distributor or retailer who agreed with a manufacturer to handle only one brand of television or bicycle would be engaged in a group boycott of other manufacturers."[18]

The competitors of Healthsource, Inc., failed to establish violation of the Sherman Antitrust Act under the rule of reason. U.S. Healthcare asserted that the exclusivity clause completely foreclosed U.S. Healthcare and any other nonstaff HMO from operation in New Hampshire. Although the number of physicians tied to Healthsource represented 25 percent of the total number of primary care physicians practicing in the state of New Hampshire, a significant number of physi-

cians were not tied to an exclusive arrangement with Healthsource. Physicians who signed into the exclusivity contract were not tied in permanently. U.S. Healthcare could have competed for Healthsource physicians by offering greater financial incentives to switch over. In addition, there is a constant stream of new physicians entering the marketplace. These physicians are a source for recruitment for any competitor. Absent the showing of a properly defined market in which Healthsource could approach monopoly size, there was no reason to consider the geographic dimension of the market.

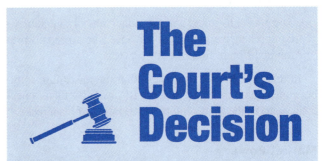

The Court's Decision

The U.S. Court of Appeals for the Eighth Circuit agreed that knowledge of financial incentives that affect a physician's decisions to refer patients to specialists is material information requiring disclosure, and it reversed a lower court's dismissal of the claim.

CHAPTER REVIEW

1. *Managed care* is the process of structuring or restructuring the health care system in terms of financing, purchasing, delivering, measuring, and documenting a broad range of health care services and products.

2. *Health maintenance organizations* (HMOs) are the most highly regulated form of *managed care organizations* (MCOs) and are health systems that are responsible for the financing and delivery of a wide range of comprehensive services to their enrolled populations.
   - *Independent practice association* (IPA) models provide care to subscribers through contracts with independent physicians.
   - *Staff models* normally contract with physicians as full-time employees.

3. Entities through which employer health benefit plans and health insurance carriers contract to purchase services for covered beneficiaries from a selected group of providers are called *preferred provider organizations* (PPOs). *Exclusive provider organizations* (EPOs) limit beneficiaries to participating providers.

4. IPAs are legal entities of physicians who have organized to negotiate contracts to provide their services. Group practices are physician groups that have only one or a small number of service delivery locations, while in a group practice without walls, physicians organize to share administrative and management costs but practice at their own locations.

5. *Management service organizations* (MSOs) provide services such as practice management, marketing, managed care contracting, billing, and personnel management for physicians. Vertically *integrated delivery systems* (IDS) provide physician and hospital services to patients. IDSs can be one organization or several affiliated organizations.

6. Federal qualification of HMOs is voluntary, and those that are federally qualified must provide or arrange for basic services for members as needed and without limitations on time, cost, frequency, extent, or nature of services provided.

7. Most state HMO laws require that an application for a certificate of authority be accompanied by a description of proposed marketing plans. A regulator must approve this plan.

8. *Utilization review* (UR) is a process through which a third-party payer assesses the medical necessity of a course of treatment. Prospective review is the determination of whether to pay for a treatment before the treatment is administered, concurrent review takes place during the treatment, and retrospective review takes place after the treatment.

9. Congress passed the *Health Care Quality Improvement Act* (HCQIA) of 1986 to encourage continued participation in peer-review and credentialing activities. The act grants immunity to persons who supply to professional review bodies information that may result in adverse decisions against a physician.

10. A fiduciary is obligated to deal fairly and honestly with plan members. The duty not to mislead is derived both from the common law of trusts and the statutory language in the *Employee Retirement Income Security Act* (ERISA) of 1974.

11. Price fixing is when two or more competitors collude to decide on the price that will be charged for services or goods. For MCOs, there is a danger that provider-controlled organizations will be seen as a horizontal conspiracy between competitors that acts as a mechanism for price fixing.

REVIEW QUESTIONS

1. Describe some of the more common models of MCOs.
2. What are the advantages and disadvantages of HMOs?
3. What is the purpose of utilization review?

NOTES

1. 107 F.3d 625 (8th Cir. 1997).
2. 42 U.S.C. § 300 (1995).
3. See 42 U.S.C. § 300e (1995) (Historical and Statutory Notes).
4. 239 Cal. Rptr. 810 (Cal. Ct. App. 1986).
5. 536 U.S. 355 (2002).
6. 808 F. Supp. 1253 (E.D. Va. 1992).
7. 600 P.2d 1060 (Cal. 1979).
8. 515 N.W.2d 645 (Neb. 1994).
9. 968 F. Supp. 757 (D.C. N.H. 1997).
10. 46 Fed. Reg. 48, 982 (1981).
11. 457 U.S. 332 (1982).
12. 1991-1 Trade Cas. (CCH) ‖ 69,339.
13. 698 F. Supp. 679 (D. Mich. 1988).
14. *Eastern States Retail Lumber Dealers Ass'n v. United States,* 234 U.S. 600 (1914).
15. 472 U.S. 284 (1985).
16. 986 F.2d 589 (1st Cir. 1993).
17. *Id.* at 592.
18. *Id.* at 594.

Tort Reform and Risk Reduction

It's Your Gavel ...

RECOVERY OF EXPENSES IN EXCESS OF MEDICAID PAYMENTS

Taylor suffered a ruptured disc during an automobile accident. On October 26, 1994, he underwent surgery at Louisiana State University Medical Center (LSUMC). After surgery, Taylor began to experience numbness and difficulty moving his lower extremities. An emergency surgery was performed to correct these problems. The procedure was unsuccessful, and Taylor's condition deteriorated to quadriplegia and he eventually became ventilator dependent. Taylor was treated at LSUMC until January 1995, at which time he was transferred to LifeCare Hospital, as a Medicaid patient, for long-term rehabilitation treatment. Taylor remained at LifeCare until his death on May 22, 1995.

Taylor's family-plaintiffs filed suit for damages. A medical review panel determined that LSUMC breached the applicable standard of care by failing to conduct or record neurological checks from the end of the first surgery until over three hours later. The plaintiffs and LSUMC reached a partial settlement for $630,000. The settlement did not include the plaintiffs' claim for medical expenses contractually written off by LifeCare pursuant to Medicaid requirements.

Evidence showed that Taylor's medical expenses at LifeCare totaled $1,110,922.82 and that Medicaid paid LifeCare $164,084.82. The difference of $946,838 was contractually written off by Life-Care as required by Medicaid. Because LifeCare accepted Taylor as a Medicaid patient, LifeCare was required by both federal and state law to accept the Medicaid payment as payment in full and was prohibited from collecting further payment from Taylor. The plaintiffs relying upon the collateral source rule claimed that contractually adjusted medical expenses are an item of damages to which they are entitled.[1]

WHAT IS YOUR VERDICT?

Given the difficulties in the present tort system, we often become victims of the failures of medicine as opposed to beneficiaries of its many successes. Physicians have lost in that they have changed, limited, or closed their practices after having spent the most vigorous years of their lives training for such work. Patients have lost in that the physicians of their choice, with whom they have developed trusting relationships, are no longer available to care for them. It is certain that the system requires sensible reform.

Pozgar

The tort system has proven to be inadequate in the prevention of medical malpractice. Damage awards as a deterrent to malpractice have failed to hold the number of claims to a reasonable level. Exorbitant jury awards and malpractice insurance premiums, costing billions of dollars annually, are bringing health care organizations ever closer to a day of reckoning with financial disaster. "The cost of the U.S. tort system for 2003 was $246 billion, or $845 per citizen or $3,380 for a family of four."[2]

Physicians who wish to practice medicine and survive have accepted the concept of practicing defensive medicine. *Defensive medicine* (self-protective) is believed to be one of the most harmful effects produced by the threat of malpractice litigation. Such medicine is practiced to forestall potential litigation and provide an advantageous legal defense should a lawsuit be instituted. Defensive medicine often results in *undertreatment,* perhaps by avoiding high-risk tests and procedures, or *overtreatment,* such as the excessive use of diagnostic tests. "The message the tort system is sending to doctors is not so much deterrence, in terms of practicing good medicine, but more just 'drive defensively,' because any patient you may see may be a litigant."[3]

It should be noted that the various states have not ignored the need for tort reform and have and continue to legislate tort reform:

> In 2005 alone, 48 state legislatures responded to fevered calls for medical liability reform through the introduction of over 400 bills to address the situation. Solutions ranged from enacting limits on noneconomic damages, to malpractice insurance reform, to gathering lawsuit claim data from malpractice insurance companies and the courts for the purpose of assessing the connection between malpractice settlements and premium rates. During the 2005 legislative session, 32 states enacted over 60 bills, and 2 more states had Supreme court rulings relating to medical liability lawsuit statutes.[4]

This chapter reviews selected schemes for tort reform and suggested programs for coping with the malpractice crisis.

ARBITRATION AND MEDIATION

Among the many factors contributing to the malpractice crisis is the high cost of litigation. Trial by jury is lengthy and expensive. If case disputes can be handled out of court, the process and expense of a lawsuit can be significantly reduced. Arbitration and mediation are basically mechanisms for simplifying and expediting the settlement of claims.

Arbitration is the process by which parties to a dispute voluntarily agree to submit their differences to the judgment of an impartial mediation panel for resolution. It is used as a means to evaluate, screen, and resolve medical malpractice disputes before they reach the courts. Arbitration can be accomplished by mutual consent of the parties or statutory provisions. A decision made at arbitration may or may not be binding, depending on prior agreement between the parties or statutory requirements.

Mediation is the process whereby a third party, the mediator, attempts to bring about a settlement between the parties of a complaint. The mediator cannot force a settlement.

STRUCTURED AWARDS

Structured awards are set up for the periodic payment of judgments by establishing a reversible trust fund for specified risks of malpractice parts of awards due plaintiffs. The purpose of a structured award is to provide compensation during a plaintiff's lifetime. It would eliminate an unwarranted windfall to the plaintiff's beneficiaries in the event of death. Some states have sought to deal with award limitations by mandating so-called structured recoveries when awards exceed a certain dollar amount.

Structured recoveries provide that money awarded to the plaintiff be placed in a trust fund and invested appropriately so that those funds will be available to the plaintiff over a long period. The rationale behind such legislation is that an immediate award of a large sum of money is not necessary for a plaintiff to be well taken care of after suffering injuries. The prudent investment of a smaller amount of money can produce a recovery commensurate with the needs and the rights of the plaintiff. This, in turn, requires a smaller cash outlay by the defendant or the defendant's insurance company, thereby holding down the costs of malpractice insurance and the ultimate cost of medical care to the consumer.

PRETRIAL SCREENING PANELS

Pretrial screening panels are designed to evaluate the merits of medical injury claims to encourage the settlement of claims outside the courtroom. "Panels render an opinion on provider liability and, in some cases, on damages. In most states, the panel's decision on the merit of the claim is admissible in court."[5] Unlike binding arbitration, the decision of a screening panel is not binding and is imposed as a condition precedent to trial, whereas arbitration is conducted in lieu of a trial. Mandatory screenings of alleged negligence cases are useful in discouraging frivolous lawsuits from proceeding to trial.

The Alaska Supreme Court in *Keyes v. Humana Hospital Alaska*[6] held that a statute creating mandatory pretrial review of medical malpractice claims by an expert advisory panel did not impermissibly infringe on the plaintiff's constitutional right to a trial by jury. The statute was a reasonable legislative response to the medical malpractice insurance crisis.

The constitutionality of a Virginia statute in *Speet v. Bacaj*[7] provided that admission of a medical review panel's opinion into evidence did not infringe on the plaintiff's right to a trial by jury as guaranteed by the Virginia Constitution.

COLLATERAL SOURCE RULE

The collateral source rule is a common-law principle that prohibits a court or jury from taking into account when setting an award that part of the plaintiff's damages covered by other sources of payment (e.g., health insurance, disability, and compensation). Several states have modified the collateral source rule so that evidence regarding other sources of payment to the plaintiff may be introduced for purposes of reducing the amount of the ultimate award to the plaintiff. The jury then would be permitted to assign the evidence such weight as it chooses. The award could be reduced to the extent that the plaintiff received compensation from other sources.

Imposition of the collateral source rule can result in recoveries to plaintiffs far in excess of their economic loss. Such excessive payments contribute significantly to the high cost of malpractice insurance and the high cost of health care to the public. When evidence regarding collateral sources of payment is allowed to be introduced to mitigate the damages payable to a plaintiff, excessive recoveries may be discouraged.

CONTINGENCY FEE LIMITATIONS

A *contingency fee* is payment for services rendered by an attorney predicated on the favorable outcome of a case. Payment is based on a preestablished percentage of the total award. Some states set this percentage by statute. Under a contingency agreement, if there is no award to the plaintiff, then the attorney receives no payment for services rendered.

Physicians argue that the contingency fee arrangement serves to encourage an inordinate number of lawsuits. Attorneys reason that if they or their clients must bear the initial cost of a lawsuit, only those with obvious merit will be brought forward. The contingency fee structure allows those unable to bear the cost of litigation to initiate a suit for damages. Limiting contingency fees on a sliding scale basis, with the percentage decreasing as the award to the plaintiff increases, and/or providing for a lesser fee if a claim is settled prior to trial, seems to have some merit.

COUNTERSUITS: FRIVOLOUS CLAIMS

Health care providers, in some instances, have filed countersuits after being named in what they believe to be malicious, libelous, slanderous, frivolous, and nonmeritorious medical malpractice suits. The threat of countersuits, however, has not been helpful in reducing the number of malpractice claims. Remedies for such actions vary from one jurisdiction to the next. For a physician to prevail in a suit against a plaintiff or plaintiff's attorney, the physician must show that the

- suit was frivolous

- motivation of the plaintiff was not to recover for a legitimate injury

- physician has suffered damages as a result of the suit

There have been arguments that defendants should be allowed to recover court costs and damage awards from both the plaintiff(s) and the attorneys for frivolous claims and counterclaims. The courts thus far have not looked favorably on countersuits for frivolous and unscrupulous negligence actions. Some state legislatures have taken limited action in this area. An Arkansas statute, for example, provides that in any civil action in which the court finds that there was a complete absence of a judicial issue of either law or fact raised by the losing party or his or her attorney, the court shall award, with certain stipulations, an attorney fee in an amount not to exceed $5,000 or 10 percent of the amount in controversy, whichever is less, to the prevailing party.[8]

In *Berlin v. Nathan*,[9] a radiologist, a surgeon, and a hospital were sued for alleged malpractice by a patient who sought $250,000 because the defendants did not diagnose a fracture of her little finger. The radiologist missed the break, but he claimed that it was not evident on the X-ray taken at the hospital and that there was no error on his part. Further, the finger was placed in a splint just as if it had been broken, so the treatment was correct regardless of the diagnosis. The radiologist countersued, so the malpractice suit and countersuit were tried together. When the jury was selected, the patient withdrew the malpractice suit, but the radiologist persisted with his case. The jury awarded the radiologist $2,000 as compensation and $6,000 in punitive damages, presumably convinced that the patient and her attorneys acted improperly in bringing the lawsuit and that the attorneys were negligent in their investigation of the patient's case before filing suit.

When the case was taken to an appellate court, the decision of the lower court was reversed on the grounds that the physician failed to plead special damages and (because the countersuit had been filed prematurely) failed to plead a favorable result in the original suit. The appellate court went on to say that a showing of special damages is essential in a case of this type in order that the public's right to free access to the court system not be impeded by the threat of counter-litigation. The court reasoned that persons who believe they have legitimate claims should not be dissuaded from using the court system solely because of the fear of liability in the event their claim is unsuccessful.

The appellate court holding in the *Berlin* case represents the majority judicial view across the country regarding countersuits. Courts generally do not find in favor of the countersuing party because they fear that persons who otherwise would bring malpractice suits will be discouraged simply because of a concern over the possibility of a countersuit.

Frivolous and unscrupulous malpractice actions have caused physicians to place limitations on their scope of practice. Many obstetricians/gynecologists, for example, have dropped the high-risk obstetrics portion of their practices to reduce their malpractice premiums. There is also an ever-increasing reluctance by physicians to perform heroic measures on accident victims because of the high risks of malpractice exposure.

JOINT AND SEVERAL LIABILITY

The doctrine of joint and several liability provides that a person causing an injury concurrently with another person can be held equally liable for the entire judgment awarded by a court. It is proposed by some that each defendant in a multidefendant action should be limited to payment for the percentage of fault ascribed to him or her. Some states have taken action to modify the doctrine. A Wyoming statute, for example, provides that each defendant to a lawsuit is liable only for that proportion of the total dollar amount of damages according to the percentage of the amount of fault attributed to him or her.[10] A Minnesota statute provides that a defendant whose fault is 15 percent or less may be jointly liable for a percentage of the whole award not greater than four times his or her percentage of fault.[11]

MALPRACTICE CAPS

The impetus for malpractice caps is due, in part, because jury awards often vary substantially from one jurisdiction to the next within the same state. As a result, negligence attorneys often prefer to try personal injury cases in those jurisdictions in which a jury is likely to grant a higher award. Different states are attempting to stem the tide of rising malpractice costs by passing laws that impose restrictions on

limiting the total dollar damages allowable in malpractice actions. Although there have been challenges to statutes limiting awards, it would appear that limitations on malpractice recoveries are not unconstitutional. The Idaho Supreme Court in *Jones v. State Board of Medicine*[12] held that the state's limitation on malpractice recoveries ($150,000) need not necessarily be unconstitutional. The court held that there was no inherent right to an unlimited amount of damages and that the state had a legitimate interest in controlling excessive medical costs caused by large malpractice recoveries, and thus the statute could be held constitutional.

The California Supreme Court in *Fein v. Permanente Medical Group*[13] found that provisions in the Medical Injury Compensation Reform Act of 1975, Section 3333.2 of the Civil Code, that limit noneconomic damages for pain and suffering in medical malpractice cases to $250,000 are not unconstitutional. The legislature did not place limits on a plaintiff's right to recover for economic damages, such as medical expenses and lost earnings resulting from an injury.

A Virginia statute that places a cap of $750,000 on damages recoverable in a malpractice action was found not to violate the Seventh Amendment separation of powers principles or the Fourteenth Amendment due process or equal protection clauses.[14]

NO-FAULT SYSTEM

A no-fault system compensates injured parties for economic losses regardless of fault. It is intended to compensate more claimants with smaller awards. A no-fault system compensates victims of medical injury whether they can prove medical negligence. Proponents of the no-fault approach cite as its advantages swifter and less-expensive resolution of claims and more equitable compensation for patients.

A no-fault system of compensation has its drawbacks. Opponents of the no-fault system are concerned about the loss of whatever deterrence effect the present tort system exerts on health care providers. The system's lower administrative costs can be an incentive to file lawsuits and, therefore, may not produce the desired outcome of reducing the incidence of malpractice claims.

PEER REVIEW

Public Law No. 92-603 of the Social Security Amendments of 1972 and Public Law No. 94-182 of the Social Security Act of 1975 created a nationwide review agency known as professional standard review organizations (PSROs) under Title XI of the Social Security Act.[15] Their purpose is to ensure that medical care provided to patients is of high quality and reflects the most appropriate and efficient use of an organization's health care services.

PSRO norms, standards, and criteria were to be used as guidelines of acceptable medical care to measure the standard of care rendered to beneficiaries of Medicare, Medicaid, and maternal and child health programs. PSROs compiled and studied physician profiles of care to determine whether services rendered in a given area were consistent with the standards of learning and skill of the average reputable physician, either nationwide or in communities similar to those under examination.

In 1982, Congress repealed the PSRO program, replacing it with the Peer Review Improvement Act.[16] Under this act, peer-review organizations (PROs) perform functions similar to those of the PSROs. Hospitals must have agreements with PROs as a condition of receiving Medicare payments under the prospective payment system, as required by the Deficit Reduction Act of 1984.[17] PROs can deny reimbursement for substandard care. They also can recommend that a practitioner be suspended from the Medicare and Medicaid programs, as well as be fined for a pattern of poor performance.

Peer-review documents generally are protected from discovery as long as they are maintained in compliance with a formalized quality assurance program. The U.S. Supreme Court in *Patrick v. Burget*,[18] by an 8–0 vote, reversed the decision of the Ninth Circuit Court of Appeals, which had held that the peer-review process was exempt from antitrust scrutiny under the so-called state action doctrine.

> Because we conclude that no state actor in Oregon actively supervises hospital peer-review decisions, we hold that the state action doctrine does not protect the peer-review activities challenged in this case from application of the federal antitrust laws. In so holding we are not unmindful of the policy argument that respondents and their amici have advanced for reaching the opposite conclusion. They contend that effective peer review is essential to the provision of quality medical care and that any threat of antitrust liability will prevent physicians from participating openly and actively in peer-review proceedings. This argument, however, essentially challenges the wisdom of applying the antitrust laws to the sphere of medical care, and as such is properly directed to the legislative branch. To the extent that Congress has declined to exempt medical peer review from the reach of the antitrust laws, peer review is immune from antitrust scrutiny only if the state effectively has made this conduct its own. The State of Oregon has not done so.[19]

Compliance with the Health Care Quality Improvement Act (HCQIA) is the only way health care organizations and their medical staffs can hope to protect credentialing and peer-review activities from antitrust liability. The Supreme Court endorsed the act in the *Patrick* opinion, holding that the HCQIA, which was enacted well after the events at issue in this case and is not retroactive, essentially immunizes peer-review action from liability if the action was taken in the reasonable belief that it was in the furtherance of quality health care.

A physician who resigned after evaluation of his suspected alcohol, drug, or emotional problem filed a complaint against the hospital and the assistant administrator for slander, coercion, intentional infliction of emotional distress, and intentional interference with his employment contract as medical director of the hospital's department of perinatology.[20] Alcohol had been detected on the physician's breath while he was performing certain medical procedures. A chemical-dependency specialist conducted interviews with members of the hospital's staff who had contact with the plaintiff. According to the witnesses, the plaintiff was subject to mood swings, became abrupt and tactless with patients, boasted of becoming intoxicated, and occasionally would leave work and return wired. The plaintiff had been described as bizarre and paranoid. In conducting the interviews with the hospital staff, the witnesses believed that something was wrong with the plaintiff, but they were reluctant to speak because of their fondness for him.

Acting on the advice of the chemical-dependency specialist, the vice president of medical staff affairs for the hospital formed a committee that met for the purpose of confronting the physician regarding the alleged behavior problem. The physician reluctantly agreed to an evaluation by a physician experienced in treating impaired physicians. The plaintiff was evaluated later that day at a nearby hospital. The record is silent as to the results of that evaluation, except to indicate that the plaintiff did not require hospitalization. The circuit court dismissed the complaint, and the physician appealed. On appeal, the appellate court held that the Hospital Licensing Act provided the defendants with absolute immunity from liability for the hospital peer-review committee's investigation of the physician's conduct.

PROFESSIONAL MISCONDUCT

Some states require the reporting of professionals found liable for medical misconduct. Medical misconduct generally includes obtaining a license fraudulently; practicing a profession fraudulently, beyond its authorized scope, with gross incompetence; practicing a profession while the ability to practice is impaired by alcohol, drugs, physical disability, or mental disability; refusing to provide professional service to a person because of such person's race, creed, color, or national origin; permitting, aiding, or abetting an unlicensed person to perform activities requiring a license and being convicted of committing an act constituting a crime.

The penalties that may be imposed on a licensee found guilty of medical misconduct include suspension of the license to practice, revocation of the license to practice, limitation on registration or issuance of any further licenses, and imposition of a fine.

The physician in *Gunduy v. Commissioner of Education*[21] appealed the commissioner of education's decision to revoke his license for being convicted under federal law on seven counts of an indictment. The physician was involved in the possession and distribution of large amounts of amphetamines and furnished false information in required reports and records. The court confirmed the commissioner's decision and noted that professionals have considerable responsibility not to abuse the trust that licensure places on them by violating the laws controlling dangerous drugs.

REGULATION OF INSURANCE PRACTICES

Many believe that the regulation of insurance practices is necessary to prevent windfall profits. Both the medical profession and the legal profession believe that insurance carriers have raised premiums disproportionately to their losses and that, despite their claims of substantial losses, they have reaped substantial profits.

REQUIRE IMPLEMENTATION OF BEST PRACTICES

Setting and following preestablished medical standards can help reduce the number of lawsuits in any given medical specialty. "Many of the specialty societies either have drafted or are drafting practice guidelines for their medical area of expertise. For example, the American Society of Anesthesiologists developed guidelines for intra-operative monitoring in 1986. During the following year, no lawsuits were brought for hypoxic injuries; in previous years hypoxic injury suits averaged six per year."[22]

RISK MANAGEMENT

The purpose of a risk-management program is to reduce the number of patient injuries and minimize the exposure of an organization to lawsuits. An effective risk-management program includes a monitoring system that identifies potential risks to patients and staff. Information gathered is used to improve patient care and treatment practices. In risk management, steps are taken on a team-effort basis to improve the quality of care and eliminate or minimize the number of accidents that become potential lawsuits. Liability insurers have been strong proponents of risk management; in many

cases, insurers have cut premiums for physicians and health care organizations who adopt risk management practices.

Risk management must include a heightened sensitivity to providing a safe environment and addressing the emotional needs of patients. The input of the provider-patient relationship cannot be overemphasized when the provider-patient relationship is intense and inescapable. Individuals, not incidents, bring lawsuits. Good relationships with patients are very important in preventing malpractice suits. Public relations for health care professionals are a challenge. It is not only good medical practice but it is also at the very core of the problem of medical malpractice.

Increasing insurance costs and general financial constraints have pressured hospitals to assume leadership in the prevention of medically related injuries. Risk-management programs should include the following components:

- a grievance or complaint mechanism designed to process and resolve as promptly and effectively as possible grievances by patients or their representatives

- a collection of data with respect to negative health care outcomes (whether they give rise to claims)

- medical care evaluation mechanisms, which shall include a tissue committee or medical audit committee to periodically assess the quality of medical care being provided

- education programs for staff personnel engaged in patient care activities dealing with patient safety, medical injury prevention, the legal aspects of patient care, problems of communication and rapport with patients, and other relevant factors known to influence malpractice claims and suits

Elements of a Risk-Management Program

Valuable components of a risk management program include

- early intervention and sympathetic care after accidental injury to a patient

- preparation of incident reports

- prompt identification and investigation of specific incidents of patient injuries and, when possible, intervention

- definition of the cause of each incident

- generation and maintenance of a risk database from which hazardous trends and areas may be identified and corrected

- evaluation of the frequency and severity of incident exposure

- formulation and implementation of corrective actions to reduce risk and exposure to liability

- training and education of employees and clinicians to assist in reducing exposure

- continuing attention of a safety committee

- use of a suggestion box

- a public relations program (employees should be trained in completing timely incident reports that document the facts and that are not used to cover up unfortunate incidents but to train personnel and identify problems)

Risk-Management Committee

A risk-management committee with representation from the organization's governing body, administration, and medical staff should be established. The committee should be chaired by a person trained in medical audits and the risk management process. The risk manager should be responsible for the development and coordination of strategic prevention programs. Information from all committees (e.g., pharmacy, transfusion, infections, safety, audit, utilization, tissue, medical records, personnel, credentials, continuing education, product review, etc.) regarding potential liability hazards should be funneled into this committee for review, evaluation, and appropriate action. This committee serves to monitor all potential hazards. The organization's attorney should be readily available for legal counsel.

Because an organization's governing body has the ultimate responsibility for adequate patient care, that group's involvement in the risk-management process is mandatory. The governing body must be just as concerned with reviewing the competence of the medical staff as it is with the financial aspects of institutional operations. Public expectations place a broad responsibility on organizations to ensure quality care whether that care involves administrative, nursing, or physician activities.

CONTINUOUS QUALITY IMPROVEMENT

Continuous quality improvement (CQI) is an approach to improving quality on a continuing basis. CQI is introduced here because of its value in reducing the risks of malpractice. This section presents the practical side and components of CQI, the success factors, the advantages and benefits, and how to implement CQI teams.

CQI is a term given to the philosophy of management introduced into the U.S. business world in 1980 by an American statistician, Dr. W. E. Deming. Deming was rediscovered by his own country when an NBC news documentary entitled "If Japan Can—Why Can't We?" was broadcast on June 24, 1980. A portion of the documentary highlighted Deming's efforts in helping to make Japanese management and products what some would call the best in the world. His concepts on improving quality, however, failed to catch the immediate attention of the business world in the United States. Through his years of research, Deming formulated step-by-step procedures for improving quality and decreasing costs. Since that time, there have been numerous variations on the CQI process of improving quality. CQI comes in a diversity of packages that contain sound business practices that have been developed over the years. The following lists the numerous labels ascribed to the quality improvement process:

- TQM: total quality management

- PM: participative management

- PI: performance improvement

- QCs: quality circles

- TQI: total quality improvement

- CQI: continuous quality improvement

- MBO: management by objectives

- IOP: improving organizational performance

CQI involves improving performance at every functional level of an organization's operation, using available resources (human and capital). It combines fundamental management techniques, innovative improvement efforts, and specialized technical skills in a structure focused on continuously improving processes. CQI relies on people and involves everyone. CQI is concerned with providing a quality product, getting to market on time, providing the best service, reducing costs, broadening market share, and organizational growth. The benefits of CQI are well documented and include reduced customer complaints and turnover; increased ability to attract new customers; and improved productivity, services, and quality.

Paradigm Shift

Most health care organizations have recognized the need for a paradigm shift from the autocratic style of management to a more humanistic participative style of management. The hierarchical autocratic organization is not appropriate for modern society's highly competitive marketplace. The fruits of the autocratic style of management, which include high staff turnover, low morale, resistance to change, limited creativity, lack of excitement and challenge, rigidity, entrenchment in the status quo, low ownership and accountability, and a passive following, have served only to slow the wheels of progress.

Selecting a CQI Process

Although many health care organizations still strive to overcome eighteenth-century European and American management philosophies that considered workers to be expendable, numerous successes have occurred through collaboration and involvement to improve the quality of care. The shift toward the concepts of CQI in the health care industry is particularly important because of The Joint Commission's emphasis on improving organizational performance. The Joint Commission provides that health care organizations must have a planned, systematic, organization-wide approach to designing, measuring, assessing, and improving their performance.

CQI Implementation

The ultimate successes of CQI require commitment by the organization's leadership. In the health care setting, leadership includes the administration, governing body, medical staff, and nursing staff. From the leadership, involvement must be expanded to include the entire organization.

The organization's plan should be designed to provide a systematic and ongoing process for monitoring and evaluating patient care, identifying opportunities for improvement, and identifying high-risk areas having the potential for adverse outcomes and increased exposure to litigation.

Steering Committee

To be successful in implementing a CQI program, an organization's leaders should establish a steering committee or coordinating council with senior leaders of the organization at the helm. This committee is responsible for providing direction, designing and implementing a CQI program, overseeing the progress of the organization's CQI program, assessing the strengths and weaknesses of the organization, determining the right strategy for the organization, creating and tracking management indicators, and providing the appropriate resources necessary to make the CQI program successful.

Training

Education in the principles of CQI must occur at every level of the organization. An effective CQI program requires

- an understanding of the organization's mission and vision
- change to be the norm, not the exception
- communications and information dissemination
- continuous evaluation, measurement, and improvement
- identification of customer requirements
- constant feedback from all levels of the organization
- self-assessment

- empowerment of a CQI team to act (If the team is not supported by the organization, it will lead to disintegration.)
- active involvement by all employees
- authority and autonomy to be commensurate with duties
- a periodic reporting mechanism to the governing body
- an annual evaluation of the organization's performance improvement plan

Facilitators

Facilitators act as helpers in the CQI process. They should know all about the brainstorming process and have an in-depth understanding about human behavior, with little or no stake in the outcome of a team's decision-making process. A good facilitator will ensure equal participation from the group members and will aid in maximizing the number of ideas from the group. The facilitator must be trained in CQI and basic management skills. The facilitator is not a boss; rather, the facilitator's role includes being a teacher/trainer and a consultant. The facilitator supports, provides oversight, helps CQI teams obtain the information and resources necessary to complete their tasks, and provides the group with direction.

Persons experienced in implementing CQI programs should train facilitators. A training agenda should include

- an historical overview of CQI concepts
- examples of the processes and principles involved
- highlights of the benefits of a CQI program
- small-group behavior, processes, and dynamics
- participative management theory
- theories of motivation
- communications skills
- body language
- methodologies for problem solving
- changing behavior
  - the stone wall
  - staying calm under confrontation
  - working with difficult people
  - minimizing the negative effects of difficult behavior
  - turning conflict into stepping stones for harmony
  - being a catalyst for changing difficult behavior
  - overcoming the fear of confrontation
  - recognizing the important difference between occasional difficult behavior and behavior that has become a lifestyle

- data collection methodologies

- cost analysis and forecasting

- statistical analysis and report writing skills

- public speaking skills

CQI Teams

CQI teams are multidisciplinary groups of individuals that meet regularly to identify opportunities for improvement, generate ideas as to how to make improvements, select and implement a preferred improvement, and audit the progress of and refine improvements. The advantages of CQI teams include

- development of a problem-solving ethic

- more effective use of an organization's resources

- increased productivity

- improvement in quality and patient satisfaction

- participation and personal pride in the organization

- improved morale and job satisfaction

- team building

- the cultivation of professional growth

- improvement of leadership performance

- improvement in market share and increased revenues

CQI Data Collection/Indicators and Screens

Volume Indicators

Volume indicators provide data that demonstrate the scope and frequency of services provided over time (e.g., admission/discharge data, number of procedures, and outpatient visits). Volume indicators also provide valuable information for monitoring the incidence of adverse outcomes (e.g., infection rates following surgical procedures, adverse drug reactions, and medication errors). The information and data gathered by an organization are of significant importance as they relate to budgeting, resource allocation, and strategic planning.

Clinical Indicators

Clinical indicators are used to screen the care provided to patients by clinical specialty. The screens are generally confined to those related to high-volume or high-risk problems that may be unique to the clinical specialty. Each specialty uses such indicators to aid in the identification of opportu-

nities for improving care practices. These opportunities are identified when collected data elements cross a preestablished threshold set by the clinical department or service. Once the threshold has been crossed, those cases are then examined and the reason for variation is determined.

Occurrence Screens

Occurrence screens are predetermined indicators used to signal the need for evaluation of some aspect of patient care. Screens may describe the processes in the delivery of care, clinical events, complications, or outcomes for which data can be collected in order to compare actual results with criteria related to the screen. Events such as unexpected deaths, returns to the surgical suite, or adverse drug reactions should prompt an investigation to determine whether the events could be traced to structural problems (e.g., availability of resources) or process problems (e.g., timeliness and skills in the delivery of health care).

Focused Reviews

Focused reviews are concentrated reviews of key areas in a department or clinical specialty determined by their high risk, high volume, or history of identified problems. Focused reviews might target a representative sample of high-volume diagnoses or procedures over a finite time period or a review of all cases of low-volume but high-risk care.

Clinical Pertinence Review of Medical Records

The clinical pertinence review of medical records is a CQI process that monitors and evaluates the clinical pertinence, completeness, accuracy, timeliness, and legibility of documentation as reflected in the medical record. The purpose of such a review is to identify opportunities for improvement in the record documentation process.

Successful CQI Programs

Listed here are a few of the many areas in which health care organizations have successfully implemented the CQI process:

- improving response time for thrombolytic therapy

- tracking and reducing employee needle sticks

- recognizing abnormal vital signs and changes in patient's condition

- improving response time (e.g., cardiopulmonary arrest)

- improving charting (charting objectively, descriptively, and clinically)

- providing patient-family education

- utilizing resources in a cost-effective manner

- improving safety

- improving patient satisfaction

- designing and implementing clinical pathways

- providing security and confidentiality of computer-generated information

- using antibiotics effectively and efficiently

- improving pain management

- developing and implementing nutritional screens and assessments

- improving patient records and pertinent documentation

- reducing the use of restraints

The implementation of CQI in health care organizations will improve the quality of patient care and reduce the untoward events that result in lawsuits. Success will come with true commitment by each organization's leadership. Such commitment requires the full participation of all caregivers. The evolution of a truly successful CQI program involves the transition from CQI as a plan to CQI as a process, and ultimately to CQI as an organizational culture.

FAILURE MODE EFFECTS ANALYSIS

A *failure mode effects analysis* is a method of identifying and preventing product and process problems before they occur (see Chapter 23).

SENTINEL EVENTS

A *sentinel event* is an unexpected occurrence involving death or serious injury or risk thereof. In the health care setting, a sentinel event is an unanticipated death or major permanent loss of function not related to the natural course of the patient's illness or underlying condition(s). Sentinel events include such things as a blood transfusion reaction, surgery on the wrong patient or body part, and leaving an unintended foreign object in a patient's body during surgery. They are sentinel because they signal the need for immediate response for investigation and systems improvement in order to prevent reoccurrence of the event.

Conduct Root Cause Analyses

A *root cause analysis* (RCA) is a chronological review of

an event to identify what, how, why, when, and where an unwanted event occurred in order to prevent reoccurrence of the event. RCAs focus on systems and processes, not individual performance.

NATIONAL HEALTH CARE REFORM

The medical malpractice crisis continues to be a major dilemma for the health care industry. Although there have been many approaches to resolving the crisis, there appears to be no one magic formula. The solution most likely will require a variety of efforts, including tort reform.

The ever-increasing proliferation of regulations by policymakers, which have been designed to control costs and improve the quality of care, has alienated health care providers and added fuel to the practice of defensive medicine.

Physicians who are on the front lines often have been excluded from the decision-making processes that threaten their autonomy and financial security. A concerted effort must be made to include them in policy development and implementation. The present system of punishment for all because of the inadequacies of the few has proven to be costly and far from productive. The key to improving quality and controlling costs is cooperation, not alienation. Policymakers have failed in this arena and must return to a commonsense approach to policy development by including those who are on the front lines of medicine.

The Court's Decision

A plaintiff may ordinarily recover reasonable medical expenses, past and future, which he incurs as a result of injury. The term "incur" is defined as "to become liable for." As a Medicaid patient, the medical expenses incurred by Taylor were those paid by Medicaid. There was no liability on the part of Taylor, and there is no liability on the part of the plaintiffs for expenses above those paid by Medicaid. The Medicaid payment to LifeCare was payment in full for Taylor's expenses.

CHAPTER REVIEW

1. *Arbitration* is a process wherein parties agree to submit their differences to the judgment of an impartial mediation panel for resolution. It is conducted in lieu of trial. Mediation is a process wherein a third party attempts to bring about a settlement between the parties.
2. *Structured awards* are placed in a trust and set up to provide compensation over a plaintiff's lifetime.
3. *Pretrial screening panels* are used to encourage out-of-court settlements. The panels give an opinion on provider liability and, in some cases, damages.
4. The *collateral source rule* is a common-law principle that prohibits a court or jury, when setting an award, from taking into account that part of the plaintiff's damages that would be covered by other sources of payment.
5. A *contingency fee* is payment for an attorney's services predicated on the favorable outcome of a case. Many believe that a limitation on such fees would limit the windfall profits of attorneys, thus reducing the economic drain on the health care system.
6. Some health care providers have filed *countersuits* after being named in what they believe to be *frivolous claims*. The threat of such suits, however, has not proven to be helpful in reducing the number of malpractice claims.
7. The concept of *joint and several liability* holds that a person who caused an injury concurrently with another person can be held equally liable for the full judgment awarded by a court. Some states require that each defendant in a multidefendant action should be limited to payment for the percentage of fault ascribed to him or her.
8. Some states are attempting to limit the rising costs of malpractice awards by setting *malpractice caps*.
9. Proponents of a *no-fault approach* to reducing the costs associated with exorbitant malpractice awards cite as its advantages swifter and less-expensive resolution of claims and more equitable compensation for patients.
10. Professional standard review organizations (PSROs) were charged with ensuring that medical care is of high quality and reflects the most appropriate and efficient use of an organization's health care services. In 1982, Congress repealed the PSRO program and replaced it with the *Peer Review Improvement Act,* under which peer review organizations (PROs) perform a similar function of ensuring quality of care.
11. Some states require *professional misconduct* reporting. The hope here is to reduce the number of lawsuits by limiting the privileges or suspending the licenses of those professionals with a propensity to lawsuits.
12. Other reforms that should prove helpful in reducing the high costs of malpractice litigation include *regulation of insurance practices* and requiring *implementation of best practice standards* for patient care.
13. *Risk management* involves the identification of potential accidents with an emphasis on claims prevention. Teams take steps to improve the quality of care and eliminate or minimize the number of accidents that could result in lawsuits.
14. *Continuous quality improvement* (CQI) is a process for improving the quality of patient care on a continuing basis.

REVIEW QUESTIONS

1. Should there be limits placed on malpractice awards? Support your opinion.
2. How does a structured award work?
3. Which of the schemes for tort reform discussed previously do you consider most helpful in addressing the malpractice insurance crisis?
4. Describe how the risk management process can be helpful in reducing the number of malpractice claims.
5. Describe the continuous quality improvement process as it applies to health care organizations.

NOTES

1. *Terrell v. Nanda,* 759 So. 2d 1026 (2d Cir. 2000).

2. *Tillinghast-Towers Perrin. U.S. Tort Costs: 2004 Update (New York, New York, 2005),* American Tort Reform Association, www.atra.org/wrap/files.cgi/7963_howtortreform.html.

3. THE ROBERT WOOD JOHNSON FOUNDATION, *The Tort System for Medical Malpractice: How Well Does It Work, What Are the Alternatives?* ABRIDGE, Spring 1991, at 2.

4. *Medical Malpractice Tort Reform,* National Conference of State Legislatures, September 5, 2006, www.ncsl.org/standcomm/sclaw/medmaloverview.htm.

5. THE ROBERT WOOD JOHNSON FOUNDATION, *Legal Reform,* ABRIDGE, Spring 1991, at 3.

6. 750 P.2d 343 (Alaska 1988).

7. 377 S.E.2d 397 (Va. 1989).

8. ARK. CODE ANN. § 16-22-309 (Michie 1987).

9. 381 N.E.2d 1367 (1978).

10. WYO. STAT. § 1-1-109 (1986).

11. MINN. STAT. § 604.02 (1988).

12. 555 P.2d 399 (Idaho 1976).

13. 695 P.2d 665 (Cal. 1985).

14. *Boyd v. Bulala,* 877 F.2d 1191 (4th Cir. 1989).

15. 472 U.S. 284 (1985).

16. Tit. XI, § 143, part B.

17. Pub. L. No. 98-369.

18. 486 U.S. 94 (1988).

19. *Id.* at 105.

20. *Cardwell v. Rockford Mem'l Hosp. Ass'n,* 539 N.E.2d 1322 (Ill. App. Ct. 1989).

21. 460 N.Y.S.2d 664 (N.Y. App. Div. 1983).

22. THE ROBERT WOOD JOHNSON FOUNDATION, *Preventing Negligence,* ABRIDGE, Spring 1991, at 8.

Patient Safety and Zero Tolerance

The Institute of Medicine (IOM) of the National Academies was chartered in 1970 as a component of the National Academy of Sciences. The November 1999 IOM report, "To Err Is Human: Building a Safer Health System" indicated that at least 44 thousand and perhaps as many as 98 thousand people die in hospitals each year as a result of preventable medical errors. Such figures rank medical errors as the eighth leading cause of death in the United States, ahead of deaths from motor vehicle accidents, breast cancer, or AIDS.

Both health care organizations and accrediting bodies are adopting a zero-tolerance policy toward poor judgment and careless mistakes by focusing on processes and not individuals. Strides are being made to ensure that desired outcomes are more closely aligned with predictability. More focus on how to do things right the first time will lessen the likelihood of having to ask why things went wrong after a medical error occurs.

This chapter focuses on the development of a corporate culture of safety with emphasis on national patient safety goals. A self-evaluation process, including a variety of safe practices, is also presented on the following pages.

DEVELOPING A CULTURE OF SAFETY

Organizations are encouraged to create and maintain a culture of safety in order to reduce the risks of patient injuries and deaths due to common mistakes. Patients expect hospitals to provide a safe environment for medical care. Although health care organizations are aware of where systems often break down, evidence suggests that they have been ineffective in preventing patient injuries that are often the result of human error or just plain carelessness. Implementation of the following suggestions will help hospitals move toward a culture of safety:

- Ensure that accountability and responsibility has been assigned for monitoring an organization's safety initiatives.

- Involve the medical staff in the development and implementation of systems that are designed to create a culture of safety.

- Educate all staff as to their individual roles in establishing and maintaining a safe environment for patients.

- Encourage patients to question their care. Provide guidelines in patient handbooks as to the kinds of questions that they should be asking caregivers (e.g., Is this a new medication; I don't recognize it. What is this medication for? Did you wash your hands (before changing my surgical dressing)? Is my nurse, Ms. X, off today?).

- Appoint a safety officer.

- Establish a patient safety committee with responsibility for oversight of the organization's patient safety program. It is a multidisciplinary committee that includes representation from administration, nursing, and medical staff.

- Set up a 24-hour-a-day dedicated safety hotline.

- Establish a voluntary event reporting system. Educate employees and patients as to reporting options (e.g., telephone, e-mail). Assure employees that there will be no retaliation for reporting patient safety concerns.

- Participate in the Institute for Healthcare Improvement's 100K Lives Campaign by committing to the implementation of its six life saving initiatives: (1) establishment of a rapid response team; (2) improvement of care for myocardial infarctions; (3) prevention of adverse drug events; (4) prevention of central-line-associated bloodstream infections; (5) prevention of surgical site infections; and (6) prevention of ventilator-associated pneumonia.

- Utilize the online tools released by Agency for Healthcare Research and Quality (AHRQ) to assist organizations in evaluating and improving safe care.

Failure Mode Effects Analysis

The health care industry's focus is on identification and reduction of medical errors. The approach is proactive in nature. Failure mode effects analysis has long been recognized as a method for identifying and preventing product and process problems before they occur. The Joint Commission adopted this concept as a standard in its accreditation process and is surveying organizational compliance with this standard. The organizations discussed here are cooperating to reduce the number of medical errors in the nation, and, in some instances, the world.

National Patient Safety Goals

The Joint Commission is striving to improve patient safety by identifying national patient safety goals in its accreditation process. Some of these goals include improving the accuracy of patient identification; effective communications among caregivers; safe use of high-alert medications; elimination wrong-site, wrong-patient, wrong-procedure surgery through the development of universal protocols; safe and effective use of clinical alarm systems; and reduction in the frequency of health care–acquired infections.

Periodically, the Joint Commission introduces national patient safety goals into its survey process. Joint Commission surveyors evaluate organizations at the time of an organization's accreditation survey, determining compliance with patient safety goals. The goals encourage compliance with safe practices in the delivery of patient care and are designed to reduce the likelihood of medical errors in the delivery of patient care. Due to the frequency of questions asked as to interpretation and implementation of the goals, along with the periodic introduction of new goals to the survey process, the Joint Commission, on its Web site at www.jcaho.org, clarifies existing goals and describes new goals.

Patient Complaint Process

The Joint Commission has implemented a patient complaint process that requires that the health care organizations it accredits educate employers and employees as to their right to report safety or quality concerns to the Joint Commission. Joint Commission policy forbids accredited organizations from taking retaliatory actions against employees for having reported quality of care concerns to the Joint Commission. Patient complaints may be reported by:

- Online (www.jointcommission.org/GeneralPublic/Complaint/)

- Fax (Office of Quality Monitoring at 630-792-5636)

- Written correspondence (Office of Quality Monitoring, The Joint Commission, One Renaissance Boulevard, Oakbrook Terrace, IL 60181)

- Telephone (800-994-6610) for questions about how to file a complaint (8:30 A.M. to 5 P.M., Central time, weekdays); NOTE: Surveyors may query staff during the survey process as to what procedures an organization has in place for addressing quality of care concerns and how employees and patients are educated as to the Joint Commission's complaint process.

National Quality Forum

The National Quality Forum (NQF) is a private, non-profit, public-benefit corporation created for the purpose of developing and implementing a national strategy for health care quality measurement and reporting. NQF is a unique public-private partnership representing all sectors of the health care industry, including consumers, employers, insurers, and health care providers. The NQF has identified 30 safe practices that it recommends for adoption in health care settings to reduce the risks of harm to patients. These practices have been endorsed by representatives of 260 of the nation's leading health care provider, purchaser, and consumer organizations. For complete information on the activities and functioning of the NQF, the reader should visit the corporation's Web site at www.qualityforum.org/.

Agency for Healthcare Research and Quality

The Agency for Healthcare Research and Quality (AHRQ) is the lead federal agency within the Department of Health and Human Services charged with improving the quality, safety, efficiency, and effectiveness of health care. Information from AHRQ's research helps people make more informed decisions and improve the quality of health care services. AHRQ collaborated with the National Quality Forum in identifying the 30 safe practices just noted. Evidence shows that such practices can prevent or reduce the number of medical errors.[1]

Institute for Healthcare Improvement

The Institute for Healthcare Improvement (IHI) is a not-for-profit organization whose mission is to improve health care throughout the world. The IHI was founded in 1991 and is based in Cambridge, Massachusetts. To reduce medical errors, health care organizations are becoming more proactive by implementing safe practices. Some hospitals have joined the IHI 100K Lives Campaign, which has a goal of saving one hundred thousand lives annually. For complete information on the activities and functioning of the IHI, the reader should visit the corporation's Web site at www.moore.org/.

The Leapfrog Group for Patient Safety

The Leapfrog Group and its members work together to reduce preventable medical mistakes and improve the quality and affordability of health care. The Leapfrog Group promotes improvements in the safe delivery of health care by collecting and providing healthcare consumers with the necessary information to make informed health care decisions. For complete information on the activities and functioning of the Leapfrog Group, the reader should visit its Web site at www.leapfroggroup.org/.

ECRI

ECRI (formerly the Emergency Care Research Institute) is a nonprofit health services research agency and a collaborating center of the World Health Organization (WHO). It is designated as an evidence-based practice center by the AHRQ. ECRI is widely recognized as one of the world's leading independent organizations committed to advancing the quality of health care. ECRI's mission is to promote the highest standards of safety, quality, and cost effectiveness in health care to benefit patient care through research, publishing, education, and consulting. For complete information on the activities and functioning of ECRI, the reader should visit its Web site at www.ecri.org/.

TOOL FOR EVALUATING SAFE PATIENT CARE

A tool for evaluating the safe delivery of patient care is presented throughout the remainder of the chapter. Each statement is meant to assist the practicing professional in evaluating a health care organization. This tool has been developed to apply to a variety of health care organizations. Each bulleted statement is meant to encourage the reader to ask more—who, how, what, why, when, and where. For example, a bulleted statement could be

- The organization has implemented a patient complaint process.

Questions that could be asked include:

1. What procedures does the organization have in place for addressing complaints?

2. How are patients made aware of the complaint process?

3. Who does the patient contact?

4. When can the patient expect a response to the complaint?

It should be noted that this tool is not exhaustive for any particular topic.

Leadership

- The governing body includes hospital, medical staff, and community representation.

- The organization's mission, vision, and values have been identified.

- The planning process relates to the organization's mission, vision, and values.

- There is a strategy that charts the direction of the organization in response to community need.

- The planning process is described in writing.

- The planning process identifies the organization's strengths and opportunities for improvement.

- Planning is conducted on a collaborative basis.

- Patient input is solicited to improve services through, for example, patient satisfaction surveys and focus groups.

- A process for setting priorities has been established.

- The organization's scope of services is defined.

- There is a process for orientation and education of new board members.

- Clinical outcomes are improving.

- The governing body has adopted a conflict-of-interest policy.

- The same level of care is delivered in all settings across the organization.

- Care is not based on ability to pay.

- A corporate compliance program has been developed and implemented.

- Accountability for the organization's leadership has been defined in writing.

- The governing body conducts self-assessments and identifies areas needing improvement.

- The governing body monitors the effectiveness of the organization's leadership.

Staff Competence

- There is a process for credentialing licensed health care practitioners.

- The National Practitioner Data Bank is utilized in the credentialing process.

- There is ongoing evaluation of each professional.

- Delineation of clinical privileges includes:

  - a description of the privileges requested

  - relevant education, training, and experience

  - limitations on privileges requested

  - evidence of competency in performing requested privileges

  - primary source verification of current licensure

  - relevant references

  - current competency is evaluated

Human Resources Process

- There is a process for verification of licensure.

- Job descriptions reflect each staff member's duties and responsibilities.

- The technical skills of each position have been determined.

- The organization has the appropriate competencies, mix, and numbers of employees.

- Recruitment, retention, development, and recognition programs have been implemented.

- There is a department-specific orientation program for employees, agency and contracted staff, and volunteers.

- The competency-review process is effective.

- Competency evaluations relate to job expectations.

- Age-specific competencies are evaluated.

- The education and training needs of staff are assessed.

Patient Education

- The patient's first contact with a staff member involves the establishment of trust, which emanates from patient recognition that the caregiver is knowledgeable and competent. Remember, patients subconsciously evaluate their caregiver's ability to care for them and decide quickly whether they will have confidence in a staff member.

- Greetings, gestures, manner of taking information, and attitude are important ingredients in establishing a good relationship with the patient.

- There is evidence of patient/family education in the patient's record.

- An assessment of the patient's readiness/willingness, ability, and need to learn is conducted.

- Education is conducted in all settings (e.g., inpatient, ambulatory, emergency department, home care) on a collaborative basis.

- Education includes medication safety; nutrition, medical equipment use; access to community resources; how to obtain further care if necessary; and responsibilities of the patient and family.

- The patient understands the care instructions.

- Follow-up and reinforcement of education is ongoing.

- There is an interdisciplinary approach to patient and family education.

- The physician plays a role in patient and family education.

- Adequate resources are available for education.

Information Technology

- The organization addresses its information technology (IT) needs.

- There is an interdisciplinary committee structure for assessing and reassessing needs.

- The pharmacy has a software package that alerts the pharmacist as to potential food-drug interactions, drug-drug interactions, drug-herbal interactions, and inappropriate dosing on a real-time basis.

- Alerts are provided to the professional staff on patient-care units (e.g., panic lab values, medication alerts).

- A physician order entry system has been implemented.

- IT needs are rationally prioritized based on patient care needs.

- The organization has committed funds for upgrading IT systems.

- IT systems security and confidentiality are maintained.

Resource Allocation

- There is a process for developing budgets (capital, human resource, and expense).

- Processes are in place for the organization to position itself for economic survival.

- Priorities are set for allocation of financial resources.

- The organization has parameters for feedback on variance reporting.

- The organization has a process for approving expenditures.

- There is aggregate data to support decision-making processes.

Performance Improvement

- The organization has a process for performance improvement (PI).

- There is a committee to coordinate PI activities.

- All staff members are educated and oriented in the PI process.

- Opportunities for improvement are identified.

- There is a methodology for establishing priorities for PI.

- It can be demonstrated that PI activities have improved the health of the community.

- Clinical databases are in place for benchmarking.

- Processes for collecting data are meaningful.

- The effectiveness the PI program is evaluated.

Communications

Abbreviations

- Abbreviations are discouraged. Where abbreviations are permitted, they must have one meaning.

- A standardized list of unapproved abbreviations, acronyms, and symbols that are not to be used are identified and published for use by staff.

- A list of unapproved abbreviations might appear somewhat like this:

Do Not Use	Do Use
U	Unit
IU	International Unit
QD or QOD	Daily/every other day
MS	Morphine Sulphate
MSO4 or MgSo4	Magnesium Sulfate
Medications	Orders
Trailing 0 (e.g. 1.0 mg of x)	Include leading 0 (e.g. 0.1 mg of x)
D/C	Discharge
< >	Less than, greater than

- Staff members are trained not to use abbreviations.

- Periodic review of unapproved abbreviations should be conducted to ensure that each approved abbreviation has only one meaning.

Illegible Handwriting

- A process should be in place for validating the correct interpretation of illegible medication orders. For assistance, check out the Web sites for the *Institute for Safe Medication Practices* (www.ismp.org/msaarticles/specialissuetable.html) and the National Coordinating Council for Medication Error Reporting and Prevention (www.nccmerp.org/dangerousabbr.htm).

- Because words are the tools of thought and communications, caregivers must express themselves clearly, both orally and in writing.

- The communication problems and errors caused by illegible handwriting can seriously impede patient care and the defense of a malpractice claim, even when the care given was appropriate.

Telephone or Verbal Orders

- Telephone or verbal orders must be written and read back to the ordering physician by the person who received the order to verify the accuracy of the written order.

- It is preferable that read-backs be documented as such on the order sheet.

- A process is in place to monitor staff to ensure that caregivers are following an organization's read-back policies.

Timely Reporting

- Critical test results and values are reported on a timely basis.

- Data is collected to measure and assess the success of timely reporting.

- Action is taken, when necessary, to improve the reporting process.

Patient Hand-off

A patient hand-off occurs, for example, when a patient is transported from a patient care unit to the radiology department for a CT scan. When handing a patient off from one caregiver to the next, the patient's identification is verified and special care need information is provided to the receiver of the patient (e.g., patient has been categorized as a high risk for falls).

Safety of Blood Transfusions

- Blood transfusion errors can be due to

  - incomplete patient blood transfusion verification

  - failure to recognize vital signs and symptoms of a transfusion reaction

  - multiple samples being cross-matched at the same time

  - a cross-match being started before an order is received

  - insufficient orientation and training for staff members

- Procedures have been adopted for the safe processing, storing, ordering, blood typing and cross-matching, and issuing of blood.

- A patient identification system has been implemented, using at least two identifiers, to ensure that the correct patient is administered the correct blood.

- Procedures have been implemented to address transfusion reactions in a timely and competent manner.

- Consent forms authorizing blood transfusion are executed.

Emergency Services

- Competencies of staff have been defined.

- Adequate staff is available to care for patients.

- Medical records are maintained for each patient treated.

- Patients are triaged, assessed, and treated within a reasonable period of time.

- Criteria for admission and discharge have been established.

- Response time by on-call physicians is timely.

- The organization has a mechanism for obtaining consultations.

- Care is timely.

- All patients are assessed and treated by a physician prior to discharge.

- The records of patients treated in other settings within the organization (e.g., ambulatory care settings) are readily available.

- Patient education is provided in the emergency department (ED) prior to discharge.

- Documentation is complete.

- Responsibility for follow-up with patients who have abnormal tests has been assigned.

- Patient perception of their care is assessed.

- Patients are safely transferred to settings appropriate to meet their care needs.

- ED staff education includes, as examples, abuse and neglect and recognizing contagious diseases.

- Informed consent is obtained when necessary.

- Advance directives are handled appropriately for end-of-life patients.

- Observation beds, as appropriate, are maintained in the ED.

- The organization has a policy for treat and divert situations.

- Isolation procedures have been established.

- There is a procedure in place for reading X-rays and other imaging studies when there is no radiologist readily available.

- Signs are conspicuously posted specifying the rights of individuals with respect to examination and treatment for emergency medical conditions.

- The organization posts notices indicating whether it participates in Medicaid programs under a state plan approved under Title XIX.

- Criteria for referral and transfer of ED patients have been defined in writing.

- Patients requiring transfer are transferred by physician order.

- The receiving facility has available space and qualified staff to treat the patient being transferred.

- The transferring facility sends all available medical records to the receiving facility.

- When patients refuse a recommended transfer

  - The organization takes reasonable steps to secure the patient's (or the person acting on the patient's behalf) written informed refusal prior to transfer.

  - The patient is informed of the risks and benefits of the transfer.

  - The means of transfer is appropriate to meet the needs of the patient during transfer.

Environmental Safety

Safety Program

- There is a designated safety officer responsible for the overall activities of the safety program.

- The safety program addresses all aspects of environmental safety.

- There is an in-house program for addressing safety complaints.

Fire Safety

- Exits are clearly marked.
  - Exit signs are clear as to direction of egress.
  - Exit signs are illuminated.
- Fire-rated doors
  - have a self-closing device
  - have a positive latching mechanism
  - are smoke-tight with vertical gaps no greater than $\frac{1}{8}$ inch and undercuts no greater than $\frac{3}{4}$ inch
- Exit corridors are not blocked with storage.
- Smoking is prohibited in the organization's facilities.
- Fire drills are conducted as often as is prescribed by regulatory agencies.
- Through-the-wall penetrations are sealed to prevent the spread of smoke.
- There is a clear space 18 inches below sprinkler heads.
- Linen and trash chutes have positive latching and are locked.
- Fire extinguishers are mounted in readily accessible locations throughout the organization.
  - Fire extinguishers are properly maintained.
  - Employees have been trained in the proper handling and use of fire extinguishers.
- Employees have been trained in proper fire evacuation procedures.
- Stairwells in buildings five stories or higher are clearly marked as to floor level at each stairwell entrance, including direction and floor of egress.
- The fire department is acquainted with the facility.

Hazardous Materials

- There is an inventory of hazardous materials.
- There is a written hazard communication program that addresses staff education needs.
- Material safety data sheets are readily available to all employees.

- Precautions are taken when handling, storing, and disposing of hazardous materials.

- Flammable liquids are kept in closed containers when not in use.

- Storage containers and piping connections are vapor and liquid tight.

- Hazardous materials are stored in a safe, secure, and ventilated environment.

- Storage rooms for flammable and combustible liquids have explosion-proof lights.

- "No smoking" signs are posted in hazardous areas.

- Reports of incidents related to spills are maintained.

Medical Equipment

- The organization maintains written criteria as to the selection of medical equipment.
- Equipment is tested prior to use.
- Responsibility for training the end user has been assigned.
- Medical equipment policies and procedures provide for
  - selecting and acquiring equipment
  - the identification, location, and evaluation of medical equipment
  - assessing and minimizing clinical and physical risks associated with medical equipment by providing preventative and corrective maintenance services
  - addressing medical equipment hazard notices and recalls
  - monitoring and reporting incidents that may have caused or contributed to an injury
  - reporting and investigating equipment management problems

Clinical Alarm Systems

- A preventative maintenance program is implemented for the testing of alarm systems.
- Alarms are activated with appropriate settings.
- Alarms are audible with respect to distances and competing background noise.
- Sound-alike alarms are eliminated or adjusted so that caregivers easily recognize the type of alarm that is sounding.

- Employees are trained to easily distinguish the sounds and significance of each alarm.
- Clinical alarms are not turned off, audible, and regularly scheduled for preventative maintenance.

Safe Use of Infusion Pumps

- Free-flow protection is mandated for all types of infusion pumps.
- Infusion pumps without free-flow protection are removed from service.

Needlesticks

- Health care workers are properly trained in the safe use and disposal of needles and sharps.
- Use devices have appropriate safety features.
- There is timely follow-up of all needlestick and sharps-related injuries.

Personal Protective Equipment

- The work environment has been assessed to determine whether there are hazards that require the use of personal protective equipment.
- Employees use properly fitted protective equipment.
- Protective goggles and face masks are worn in hazardous areas while working with hazardous materials, including all body fluids.
- Hard hats are worn where there is danger of falling objects.

Security

- Security issues have been addressed throughout the organization.
- Sensitive areas have been identified.
  - Nursery, operating rooms, pediatrics, and the emergency department are all security areas.
  - Appropriate precautions are taken to protect patients, staff, and visitors.

Infant Security

- Infant/child abduction policies and procedures have been established.

- Newborns are footprinted.
- An organization-approved identification band is attached to mothers and infants.
- Identification badges for mother and infant match.
- All staff members have current color photo identification badges.
- Staff and parents are educated as to security procedures.
- Infant abduction drills are conducted.
- An electronic security alarm system has been installed.
- Security cameras and monitors have been installed.

Utilities

- A biomedical technician is included in the selection and purchase of all medical equipment.
- Procedures to be followed in the event of a loss of water, power, medical gas, heat, cooling, and so forth have been established.
- Equipment testing is documented.
- An effective preventive maintenance program has been implemented.
- Outside maintenance contracts are monitored.
- Employees who handle medical gases are trained to identify and handle medical gas cylinders.
- Medical-grade gas products are stored separately from industrial-grade products.
- Full gas cylinders are separated from empty cylinders.
- Cryogenic cylinders with improper fittings are returned to the supplier.
- Medical gas connections and hook-ups are checked by a qualified person.
- Effective security measures include combination locks, cameras, security rounds, mirrors, visitor control/identification tags, alarms, wristband/ankle/umbilical cord alarms, closed units, and staff education.
- Electrical panels are secure/locked, labeled, and provided with preventive maintenance.
- Emergency generators are properly tested.
- Primary and secondary shutoff valves for utility systems are properly tagged for identification purposes.
- Air intake is maintained at a safe distance from the nearest exhaust.
- Air-handling systems are monitored for efficiency.
- Air filters are replaced as necessary.

• There is a reliable and adequate emergency power system able to provide electricity to all critical areas.

Reducing Risks of Patient Falls

• Patients are assessed and reassessed for the risk of falling.

• Action is taken to address identified risks.

• A fall-reduction program is implemented.

• The patient-falls program is periodically reevaluated as to the effectiveness of the program.

• Improvements to the fall-reduction program are implemented as necessary.

Emergency Preparedness

• An emergency preparedness director has been appointed

• The organization has an emergency preparedness plan for both internal and external disasters.

• The plan has been developed in cooperation with local and national emergency preparedness programs.

• The organization identifies its vulnerabilities (e.g., equipment, supplies, staff, communications) and implements improvements.

• The plan is periodically practiced to determine the organization's readiness for a variety of disasters (e.g., earthquake, hurricane, act of terrorism).

Patient Identification

• All employees receive the proper training.

• Monitoring is conducted to assure that patient identification procedures are consistently followed.

• The patient's wristband is checked for identification prior to rendering treatment.

• Take note of two identifiers before treatment (patient's name, birth date, medical record number, etc.) and match the information on the wristband to the patient's medical chart.

• When possible prior to rendering care, ask patient to identify him- or herself, including his or her date of birth.

• Avoid using the patient's room number and bed location as an identifier.

• Consider using photo identification bracelets.

Infection Rates

The Centers for Disease and Control of Infections has estimated that nearly two million patients annually contract a hospital-acquired infection. The medical care required as a result of treating the infections and the lawsuits stemming from them costs the nation billions of dollars annually.

• Compliance with the Centers for Disease Control (CDC) recommendations:

  - hand hygiene guidelines

  - use of recommended soaps

  - use alcohol-based hand rubs

  - follow recommended equipment-cleaning procedures

• Ventilation systems are maintained. Infections are of particular concern with patients who are immunosuppressed. Organisms of concern include *Aspergillus*, a mold that causes lung infections, which lies dormant in spores and is often found in ventilation systems. It is particularly harmful to individuals such as bone transplant patients, whose autoimmune systems are compromised.

• Ventilation systems are monitored.

  - appropriate air exchanges as recommended

  - monitoring need for filter changes

  - safe air supply and return cleaning practices for ducts and vents

  - selection of filters (hepa filtration and ultra violet light)

• Torn stretcher and operating room pads are replaced. Mattress pads are often contaminated with a variety of bacteria that have evolved from the seepage of body fluids into mattress pads. As a result, harmful bacteria can be transferred from one patient to the next. Other organisms of concern include *e. coli*, methicillin-resistant *staphylococcus aureus, salmonella*, and *clostridium sordellii*.

• Clinical guidelines have been adopted. For example, appropriate protocols for the prevention of central venous catheter-associated bloodstream infections have been adopted.

• Surveillance rounds are conducted and infection risks have been identified and eliminated.

• Appropriate temperature and humidity levels are maintained.

  - High humidity increases the risks of nosocomial infections.

  - Low humidity increases the risk of static electricity in the operating suite.

• Orientation, education, and good practices are continuously improved.

• Patients are assessed upon admission.

- Patients at risk for developing pressure ulcers are assessed.

- Protocols to prevent development of pressure ulcers are followed.

- Food products are labeled as to contents and expiration dates.

- Infection-control policies and procedures include gowning, masks, and glove changes between patients.

- Furniture, equipment, and toys are disinfected with appropriate germicidal solutions.

- Equipment-associated infections are tracked.

- Nosocomial infections for each patient care unit are tracked.

- Prophylactic-recommended antibiotics are used on a timely basis.

- All identified cases of unidentified death or major permanent loss of function with a health care setting–associated infection are managed as sentinel events.

Laboratory Services

- The lab is appropriately accredited.

- Panic values are reported promptly.

- Therapeutic ranges are closely monitored.

- Blood levels for toxicity are closely followed.

- Data vital to evaluating a patient's nutritional status is provided.

- Culture and sensitivity studies are conducted.

- Performance improvement activities are conducted with other disciplines on a collaborative basis.

- The laboratory, pharmacy, and dietary staff work collaboratively to improve patient care.

- Test results that do not fit a patient's clinical picture or expected outcomes are addressed by the patient's physician(s).

- Lab personnel review test results for drug interactions through testing procedures (e.g., patients can produce antibodies to drugs that can cross-react with lab tests).

- The suspected/working diagnosis is available when tests are ordered.

- Autopsy criteria have been developed.

- Pre- and postoperative pathology report discrepancies are addressed.

- Approval of the medical staff is obtained prior to approving and signing contracts with reference laboratories.

- Clinical patient information not reflected in lab results is intensely reviewed.

Surgical Specimens

- Second reads are conducted, as appropriate.

- Procedures are implemented to reduce the risk of surgical specimen mix-ups.

- Specimens are properly jarred and labeled at the surgical table.

- Specimens do not leave one's possession until labeled.

- A strict chain of custody for each specimen is maintained. For instance, at one hospital, a pathologist actually goes into the operating suite where a surgical procedure is under way. This pathologist jars, labels, and identifies the specimen(s); performs frozen section(s); and then returns to the surgical suite to describe his or her findings to the operating surgeon, thus maintaining a chain of custody of the specimen(s).

Medication Safety

- Drugs are safely stored, ordered, and distributed.

- Computer software that can aid in the reduction of human errors (e.g., drug-drug and food-drug interactions can be reduced by use of technology to help in identifying potential interactions) is used.

- Potentially dangerous look-alike drugs are separated in the pharmacy to prevent mix-ups.

- There is a nonpunitive approach to reporting medication errors.

- Concentrated electrolytes are tightly controlled.

- All medications are labeled by including the drug, dosage, and expiration date.

- Medications are reconciled across the continuum of care.

- A process is implemented for obtaining and documenting a complete listing of a patient's current medications upon admission to the organization (e.g., inpatient setting).

- A determination as to which medications should be continued during the patient's stay is determined by the attending physician.

- Upon discharge, the attending physician instructs the patient as to which drugs he or she should continue taking and which drugs should be discontinued.

- A complete list of drugs is made available to the next provider when the patient is transferred to another setting, service, practitioner, or level of care within or outside the organization.

- There are procedures for obtaining medications that are not included in the hospital's formulary.

- Risk-reduction activities are in place to reduce the likelihood of adverse drug reactions and medication errors.

- Appropriate disciplines have been credentialed to prescribe medications.

- Controlled substances are monitored, inventoried, and wasted according to protocol.

- There is a mechanism for monitoring the effect of medications on patients.

- Responsibility for ensuring the integrity of crash carts has been assigned.

- The organization maintains the appropriate equipment on crash carts for treating both children and adults.

- Staff members are appropriately trained in the testing and use of equipment contained in or on the crash cart.

- Staff members who participate in codes are periodically tested for competency.

- At a minimum, pharmacists periodically attend codes for observation and educational purposes.

- Mechanisms are in place for reviewing medications administered during a code.

- Medications are dispensed in unit dose or unit-of-use form whenever feasible.

- The variety of drug concentrations is easily identified and standardized when feasible.

- There is a mechanism in place for approving and overseeing the use of investigational drugs.

- Investigational drug protocols and criteria have been developed and approved.

- Look-alike medications are repackaged or relabeled, as necessary, in the pharmacy.

- The organization has a process for monitoring, tracking, and trending medication errors. The information gathered is utilized to reduce the likelihood of medication errors.

- Causes and trends of medication errors are tracked.

- The organization has processes in place to reduce the likelihood of transcription errors.

- Consent is obtained for the use of investigational drugs and high-risk medications.

- Regular medication safety rounds are conducted by a pharmacist in all sites where medications are stored.

- There is a protocol for monitoring patients on multiple medications.

- A medication log is maintained for the tracking and dispensing of sample drugs.

- There is a process for evaluating high-risk, high-volume, problem-prone, and high-cost medications.

- A multidisciplinary team has been established to improve medication use.

- Educational processes have been implemented to reduce the likelihood of medication errors.

Patient Assessments

- There is a process for assessing patient care needs.

- The organization has a policy for conducting screenings and assessments.

- Second opinions are obtained as necessary; literature is searched; and other resources are used to provide current, timely, and accurate diagnoses and treatment of patients.

- The organization has a policy for nutritional care.

- A diet manual has been developed and approved.

- The criteria for nutritional screens have been developed and approved.

- The dietitian participates in determining screening criteria.

- Nutritional screens are performed by a dietitian or an appropriately trained nurse.

- Patients are periodically reassessed for nutritional needs as determined by the patient's condition.

- The potential for food-drug interactions is monitored.

- Patients on special diets are monitored to ensure that they have the appropriate food tray.

- The organization's mechanism for ordering, preparing, dispensing, administering, and monitoring total parenteral nutrition is defined by the medical staff.

- Provision is made to ensure that each patient receives appropriate assistance with feeding.

- Functional screens have been developed and implemented.

- Full assessments, as necessary, are conducted within established time frames.

- Patient/family education is provided by appropriate staff.

Patient Care Unit

- Patient satisfaction surveys are evaluated for purposes of improving patient care.

- Patient rights and privacy are addressed.

- Confidentiality issues are addressed.

Patient Rights

- Organizations adhere to federal and state laws that address advance directives.

- Documentation of a patient's preferences for health care is placed in the patient's chart.

- Consultation is held with the patient's designated advocate regarding his or her understanding of the patient's wishes in the event the patient becomes unable to articulate his or her own decisions.

- Patients who have no advance directive are provided an opportunity to execute one.

- Patients and staff are educated as to the existence and functions of the organization's ethics committee.

- A procedure has been adopted regarding how the committee can be accessed for consultation.

- Patients are provided a statement of their rights and responsibilities upon admission.

- Patients have a right to review their medical records.

Surgery and Invasive Procedures

- Patients are informed of the risks, benefits, and alternatives to anesthesia, surgical procedures, and the administration of blood or blood products.

- Consent forms are executed and placed in the patient's record.

- Hand-washing protocols are strictly enforced.

- Antibiotics are administered prior to surgery to reduce the likelihood of patients developing postsurgical infections.

- Responsibility has been assigned for ensuring that appropriate equipment, supplies, and staffing are available prior to the administration of anesthesia.

- A pertinent and thorough history and physical has been completed and reviewed prior to surgery.

- Supporting documentation has been reviewed by the surgeon and anesthesiologist prior to surgery (e.g., labs, EKGs, imaging studies).

- A process exists by which there is correlation of pathology and imaging findings.

- A preanesthesia assessment has been conducted.

- The surgeon has been credentialed to perform the surgical procedure that he or she is about to perform.

- Annual competency evaluations are required for all individuals working in the surgical environment.

- Vital signs, airway, and surgical site assessments are continuously monitored.

- Medical equipment is properly maintained.

- IV lines and tubes (e.g., suction and feeding) are properly placed.

- Postoperative care on patient units is provided through the use of appropriate assessments and protocols.

- A procedure for instrument and sponge counts prior to closing the surgical site has been implemented.

- Surgical equipment is properly cleaned and stored following each procedure.

- Surgical site infections are closely tracked.

- Processes are in place to follow up with patients who have postoperative infections.

Wrong Site Surgery

- A process has been implemented to clearly mark the correct surgical site.

- If the actual site cannot be marked, a mark is placed in close proximity of the surgical site.

- There is documentation in the medical record that records the correct procedure, site, and patient.

- Both the operating physician and patient are involved in the preoperative marking process.

- An informed consent form has been signed and it describes the site and procedure to be performed.

- The patient's medical record is available to help determine the correct site prior to the start of surgery.

- Imaging studies are available for review prior to surgery to help determine the correct surgical site.

- There is verbal verification of the correct site by each member of the team in the operating room prior to induction of anesthesia.

- Observation confirms that the correct site has been marked, with the patient's participation.

- Anesthesia is not administered until the operating surgeon is in the operating suite.

- The surgical team (all disciplines) conducts a "time out" prior to the start of surgery to confirm the correct patient, correct site, and correct procedure.

- A verification checklist that includes all documents referencing the operative site has been implemented.

Spiritual Care Services

- The spiritual needs of patients are addressed.

- Patients know such services are available and how to access them.

- Organizational policies and procedures address the psychosocial, spiritual, and cultural variables that influence one's understanding and perception of illness.

- Referrals are made by caregivers for spiritual assessment, reassessment, and follow-up.

- Documentation is placed in the patient's medical record to indicate that the patient's spiritual needs have been addressed.

REVIEW QUESTIONS

1. What is this chapter referring to when it speaks of a zero-tolerance policy?

2. Why are organizations encouraged to create a culture of safety?

3. Describe steps hospitals can take in order to achieve a culture of safety.

4. What is the purpose of the Joint Commission's *national patient safety goals*?

5. What is the purpose of the Joint Commission's *complaint process*?

6. What is the mission of the National Quality Forum?

7. What is the mission of the Agency for Healthcare Research and Quality?

8. What is the mission of The Leapfrog Group for Patient Safety?

9. What is the mission of the Institute for Healthcare Improvement?

NOTES

1. *30 Safe Practices for Better Health Care. Fact Sheet.* AHRQ Publication No. 05-P007, March 2005. Agency for Healthcare Research and Quality, Rockville, MD. http://www.ahrq.gov/qual/30safe.htm.

Worldwide Search

Knowledge is of two kinds. We know a subject our-selves, or we know where we can find information upon it.

Samuel Johnson (1709–1784)
English author and lexicographer

INTRODUCTION

This chapter is designed to assist the reader in conduct-ing a worldwide search of ethics health care and law-related topics through the effective use of the Internet. "The World Wide Web (WWW) is the universe of network-accessible information, an embodiment of human knowledge," accord-ing to the organization that Web inventor Tim Berners-Lee helped found, the World Wide Web Consortium.

This chapter provides helpful Web sites to readers search-ing for best practices. It is a journey to the far corners of the earth in search of answers to difficult issues. This chapter is written for those individuals unwilling to accept an end without a fight; it recognizes that the answers to difficult disease processes may lead the reader to exotic lands in search of a remedy. Sometimes the issue(s) may be so over-whelming that it would seem easy to give up. Don't do it; the answer may be a click away.

This is the beginning of a new adventure. Enjoy the trip by first taking a comfortable journey to the National Library of Medicine's Web site at www.nlm.nih.gov/. The library, located on the grounds of the National Institutes of Health in Bethesda, Maryland, is the world's largest medical library. There are more than 6 million items, including books, jour-nals, photographs, and images in its collection.

Before the journey begins, consider the following observa-tions made during travels to hospitals throughout the nation.

Possible Treatment Options: What and Where Are They?

Patients are not always aware of the various treatment options for their medical conditions. Unique experiences and successes of physicians and hospitals from different parts of the country often remain unnoticed. Thus, physi-cians are left in the dark as to who is doing what and where varying combinations of treatment programs might be help-ful in treating their patients. For example:

> In Florida, a physician described a case in which a mus-cular dystrophy (MS) patient came to the hospital in a wheelchair needing wound care. After 42 wound care treatments in a hyperbaric chamber, the patient left with a cane, not in a wheelchair.

> In New Jersey, a physician described how he developed a "cocktail of medications" for MS patients.

> A physical therapist in New Hampshire described equip-ment that has helped both MS patients and stroke victims learn to walk again without the assistance of a cane.

These observations may not lead to a formula for the suc-cessful treatment of MS patients, but the message is unmis-takable; there needs to be a repository for the compilation and sharing of unexpected successful outcomes.

Evaluating Web Sites

When evaluating health care Web sites on the Internet, look for the symbol of the HON code of conduct for health care at the bottom of Web pages. Health On the Net Foun-dation is the leading organization promoting and guiding the deployment of useful and reliable online medical and health information and its appropriate and efficient use. Created in

1995, HON is a nonprofit, nongovernmental organization, accredited to the Economic and Social Council of the United Nations. For more information on the HON Foundation, go to www.hon.ch.

Search Engines and Browsers

A *search engine* is a program that searches the World Wide Web for Web sites and creates a catalog of information about those sites. The search engine that one chooses to use will search its catalogue for the occurrences of the text being searched. A majority of search engines are subject and keyword engines. Not all search engines access all possible Internet Web sites, therefore, it may be necessary to use different search engines to conduct a successful search. Listed here are some of the more popular search engines in use:

Altavista	www.altavista.com/
America Online	www.aol.com/
Ask Jeeves	www.ask.com/
Dogpile	www.dogpile.com/
Excite	www.excite.com
Expedia	www.expedia.com
Google	www.google.com/
InfoSpace	www.infospace.com/
Internet Explorer	www.microsoft.com/ windows/ie/default.asp
Lycos	www.lycos.com/
Mamma	www.mamma.com/
Medscape	www.medscape.com
Northern Light	www.northernlight.com
Overture	www.content.overture.com/
WebMD	www.webmd.com/
Yahoo	www.yahoo.com/

Search Tips

- Review the search tips that various search engines provide.

- Use quote marks around phrases to ensure adjacency of words.

- Use a variety of search engines if you are having difficulty locating a particular topic.

- Domain names describe the location of the server where the information being sought is stored.

- Knowing domain names where files are stored is helpful when conducting random searches for information. Domain Web sites include the following:

  .com: commercial organizations (businesses)

  .edu: educational organizations

  .gov: government agencies

  .mil: military

  .org: miscellaneous organizations

  .net: network providers

- A path name follows the domain name and identifies the location of an item on the server.

Telemedicine

Telemedicine is the delivery of health care services by means of telecommunications technology (e.g., fax, telephone, Internet, interactive audiovisual transmissions). It is a means for connecting remote areas of the nation and world with various forms of modern communications. The use of telemedicine brings modern health care to remote areas of the nation and the world. Telecommunications links the United States with the world. Telecommunications includes *teleradiology,* the interpretation of imaging procedures at a site remote from the patient and where the diagnostic procedure was performed. *Telepathology* involves the interpretation of slides at a location far from where the slides are prepared. EEGs and EKGs can also be transmitted almost anywhere in the world. *Teleeducation* is a tremendous learning tool for linking lectures and formal education programs to multiple sites.

The possibilities of telemedicine are endless. The benefits include improving access to high-tech care in remote areas of the nation and the world as well as reducing the transportation hardships for patients. Patients can remain in their community and still have access to the marvels of modern medicine. Global telemedicine has arrived to provide:

- worldwide medical consultations

- continual access to updated physiological data about patients in remote areas

- electronic medical records

- remote review of imaging studies

- remote examination of patients

- remote consultations

Telemedicine Web Sites

AMD Telemedicine	www.amdtelemedicine.com/
American Telemedicine Association	www.atmeda.org/
Association of Telehealth Service Providers	www.atsp.org/
Biohealthmatics.com	www.biohealthmatics.com/ healthinformatics/ telemedicine/telemed.aspx
Healthweb Telemedicine	www.healthweb.org/ telemedicine/
Personal MD	www.personalmd.com
The Radlinx Group	www.radlinxgroup.com/

Quackwatch

Quackwatch (www.quackwatch.com), is a Web site guide to health care fraud, quackery, and intelligent decisions. It includes questionable products, services, advertisements, and theories. It also covers education, consumer protection, research, additional links to other Web sites, and legal and political activities, as well as sources not recommended for health advice.

ETHICS-RELATED WEB SITES

Advance Directives	www.mindspring.com/ ~scottr/will.html
Bioethics	www.bioethics.net
Biotech and Health Care Ethics	www.scu.edu/ethics/ practicing/focusareas/ medical/
The Ethics Institute	www.ethics.uu-nl/old/index. html
Doctor's Ethics?	www.spcp4u.org/ NODOCTORSETHICS.html
National Advisory Board on Health Care Ethics	www.etene.org/e/index.shtml
National Center for Bio-technology Information	www.ncbi.nlm.nih.gov/
Questia-Medical Ethics	www.questia.com/library/ science-and-technology/ health-and-medicine/ medical-ethics.jsp
TransWeb.org	www.transweb.org

Professional Codes of Ethics

Administrator

American College of Health Care Executives	www.ache.org/

Dietitian

American Dietetic Associ-ation Code of Ethics	www.eatright.org/cps/rde/ xchg/ada/hs.xsl/home_347_ ENO_HTML.htm

Laboratory Technologist

College of Medical Laboratory Technologists of Ontario	www.cmlto.com/ government_policy/ code_of_ethics/

Nurse, RN

American Nurses Association	http://ana.org/
The Center for Ethics & Human Rights	www.nursingworld.org/ ethics/ecode.htm
International Council of Nurses Code of Ethics for Nurses	www.icn.ch/icncode.pdf

Pharmacist

Code of Ethics for Pharmacists	www.aphanet.org/AM/ Template.cfm?Section= Search&template=/CM/ htmlDisplay.cfm& ContentID=2809

Physical Therapist

American Physical Therapist Association	www.apta.org/AM/Template. cfm?Section=Home& ContentID=21760& Template=/CM/ ContentDisplay.cfm

Physician

PDA Code of Medical Ethics	www.ama-assn.org/ama/ pub/category/8288.html

Radiologic Technologist

American Society of Radiologic Technologists	www.asrt.org/content/RTS/ CodeofEthics/Code_Of_ Ethics.aspx

Respiratory Therapist

North Carolina Respiratory Care Board Code of Ethics	www.ncrcb.org/ code_ethics.html

LEGAL-RELATED WEB SITES

American Bar Association	www.abanet.org/
American Society of Law, Medicine, and Ethics	www.aslme.org
Answers to Your Legal Questions	www.legalscholar.com
Federal Law	www.thecre.com/fedlaw/ default.htm
FindLaw	www.findlaw.com
Guide to Law	www.loc.gov/law/guide
Health Law Resource	www.netreach.net/ ~wmanning/
Healthcare Law Net	www.healthcarelawnet.com/
Law.com	www.law.com
Legal Information	www.law.cornell.edu/ soj.html
Legal Research	bender.lexisnexis.com/ bender/us/catalog?action= home
LexisNexis	www.lexisnexis.com
National Court Reporters Association	www.ncraonline.org
NoLo	www.nolo.com
U.S. Courts/Links	www.uscourts.gov/ allinks.html#7th
Westlaw	www.westlaw.com
Wrong Diagnosis	www.wrongdiagnosis.com/

GOVERNMENT-RELATED WEB SITES

Agency for Healthcare Research and Quality	www.ahrq.gov/news/
Antitrust Division Manual	www.usdoj.gov/atr/foia/ divisionmanual/ch2.htm#a1
Centers for Disease Control and Prevention	www.cdc.gov
Centers for Medicare and Medicaid Services	www.cms.hhs.gov/ default.asp
NLM Gateway, Resources of the National Library of Medicine	gateway.nlm.nih.gov/ gw/Cmd
Government Manual	www.gpoaccess.gov/ gmanual/index.html
MedlinePlus	www.Medlineplus.gov
National Center for Health Statistics	www.cdc.gov/nchs
National Institute of Medicine	www.iom.edu
National Institutes of Health	www.nih.gov
National Library of Medicine	www.nlm.nih.gov/
PubMed	www.ncbi.nih.gov/entrez/ query.fcgi
U.S. Department of Justice	www.usdoj.gov/
U.S. Food and Drug Administration	www.fda.gov
U.S. Department of Health and Human Services	www.hhs.gov/

MEDICAL-RELATED WEB SITES

Health Insurance Portability and Accountability Act	http://cms.hhs.gov/hipaa/
U.S. Department of Health and Human Services	www.os.dhhs.gov/ocr/hipaa/
Summary of HIPAA	http://hipaadvisory.com

Accreditation and Regulatory Agencies

The Joint Commission	www.jointcommission.org/

Associations

American College of Healthcare Executives	www.ache.org
American Hospital Association	www.aha.org
American Medical Association	www.ama-assn.org
American Nurses Association	www.ana.org
World Health Organization	www.who.int

Best Practices/Evidence-Based Medicine/ Clinical Practice Guidelines

Advisory Board Company	www.advisoryboardcompany .com/
Agency for Healthcare Policy and Research	www.ahcpr.gov/clinic/ cpgsix.htm
Agency for Healthcare Research and Quality	www.ahrqpubs@ahrq.gov
Best 4health.org	www.best4health.org
Care Plans	www.careplans.com
Centre for Evidence-Based Medicine	www.cebm.net
Clinical Pathways	www.openclinical.org/ clinicalpathways.html
Health Care Professionals Network	www.wlm-web.com/hcnet
Institute for Safe Medication Practices	www.ismp.org
MDConsult	www.mdconsult.com
National Guideline Clearing House	www.guideline.gov
National Pathways Association	www.the-npa.org.uk/

Sample Bylaws, Policies, & Procedures	www.hcwp.org/meddirfm
SF=36.org	www.sf36.com

Cancer Care

American Cancer Society	www.cancer.org
Association of Cancer, Online Resources	www.acor.org
Cancer Links	www.cancerlinks.org
National Cancer Institute	www.nci.nih.gov

Clinical Trials

CancerNet (National Cancer Institute)	www.cancernet.nci.nih.gov
Clinical Trials Listing Service	www.centerwatch.com
International Clinical Trial Management	www.medisearch-int.com/ ictm.html
National Cancer Institute Clinical Trials	http://www.cancer.gov/ clinicaltrials

Complex Patient Care

Rarediseases.com	www.rarediseases.com

Disasters/Bioterrorism

Disaster Center	www.disastercenter.com
U.S. Department of Defense	www.defenselink.mil

Hospitals and Physician Finders

American Board of Medical Specialties	www.abms.org
American Medical Association DoctorFinder	www.ama-assn.org/aps/ amahg.htm
America's Best Hospitals	www.usnews.com/usnews/ health/best-hospitals/ tophosp.htm
Besthospitals.com	www.besthospitals.com

Children's Hospitals Around the World	www.pediheart.org/general/hospitals.htm
Choice Trust/Check Physician Credentials	
HealthGrades.com	www.healthgrades.com
Hospital Connect	www.hospitalconnect.com
National Association of State Mental Health Program Directors	www.nasmhpd.org
National Practitioner Data Bank	www.npdb-hipdb.com

Journals

Journal of the American Medical Association	www.jama.com
New England Journal of Medicine	www.nejm.com
Scientific American	www.scientificamerican.com

Library Resources

American Library Association	www.ala.org
Library Spot	www.libraryspot.com
National Library of Medicine	www.nlm.nih.gov/

News

BBC	www.bbc.com
CNN.com: Health	www.cnn.com/HEALTH/index.html
Reuters Health	www.reutershealth.com
USA Today Health	www.usatoday.com/news/health/healthdigest.htm

Nursing

American Nurses	www.ana.org
National League for Nursing	www.nln.org

U.S. Department of Labor, Nursing	www.stats.bls.gov/oco/ocos083.htm

Pain Management

American Academy of Pain Medicine	www.painmed.org
American Pain Foundation	www.painfoundation.org

Pharmacy

American Pharmacists Association	www.aphanet.org
Virtual Library Pharmacy	www.pharmacy.org

Preventative Care

Alternative Medicine	www.askdrweil.com
HealthWorld Online	www.healthy.net
Life Extension Foundation	www.lef.org

Resources/Research

Healthfinder	www.healthfinder.gov
Intelihealth	www.intelihealth.com
MDChoice.com	www.mdchoice.com/pt/index.asp
MedlinePlus	www.medlineplus.gov
Medscape	www.medscape.com
Virtual Hospital Information for Patients	www.vh.org/Patients/Patients.html

Schools

Allied Health Schools	www.allalliedhealthschools.com/
Medterms™ online medical directory	www.medterms.com/script/main/hp.asp
Nursing Schools Guide	www.allnursingschools.com/

Spiritual

		International Union Against Cancer	www.uicc.org
Religions of the World	emuseum.mnsu.edu/cultural/religion/	World Health Network	www.worldhealth.net/p/1.html
Search "Hospital Spiritual"	www.dayspring.com/	World Health Organization	www.who.int

INTERNATIONAL MEDICAL-RELATED WEB SITES

		World Medical Association	http://www.wma.net/e/
Cancer Index	www.cancerindex.org/clinks5o.htm		

REVIEW QUESTIONS

1. What is the importance of HON?

2. What is a search engine?

3. What is Telemedicine?

4. What is Quackwatch (www.quackwatch.com)?

Journey to Excellence

Excellence can be attained if you . . .
Care more than others think is wise.
Risk more than others think is safe.
Dream more than others think is practical.
Expect more than others think is possible.

Author Unknown

A PATIENT'S ILLNESS: A DIFFICULT JOURNEY

During the past five years, I have filled out numerous standardized forms requiring answers to questions that have been repeatedly asked by a wide variety of physician specialists and other caregivers. I've been told that my most recent specialist had great credentials. He came highly recommended. I was hopeful as I drove to his office during the early morning rush hour in a major metropolitan city. I would finally meet someone who cared and would understand my disease processes. As I walked into his office, I noted that my medical chart was lying on the desk in front of him. Its placement on his desk gave me some comfort in thinking that he had actually read the answers to the questions his staff said he wanted answered several weeks prior to my appointment, because he needed time to familiarize himself with my case. I soon realized shortly into the conversation that he had not reviewed my medical chart. The forms that I so had painstakingly completed, hoping for some answer to what I was experiencing because of this illness, had not been read. He inquired about what medications I was taking. My husband had accompanied me that

day and noticed that the list of medications was lying in front of him. The doctor asked me: "What is your pain on a scale of 1 to 10?" I thought for a moment. How do I answer that? "I am off your scale. I cannot remember not being in pain for the past five years. I sometimes wonder how it feels to be free of pain. I don't know that feeling anymore." Hello, is anyone out there?

I was eventually admitted to the hospital for the first time, my nerve endings felt frayed, my stomach was churning, worries were multiplying, and my thoughts turned to, "Is it time to get more bad news?" I was extremely ill. The sitting area in the admissions office was uncomfortable and uninviting. Privacy was minimal and soft music was nonexistent. I wondered what was going to happen to me. I had been an independent person all my life, always in control, never sick, and not dependent on even an aspirin.

Things got worse when I was finally admitted to a room. Now I had to stay in an alien room staring at drab, nondescript walls and was dependent upon people who hardly have the time to dispense medications. Most physicians and other staff were rushing about engaged in their everyday tasks. No one seemed to have time for me.

Confusion set in, I became anxious from the fear of being in a strange place. Unfamiliar people looked at me and touched me and repeatedly asked me the same questions over and over again. The questioning seemed never ending. I wondered, "Do these people ever talk to each other?" While I was being peppered with unending questions, some so technical, I couldn't respond, I in turn was not receiving answers. The surroundings were sterile and unfriendly, adding to my uneasy feelings.

Why can't health care facilities be more patient friendly to those they serve? Why must I worry about complaining and fear of retribution? Provisions should be made for a serene environment, with calming colors and carefully chosen people to gently ease answers from a frightened sick patient. More attention should be given to making a patient's room a calm and inviting place, which would help to soothe and carry the patient through troubling times.

Who will step up and make things better for the patient? Who is willing to search the world to help manage my pain? Who will take the Journey to Excellence? Will you?

Anonymous

THE JOURNEY

Accept the challenges so that you may feel the exhilaration of victory.

Author Unknown

Following 14 years of surveying, educating, and consulting in more than 600 hospitals across the nation, the patient's message above and on the previous page is a reminder to all that health care must address the concerns of this person and every other individual who will someday feel her loneliness and her pain in battling the complexity of her diseases. This patient's message brings the reader to this journey, one that requires all health care professionals to continuously work together and seek new ways to improve the quality of patient care. Progress lies with those who have the vision to see and act on numerous opportunities for improving health care.

Assign Responsibility and Accountability for Change

A strategic alliance is a mutually satisfying relationship, grounded in a strong commitment to all stakeholders.

Author Unknown

The journey to excellence begins with the assignment of responsibility and accountability for charting a path to excellence. This journey requires leadership by an executive who is comfortable in any setting—an executive who has

the passion, creativity, knowledge, and determination to fulfill a project's mission and vision. The leader must be committed to the selection of those who believe in the limitless potential to carry a project forward as a team. The visionaries and the innovators need to be identified and their energies given focus and direction. A proactive leadership must assume responsibility for its mandate to provide quality health care for the community.

Implement a Health Care War Room

The loftier your goals, the higher the risk, the greater your glory

Author Unknown

The health care war room is designed for and dedicated to brainstorming, strategizing, and storyboarding courses of action. The war room encourages far-reaching dreams with the belief that they can become reality. A health care organization may meet all the standards of patient care and may employ the best health care professionals in the country, but still fail in its ultimate mission to provide the best of health care. The health care war room is not just about doing the right thing, but is about doing the right thing well.

In the war room ideas are formed, prioritized, and assigned to a team member who has the leadership skills, abilities, knowledge, vision, and passion to turn a dream into reality. This person is a *rainmaker*. The doors of the war room are always open to all departments within the organization, and resources are readily available to aid in making positive changes. In this room, all caregivers have a unique opportunity to present ideas that otherwise may never have been taken seriously.

While the main resources of the war room are the people with ideas and plans, the room should also harbor state of the art technology, such as computers with high-speed Internet capabilities, telephone lines, conferencing equipment, and electronic subscriptions to worldwide medical journals. Great effort should be taken to keep equipment and subscriptions updated and maintained.

Medical librarians are helpful assets to the war room as individuals who can organize materials and schedule maintenance while also training others how to navigate through the maze of resources. The medical librarian searches and collects much of the information that visionaries need to design and effectuate change.

The war room must be conducive to brainstorming with sleeves rolled up, all in a comfortable, inviting setting, with pleasant decor free of cell phones and pagers. Executives interested in setting up a war room should consider hiring an interior designer to help create an environment suited to creative, free thinking. In the war room, tangible change happens, and the organization watches unlikely ideas unfold and succeed.

IDEAS FOR GETTING STARTED

The journey to excellence is not an easy path to follow:

> . . . *There is nothing more difficult to take in hand, more perilous to conduct, or more uncertain in its success, than to take the lead in the introduction of a new order of things. Because the innovator has for enemies all those who have done well under the old conditions, and lukewarm defenders in those who may do well under the new. This coolness arises partly from fear of the opponents, who have the laws on their side, and partly from the incredulity of men, who do not readily believe in new things until they have had a long experience of them.*
>
> Niccolo Machiavelli (*The Prince*, 1513)

The topics described here are but a few of the many to help get the war room up and running. They are offered as first-agenda items for the first war room's leadership meeting and topics for generating even better ideas. They include some practices that have been implemented successfully by other organizations. These topics are not presented as being the only solutions to how a war room could be started and utilized effectively to deliver the best health care to the most people. They are not the end—they are merely the means to a new beginning.

Encourage Ambassadors Worldwide

> *The structure of world peace cannot be the work of one man, or one party, or one nation. . . . It must be a peace which rests on the cooperative effort of the whole world.*
>
> Eleanor Roosevelt

Eleanor Roosevelt's words apply to the world of health care. The structure of a world class health care system cannot be the work of one man or one nation. It must be a system that depends on the cooperative effort of the world community. Leaders should encourage employees to contact other caregivers in their discipline from around the world. Employees could begin by inquiring about the way in which another professional addresses a specific issue. From there, a professional relationship may ensue. This gives the two a type of informal partnership to learn what works in one another's country and how to best apply the treatments and procedures in their home countries. Such sharing of information will create worldwide ambassadors for health care, leading to a melding of resources and knowledge for the most effective care of patients.

Hospitals that implement such a program should then share the program's findings with their local community by publishing a hospital newsletter highlighting the most interesting and informative results. Community members would then become more motivated to become involved in their hospitals.

Professional Exchange Program

This concept involves an exchange program whereby international host families would sponsor a health care professional in their home for two or more weeks. The professional would work in a foreign university hospital setting to learn the practices used in that health care setting, while also sharing with the host hospital best practices from his or her hospital. Thus, the program would provide a different cultural environment in which caregivers can learn of the others' best practices.

Partners in Education

Partners in health care education programs, created by hospital-school partnerships, support and enrich student learning by introducing students to opportunities in the health care professions. Partners in education can take the form of a school lunch program whereby health care professionals (e.g., nurses, pharmacists, physical therapists, physicians) from a local community hospital are matched with students from a local middle school or high school who have an interest in a particular health career. Hospital employee volunteers are matched with one or more students for a semester and have lunch with them during a set day and time each week. Students may even choose to learn about a different discipline the following semester. The earlier this process begins, the greater the opportunity a student has to discover a successful career path.

Best Practices

The journey to excellence involves searching for best practices worldwide. It is a journey to the far corners of the earth in search of answers to difficult health care issues. It is the "worldwide search" to improve the quality of life on a global basis. It involves providing information to those individuals unwilling to accept an end without a fight. It recognizes that the answers to complex disease processes may lead the reader to exotic lands in search of a remedy. Although many issue(s) may seem overwhelming, the answer to many health care issues may be a click away.

Focus on Preventative Medicine

Physicians are often so busy treating immediate symptoms, diseases, conditions, and injuries that preventative care is often not addressed. By committing more time to preventative medicine, the risks of early onset of disease can be reduced. Preventative care should address balancing the biological, psychological, social, and spiritual needs of each individual. The war room should be a place that encourages leaders to spend more time focusing on preventative medicine.

Streamline Data Collection and Evaluation

It's better to have no data than to have data that leads to the wrong conclusions.

Author Unknown

Over the years, health care organizations have collected an enormous amount of data that are costly and time consuming to collect and have little clinical value. Collecting data on cesarean section rates for nearly half a century, for example, has done little to improve the quality of health care. The collection of data must be meaningful and lead to improved patient outcomes. With limited financial resources, data gathering should have a recognizable clinical payoff for the patient.

Information Technology: Returning to the Mission of Caring

Health care organizations must improve their information technology systems by developing a computerized medical record that provides access to best practices, as well as computer-assisted diagnosis and treatment information. The tremendous amount of paperwork required of caregivers can be reduced, allowing more time for direct patient care.

Many skilled nurses claim they spend up to two hours of an eight-hour shift documenting in patient records. Getting the nurse back to the patient's bedside and away from the computer or pen will require some reengineering. The medical record has become a cumbersome compilation of illegible notes from many health care disciplines. It has become an unfriendly and far-from-effective communications tool in the care and treatment of patients. Its purpose has shifted from being a useful communications tool between caregivers to becoming a tool for satisfying regulatory bodies. The proverbial wheel is broken, so reinventing the health care record wheel is a must, requiring serious attention by the health care industry and regulatory bodies, in order to provide patients with increased beside care.

Caring for the Whole Person

Bedside care involves more than recordkeeping. Imagine for a moment Patient A's and Patient B's experiences as described here.

Patient A

See: Your favorite scenes from Africa are on a large, flat screen TV; you have a private room.

Hear: Your favorite music by Enya plays in the background; the corridors are quiet.

Smell: You have fresh flowers and the bathroom is clean with no harsh chemical odors.

Taste: You have your favorite foods and bottled water.

Touch: Your pain is controlled, the room is the right temperature, and you have had caring caregivers and family.

Patient B

See: The walls are cracked, the paint is peeling, and mold is growing in the vents.

Hear: The corridor is noisy. You have no visitors, but your roommate has eight of them.

Smell: A sewage plant is nearby and the wind from its direction is blowing in your open window.

Taste: You are on a liquid diet; your water is warm and has a weird taste.

Touch: Your pain is unrelenting, the room is hot, and you have no one to talk to.

Two patients, two very different experiences. Clearly, the health profession must do more to better address the five senses. Each sense has many components. For example, the sense of touch includes physical, psychological, social, and spiritual elements, each of which needs to be addressed. The physical aspect includes the effective control of a patient's pain. The social aspect involves family, caregivers, visitors, friends, and spiritual guidance. Hospitals may not be able to do everything they would like for their patients, but they can better address their sensory needs.

ADOPT A HOSPITAL

Highways and rivers are adopted; why not adopt a hospital? Creating change on a grand scale requires financial backing by mission-driven individuals and corporations. With fewer than 6,000 hospitals in the United States, the health care system would grow strong and mighty with an Adopt a Hospital sponsorship from the nation's wealthiest people and corporations such as Google, IBM, Intel, and Microsoft.

Fundraising is everybody's job and everybody has a role to play. Seniors can knit, crochet, and sell their items in a gift or thrift shop. Young people can organize a car wash. Volunteers can have bake sales, sell raffle tickets, or sponsor dinner dances. The possibilities are endless.

POST YOUR DREAM BOARDS

The way to predict the future is to create it. Vision is the gift to see or do what others only dream.

Author Unknown

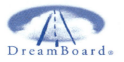

To help make a dream become reality, it is important for others to understand the dream. This can be accomplished effectively by graphically displaying the vision on an oversized dream board easily visible to all who pass by. The dream board should be displayed in high-traffic areas such as emergency department waiting area, intensive care unit, oncology unit, rehabilitation unit, or wellness center. Dreams fulfilled should be displayed in what might be termed the "hall of dreams," celebrating the successes of those who worked hard to achieve them. The first dream board under the above logo was developed by Sally Wern Comport, principal, Art At Large Inc. (http://www.artatlargeinc.com) and is on display in the Huntington Hospital lobby in Huntington, New York. It was commissioned by one of New York State's finest chief executive officers, J. Ronald Gaudreault.

REVIEW QUESTIONS

1. What message is the author attempting to convey in this chapter?

2. Discuss the ideas for getting started.

3. What are dreamboards?

Glossary

Abandonment: Unilateral severance by the physician of the professional relationship between him- or herself and the patient without reasonable notice at a time when the patient still needs continuing care.

Abortion: Premature termination of pregnancy at a time when the fetus is incapable of sustaining life independent of the mother.

Admissibility (of evidence): Refers to the issue of whether a court, applying the rules of evidence, is bound to receive or permit introduction of a particular piece of evidence.

Advance directives: Written instructions expressing one's health care wishes in the event that he or she becomes incapacitated and is unable to make such decisions.

Adverse drug reaction: Unusual or unexpected response to a normal dose of a medication; an injury caused by the use of a drug in the usual, acceptable fashion.

Affidavit: A voluntary statement of facts, or a voluntary declaration in writing of facts, that a person swears to be true before an official authorized to administer an oath.

Agent: An individual who has been designated by a legal document to make decisions on behalf of another individual; a substitute decision maker.

Americans with Disabilities Act (ADA): Federal act that bars employers from discriminating against disabled persons in hiring, promotion, or other provisions of employment.

Appellant: Party who appeals the decision of a lower court to a court of higher jurisdiction.

Appellee: Party against whom an appeal to a higher court is taken.

Artificial nutrition and hydration: Providing food and liquids when a patient is unable to eat or drink, such as intravenous feedings.

Assault: Intentional act that is designed to make the victim fearful and produces reasonable apprehension of harm.

Attestation: Act of witnessing a document in writing.

Autonomy: Right of an individual to make his or her own independent decisions.

Battery: Intentional touching of one person by another without the consent of the person being touched.

Beneficence: Describes the principle of doing good, demonstrating kindness, and helping others.

Best evidence rule: Legal doctrine requiring that primary evidence of a fact (such as an original document) be introduced or that an acceptable explanation be given before a copy can be introduced or testimony given concerning the fact.

Borrowed servant doctrine: Refers to a situation in which an employee is temporarily placed under the control of someone other than his or her primary employer. It may involve a situation in which an employee is carrying out the specific instructions of a physician. The traditional example is that of a nurse employed by a hospital who is "borrowed" and under the control of the attending surgeon during a procedure in the operating room. The temporary employer of the borrowed servant can be held responsible for the negligent acts of the borrowed servant under the doctrine of *respondeat superior*. This rule is not easily applied, especially if the acts of the employee are for the furtherance of the objectives of the employer. The courts apply a narrow application if the employee is fulfilling the requirement of his or her position.

Captain-of-the-ship doctrine: A doctrine making the physician responsible for the negligent acts of other professionals because he or she had the right to control and oversee the totality of care provided to the patient.

Cardiopulmonary resuscitation: A lifesaving method used by caregivers to restore heartbeat and breathing.

Case citation: Describes where a court's opinion in a particular case can be located. It identifies the parties in the case, the text in which the case can be found, the court writing the opinion, and the year in which the case was decided. For example, the citation *Bouvia v. Superior Court (Glenchur),* 225 Cal. Rptr. 297 (Ct. App. 1986), is described as follows:

- *Bouvia v. Superior Court (Glenchur)* identifies the basic parties involved in the lawsuit.
- 225 Cal. Rptr. 297 identifies the case as being reported in volume 225 of the California Reporter at page 297.
- Ct. App. 1986 identifies the case as being in the California Court of Appeals in 1986.

Case law: Aggregate of reported cases on a particular legal subject as formed by the decisions of those cases.

Certiorari: Writ that commands a lower court to certify proceedings for review by a higher court. This is the common method of obtaining review by the U.S. Supreme Court.

Charitable immunity: Legal doctrine that developed out of the English court system that held charitable institutions blameless for their negligent acts.

Civil law: Body of law that describes the private rights and responsibilities of individuals. The part of law that does not deal with crimes; it involves actions filed by one individual against another (e.g., actions in tort and contract).

Clinical privileges: On qualification, the diagnostic and therapeutic procedures that an institution allows a physician to perform on a specified patient population. Qualification includes a review of a physician's credentials, such as medical school diploma, state licensure, and residency training.

Closed-shop contract: Labor-management agreement that provides that only members of a particular union may be hired.

Common law: Body of principles that has evolved and continues to evolve and expand from court decisions. Many of the legal principles and rules applied by courts in the United States had their origins in English common law.

Complaint: In a negligence action, the first pleading that is filed by the plaintiff's attorney. It is the first statement of a case by the plaintiff against the defendant and states a cause of action, notifying the defendant as to the basis for the suit.

Congressional Record: Document in which the proceedings of Congress are published. It is the first record of debate officially reported, printed, and published directly by the federal government. Publication of the *Record* began March 4, 1873.

Consent: *See informed consent.*

Criminal negligence: Reckless disregard for the safety of others. It is the willful indifference to an injury that could follow an act.

Defamation: Injury of a person's reputation or character caused by the false statements of another made to a third person. Defamation includes both libel and slander.

Defendant: In a criminal case, the person accused of committing a crime. In a civil suit, the party against whom the suit is brought, demanding that he or she pay the other party legal relief.

Demurrer: Formal objection by one of the parties to a lawsuit that the evidence presented by the other party is insufficient to sustain an issue or case.

Deposition: A method of pretrial discovery that consists of statements of fact taken by a witness under oath in a question-and-answer format as it would be in a court of law with opportunity given to the adversary to be present for cross-examination. Such statements may be admitted into evidence if it is impossible for a witness to attend a trial in person.

Directed verdict: When a trial judge decides either that the evidence and/or law is clearly in favor of one party, the judge may direct the jury to return a verdict for the appropriate party. The conclusion of the judge must be so clear and obvious that reasonable minds could not arrive at a different conclusion.

Discharge summary: That part of a medical record that summarizes a patient's initial complaints, course of treatment, final diagnosis, and suggestions for follow-up care.

Discovery: To ascertain that which was previously unknown through a pretrial investigation; it includes testimony and documents that may be under the exclusive control of the other party.

Do not resuscitate (DNR): Directive of a physician to withhold cardiopulmonary resuscitation in the event that a patient experiences cardiac arrest.

Durable power of attorney: Legal instrument enabling an individual to act on another's behalf. In the health care setting, a *durable power of attorney for health care* is the authority to make medical decisions for another.

Ethical dilemma: A situation that forces a person to make a decision that involves breaking some ethical norm or contradicting some ethical value. The effect of an action may put others at risk, harm others, or violate another person's rights.

Ethicist: One who specializes in ethics.

Ethics: A set of principles of right and wrong conduct; a theory or system of moral values, of what is right and what is wrong. Ethics is a system of values that guides behavior in relationships among people in accordance with certain social roles.

Ethics committee: A committee created to deal with ethical problems and dilemmas in the delivery of patient care.

Euthanasia: A Greek word meaning "the good death." It is an act conducted for the purpose of causing the merciful death of a person who is suffering from an incurable condition, such as providing a patient with medications to hasten his or her death.

Evidence: Proof of a fact, which is legally presented in a manner prescribed by law, at trial.

Expert witness: Person who has special training, experience, skill, and knowledge in a relevant area and who is allowed to offer an opinion as testimony in court.

Futility: Having no useful result. Futility of treatment, as it relates to medical care, occurs when the physician recognizes that the effect of treatment will be of no benefit to the patient. Morally, the physician has a duty to inform the patient when there is little likelihood of success.

Good Samaritan laws: Laws designed to protect those who stop to render aid in an emergency. These laws generally provide immunity for specified persons from a civil suit arising out of care rendered at the scene of an emergency, provided that the one rendering assistance has not done so in a grossly negligent manner.

Grand jury: Jury called to determine whether there is sufficient evidence that a crime has been committed to justify bringing a case to trial.

Grievance: The process undertaken to resolve a labor-management dispute when there is an allegation by a union member that management has failed in some way to meet the terms of a labor agreement.

Guardian: Person appointed by a court to protect the interests of and make decisions for a person who is incapable of making his or her own decisions.

Health: According to the World Health Organization, "[a] state of complete physical, mental, and social well-being and not merely the absence of disease or infirmity."

Health Care Financing Administration (HCFA): Federal agency that coordinates the federal government's participation in the Medicare and Medicaid programs.

Health care proxy: Document that delegates the authority to make one's own health care decisions to another, known as the health care agent, when one has become incapacitated or is unable to make his or her own decisions.

Hearsay rule: Rule of evidence restricting the admissibility of evidence that is not the personal knowledge of the witness.

Holographic will: A will hand written by the testator.

Home health agency: An agency that provides home health services. Home health care involves an array of services provided to patients in their homes or foster homes because of acute illness, exacerbation of chronic illness, and disability. Such services are therapeutic and/or preventative.

Home health care: Home health care is an alternative for those who fear leaving the secure environment of their home. Such care is available through home health agencies. These agencies provide a variety of services for the elderly living at home. Such services include part-time or intermittent nursing care; physical, occupational, and speech therapy; medical social services, home health aide services, and nutritional guidance; medical supplies other than drugs and biologicals prescribed by a physician; and the use of medical appliances.

Hydration: Intravenous addition of fluids to the circulatory system.

In loco parentis: Legal doctrine that permits the courts to assign a person to stand in the place of parents and possess their legal rights, duties, and responsibilities toward a child.

Incompetent: Individual determined by a court to be incapable of making rational decisions on his or her own behalf.

Independent contractor: One who agrees to undertake work without being under the direct control or direction of an employer.

Indictment: Formal written accusation presented by a grand jury, charging a person therein named with criminal conduct.

Informed consent: Legal concept that provides that a patient has the right to know the potential risks, benefits, and alternatives of a proposed procedure prior to undergoing a particular course of treatment. Informed consent implies that a patient understands a particular procedure or treatment, including the risks, benefits, and alternatives; is capable of making a decision; and gives consent voluntarily.

Injunction: Court order either requiring a person to perform a certain act or prohibiting the person from performing a particular act.

Interrogatories: List of questions sent from one party in a lawsuit to the other party to be answered under oath.

Judicial notice: An act by which a court, in conducting a trial or forming a decision, will of its own motion and without evidence, recognize the existence and truth of certain facts bearing on the controversy at bar (e.g., serious falls require X-rays).

Jurisdiction: Right of a court to administer justice by hearing and deciding controversies.

Larceny: Taking another person's property without consent with the intent to permanently deprive the owner of its use and ownership.

Liability: As it relates to damages, an obligation one has incurred or might incur through a negligent act.

Libel: False or malicious writing that is intended to defame or dishonor another person and is published so that someone other than the one defamed will observe it.

Life support: Medical intervention(s) designed to prolong life (e.g., respirator, kidney dialysis machine, tube feedings).

Living will: A document in which an individual expresses in advance his or her wishes regarding the application of life-sustaining treatment in the event that he or she is incapable of doing so at some future time. A living will describes in advance the kind of care one wants to receive or does not wish to receive in the event that he or she is unable to make decisions for himself or herself. A living will takes effect when a person is in a terminal condition or permanent state of unconsciousness.

Malfeasance: Execution of an unlawful or improper act.

Malpractice: Professional misconduct, improper discharge of professional duties, or failure to meet the standard of care of a professional that results in harm to another; the negligence or carelessness of a professional person, such as a nurse, pharmacist, physician, or accountant.

Mandamus: Action brought in a court of competent jurisdiction to compel a lower court or administrative agency to perform—or not to perform—a specific act.

Medicaid: Medical assistance provided in Title XIX of the Social Security Act. Medicaid is a state-administered program for the medically indigent.

Medicare: Medical assistance provided in Title XVIII of the Social Security Act. Medicare is a health insurance program administered by the Social Security Administration

for persons aged 65 years and older and for disabled persons who are eligible for benefits. Medicare Part A benefits provide coverage for inpatient hospital care, skilled nursing facility care, home health care, and hospice care. Medicare Part B benefits provide coverage for physician services, outpatient hospital services, diagnostic tests, various therapies, durable medical equipment, medical supplies, and prosthetic devices.

Misdemeanor: Unlawful act of a less-serious nature than a felony, usually punishable by a jail sentence for a term of less than one year and/or a fine.

Misfeasance: Improper performance of an act.

Negligence: Omission or commission of an act that a reasonably prudent person would or would not do under given circumstances. It is a form of heedlessness or carelessness that constitutes a departure from the standard of care generally imposed on members of society.

Non compos mentis: "Not of sound mind"; suffering from some form of mental defect.

Nonfeasance: Failure to act, when there is a duty to act, as a reasonably prudent person would in similar circumstances.

Nuncupative will: Oral statement intended as a last will made in anticipation of death.

Ombudsman: Person who is designated to speak and act on behalf of a patient/resident, especially in regard to his or her daily needs.

Opined: To give or express as an opinion.

Perjury: Willful act of giving false testimony under oath.

Plaintiff: Party who brings a civil suit seeking damages or other legal relief.

Privileged communication: Statement made to an attorney, physician, spouse, or anyone else in a position of trust. Because of the confidential nature of such information, the law protects it from being revealed even in court. The term is applied in two distinct situations. First, the communications between certain persons, such as physician and patient, cannot be divulged without the consent of the patient. Second, in some situations, the law provides an exemption from liability for disclosing information for which there is a higher duty to speak, such as statutory reporting requirements.

Probate: A judicial proceeding that determines the existence and validity of a will.

Probate court: A court with jurisdiction over wills. Its powers range from deciding the validity of a will to distributing property.

Process: A series of related actions to achieve a defined outcome.

Prognosis: Informed judgment regarding the likely course and probable outcome of a disease.

Proximate: In immediate relation with something else. In negligence cases, the careless act must be the proximate cause of injury.

Real evidence: Evidence furnished by tangible things (e.g., medical records and equipment).

Rebuttal: Giving of evidence to contradict the effect of evidence introduced by the opposing party.

Release: Statement signed by one person relinquishing a right or claim against another.

Remand: Referral of a case by an appeals court back to the original court, out of which it came, for the purpose of having some action taken there.

Res gestae: "The thing done"; all the surrounding events that become part of an incident. If statements are made as part of the incident, they are admissible in court as res gestae despite the hearsay rule.

Res ipsa loquitur: "The thing speaks for itself"; a doctrine of law applicable to cases in which the defendant had exclusive control over the thing that caused the harm and where the harm ordinarily could not have occurred without negligent conduct.

Res judicata: "The thing is decided"; that which has been acted on or decided by the courts.

Respondeat superior: "Let the master answer"; an aphorism meaning that the employer is responsible for the legal consequences of the acts of the servant or employee who is acting within the scope of his or her employment.

Slander: False oral statement, made in the presence of a third person, that injures the character or reputation of another.

Standard of care: Description of the conduct that is expected of an individual in a given situation. It is a measure against which a defendant's conduct is compared.

Stare decisis: "Let the decision stand"; the legal doctrine that prescribes adherence to those precedents set forth in cases that have been decided.

Statute of limitations: Legal limit on the time allowed for filing suit in civil matters, usually measured from the time of the wrong or from the time when a reasonable person would have discovered the wrong.

Statutory law: Law that is prescribed by legislative enactments.

Stipulation: Agreement, usually in writing, by attorneys on opposite sides of an issue as to any matter pertaining to the proceedings. A stipulation is not binding unless agreed on by the parties involved in the issue.

Subpoena ad testificandum: Court order requiring one to appear in court to give testimony.

Subpoena duces tecum: Court order that commands a person to come to court and to produce whatever documents are named in the order.

Subrogation: Substitution of one person for another in reference to a lawful claim or right.

Summary judgment: Generally, an immediate decision by a judge, without jury deliberation.

Summons: Court order directed to the sheriff or other appropriate official to notify the defendant in a civil suit that a suit has been filed and when and where to appear.

Surrogate decision maker: Individual who has been designated to make decisions on behalf of an individual determined incapable of making his or her own decisions.

Testimony: Oral statement of a witness given under oath at trial.

The Joint Commission: A not-for-profit independent organization dedicated to improving the quality of health care in organized health care settings. The major functions of the Joint Commission include developing organizational standards, awarding accreditation decisions, and providing education and consultation to health care organizations.

Tort: Civil wrong committed by one individual against another. Torts may be classified as either intentional or unintentional. When a tort is classified as a criminal wrong (e.g., assault, battery, and false imprisonment), the wrongdoer can be held liable in a criminal and/or civil action.

Tort-feasor: Person who commits a tort.

Trial court: Court in which evidence is presented to a judge or jury for decision.

Union-shop contract: Labor-management agreement making continued employment contingent on joining the union.

Venue: Geographic district in which an action is or may be brought.

Verdict: Formal declaration of a jury's findings of fact, signed by the jury foreperson and presented to the court.

Waiver: Intentional giving up of a right, such as allowing another person to testify to information that ordinarily would be protected as a privileged communication.

Will: Legal declaration of the intentions that a person wishes to have carried out after death concerning property, children, or estate. A will designates a person or persons to serve as the executor(s) responsible for carrying out the instructions of the will.

Witness: Person who is called to give testimony in a court of law.

Writ: Written order that is issued to a person or persons requiring the performance of some specified act or giving authority to have it done.

Wrongful birth: Applies to the cause of action of the parents who claim that the negligent advice or treatment deprived them of the choice of aborting conception or of terminating the pregnancy.

Wrongful life: Refers to a cause of action brought by or on behalf of a defective child who claims that but for the defendant (e.g., a laboratory's negligent testing procedures or a physician's negligent advice or treatment of the child's parents), the child would not have been born.

Index